AF413037

2002
YEAR BOOK OF
OBSTETRICS, GYNECOLOGY, AND WOMEN'S HEALTH®

The 2002 Year Book Series

Year Book of Allergy, Asthma, and Clinical Immunology™: Drs Rosenwasser, Boguniewicz, Milgrom, Routes, and Spahn

Year Book of Anesthesiology and Pain Management™: Drs Chestnut, Abram, Black, Lang, Roizen, Trankina, and Wood

Year Book of Cardiology®: Drs Schlant, Gersh, Graham, Kaplan, and Waldo

Year Book of Critical Care Medicine®: Drs Dellinger, Parrillo, Balk, Bleck, Carcillo, and Royster

Year Book of Dentistry®: Drs Zakariasen, Boghosian, Dederich, Hatcher, Horswell, and McIntyre

Year Book of Dermatology and Dermatologic Surgery™: Drs Thiers and Lang

Year Book of Diagnostic Radiology®: Drs Osborn, Birdwell, Dalinka, Groskin, Maynard, Oestreich, Pentecost, and Ros

Year Book of Emergency Medicine®: Drs Burdick, Cone, Cydulka, Hamilton, Loiselle, and Niemann

Year Book of Endocrinology®: Drs Mazzaferri, Fitzpatrick, Horton, Kannan, Kennedy, Kreisberg, Meikle, Molitch, Morley, Osei, Poehlman, and Rogol

Year Book of Family Practice®: Drs Bowman, Dexter, Gilchrist, Morrison, Neill, and Scherger

Year Book of Gastroenterology™: Drs Lichtenstein, Ginsberg, Katzka, Kochman, Morris, Nunes, Rosato, and Stein

Year Book of Hand Surgery®: Drs Berger and Ladd

Year Book of Medicine®: Drs Barkin, Frishman, Jett, Klahr, Loehrer, and Mazzaferri

Year Book of Neonatal and Perinatal Medicine®: Drs Fanaroff, Maisels, and Stevenson

Year Book of Neurology and Neurosurgery®: Drs Bradley, Gibbs, and Verma

Year Book of Nuclear Medicine®: Drs Gottschalk, Blaufox, Coleman, Strauss, and Zubal

Year Book of Obstetrics, Gynecology, and Women's Health®: Drs Mishell, Kirschbaum, and Miller

Year Book of Oncology®: Drs Loehrer, Eisenberg, Glatstein, Gordon, Johnson, Pratt, and Thigpen

Year Book of Ophthalmology®: Drs Wilson, Cohen, Eagle, Grossman, Laibson, Maguire, Nelson, Penne, Rapuano, Sergott, Shields, Spaeth, Steinmann, Tipperman, Ms Gosfield, and Ms Salmon

Year Book of Orthopedics®: Drs Morrey, Beauchamp, Peterson, Swiontkowski, Trigg, and Yaszemski

Year Book of Otolaryngology-Head and Neck Surgery®: Drs Paparella, Holt, Keefe, and Otto

Year Book of Pathology and Laboratory Medicine®: Drs Raab, Bejarano, Bissell, Silverman, and Stanley

Year Book of Pediatrics®: Dr Stockman

Year Book of Plastic and Aesthetic Surgery™: Drs Miller, Bartlett, Garner, McKinney, Ruberg, Salisbury, and Smith

Year Book of Psychiatry and Applied Mental Health®: Drs Talbott, Ballenger, Frances, Jensen, Markowitz, Meltzer, and Simpson

Year Book of Pulmonary Disease®: Drs Jett, Hunt, Maurer, Peters, Phillips, and Ryu

Year Book of Rheumatology, Arthritis, and Musculoskeletal Disease™: Drs Panush, Hadler, Hellmann, Lahita, Lane, and Le Roy

Year Book of Sports Medicine®: Drs Shephard, Alexander, Cantu, Kohrt, Nieman, and Shrier

Year Book of Surgery®: Drs Copeland, Bland, Cerfolio, Daly, Deitch, Eberlein, Howard, Luce, and Seeger

Year Book of Urology®: Drs Andriole and Coplen

Year Book of Vascular Surgery®: Dr Porter

2002

Year Book of OBSTETRICS, GYNECOLOGY, AND WOMEN'S HEALTH

Editors

Daniel R. Mishell, Jr, MD

The Lyle G. McNeile Professor and Chairman, Department of Obstetrics and Gynecology, Keck School of Medicine, University of Southern California School of Medicine, Women's and Children's Hospital, Los Angeles County and University of Southern California Medical Center, Los Angeles, Calif

Thomas H. Kirschbaum, MD

Professor of Obstetrics and Gynecology, Maternal-Fetal Medicine Division, Department of Obstetrics and Gynecology, University of Alabama at Birmingham, Ala

David Scott Miller, MD

Director and Dallas Foundation Chair in Gynecologic Oncology, Professor of Obstetrics and Gynecology, University of Texas Southwestern Medical Center at Dallas; Medical Director of Gynecologic Oncology, Parkland Health and Hospital System, Dallas, Tex

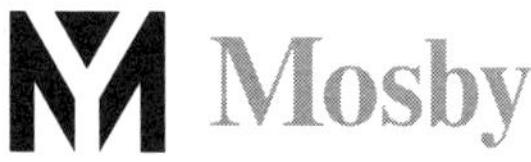

St. Louis Baltimore Boston Carlsbad Naples New York Philadelphia Portland London
Madrid Mexico City Singapore Sydney Tokyo Toronto Wiesbaden

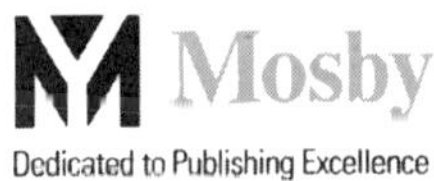

Dedicated to Publishing Excellence

Executive Publisher, Periodicals: Cynthia Baudendistel
Managing Editor: Colleen Cook
Manager, Continuity Production: Idelle L.Winer
Supervisor, Continuity Production: Joy Moore
Composition Specialist: Betty Dockins
Production Editor: Donna M. Skelton
Illustrations and Permissions Coordinator: Chidi C. Ukabam

Printed in the United States of America
Composition by Thomas Technology Solutions, Inc.
Printing/binding by Maple-Vail

Editorial Office:
Mosby, Inc.
11830 Westline Industrial Drive
St. Louis, MO 63146
Customer service: hhspcs@harcourt.com

International Standard Serial Number: 1090-798X
International Standard Book Number: 0-8151-2207-1

Contributing Editors

Raquel D. Arias, MD

Associate Dean of Women, Associate Professor of Obstetrics and Gynecology, Keck School of Medicine, University of Southern California; Women's and Children's Hospital, Los Angeles County and University of Southern California Medical Center, Los Angeles, Calif

Richard C. Bump, MD

Clinical Professor of Obstetrics and Gynecology, Indiana University School of Medicine, Indianapolis, Indiana

William H. Hindle, MD

Professor Emeritus, Department of Obstetrics and Gynecology, University of Southern California, Keck School of Medicine; Founder, Breast Diagnostic Center, Women's and Children's Hospital, Los Angeles County and University of Southern California Medical Center, Los Angeles, Calif

Table of Contents

Journals Represented

Mosby and its editors survey approximately 500 journals for its abstract and commentary publications. From these journals, the editors select the articles to be abstracted. Journals represented in this YEAR BOOK are listed below.

Acta Cytologica
Acta Obstetricia et Gynecologica Scandinavica
Acta Paediatrica
American Journal of Clinical Nutrition
American Journal of Clinical Oncology
American Journal of Emergency Medicine
American Journal of Epidemiology
American Journal of Obstetrics and Gynecology
American Journal of Perinatology
American Journal of Public Health
American Journal of Reproductive Immunology
American Journal of Roentgenology
American Journal of Surgery
American Surgeon
Anesthesia and Analgesia
Annals of Internal Medicine
Annals of Surgery
Archives of Disease in Childhood. Fetal and Neonatal Edition
Archives of Internal Medicine
Australian and New Zealand Journal of Obstetrics and Gynaecology
British Journal of Cancer
British Journal of Obstetrics and Gynaecology
British Journal of Urology International
Canadian Journal of Anesthesia
Canadian Medical Association Journal
Cancer
Cancer Journal
Chest
Circulation
Clinical Endocrinology (Oxford)
Contraception
Diabetes
Diabetic Medicine
European Journal of Surgical Oncology (London)
Fertility and Sterility
General Hospital Psychiatry
Gynecologic Oncology
Human Reproduction
Hypertension
International Journal of Gynecological Cancer
International Journal of Radiation, Oncology, Biology, and Physics
Journal of Clinical Endocrinology and Metabolism
Journal of Clinical Epidemiology
Journal of Clinical Investigation
Journal of Clinical Oncology
Journal of General Internal Medicine

Journal of Maternal-Fetal Medicine
Journal of Reproductive Medicine
Journal of Rheumatology
Journal of Sex and Marital Therapy
Journal of Surgical Oncology
Journal of Ultrasound in Medicine
Journal of Urology
Journal of the American Board of Family Practice
Journal of the American College of Cardiology
Journal of the American College of Surgeons
Journal of the American Medical Association
Journal of the National Cancer Institute
Journal of the Society for Gynecologic Investigation
Lancet
Maturitas
Menopause: The Journal of The American Menopause Society
Metabolism: Clinical and Experimental
Nature Medicine
New England Journal of Medicine
Obstetrics and Gynecology
Pediatric Research
Pediatrics
Plastic and Reconstructive Surgery
Prenatal Diagnosis
Science
Thrombosis and Haemostatis
Ultrasound in Obstetrics and Gynecology
Urology

STANDARD ABBREVIATIONS

The following terms are abbreviated in this edition: acquired immunodeficiency syndrome (AIDS), cardiopulmonary resuscitation (CPR), central nervous system (CNS), cerebrospinal fluid (CSF), computed tomography (CT), deoxyribonucleic acid (DNA), electrocardiography (ECG), health maintenance organization (HMO), human immunodeficiency virus (HIV), intensive care unit (ICU), intramuscular (IM), intravenous (IV), magnetic resonance (MR) imaging (MRI), and ribonucleic acid (RNA) and ultrasound (US).

NOTE

The YEAR BOOK OF OBSTETRICS, GYNECOLOGY, AND WOMEN'S HEALTH is a literature survey service providing abstracts of articles published in the professional literature. Every effort is made to assure the accuracy of the information presented in these pages. Neither the editors nor the publisher of the YEAR BOOK OF OBSTETRICS, GYNECOLOGY, AND WOMEN'S HEALTH can be responsible for errors in the original materials. The editors' comments are their own opinions. Mention of specific products within this publication does not constitute endorsement.

To facilitate the use of the YEAR BOOK OF OBSTETRICS, GYNECOLOGY, AND WOMEN'S HEALTH as a reference tool, all illustrations and tables included in this publication are now identified as they appear in the original article. This change is meant to help the reader recognize that any illustration or table appearing in the YEAR BOOK OF OBSTETRICS, GYNECOLOGY, AND WOMEN'S HEALTH may be only one of many in the original article. For this reason, figure and table numbers will often appear to be out of sequence within the YEAR BOOK OF OBSTETRICS, GYNECOLOGY, AND WOMEN'S HEALTH.

Introduction

The YEAR BOOK OF OBSTETRICS, GYNECOLOGY, AND WOMEN'S HEALTH contains abstracts of the most clinically relevant scientific articles published during the preceding year in the area of women's health, followed by editorial comments discussing the relevance of each article for the reader. Topics covered include care of the pregnant, parturient and postpartum woman and abnormalities of the female genital tract. Articles reviewed include those involving endocrinologic disorders and infertility as well as benign and malignant neoplasias. Other areas covered include breast disease, disorders of the urinary tract, contraception, and surveillance and treatment of the post-menopausal woman.

Throughout the year, the editors of the YEAR BOOK OF OBSTETRICS, GYNECOLOGY, AND WOMEN'S HEALTH periodically review articles published in medical journals focusing upon obstetrics, gynecology, and other areas of women's health, as well as relevant articles appearing in other medical journals. The editors select those articles that provide the most pertinent clinical information for clinicians, and write comments discussing the relevance of the findings for the reader. Once abstracts are written, they are sent to the editor who selected the article for placement in the YEAR BOOK for final review.

By reading the YEAR BOOK, clinicians with limited time will gain knowledge of the most important articles on women's health published in the previous year. As in past years, Dr Thomas H. Kirschbaum reviewed the field of maternal fetal medicine for articles in this volume. Dr David Scott Miller, an oncologist, and Dr Raquel D. Arias reviewed and selected articles on gynecologic oncology and pelvic surgery, and I have reviewed and selected articles in the areas of reproductive endocrinology, infertility, menopause, contraception, and gynecologic infection. Drs William H. Hindle and Richard C. Bump are contributing editors in the areas of breast disease and gynecologic urology, respectively.

During the past year, after receiving numerous scientific journals the authors selected 318 articles from 74 journals for publication in this volume of the YEAR BOOK.

We believe that reading this volume will enhance each clinicians' knowledge of advances in women's health. We welcome suggestions to improve our efforts in providing clinically relevant information to our readers.

Daniel R. Mishell, Jr, MD

OBSTETRICS

1 Maternal-Fetal Physiology

Gene Knockout Mice in the Study of Parturition

Gross G, Imamura T, Muglia LJ (Washington Univ, St Louis)
J Soc Gynecol Investig 7:88-95, 2000   1–1

Background.—The mechanism that controls the timing of labor onset has not been established. Many researchers have studied parturition in experimental mouse models. The consequences of targeted inactivation in mice of molecules implicated in parturition were examined in a review of current literature.

Methods and Findings.—The authors reviewed published studies of gene knockout mice with mutations in neuropeptides, prostaglandin synthetic enzymes and receptors, and other molecules that have been implicated in parturition. Mice with gene mutations at multiple levels of the prostaglandin synthetic pathway have been used to show the central role of prostaglandins in murine labor (Fig 1). Novel molecules such as steroid 5α-reductase appear to play a crucial role in labor progression. The deficiency of neuropeptides such as oxytocin and corticotropin-releasing hormone has been found to have little effect on parturition.

Conclusions.—Molecular genetic analyses in murine models provide insight into the molecules essential to parturition in mice. The importance of these molecules in human parturition now needs to be extrapolated.

► This is an interesting application of the production of gene knockout mice in studying the regulation of the onset of labor. The technique involves insertion of a mutated disrupted gene into a pluripotential embryonic stem cell, incorporating a segment of DNA known to be complementary or homologous to DNA segments adjoining the site of the normal gene. In this way, homologous DNA recombination fixes the disrupted knockout gene as a replacement to the normal gene in its approximately normal chromosome site. Simultaneous injection of a vector containing, for example, a neomycin-resistant gene as a random integration product, allowing stem cell growth in neomycin-containing medium which facilitates growth of cells bearing the knockout gene, but, to aid identification in culture, a second agent is inserted (FIAU), which generates a toxic metabolite for the old gene. Cell clusters

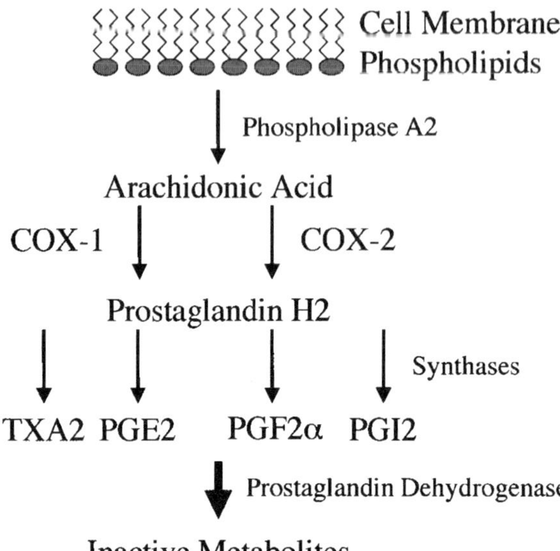

FIGURE 1.—Prostaglandin (PG) synthetic pathway. Arachidonic acid released from cell membrane phospholipids, primarily by the action of PLA2, serves as substrate for cyclooxygenase (COX)-1 or -2 (ie, PGH synthase-1 or -2). The COXs catalyze the first committed step in PG biosynthesis. PGH2 is then converted by specific synthases ro thromboxane A2 (TXA2), PGE2, PGF2α, and PG12. Each of these PGs acts on a cognate G protein-coupled receptor to exert its biologic action, or is inactivated by the action of PG dehydrogenase. (Reprinted by permission of the publisher from Gross G, Imamura T, Muglia LJ: Gene knockout mice in the study of parturition. *J Soc Gynecol Investig* 7:88-95. Copyright 2000 by Elsevier Science Inc.)

found in culture homozygous or heterozygous for the knockout gene are then inserted into normal mouse blastocysts and implanted in pseudo-pregnant surrogate mothers. Biologic testing and controlled mating allow the generation of populations of mice in which the chosen gene is specifically inactivated and the impact of lack of that gene on reproductive phenomena can be observed.

The feasibility of the procedure is being explored in mice before being applied to more complex mammals although there are some differences from the human with respect to the mechanics of the onset of labor. The mouse produces sex steroids during pregnancy from the corpus luteum, not the placenta as does the human. Maternal glucocorticoids show little in-crease in blood concentration in the human during pregnancy and before the onset of labor but are elevated in the mouse until close to term. Prosta-glandin E2 is produced in the mouse decidua, not the amnion, and prosta-glandins act primarily by producing luteolysis, not through direct action on myometrial contractility. Both species show the same increases in myome-trial oxytocin receptors and gap junction formation in smooth muscle fibers of the uterus close to term. The general pattern of sequence of changes defined by Liggins in the onset of ungulate labor (fetal endocrine changes, altered placental steroidogenesis, release of arachidonic acids, and prostaglandin production) applies to other species and supports the importance of comparative studies such as this.

When the gene for oxytocin production in mother and fetus is knocked out, labor occurs normally with normal litter size. Lactation, through lack of the milk let down effects of oxytocin, fails to occur. This observation makes it easy to understand the general ineffectiveness of atosiban, an oxytocin receptor antagonist, in blocking preterm labor (see the 2000 YEAR BOOK OF OBSTETRICS, GYNECOLOGY, AND WOMEN'S HEALTH, Abstract 3–7). When corticotrophin-releasing hormone (cRH) production is blocked by knockout, the increase in messenger RNA and protein ACTH as well as adrenocortical hormone concentrations fails to occur during pregnancy. This has no effect on litter size or the onset of labor, but the newborns die of pulmonary insufficiency due to the absence of the pulmonary maturation effects of adrenocortical hormone. Knockout of phospholipase A2, which makes arachidonic acid stored as a glycerophospholipid in the placenta available for prostaglandin synthesis, results in delayed onset of labor and incidents of perinatal death, making clear the essential role of prostaglandins in determining labor onset in this species. Knockout of cyclooxygenase-1 enzyme, essential in the production of prostaglandin in the presence of adequate arachidonic acid, prevents the onset of labor by inhibiting luteolysis, and knockout of cyclooxygenase-2 enzyme impairs ovulation and implantation, resulting in infertility. The gene for ovarian relaxin production appears to have no effect when inactivated out on labor onset or parturition.

In brief, this fascinating study helps confirm the role of prostaglandin species in determining the onset of labor in mice and supports prior evidence for lack of importance of oxytocin and CRH. (See 1988 YEAR BOOK, pp 41-42, 1989 YEAR BOOK, pp 23-24, and 1998 YEAR BOOK, pp 32-33.) More than that, it illustrates the use of an exquisitely specific and demanding technique in dissecting the role of specific proteins and enzymes in the complex biological interactions underlying the onset of labor.

T. H. Kirschbaum, MD

Hormonal Regulation of Neonatal Weight: Placental Leptin and Leptin Receptors

Schulz S, Häckel C, Weise W (Otto-von-Guericke Univ, Magdeburg, Germany)

Br J Obstet Gynaecol 107:1486-1491, 2000   1–2

Background.—The mechanisms regulating maternal and fetal weight during pregnancy are not well understood. Whether umbilical and maternal leptin concentrations are associated with birth weight, placental weight, and maternal weight was studied.

Methods.—Thirty-one mother-newborn pairs were included in the prospective observational study. Serum levels of leptin and soluble receptors were analyzed, and placental tissue was assayed for leptin receptors.

Findings.—The mean leptin level in umbilical cord venous blood was 7.1 ng/mL, which was significantly lower than in maternal blood, at 22.5 ng/mL. Umbilical cord leptin levels were significantly associated with birthweight and placental weight but not with maternal leptin (Fig 1). Maternal leptin levels were related to maternal weight only. Trophoblasts in chorionic villous tissue stained strongly positive for leptin receptor-like

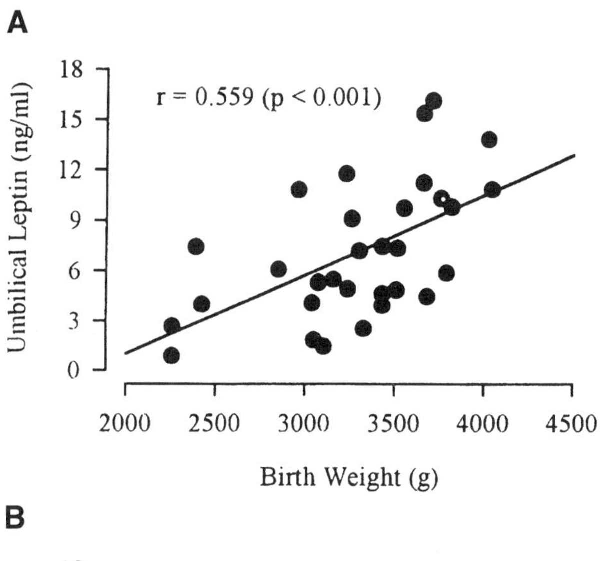

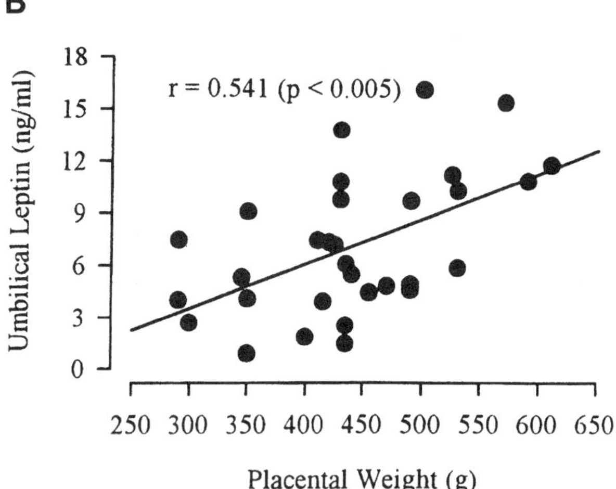

FIGURE 1.—Correlation between serum leptin concentrations and various parameters in 31 healthy mother infant pairs; (**A**) positive correlation between umbilical leptin and birthweight; (**B**) positive correlation between umbilical leptin and placental. (Courtesy of Schulz S, Häckel C, Weise W: Hormonal regulation of neonatal weight: Placental leptin and leptin receptors. *Br J Obstet Gynaecol* 107:1486-1491. Copyright 2000 by Elsevier Science, publisher.)

immunoreactivity. In addition, placental tissue contained 2 membrane-bound isoforms of a leptin receptor. A soluble leptin receptor migrating as broad band at M_r 97,000 daltons was identified in both umbilical and maternal serum.

Conclusions.—Circulating leptin concentrations appear to provide a growth-promoting signal for fetal development in late pregnancy. Membrane-bound leptin receptor may be involved in autocrine regulation of placental leptin production. The soluble receptor form may act as a transport vehicle for leptin to fetal tissues.

▶ In simultaneously measuring maternal and newborn leptin concentrations and relating them to maternal and fetal weights, as well as determining leptin receptor mRNA in term placentas, these authors have provided some clarifications in this interesting and evolving field. Leptin serum concentrations were measured by using radioimmunoassay on maternal and umbilical blood obtained simultaneously in normal term deliveries, and mRNA for the leptin receptor (OB-R) measured in maternal and newborn blood as well as placental homogenates, employing Western blots. Confirming the results of others, they found no correlation between maternal and fetal leptin blood concentrations at term, but their results show a strong correlation of cord blood leptin with both newborn and placental weight (see 1999 YEAR BOOK OF OBSTETRICS, GYNECOLOGY, AND WOMEN'S HEALTH, pp 13-15 and 14-16). Maternal blood leptin concentration correlated well with maternal weight at the onset and end of pregnancy but was unrelated to newborn birthweight. There was only a modest association of umbilical blood leptin concentration with maternal weight at term. Soluble OB-R was found in both maternal and cord blood and was similar in concentration among various newborns but showed wide individual variations among mothers. Messenger RNA for OB-R was found in placental tissue homogenates and, with the use of immunohistochemistry and antibodies specific to all 6 of its isoforms, was found localized to trophoblastic cells.

These data strongly support a regulatory role of fetal leptin for fetal growth acting independently of maternal leptin. Maternal leptin, although present in high concentration, appears to play a role only in maternal weight determination and weight gain. The likelihood that fetal leptin is, in the third trimester, derived largely from placental production is supported by the relationship between cord blood leptin and placental weight, high mRNA concentration for OB-R in placental tissue, persistently positive umbilical venous-arterial concentration differences in newborn cord blood, and the rapid decline of maternal leptin immediately after delivery. The authors' findings bring some clarification of the sometimes conflicting results reported earlier in this developing story of reproductive weight regulation.

T. H. Kirschbaum, MD

Effects of Altitude *Versus* Economic Status on Birth Weight and Body Shape at Birth

Giussani DA, Phillips PS, Anstee S, et al (Univ of Cambridge, England; Univ of Southampton, England)
Pediatr Res 49:490-494, 2001

1–3

Background.—Limited fetal growth results from reduced maternal nutrient intake and oxygen delivery to the fetal circulation. Hypoxia of the mother or fetus occurs most commonly during the hypobaric hypoxia of pregnancy at high altitude, and some reports have noted reduced birth weight occurring with increasing altitude, although additional socioeconomic factors may also be at work. The effects of high altitude on fetal growth were evaluated, and birth weight and body shape were compared in infants born in wealthy and impoverished communities in La Paz and Santa Cruz, Bolivia, the highest and lowest most populated cities of that country.

Methods.—Pregnancy records were reviewed from both high-income and low-income families in each of the 2 cities. Data particularly noted included birth weight, body (crown-heel) length, and head circumference. Four groups were identified: high-income high-altitude (100 infants), high-income low-altitude (100 infants), low-income high-altitude (100 infants), and low-income low-altitude (100 infants).

Results.—The mean birth weights of infants from La Paz were significantly lower than those of infants from Santa Cruz in both income groups, with even low-income Santa Cruz babies weighing more than high-income La Paz babies (Fig 1). The mean birth weight of babies born to low-income families in Santa Cruz was less than that of high-income Santa Cruz babies. Lower mean birth weights were noted in high-income families from La Paz than in La Paz low-income families. Body length declined with low income and altitude. Head circumference in high-income La Paz babies was greater than that in low-income La Paz babies. The ratio of head circumference to birth weight was lower in Santa Cruz babies than in La Paz babies, regardless of income level. Higher income level was linked to increased head circumference and to birth weight ratio at high altitude, but this association did not hold true at low altitude. The cumulative frequency distribution curve was shifted to the left in babies from high altitude compared with those from low altitude without reference to economic status. Cumulative frequency distribution of high-income La Paz babies was shifted to the left relative to those from low-income families. For Santa Cruz babies, the low-income group was shifted to the left in relation to the high-income group. Low birth weight occurred in a greater percentage of La Paz babies than Santa Cruz babies of either economic group.

Conclusions.—It appears that high altitude not associated with undernutrition yields decreased birth weight. The mechanism by which infants

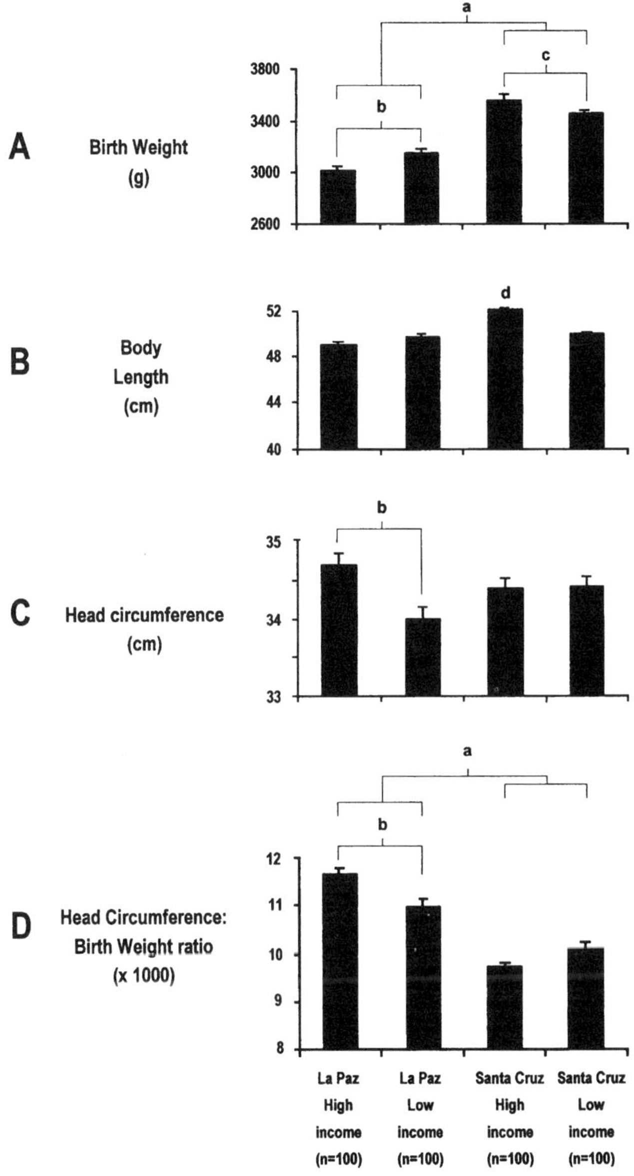

FIGURE 1.—Birth weights and measurements in Bolivian babies. Values are mean ± SEM of 100 babies taken from economically divergent populations in La Paz (3649 m above sea level) and Santa Cruz (437 m above sea level). Significant differences are [a]$P < 0.05$, La Paz *vs* Santa Cruz; [b]$P < 0.05$, La Paz-high income *vs* La Paz-low income; [c]$P < 0.05$, Santa Cruz-high income *vs* Santa Cruz-low income; [d]$P < 0.05$, Santa Cruz-high income *vs* all. ANOVA plus Dunn's or Tukey test. (Courtesy of Giussani DA, Phillips PS, Anstee S, et al: Effects of altitude *versus* economic status on birth weight and body shape at birth. *Pediatr Res* 49:490-494, 2001.)

born at higher altitudes have decreased rates of fetal growth and altered body shape at birth has not been clarified.

▶ Two classes of nutrients, oxygen and food-derived products, are essential for fetal growth; of the two, the oxygen requirement has seemed more compelling. Oxygen exists in low concentration in fetal blood, and storage in hemoglobin and myoglobin is relatively scant. Fetal oxygen consumption amounts to 5 to 6 mL/K/min at STP and placental consumption in vitro is roughly 12 to 14 mL/K/min. Both tissues increase requirements roughly exponentially in the third trimester when the predominant accretion of fetal mass occurs, howsoever important processes of embryonic differentiation and fetal development are in earlier gestation. This study uses epidemiologic data derived from hospital records of facilities located in predominantly low- and high-income regions from 2 major cities in Bolivia with differing altitudes. La Paz has an ambient air partial pressure of oxygen (pO_2) of approximately 91 mm Hg, and Santa Cruz has an ambient pO_2 of roughly 140.5 mm Hg, assuming vapor pressure of water at about 50 mm Hg. The 55% difference in pO_2 is enough to stimulate erythropoetin production and other accommodations to hypoxemia in La Paz. Although ethnic, dietary, and immediate environmental differences exist between high- and low-altitude populations, and dietary heterogeneity exists within high- and low-income populations, the authors ignore these uncontrolled variables and make no direct appraisals of dietary intake.

Clearly, altitude is important in its association with decreased body weight independent of apparent socioeconomic status, but at high altitude, babies from low-income groups were significantly heavier than those from high-income groups, presumably a reflection of uncontrolled intragroup variability. Body shape is relatively little affected by altitude, with 2 exceptions. Infants, at least those from high-income groups, born in La Paz have larger head circumferences, and the ratio of head circumference to body weight is greater in La Paz than in Santa Cruz. It is not clear why babies of high-income lowland families are longer at birth than all others, but it is likely a reflection of unwarranted population assumptions of comparability.

Although the Barker hypothesis (see Abstracts 5–1 and 10–11) deals predominantly with nutrients of foodstuff origin, the group has demonstrated that nutrient oxygen, at least at such extremes as compared here, is the more important in terms of birth weight and head circumference. No data from which mechanistic relationships can be inferred are provided here.

T. H. Kirschbaum, MD

The Fetal and Childhood Growth of Persons Who Develop Type 2 Diabetes

Forsén T, Eriksson J, Tuomilehto J, et al (Dept of Health and Disability, Helsinki; Univ of Southampton, England)
Ann Intern Med 133:176-182, 2000

1–4

Background.—Low birth weight is associated with an increased risk of type 2 diabetes mellitus (DM) in later life. Some researchers have hypothesized that type 2 DM may be the result of fetal adaptations to malnourishment, including alterations in insulin and glucose metabolism. The risk of type 2 DM is also higher in persons who are obese, and evidence suggests that obese adults who were obese as children are at greater risk of developing type 2 DM than obese adults who were normal-weight children. Thus, adults who have type 2 DM develop may show a particular pattern of low weight at birth with increased growth during childhood. This hypothesis was examined in a cohort of 7086 Finnish adults for whom detailed height and weight records throughout childhood were available.

Methods.—Height and weight data were abstracted from detailed birth and school records of 3693 men and 3447 women born at one hospital in Helsinki between 1924 and 1933 and who still lived in Finland as of 1971. These records were linked to a national database containing all persons receiving medications for type 2 DM. Differences in height, weight, and body mass index (BMI) at birth and through childhood were compared

TABLE I.—Cumulative Incidence of Type 2 DM According to Size at Birth

Size at Birth	Men	Women	All
	% (*n*)		%
Birthweight			
≤2500 g	8.3 (145)	10.0 (190)	9.3
2501-3000 g	10.9 (552)	5.3 (704)	7.7
3001-3500 g	7.7 (1318)	5.1 (1411)	6.4
3501-4000 g	7.5 (1153)	5.2 (879)	6.5
>4000 g	5.9 (444)	4.4 (248)	5.3
P value for trend	0.002	0.08	<0.005
Length at birth			
≤48 cm	10.5 (497)	6.4 (719)	8.1
48.1-49.0 cm	7.9 (518)	4.7 (593)	6.2
49.1-50.0 cm	8.1 (993)	5.4 (1071)	6.7
50.1-51.0 cm	8.1 (749)	5.1 (588)	6.8
>51.0 cm	6.1 (841)	4.9 (449)	5.7
P value for trend	0.009	0.11	0.002
Placental weight			
≥450 g	11.2 (251)	10.1 (257)	10.6
451-550 g	7.7 (845)	5.5 (855)	6.6
551-650 g	8.6 (1181)	4.9 (1106)	6.8
651-750 g	6.7 (836)	4.9 (789)	5.8
>750 g	6.9 (496)	4.5 (418)	5.8
P value for trend	0.05	0.02	0.002

(Courtesy of Forsén T, Eriksson J, Tuomilehto J, et al: The fetal and childhood growth of persons who develop type 2 diabetes. *Ann Intern Med* 133:176-182, 2000.)

TABLE II.—Cumulative Incidence of Type 2 DM According to BMI at 11 Years of Age

Body Mass Index	Men	Women	All
kg/m^2	% (n)		%
≤15.3	7.7 (675)	4.2 (804)	5.8
15.4-15.9	9.0 (690)	3.9 (571)	6.7
16.0-16.6	7.0 (790)	4.7 (695)	5.9
16.7-17.4	7.8 (798)	5.2 (560)	6.7
>17.4	8.3 (659)	8.4 (802)	8.4
P value for trend	0.2	<0.001	<0.001

(Courtesy of Forsén T, Eriksson J, Tuomilehto J, et al: The fetal and childhood growth of persons who develop type 2 diabetes. *Ann Intern Med* 133:176-182, 2000.)

among the 471 adults (6.6%; 286 men and 185 women) who developed type 2 DM and the 6615 adults who did not.

Results.—The cumulative incidence of type 2 DM was 7.9% in men and 5.4% in women. In the entire cohort, the cumulative incidence of type 2 DM increased significantly with lower birth weight (in grams), shorter length at birth (in centimeters), and lower placental weight (in grams) (Table I). Odds ratios (ORs) for development of type 2 DM ranged from 1.07 to 1.13 for each 1-U decrease in these variables. Note that the associations between all 3 variables and type 2 DM were significant in men, but only the association between type 2 DM and placental weight was significant in women. At 7 years of age, the mean weights and heights of children who subsequently had type 2 DM develop were similar to those of children who did not have type 2 DM develop. Between 7 and 15 years of age, however, growth in the children who later had type 2 DM develop was significantly higher than that in their peers who did not have type 2 DM develop. The OR for developing type 2 DM was 1.39 for each 1 SD increase in weight between 7 and 15 years of age; the OR increased to 1.83 when analyses were restricted to persons with a birth weight less than 3000 g. BMI during childhood was not significantly associated with the development of type 2 DM in men but was strongly associated with the risk of type 2 DM in women (Table II). Additionally, having a mother who had a high BMI during pregnancy was significantly associated with more rapid growth during childhood and with a greater risk of type 2 DM. The OR for developing type 2 DM was 1.42 for each 10-kg/m² increase in the mother's BMI during pregnancy.

Conclusions.—These findings are consistent with the hypothesis that low rates of fetal growth in utero predispose a person to the development of type 2 DM as adults. Placental size was significantly reduced in the persons who later had type 2 DM develop, which further supports a link between type 2 DM and fetal undernutrition. The risk of type 2 DM was even greater when a low birth weight was combined with rapid growth between 7 and 15 years of age.

▶ The possibility that infants born smaller and lighter than expected by gestational age may have undergone a series of fetal physiologic adjustments in utero that predispose them to an increased likelihood of insulin resistance, late-onset diabetes, hypertensive disease, atherosclerosis, and arteriosclerotic heart disease in later life has come to be known as the Barker hypothesis. This study of 7086 Finnish men and women born between 1924 and 1933, subject to carefully preserved newborn data, attempts to link newborn length, body and placental weight, and patterns of BMI reflected in school records with a subsequent diagnosis of type 2 diabetes. The diagnosis of diabetes is presumed, in 513 cases, from evidence of oral antidiuretic drug or insulin use registered in Finnish Social Insurance Agency and cross-registered for hospital admissions related to diabetes in The Nutritional Hospital Discharge Registry. Review of hospital records allowed the presumptive diagnosis of type 1 diabetes in 42 persons and of late onset type 2 diabetes in 471. Analyses were based on multivariate logistic regression against the presumed occurrence of type 2 diabetes.

As is often the case with this undertaking (see 2001 YEAR BOOK OF OBSTETRICS, GYNECOLOGY, AND WOMEN'S HEALTH, pp. 14-16 and 132-133), changes are evaluated in terms of trends with few discrete significant relations identified. Birth size expressed as a derived function of BMI was not significantly inversely related to diabetes in women, but a significant trend was noted among men. Ignoring sex, risk ratios ranging from 1.04 to 1.13 were said to be significant for unit changes in length, ponderal index, and placental weight, but whether equally so in men and women is unrecorded. Differences between men and women from ages 7 to 15 years were 0.1 to 0.3 of a SD, but means and SDs were not provided. Girls grew faster in BMI than did boys during this time, but BMI changes boys were not related to type 2 diabetes in later life. When rates of BMI were pooled for sex, increases were said to be related to diabetes in later life. No significant relations to maternal body measurements or social class and home crowding, in data maintained by the Finnish Central Statistic Office, were noted.

This is a reasonably familiar exploration of the Barker hypothesis. There are nonhomogeneous trends seen in some, but not all, subsets of patients, and differences are miniscule among them. Little security is offered or can exist for diagnostic entities established 60 to 75 years ago. Derived variables, not primary data, are provided by the authors and, as noted, contrary data and opinions exist. It remains a fascinating possibility that the fetus is imprinted by elements of life in utero in a way that has an impact on later life. It's that possibility that keeps this effort alive despite the softness of the data analysis used.

T. H. Kirschbaum, MD

Diabetic Endothelial Dysfunction: The Role of Poly(ADP-Ribose) Polymerase Activation

Garcia Soriano F, Virág L, Jagtap P, et al (Inotek Corp, Beverly, Mass; Univ of Medicine and Dentistry New Jersey, Newark; Ohio State Univ, Columbus; et al)
Nat Med 7:108-113, 2001

1–5

Introduction.—Retinopathy, nephropathy, neuropathy, and accelerated atherosclerosis commonly occur in patients with diabetes. These vascular alterations follow the loss of endothelial function. The loss of endothelial function in patients with diabetes was analyzed to determine if it is dependent upon the activation of the poly(ADP-ribose) polymerase (PARP) pathway within the vasculature. PARP is a profuse nuclear enzyme of eukaryotic cells that has been implicated in response to DNA injury.

Findings.—Ex vivo experiments revealed the loss of endothelial function from streptozotocin-treated mice, as determined by the relaxant respon-

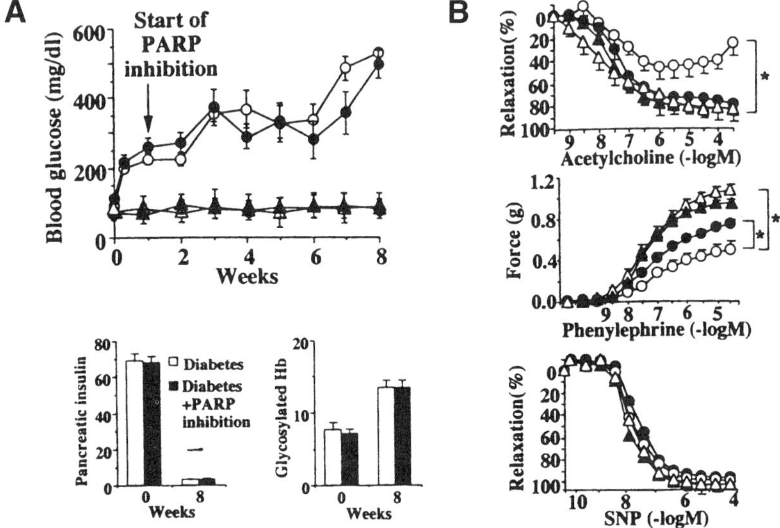

FIGURE 1.—Reversal of diabetes-induced endothelial dysfunction by pharmacological inhibition of PARP. Symbols used for the respective groups: animals which received no streptozotocin injection (*white triangle*), nondiabetic control animals at 8 weeks treated with PJ34 between weeks 1 and 8 (*black triangle*), diabetic animals at week 8 treated with vehicle (*white circle*), diabetic animals at week 8 treated with PJ34 between weeks 1 and 8 (*black circle*). A, Blood glucose levels, pancreatic insulin content (ng insulin/mg pancreatic protein) and blood glycosylated hemoglobin (Hb) (expressed as % of total Hb) at 0-8 weeks in nondiabetic control male BALB/c mice, and at 0-8 weeks after streptozotocin treatment (diabetic) in male BALB/c mice PARP inhibitor treatment, starting at 1 week after streptozotocin and continuing until the end of week 8, is indicated by the *arrow*. Pancreatic insulin and glycated hemoglobin levels content are shown at 8 weeks in vehicle-treated and streptozotocin-treated animals, in the presence or absence of PJ34 treatment. B, Acetylcholine-induced, endothelium-dependent relaxations; phenylephrine-induced contractions; and SNP-induced endothelium-independent relaxations. *P < .05 for vehicle-treated diabetic versus PJ34-treated diabetic mice (n = 8 per group). (Courtesy of Garcia Soriano F, Virág L, Jagtap P, et al: Diabetic endothelial dysfunction: The role of poly(ADP-ribose) polymerase activation. *Nat Med* 7:108-113, 2001.)

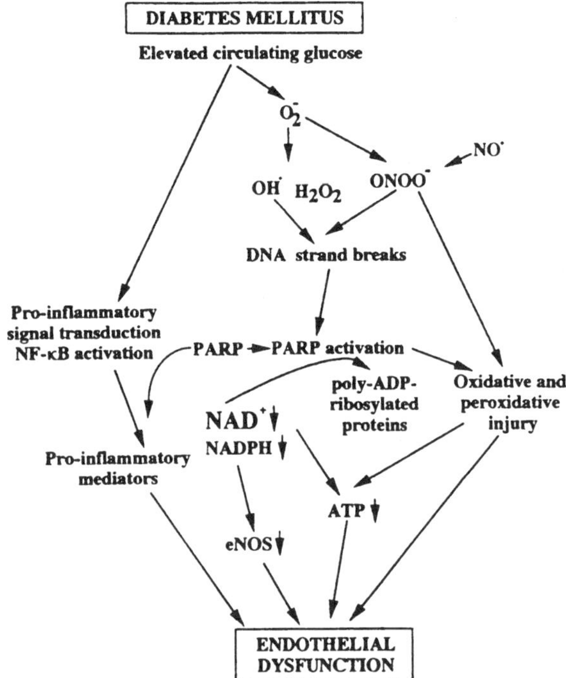

FIGURE 6.—Proposed scheme for the potential mechanisms of intravascular PARP activation and related endothelial dysfunction in diabetes mellitus. *Abbreviations*: *PARP*, Poly(ADP-ribose) polymerase; *NAD*, nicotinamide adenine dinucleotide; *NADPH*, nicotinamide adenine dinucleotide phosphate. (Courtesy of Garcia Soriano F, Virág L, Jagtap P, et al: Diabetic endothelial dysfunction: The role of poly(ADP-ribose) polymerase activation. *Nat Med* 7:108-113, 2001.)

siveness of precontracted rings to the endothelium-dependent vasodilator, nitric oxide-liberating hormone acetylcholine (Fig 1). Activation of PARP was important in the pathogenesis of endothelial dysfunction in patients with diabetes (Fig 6). Chronic treatment with PJ34 was used to inhibit PARP activation. This delayed treatment regimen averted vascular PARP activation. The destruction of islet cells with streptozotocin in mice produced hyperglycemia, intravascular oxidant production, DNA strand breakage, PARP activation, and a selective loss of endothelium-dependent vasodilation. Treatment with a novel potent PARP inhibitor, beginning at the time of islet destruction, maintained normal vascular responsiveness, in spite of the persistence of severe hyperglycemia. Endothelial cells incubated in high glucose inhibited production of reactive nitrogen and oxygen species, consequent single-stranded DNA breakage, PARP activation, and associated metabolic and functional impairment. Basal and high-glucose-induced nuclear factor-κB activation were restrained in the PARP-deficient cells.

Conclusion.—It may be that PARP is a novel drug target for the therapy of diabetic endothelial dysfunction.

▶ The search for the mechanism of endothelial dysfunction in preeclampsia has been joined by those interested in evidence of endothelial dysfunction in diabetes mellitus, which sometimes precedes structural vascular injury in renal, retinal, coronary, and other organ systems (see 1991 YEAR BOOK OF OBSTETRICS, GYNECOLOGY, AND WOMEN'S HEALTH, pp 45-46 and 2001 YEAR BOOK, pp 49-50). This series of experiments demonstrates 1 of the mechanisms that might be involved. The experimental model is the mouse rendered diabetic by treatment with streptozotocin, an agent that selectively destroys pancreatic islet cells. The authors demonstrate that the resultant hyperglycemia leads to a loss of vasodilatory responsiveness to nitric oxide-generating acetylcholine, due in turn, to a production of hydroxyl radicals, H_2O_2, and peroxynitrite. Part of the evidence for that claim is the ability of treatment with L-NAME, an inhibitor of nitric oxide synthesis and of nitrite and free radical oxidative stress, to prevent it. Left unopposed, the oxygen-free radicals result in nitrotyrosine deposition and generate single-stranded DNA with broken DNA strands, both demonstrable with cytohistochemistry (see Figure 2 in the original article). DNA injury results in induction of poly(ADP ribose) polymerase (PARP), which functions to consume cellular energy by transferring ribose ADP units from oxidized nicotinamide adenine dinucleotide (NAD^+) to damaged nuclear proteins. This step essentially reverses normal oxidative metabolism in which acetyl-CoA yields NAD hydride (NADH), which in turn, through oxidative phosphorlyation, generates ATP. In the process, NADH transfers 2 high-energy electrons to ADP to form ATP and releases a proton. Reversing this sequence through the action of PARP depletes cellular ATP, the dominant reservoir of cellular energetics, and simultaneously stimulates the endothelial isoform of nitric oxide synthase (eNOS) to increase nitric oxide synthesis. Together, these changes result in endothelial injury through reduction in mitochondrial function and cellular oxidative metabolism. The role of PARP in the process is proven through use of a PARP inhibitor, PJ34, which partially restores the ability of acetylcholine to produce reactive vasodilation. As Figure 2 shows, the results are PARP inhibition and the return of vascular activity to acetylcholine, despite persistent nitrotyrosine staining and DNA breaks as evidence of partial nitrate and oxygen radical injury. The result illustrated in Figure 6 is endothelial injury in induced diabetes, possibly occurring in spontaneous human diabetes and, perhaps, in preeclampsia. As Figure 1 shows, PARP inhibition by PJ34 selectively improves the response of aortic segments to the vascular effects of acetylcholine, indicating improved ex vitro endothelial cell function.

The hypothetical origin of such a sequence in preeclampsia is obscure, but the insulin resistance noted in women with preeclampsia may well be involved (see 1998 YEAR BOOK, pp 123-125). Although there are other possible biochemical pathways leading to endothelial injury in diabetes and yet to be delineated, this is an example of a series of steps in basic research that leads to new opportunities to understand and reverse the endovascular pathology of diabetes.

T. H. Kirschbaum, MD

Maternal Plasma Vascular Endothelial Growth Factor Concentrations in Normal and Hypertensive Pregnancies and Their Relationship to Peripheral Vascular Resistance
Bosio PM, Wheeler T, Anthony F, et al (Univ of Southampton, England)
Am J Obstet Gynecol 184:146-152, 2001   1–6

Introduction.—Vascular endothelial growth factor (VEGF) concentrations are increased in the plasma or serum of women with preeclampsia. It is not known why this occurs. Maternal plasma VEGF concentrations during normal and hypertensive pregnancies were measured. Their relationship with maternal total peripheral resistance values were compared in the first longitudinal examination of maternal plasma VEGF concentrations during pregnancy.

Methods.—Plasma concentrations of total immunoreactive VEGF and total peripheral resistances were determined serially throughout the pregnancy of 20 females with preeclampsia, 24 with gestational hypertension, and 26 normotensive control women. The relationship between VEGF levels in these groups and total peripheral resistance was analyzed.

Results.—At 10 to 14 weeks' gestation, plasma VEGF concentrations in all patients were 4 to 5 times greater than levels measured postpartum (P < .0001). The mean VEGF concentrations were similar in control and gestational hypertension groups and remained stable until 34 to 36 weeks gestation, when levels rose a further 1.3-fold (P < .01). The VEGF concentrations in patients in the preeclampsia group were higher at 28 to 32 weeks' gestation (P = .002) and at 34 to 36 weeks' gestation (P < .001). The VEGF concentrations were also higher during the 4 weeks preceding the diagnosis of preeclampsia (P < .05). An association was noted between VEGF concentrations and elevated total peripheral resistance seen during the clinical disorder in the preeclampsia group and not in the other 2 groups (Fig 1).

Conclusion.—Maternal plasma VEGF concentrations increased before the clinical onset of preeclampsia and were further increased during the vasoconstriction state that occurs in preeclampsia. It may be that the hyperdynamic circulation that characterizes the latent phase of preeclampsia produces vascular sheer stress, which then increases the levels of circulating VEGF. Because VEGF acts as a vasodilator, its increase may demonstrate an unsuccessful vascular rescue response.

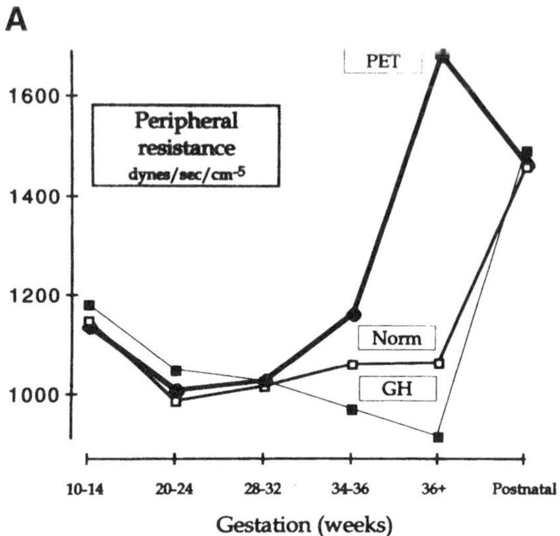

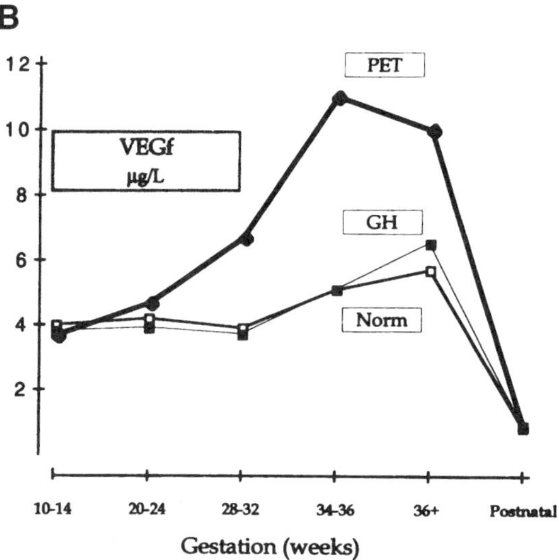

FIGURE 1.—Mean total peripheral resistances (A) and levels of VEGF (B) throughout pregnancy and 6 to 8 weeks postpartum in normotensive control group (*Norm; open squares*), gestational hypertension group (*GH, filled squares*), and preeclampsia group (*PET; filled diamonds*). (Courtesy of Bosio PM, Wheeler T, Anthony F, et al: Maternal plasma vascular endothelial growth factor concentrations in normal and hypertensive pregnancies and their relationship to peripheral vascular resistance. *Am J Obstet Gynecol* 184:146-152, 2001.)

▶ VEGF is a cytokine with receptors confined to endothelium, responsible for endothelial growth and repair and, by means of stimulating increased nitric oxide production and arteriolar vasodilation. This longitudinal study of 20 women with preeclampsia, 24 women with gestational hypertension

(hypertension during pregnancy in the absence of proteinuria), and 26 normal control pregnant patients explores its possible role in preeclampsia. Blood sampling for radioimmunoassay for VEGF was done on 5 occasions through pregnancy and maternal peripheral vascular resistance calculated from echocardiography and Doppler estimates of cardiac output, together with standard clinical blood pressure measurements. VEGF was found to increase in concentration in the maternal plasma of preeclamptic women, paralleling the increase in calculated peripheral vascular resistance prior to delivery. Presumably, the increased endothelial shear stress associated with vasoconstriction in preeclampsia stimulates endothelial VEGF (see Abstract 4–10) apparently a means of increasing endothelial nitric oxide with a possible role in implementing vasodilatation and ameliorating the effects of preeclamptic vasoconstriction. Evidence of overlap of VEGF concentration in preeclamptic and normotensive gravidas suggest that VEGF is a result, not a cause, of the increased peripheral vascular resistance of preeclampsia.

T. H. Kirschbaum, MD

A Longitudinal Study of Maternal Plasma Insulin-Like Growth Factor Binding Protein-1 Concentrations During Normal Pregnancy and Pregnancies Complicated by Pre-Eclampsia
Anim-Nyame N, Hills FA, Sooranna SR, et al (Chelsea & Westminster Hosp, London; Queen Charlotte's & Chelsea Hosp, London)
Hum Reprod 15:2215-2219, 2000   1–7

Background.—The decidualized endometrial stroma produces insulin-like growth factor binding protein-1 (IGFBP-1), which may take part in implantation, possibly reducing trophoblast invasion. Higher-than-normal circulating levels are found in pregnancies complicated by preeclampsia and intrauterine growth restriction (IUGR). This longitudinal study was done to elucidate the role of IGFBP-1 during placentation and the development of pre-eclampsia.

Methods.—Ten women studied went on to develop preeclampsia; 12 others with similar age, body mass index, and gestational age who did not develop preeclampsia were used for comparison. Plasma concentrations of maternal IGFBP-1 were measured at 16, 20, 24, 28, 32, and 36 weeks of gestation.

Results.—The normal women had no change in IGFBP-1 concentrations, but the women who developed preeclampsia had values that increased progressively. Compared with the normal pregnancies, levels in the preeclamptic women were significantly lower at weeks 16, 20, and 24; they were similar at weeks 28 and 32, and significantly higher by week 36.

Conclusions.—IGFBP-1 levels were significantly lower in early pregnancy for women who went on to develop pre-eclampsia than for women who did not. This is well before the development of pre-eclampsia, making it unlikely that IGFBP-1 leads to preeclampsia by inducing the inhibition of IGF activity.

▶ IGF-1 and -2 are polypeptide somatomedins that affect implantation and placentation (IGF-1) and infant nutrition as measured by birth weight (IGF-2). The reader may wish in this connection to review the 1992 Year Book of Obstetrics, Gynecology, and Women's Health, pp 122-124; 1995 Year Book, pp 123-124; 1996 Year Book, pp 17-21; 1998 Year Book, pp 3-8 and pp 218-220; and 1999 Year Book, pp 163-166. The activities of these substances are influenced in a complex way by a series of 7 binding proteins, differentially localized within the reproductive tract, which may act by facilitation or inhibition upon ligand binding. Binding proteins to IGF-1, produced in its decidual origin, are felt to have the capacity to inhibit IGF-1 in its role in facilitating trophoblastic invasion into decidualized endometrial stroma in the course of early implantation. Such inhibition might explain the superficial implantation associated with preeclampsia and some cases of intrauterine growth retardation (see 1994 Year Book, pp 59-60). Since the fundamental organization of implantation is established as early as 18 days postconception, and placental and fetal differentiation completed by 10 to 12 weeks' gestational age, increased IGFBP-1 should be noted in early pregnancy, certainly by 16 weeks, if it is to play a role in the superficial penetration and implantation of the trophoblast associated with the development of pregnancy hypertension. Two cross-sectional studies of maternal IGFBP-1 activity in human blood reached opposing conclusions regarding the early timing of changes. This study uses longitudinal data collection in 10 women destined for preeclampsia and 12 ultimately normotensive women with sampling at 16, 20, 24, 28, 32, and 36 weeks' gestational age. Regrettably, studies were not confined to primigravidas, but the results clearly show low concentrations of IGFBP-1 in the first trimester of pregnancy, increasing progressively thereafter. Although contrary data may emerge, these data fail to support a putative role for excessive IGF binding protein 1 in the vascular pathology of pregnancy-induced hypertension.

T. H. Kirschbaum, MD

Conditioned Medium From Hypoxic Cytotrophoblasts Alters Arterial Function
Gratton RJ, Gandley RE, Genbacev O, et al (Univ of Pittsburgh, Pa; Univ of California, San Francisco)
Am J Obstet Gynecol 184:984-990, 2001   1–8

Objective.—Preeclampsia appears to arise from vascular endothelium and smooth muscle abnormalities. The placenta seems to be involved in mediating these changes by impairing cytotrophoblast invasion into the uterine decidua, myometrium, and spiral arteries. Cytotrophoblasts, under low oxygen tension, may release substances to affect vascular behavior. Vascular contractility, relaxation capacity, and oscillatory behavior of isolated resistance-sized mesenteric arteries were tested after incubation in conditioned medium from first-trimester human cytotrophoblasts maintained in hypoxic culture conditions.

Methods.—Arterial segments from the mesentery of pregnant rats were incubated in standard or hypoxic conditions with cytotrophoblasts isolated from pooled first-trimester human placentas. The vascular response of arterial segments equilibrated in HEPES physiologic saline solution to phenylephrine (receptor dependent) and potassium (receptor independent), the relaxation response to methacholine, and vasomotion amplitudes were determined.

Results.—Vascular response to phenylephrine was increased after incubation in hypoxia media. The response to potassium was significantly greater in arteries incubated in hypoxia media. Relaxation response to methacholine was blunted by incubation in hypoxia media compared with arteries incubated in control medium.

Conclusion.—These results indicate that there is relative hypoxia within the placenta in preeclampsia. There appears to be a link between the abnormal placentation and the maternal vascular abnormality. Low oxygen tension may facilitate changes in trophoblast function.

▶ These very productive scientists are approaching an important issue: whether hypoxic cytotrophoblasts during preeclampsia produce substances that result in the increased systemic vascular resistance in preeclampsia. The longstanding collaboration between the University of California at San Francisco and the University of Pittsburgh has a splendid record in studies of the nature of trophoblastic integrins and connexins linking trophoblast to decidua (see 1994 YEAR BOOK OF OBSTETRICS, GYNECOLOGY, AND WOMEN'S HEALTH, pp 59-60), the normal progression of expression of adhesion molecules with normal and pathologic trophoblastic invasion and maturation in decidual interactions (see 1998 YEAR BOOK, pp 18-21 and pp 50-51), and trophoblastic apoptosis in preeclamptic placentas (see 2001 YEAR BOOK, pp 119-123).

Here, using cell cultures of human cytotrophoblasts exposed to control gas phase consisting of 95% air versus a hypoxic phase (2% oxygen, 93% nitrogen, 5% carbon dioxide), samples of conditioned media were collected. The test system in which vessel reactions were compared consisted of cannulated segments of pregnant rat mesenteric vessels 0.25 to 0.35 cm in diameter in a system that allows perfusion and internal pressure to be monitored and vessel wall thickness and luminal diameters to be measured electronically. The effects of the medium from hypoxic cell cultures was to increase contractility stimulated by a β-adrenergic agent and by potassium depolarization, to decrease the observed relaxation of preconstructed vessel segments on exposure to a choline ester, and to increase the amplitude of arrhythmic contractility compared with controls.

Within the test system, they have proven the ability of hypoxic trophoblasts to effect changes in vascular behavior in a paracrine fashion. This is, however, preliminary work in the sense that the experiments should be repeated with human vascular tissue and by using hypoxic perfusate PO_2 as an independent variable. The PO_2 within the intervillous space appears to be heterogenous, and the size of its roduction in preeclampsia is incompletely measured. Two percent oxygen yields a PO_2 of about 14 mm Hg, clearly less than measurements performed in the human uterus at or past 10 weeks' gestation.[1] The authors choice of PO_2, which allows maintenance of cell culture without apoptosis, may not suffice to depict a trophoblastic response to hypoxia in vivo. This is, however, an important step and their future work should be eagerly anticipated.

T. H. Kirschbaum, MD

Reference

1. Rodesch CF, Simon P, Donner C: Oxygen measurements in endometrial and trophoblastic tissues during early pregnancy. *Obstet Gynecol* 80:283, 1992.

Delayed Hypotension and Subendocardial Injury After Repeated Umbilical Cord Occlusion in Near-Term Fetal Lambs
Gunn AJ, Maxwell L, de Haan HH, et al (Univ of Auckland, New Zealand)
Am J Obstet Gynecol 183:1564-1572, 2000   1–9

Introduction.—Repeated brief episodes of total umbilical cord occlusion in the fetal sheep leads to the progressive evolution of cardiovascular compromise and cerebral injury. The cardiac disease condition after a recovery of 3 days was assessed in near-term fetal sheep to determine (1) whether pathologically defined cardiac damage occurs in fetuses that survive clinically relevant asphyxia and (2) whether cardiac dysfunction is associated with the extent or severity of cardiac disease changes.

Methods.—Instrumentation was implanted in near-term fetal sheep who underwent either sham occlusions or repeated brief umbilical cord occlusions (8 and 12 animals, respectively). The occlusions were continued until the onset of severe (less than 20 mm Hg) or sustained hypotension. After 3 days of recuperation from the occlusions, the sheep were killed, and the fetal hearts were prepared for analysis.

Results.—Repeated umbilical cord occlusions produced a severe metabolic acidosis (pH, 6.84; lactate concentration, 14.1 mmol/L) with increased hypotension during occlusions, which were halted after a mean of 128 min. After occlusions, the mean arterial pressure revealed a delayed fall, which resolved after 12 hours (Fig 4). Ultrastructural evaluation identified evidence of subendocardial injury, with dilatation of sarcoplasmic reticulum, margination and clumping of nuclear chromatin, and mitochondrial swelling (Fig 2). The most severe morphologic changes, including electron-dense mitochondrial inclusions, were observed in the fetuses with delayed recovery of the fetal heart rate after the final occlusion (Fig 6).

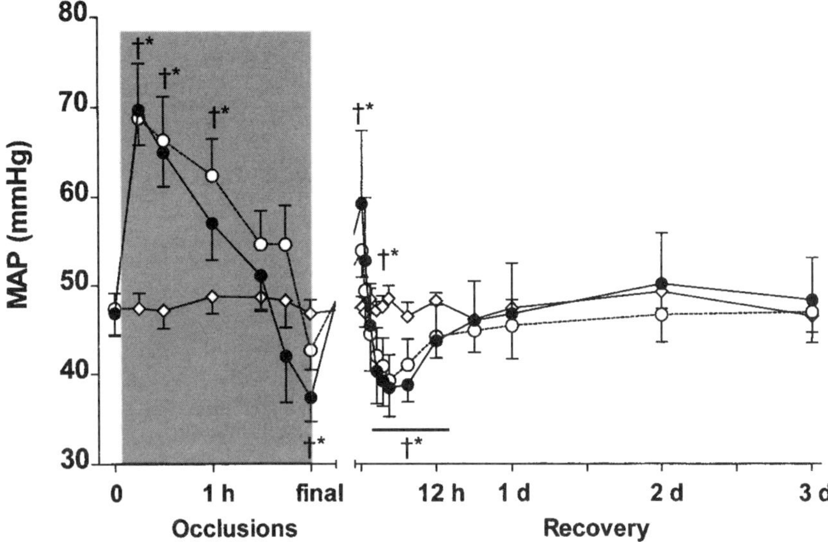

FIGURE 4.—Time sequences of changes in fetal mean arterial pressure (MAP), showing average MAP during occlusions and then during postinsult recovery period. Overall sequence of changes in MAP was not different between the fetuses showing moderate to severe subendocardial changes (*closed circles*; n = 4) and fetuses showing mild subendocardial changes (*open circles*; n = 8). Sham control fetuses (*open diamonds*; n = 8) showed no significant changes. From 60 minutes onward nadir of MAP at end of each occlusion was significantly lower than baseline MAP. *Asterisk*, $P < .05$, compared with sham control group. *Dagger*, $P < .05$, Wilcoxon matched-pairs signed rank test for both groups combined compared with first occlusion. *Shaded region*, Period of occlusions; subsequent *unshaded region*, 3-day recovery period. *Data points*, Mean; *error bars*, SEM. (Courtesy of Gunn AJ, Maxwell L, de Haan HH, et al: Delayed hypotension and subendocardial injury after repeated umbilical cord occlusion in near-term fetal lambs. *Am J Obstet Gynecol* 183:1564-1572, 2000.)

Conclusion.—Subendocardial injury results from severe repeated intrauterine asphyxia in the late-gestation fetus, and this may contribute to cardiovascular compromise and the development of late decelerations.

▶ In their extensive experience in the documentation of the effects of intrauterine asphyxia on fetal lambs, these authors have attempted to simulate the effects of repeated cord compromise as though it occurred from latent cord prolapse, nuchal, or short umbilical cords. Employing cord occlusion in utero an average of once every 2½ minutes, they continued serial occlusions until fetal arterial blood pressure had either declined by 20 mm Hg from baseline or failed to return to the baseline after release of occlusion. As reported earlier (see 1998 YEAR BOOK OF OBSTETRICS, GYNECOLOGY, AND WOMEN'S HEALTH, pp 86-89 and 150-153), the fetuses at 0.9 term (term is 142 days) developed combined metabolic and respiratory acidosis with umbilical artery pHs in the range of 6.8 to 6.9 and evidence of cardiovascular and cerebral injury. Such changes in cerebral function and respiratory metabolism have been reported here extensively (see 1990 YEAR BOOK, pp 206-207; 1992 YEAR BOOK, pp 189-191, and 1993 YEAR BOOK, pp 123-124); here the focus is on related cardiac pathology.

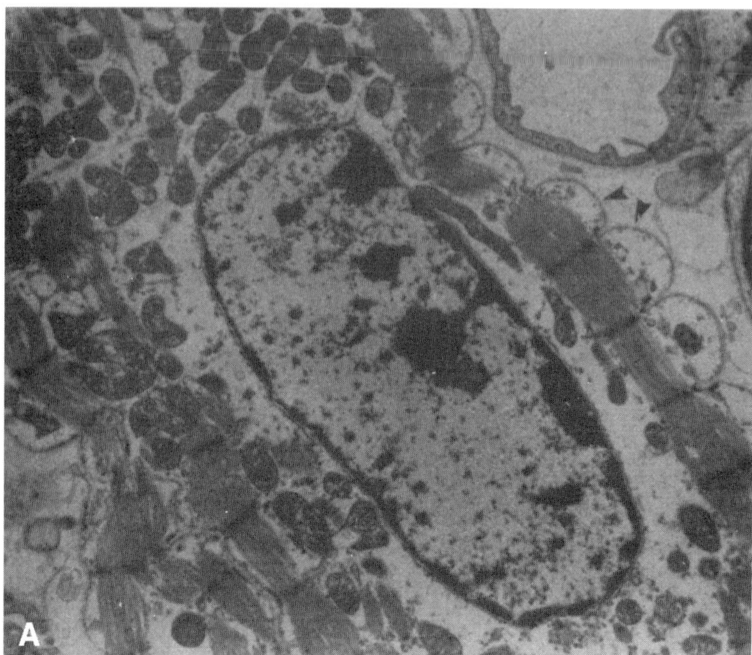

FIGURE 2.—Transmission electron photomicrograph of subendocardial myocardium from asphyxiated fetuses. A, Mild myocardial injury, showing focal mitochondrial swelling, subsarcoplasmic blebbing (*arrowheads*), and clearing of cytoplasm. (Courtesy of Gunn AJ, Maxwell L, de Haan HH, et al: Delayed hypotension and subendocardial injury after repeated umbilical cord occlusion in near-term fetal lambs. *Am J Obstet Gynecol* 183:1564-1572, 2000.)

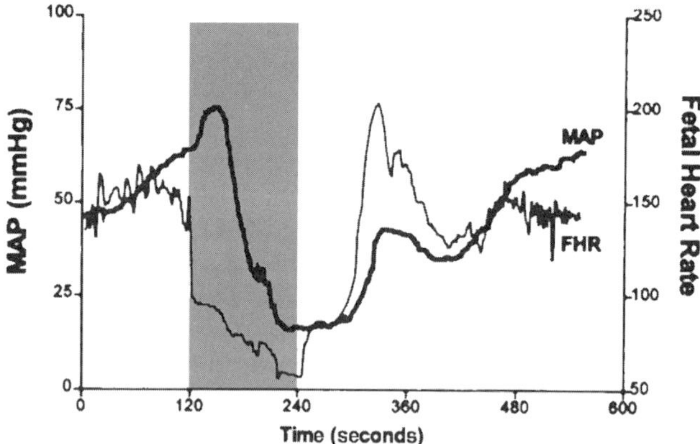

FIGURE 6.—Examples of changes in fetal heart rate (FHR) (*thin line*) and mean arterial pressure (MAP) (*thick line*) during final 2-minute episode of umbilical cord occlusion (*shaded area*) in fetus that showed extensive subendocardial changes 3 days after recovery. Note that both FHR and MAP took several minutes to fully recover. (Courtesy of Gunn AJ, Maxwell L, de Haan HH, et al: Delayed hypotension and subendocardial injury after repeated umbilical cord occlusion in near-term fetal lambs. *Am J Obstet Gynecol* 183:1564-1572, 2000.)

In general, the occurrence of fetal cardiac injury was reflected by fetal hypotension during or after a period of cord occlusion, but only the time required for recovery to normal fetal heart rate after the occlusion correlated with the severity of cardiac injury. When necropsy was done 3 days after the last occlusion, 11 of 12 fetuses showed biventricular subendocardial capillary and intramyocardial vacuolization. In 3 of 12 cases, similar lesions were seen in the septal myocardium. Transmission electron microscopy showed myofibrillary separations, subsarcoplasmic blebbing, chromatin clumping and margination, and both mitochondrial swelling and disruption.

The authors demonstrate that potentially reversible structural myocardial changes can occur in fetuses exposed to periodic cord occlusion, not explicable on the basis of acidosis and metabolic derangement, as demonstrated in their earlier work. Persistent hypotension tended to persist nearly 36 hours after cessation of asphyxia (see Fig 4), and acutely for as long as 6 minutes after the termination of an occlusion episode (see Fig 6), indicating cardiac dysfunction independent of simple interruption of umbilical vein metabolic effects. Further, the cardiovascular changes persist for at least 72 hours after the last occlusion episode. This means that fetal cardiac injury following severe repeated cord occlusion can influence fetal heart rate patterns and cardiovascular function for long periods after transient but repeated cord occlusion. Though it is not entirely safe to assume the same changes would be seen in the human fetus, these authors have in the past been able to point the way to human pathology, based on their work in experimental animals.

T. H. Kirschbaum, MD

Fetal Parathyroids Are Not Required to Maintain Placental Calcium Transport

Kovacs CS, Manley NR, Moseley JM, et al (Mem Univ of Newfoundland, St John's, Canada; Med College of Georgia, Augusta; Univ of Melbourne, Fitzroy, Victoria, Australia; et al)
J Clin Invest 107:1007-1015, 2001   1–10

Background.—Parathyroid hormone–related protein (PTHrP) contributes significantly to normal fetal-placental calcium homeostasis, and its absence produces hypocalcemia, hyperphosphatemia, and reduced placental calcium transfer. Parathyroid hormone (PTH) cannot compensate sufficiently for the lack of PTHrP, but PTH also has a role in fetal blood calcium regulation. The role of fetal parathyroid glands in fetal blood homeostasis in mice was addressed.

Methods.—The *Hoxa3* knockout mouse and other mouse models were used. The *Hoxa3*-null fetuses do not have a parathyroid gland; absence of PTH was confirmed by immunoradiometric assay. Samples collected included fetal blood, amniotic fluid, maternal blood, and various fetal tissues (head, neck, lung, liver, umbilical cord, placenta). Ionized calcium levels were determined, as well as placental calcium transfer and plasma PTHrP levels. Other tests included riboprobe and DNA probe labeling, Northern blot analysis, in situ hybridization, and immunohistochemical evaluations.

Results.—*Hoxa3* mutants and their heterozygous siblings had normal rates of placental calcium transfer and plasma PTHrP levels. The plasma PTHrP levels found in *Pthr1*-null fetuses were 11-fold higher than those found in their littermates. Liver and placenta were the sites of increased expression of PTHrP in *Pthr1*-null fetuses.

Conclusions.—*Hoxa3*-null fetuses lack PTH, have reduced levels of ionized calcium (as well as magnesium), and have higher levels of serum phosphate, but their plasma PTHrP levels and rate of placental calcium transfer were normal. Thus, both PTHrP and PTH are required for normal fetal calcium homeostasis, with the lack of either of them leading to disrupted calcium metabolism.

▶ PTHrP is a peptide comprising 173 amnio acids or more, produced by a wide range of tissues functioning in paracrine fashion. It has considerable structural homology with parathormone (PTH), an 84 amino acid peptide, and, although each has its own discrete gene, the 2 have likely evolved from a single ancestral gene. Known to be heavily expressed in the presence of tumor aggregates, PTHrP has been recognized to cause hypercalcemia in some tumor patients, but this group's work has defined its role in fetal calcium balance and its regulation through use of gene knockout preparations.

For a description of the technique, see Abstract 1–1. Briefly, it involves plasmid insertion of a chosen inactivated gene segment together with neighboring normal complimentary DNA into embryonic stem cells. Using marker DNA segments, the incorporated DNA segments are identified in culture and inserted into blastocysts. Individuals expressing the absence of function of the "knockout gene" are identified by phenotype, and controlled mating for several generations yields a homogeneous group of individuals with the altered genotype. For obvious reasons, this work cannot be done in the human and the animal of dominant choice is the mouse. Using these preparations, these investigators studied the absence of parathyroid tissue in homozygous PTH knockouts (*Hoxa3*-null) and PTHrP receptor knockouts (*Pthr1*-null) mice, hoping to define the role of PTHrP and its fetal sources in fetal calcium metabolism.

The *Hoxa3* mice show undetectable PTH, proving the absence of parathyroid tissue. The fetal serum calcium level is lower than the maternal level and phosphate concentration is increased in concentration whereas amniotic fluid calcium level is reduced, reflecting renal tubular reabsorption of calcium to attempt homeostasis for the lack of PTH. The fetuses die soon after birth with absence of thyroid and thymus and a bone disorder similar to chondrodysplasia, demonstrating the need for PTH to sustain fetal development when homozygous PTH knockout is accomplished. In pregnant mice, fetal calcium concentration roughly equals maternal calcium concentration; maternal PTHrP is reduced but unaltered in the fetal blood. Placental calcium transfer measured by determination of ratios of [45]Ca to ^{51}Cr in fetal blood 5 minutes after fetal injection is found to be normal in *Hoxa3*-null mice.

Northern blots and immunocytochemistry demonstrate the origin of PTHrP to be fetal liver and placenta; the protein has also been seen in pancreas, brain, lung, heart, breast tissue, muscle, and endothelium. PTHrP appears to play an essential role in fetal animals in maintaining maternal-to-fetal placental active calcium transport and probably in other fetal developmental processes as well. It is becoming clear that both PTH and PTHrP are essential for fetal calcium homeostasis; the lack of either interferes with normal metabolism, but only the lack of PTHrP reduces placental calcium transfer from mother to fetus.

T. H. Kirschbaum, MD

A New Concept of the Significance of Regional Distribution of Prostaglandin H Synthase 2 Throughout the Uterus During Late Pregnancy: Investigations in a Baboon Model

Wu WX, Ma XH, Smith GCS, et al (Cornell Univ, Ithaca, NY; Univ of Glasgow, Scotland)
Am J Obstet Gynecol 183:1287-1295, 2000 1–11

Introduction.—The endocervical application of exogenous synthetic prostaglandin E_2 (PGE_2) is effective in softening and preparing the cervix

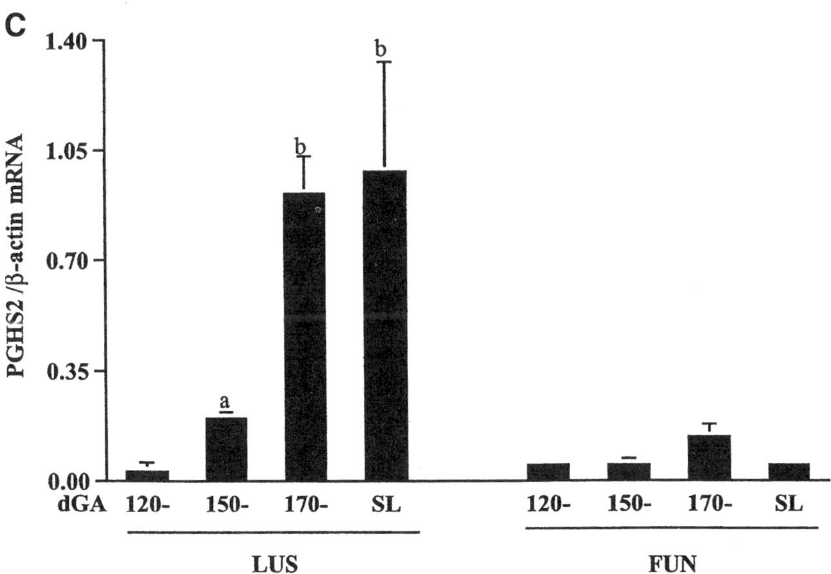

FIGURE 5C.—Densiometric analysis of ratio of messenger RNA for PGHS2 to that for gene for beta-actin in lower uterine segment and uterine fundus from baboons during late gestation and during spontaneous labor. Letters *a* and *b*, *P* < .05, compared with groups with different letters or no letters. *Bar Heights*, mean; *error bars*, SEM. *Abbreviations*: *dGA*, Days of gestation; *LVS*, lower uterine segment; *FVN*, uterine fundus, *SL*, spontaneous labor. (Courtesy of Wu WX, Ma XH, Smith GCS, et al: A new concept of the significance of regional distribution of prostaglandin H synthase 2 throughout the uterus during late pregnancy: Investigations in a baboon model. *Am J Obstet Gynecol* 183:1287-1295, 2000.)

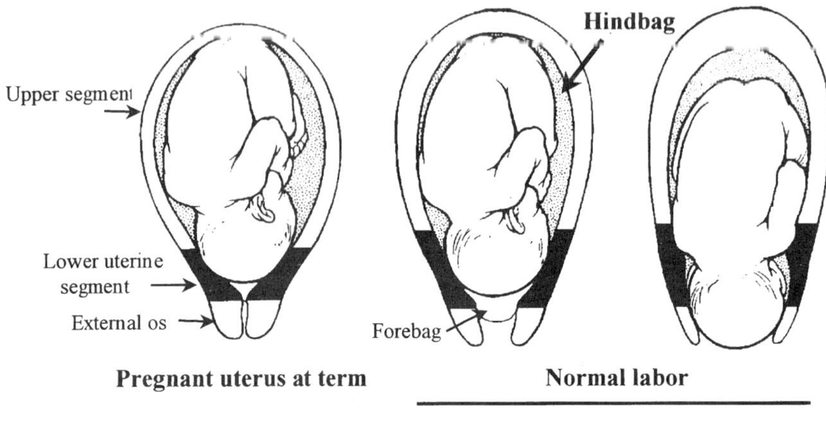

FIGURE 7.—Diagram of relationship of fetus to cervix and lower and upper uterine segments during late gestation, when fetal head engages, and as labor advances. Note pressure and stretching effects of fetal presenting part on lower uterine segment and cervix. Also note how lower uterine segment is taken up into upper uterus as labor progresses. (Courtesy of Wu WX, Ma XH, Smith GCS, et al: A new concept of the significance of regional distribution of prostaglandin H synthase 2 throughout the uterus during late pregnancy: Investigations in a baboon model. *Am J Obstet Gynecol* 183:1287-1295, 2000.)

and in inducing labor. It is likely that increased local prostaglandin activity occurs in the tissues of the lower uterine segment and cervix at the end of gestation, long before onset of labor. Understanding this dynamic could help explain the various interactive roles of different intrauterine tissues in the processes that precede, promote, and complete labor. Regional differences in prostaglandin H synthase 2 (PGHS2) messenger RNA (mRNA) expression in various uterine tissues were examined in pregnant baboons to determine prostaglandin production capability.

Methods.—PGHS2 mRNA expression was evaluated via reverse transcriptase-polymerase chain reaction or Northern blot analysis in the uterine fundus, lower uterine segment, cervix, amnion, chorion, and placenta during late pregnancy and spontaneous term labor in the pregnant baboon. Myometrial electromyography showed a clear relation of the findings to uterine contractile activity.

Results.—A marked increase in PGHS2 mRNA expression was noted during late gestation and during labor in the lower uterine segment, cervix, and decidua. An increase in amniotic PGHS2 mRNA was observed during labor, compared with no change in the uterine fundus, chorion, and placenta during late gestation and labor (Fig 5).

Conclusion.—The observed increased lower uterine segment and cervical PGHS2 abundances would stimulate lower uterine segment elongation and cervical effacement (Fig 7). Engagement of the fetal presenting part would stimulate local PGHS2 expression and obstruct diffusion of high forebag prostaglandin to the remaining uterus, as reported earlier in human pregnancy. This information supports a new conceptual mechanistic framework for preparatory changes in the lower uterine segment and cervix before labor as precisely related to myometrial contractility changes.

▶ It was the late Paul C. MacDonald and his colleagues in Dallas who first pointed out the high concentrations of PGE_2 and PGF_2 alpha metabolites in the amniotic fluid forewaters compared with the hind waters in women in labor (see 1994 YEAR BOOK OF OBSTETRICS, GYNECOLOGY, AND WOMEN'S HEALTH, pp 19-21). They attributed their finding to inflammatory changes in the forward amniotic compartment from adjoining vaginal microorganisms and decidual disruption coincident with, and possibly, stimulating spontaneous labor.

To explore the possibility that there are regional differences in the availability of prostaglandin H synthase 2 (PGHS2), an inducible isoform that is a major determinant of prostaglandin synthesis in the uterus, comparisons were made among section hysterectomy specimens done in 9 gravid baboons prior to labor and 5 animals in spontaneous labor with typical uterine contractions. Samples of uterine fundus, lower uterine segment as well as amnion, chorion, placenta, and cervix were obtained.

Analysis was by reverse transcription PCR for PGHS2 mRNA and quantification done as previously described using the TaqMan procedure (see 2000 YEAR BOOK, pp 22-25). Amplification products were cloned and sequenced, and high order homology with human PGHS2 gene confirmed. Finally, antisense probes were synthetized for mRNA assays. The results demonstrated a progressive roughly 40-fold increase in PGHS2 mRNA in the lower uterine segment during the interval from 120 days to the onset of labor at 180 days, while at the same time there was no significant increase in fundal derived PGHS2 messenger. The consequent increase in PGHS2 synthase helps explain the high concentration of PG metabolites preferentially in the forebag, the softening and preparation of the lower cervix in advance of labor, and, perhaps, just as local cervical application of PGE2 at term does, stimulation of the onset of labor. Increasing estrogen concentration just prior to the onset of primate labor likely plays a role in the increase in PGHS2 activity facilitated by myometrial stretch. In view of the ready inactivation of prostaglandins by the dehydrogenase activity of the chorion, autocrine or paracrine production from locally intense synthetase activity in the lower uterus would seem to be a necessity for these findings.

This is an important well constructed addition to what is known about the production of uterotonic activity in the gravid primate uterus. It is another fine contribution from this talented group.

T. H. Kirschbaum, MD

2 Maternal Complications In Pregnancy

Broad-Spectrum Antibiotics for Preterm, Prelabour Rupture of Fetal Membranes: The ORACLE I Randomised Trial
Kenyon SL, for the ORACLE Collaborative Group (Leicester Royal Infirmary, England)
Lancet 357:979-988, 2001   2–1

Objective.—Preterm, prelabor rupture of the fetal membranes (PPROM) occurs in 2.0% to 3.5% of pregnancies, results in preterm birth in 30% to 40% of cases, and leads to death, neonatal disease, and long-term disability. Although administration of antibiotics has been shown to improve neonatal health, long-term outcome results were inconclusive. Whether the effects of antibiotics on neonatal outcomes are beneficial was investigated in a multicenter, randomized, placebo-controlled study.

Methods.—Between July 1994 and June 2000, 4826 women with PPROM were randomly assigned to receive 250 mg erythromycin (n = 1197), co-amoxiclav (250 mg amoxicillin plus 125 mg clavulanic acid, n = 1212), both regimens (n = 1192), or placebo (n = 1225) 4 times daily for 10 days or until delivery. Adverse events were monitored. The composite primary outcome included neonatal death, chronic lung disease, or major cerebral anomaly.

Results.— There were 4809 women who completed the study. Twelve adverse events were reported. Women taking erythromycin had significantly prolonged pregnancies compared with women taking placebo. Women taking erythromycin had a lower rate of antibiotic prescriptions (Table 2). There was no difference between groups with respect to the number of babies born with necrotizing enterocolitis. Fewer babies of mothers taking erythromycin had the composite primary outcome (Table 3). Significantly fewer women with singleton pregnancies taking erythromycin had the composite outcome. Fewer women taking co-amoxiclav delivered within 48 hours and within 7 days. The incidence of babies with

TABLE 2.—Maternal Outcomes of Women With pPROM Randomly Assigned Erythromycin

	Erythromycin Only (n=1190)	Placebo Only (n=1225)	p	Any Erythromycin (n=2379)	No Erythromycin (n=2430)	p
Delivery within 48 h	414 (34·8%)	498 (40·7%)	0·004	786 (33·0%)	865 (35·6%)	0·062
Delivery within 7 days	725 (60·9%)	775 (63·3%)	0·23	1372 (57·7%)	1470 (60·5%)	0·05
Gestational age at delivery						
Median (range) gestation (days)	236 (150-300)	236 (142-293)	..	237 (129-300)	236 (142-300)	..
<37 weeks	1006 (84·5%)	1041 (85·0%)	0·76	2024 (85·1%)	2066 (85·0%)	0·95
<26 weeks	48 (4·0%)	59 (4·8%)	..	101 (4·2%)	107 (4·4%)	..
26-28* weeks	92 (7·7%)	113 (9·2%)	..	189 (7·9%)	220 (9·1%)	..
29-31* weeks	220 (18·5%)	231 (18·9%)	..	425 (17·9%)	446 (18·4%)	..
32-36* weeks	646 (54·3%)	638 (52·1%)	0·39	1309 (55·0%)	1293 (53·2%)	0·44
Mode of delivery						
Spontaneous vaginal	733 (61·6%)	746 (60·9%)	..	1485 (62·4%)	1501 (61·8%)	..
Forceps/Ventouse	71 (6·0%)	72 (5·9%)	..	143 (6·0%)	127 (5·2%)	..
Vaginal breech	51 (4·3%)	50 (4·1%)	..	109 (4·6%)	113 (4·7%)	..
Caesarean section	335 (28·2%)	357 (29·1%)	0·96	642 (27·0%)	689 (28·4%)	0·53
Median (range) days in hospital	4 (0-38)	4 (0-61)	0·80	4 (0-44)	4 (0-183)	0·68
Maternal antibiotic prescription	293 (24·6%)	330 (26·9%)	0·19	586 (24·6%)	640 (26·3%)	0·17
Maternal antibiotic prescription within 14 days	241 (20·3%)	262 (21·4%)	0·49	447 (18·8%)	501 (20·6%)	0·11

*Number of days.

(Courtesy of Kenyon SL, for the ORACLE Collaborative Group: Broad-spectrum antibiotics for preterm, prelabour rupture of fetal membranes: The ORACLE I randomised trial. *Lancet* 357:979-988, 2001. Copyright by The Lancet Ltd.)

TABLE 3.—Neonatal Outcomes of Babies Born to Women With pPROM Randomly Assigned Erythromycin

	Erythromycin Only (n=1190)	Placebo Only (n=1225)	p	Any Erythromycin (n=2397)	No Erythromycin (n=2430)	p
Birthweight (g)						
Mean (SD)	2102 (766)	2072 (769)	0·32	2112 (768)	2078 (762)	0·12
Median (range)	2070 (440-4420)	2055 (240-4366)	..	2090 (180-4710)	2055 (230-4488)	..
<2500	863 (72·5%)	880 (71·8%)	0·70	1704 (71·6%)	1757 (72·3%)	0·60
<1500	255 (21·4%)	284 (23·2%)	0·30	505 (21·2%)	555 (22·8%)	0·18
Admission to NICU/SCBU	836 (70·3%)	880 (71·8%)	0·39	1654 (69·5%)	1728 (71·1%)	0·23
Total babies ventilated	251 (21·1%)	283 (23·1%)	0·23	495 (20·8%)	537 (22·1%)	0·28
Total babies in >21% O_2	370 (31·1%)	436 (35·6%)	0·02	742 (31·2%)	819 (33·7%)	0·06
At 48 h	302 (25·4%)	358 (29·2%)	0·03	607 (25·5%)	674 (27·7%)	0·08
At 7 days	153 (12·9%)	181 (14·8%)	0·17	311 (13·1%)	349 (14·4%)	0·19
At 14 days	119 (10·0%)	140 (11·4%)	0·26	233 (9·8%)	275 (11·3%)	0·09
At 28 days	95 (8·0%)	116 (9·5%)	0·20	192 (8·1%)	228 (9·4%)	0·11
RDS confirmed by radiography	236 (19·8%)	266 (21·7%)	0·25	478 (20·1%)	507 (20·9%)	0·51
Treatment with exogenous surfactant	176 (14·8%)	217 (17·7%)	0·05	344 (14·4%)	399 (16·4%)	0·06
O_2 dependence >28 days	94 (7·9%)	114 (9·3%)	0·22	188 (7·9%)	225 (9·3%)	0·09
O_2 at 36 weeks post conception	66 (5·5%)	76 (6·2%)	0·49	133 (5·6%)	145 (6·0%)	0·58
Positive blood culture						
Overall	68 (5·7%)	100 (8·2%)	0·02	151 (6·3%)	182 (7·5%)	0·12
If born within 14 days	61 (5·1%)	85 (6·9%)	0·06	119 (5·0%)	148 (6·1%)	0·10
Necrotising enterocolitis						
Suspected or proven	25 (2·1%)	33 (2·7%)	0·34	67 (2·8%)	83 (3·4%)	0·23
Proven	11 (0·9%)	6 (0·5%)	0·20	31 (1·3%)	30 (1·2%)	0·83
Abnormal cerebral ultrasonography	50 (4·2%)	61 (5·0%)	0·36	96 (4·0%)	107 (4·4%)	0·53
Deaths	70 (5·9%)	82 (6·7%)	0·41	147 (6·2%)	161 (6·6%)	0·53
Composite primary outcome	151 (12·7%)	186 (15·2%)	0·08	318 (13·4%)	349 (14·4%)	0·32

Abbreviations: *NICU*, Neonatal intensive care unit; *SCBU*, special care baby unit; *RDS*, respiratory distress syndrome.

(Courtesy of Kenyon SL, for the ORACLE Collaborative Group: Broad-spectrum antibiotics for preterm, prelabour rupture of fetal membranes: The ORACLE I randomised trial. *Lancet* 357:979-988, 2001. Copyright by The Lancet Ltd.)

necrotizing enterocolitis was 4 times higher in women taking co-amoxiclav than in women taking placebo and 2.5 times higher than in women taking no-amoxiclav.

Conclusion.—Erythromycin treatment of PPROM resulted in prolonged pregnancy, a lower incidence of neonatal death and surfactant and oxygen use, and a lower incidence of necrotizing enterocolitis. Treatment of PPROM with co-amoxiclav was associated with an increased incidence of necrotizing enterocolitis.

▶ The ORACLE study, sponsored by the British Medical Research Council, using data collected for 6 years beginning in 1994, is a prospective randomized clinical trial of the efficacy of antibiotic therapy in patients with PPROM largely from Britain but also from continental Europe, South America, Australia, South Africa, and SriLanka. Entry required the diagnosis of PPROM before 37 weeks of gestation. Remarkably, of 4826 women enrolled, 99.6% completed the study with apparently 96.8% achieving compliance with drug dosage. Four groups were designated comparing erythryomycin with amoxicillin and clavulanic acid (co-amoxiclav) and an untreated placebo group. Extensive outcome data are reported, including the primary measurements, the incidence of perinatal death, pulmonary hypoplasia, and central nervous system abnormality on neonatal ultrasound. Mean gestational age at entry was 32 weeks.

As demonstrated (see 1997 YEAR BOOK OF OBSTETRICS, GYNECOLOGY, AND WOMEN'S HEALTH, pp 33-37 and 1999 YEAR BOOK, pp 159-160) previously, use of either or both antibiotics prolonged the latent period between preterm rupture of membranes and the onset of labor and reduced the number of infants requiring oxygen in the first 48 hours of life and the requirement for oxygen past 28 days. The incidence of maternal postpartum infection and positive neonatal blood cultures was also reduced with antibiotics. Results with co-amoxiclav were similar but were associated with a 4 times greater incidence of necrotizing enterocolitis. No impact of antibiotic therapy was noted on central nervous system US, perinatal death, chronic pulmonary disease, or RDS. This study confirms the effect of erythromycin on latency after PPROM and is associated with only 4 infants requiring surfactant or oxygen during the first 48 hours of life, but little long-term benefit. The increased risk of necrotizing enterocolitis with co-amoxiclav is not seen with erythomycin; at least in this comparison, erythromycin is the better choice for the indication. Remote outcomes, more often a result of neonatal therapy than obstetric events, are not highly dependent on predelivery antibiotic therapy.

T. H. Kirschbaum, MD

Broad-Spectrum Antibiotics for Spontaneous Preterm Labour: The ORACLE II Randomised Trial

Kenyon SL, for the ORACLE Collaborative Group (Leicester Royal Infirmary, England)

Lancet 357:989-994, 2001   2–2

Objective.—Preterm births account for 75% to 90% of all neonatal deaths not caused by congenital malformations and half of childhood disabilities. Whether the use of antibiotics in women in spontaneous preterm labor improves neonatal outcomes is controversial. Results of a randomized trial of antibiotics for spontaneous preterm labor are reported.

Methods.—Between July 1994 and June 2000, 6295 women in spontaneous preterm labor with intact membranes and without infection were randomly assigned to receive 250 mg erythromycin (n = 1611), 325 mg co-amoxiclav (250 mg erythromycin plus 125 mg clavulanic acid) (n = 1550), both (n = 1565), or placebo (n = 1569) 4 times daily for 10 days or until delivery. The primary composite outcome measure was neonatal death, major adverse outcome, or major cerebral abnormality. The end point was hospital discharge.

Results.—A total of 6241 women were included in the analysis (Table 1). There was no evidence that the use of any antibiotic prolonged pregnancy or improved neonatal health. There was no significant difference between antibiotic regimens with respect to the number of babies venti-

TABLE 1.—Baseline Characteristics

	Erythromycin Only (n=1600)	Co-amoxiclav Only (n=1534)	Erythromycin and Co-amoxiclav (n=1551)	Placebo Only (n=1556)
Mean (SD) age (years)	26·5 (6·1)	26·1 (5·7)	26·3 (5·7)	26·7 (5·7)
Gestational age at entry				
Median (range) gestation (days)	219 (137-258)	219 (139-256)	220 (144-258)	219 (126-258)
<26 weeks	133 (8·3%)	121 (7·9%)	140 (9·0%)	114 (7·3%)
26-28 weeks	287 (17·9%)	301 (19·6%)	265 (17·1%)	313 (20·1%)
29-31 weeks	494 (30·9%)	456 (29·7%)	478 (30·8%)	468 (30·1%)
32-36 weeks	745 (46·6%)	698 (45·5%)	735 (47·4%)	718 (46·1%)
Cervical dilatation (cm)				
Unknown	292 (18·3%)	254 (16·6%)	274 (17·7%)	277 (17·8%)
0-1	885 (55·3%)	839 (54·7%)	907 (58·5%)	894 (57·5%)
>1-2	252 (15·8%)	284 (18·5%)	236 (15·2%)	241 (15·5%)
>2	171 (10·7%)	157 (10·2%)	134 (8·6%)	144 (9·3%)
Drugs prescribed				
β-agonists	671 (41·9%)	648 (42·2%)	624 (40·2%)	634 (40·7%)
Steroids	1246 (77·9%)	1251 (81·6%)	1248 (80·5%)	1277 (82·1%)
Indomethacin	143 (8·9%)	139 (9·1%)	144 (9·3%)	143 (9·2%)
Nifedipine	95 (5·9%)	105 (6·8%)	98 (6·3%)	101 (6·5%)
Others	190 (11·9%)	197 (12·8%)	209 (15·5%)	204 (13·1%)

(Courtesy of Kenyon SL, for the ORACLE Collaborative Group: Broad-spectrum antibiotics for spontaneous preterm labour: The ORACLE II randomised trial. *Lancet* 357:989-994, 2001. Copyright The Lancet Ltd.)

TABLE 5.—Neonatal Outcomes of Babies Born to Women With Preterm Labour Randomly Assigned Erythromycin

	Erythromycin Only (n=1600)	Placebo Only (n=1556)	p	Any Erythromycin (n=3151)	No Erythromycin (n=3090)	p
Birthweight (g)						
Mean (SD)	2823 (788)	2857 (775)	0·22	2837 (791)	2850 (792)	0·52
Median (range)	2950 (450-5120)	2980 (570-5127)	. .	2970 (275-5300)	2970 (440-5520)	. .
<2500	468 (29·3%)	419 (26·9%)	0·15	894 (28·4%)	867 (28·1%)	0·78
<1500	121 (7·6%)	107 (6·9%)	0·46	235 (7·5%)	229 (7·4%)	0·94
Admission to NICU/SCBU	424 (26·5%)	380 (24·4%)	0·18	813 (25·8%)	783 (25·3%)	0·67
Total babies ventilated	126 (7·9%)	121 (7·8%)	0·92	252 (8·0%)	240 (7·8%)	0·72
Total babies in >21% O_2	216 (13·5%)	207 (13·3%)	0·87	426 (13·5%)	410 (13·3%)	0·77
At 48 h	185 (11·6%)	178 (11·4%)	0·91	372 (11·8%)	348 (11·0%)	0·50
At 7 days	86 (5·4%)	88 (5·6%)	0·73	173 (5·5%)	173 (5·6%)	0·85
At 14 days	64 (4·0%)	63 (4·0%)	0·94	123 (3·9%)	125 (4·0%)	0·77
At 28 days	52 (3·3%)	49 (3·1%)	0·87	96 (3·0%)	96 (3·1%)	0·89
RDS confirmed by chest radiography	133 (8·3%)	138 (8·9%)	0·58	272 (8·6%)	265 (8·6%)	0·94
Treatment with exogenous surfactant	89 (5·6%)	88 (5·7%)	0·91	179 (5·7%)	170 (5·5%)	0·75
O_2 dependence >28 days	51 (3·2%)	48 (3·1%)	0·87	93 (3·0%)	94 (3·0%)	0·83
O_2 at 36 weeks post conception	36 (2·3%)	29 (1·9%)	0·45	78 (2·5%)	53 (1·7%)	0·04
Positive blood culture						
Overall	34 (2·1%)	31 (2·0%)	0·79	68 (2·2%)	59 (1·9%)	0·43
If born within 14 days	24 (1·5%)	25 (1·6%)	0·81	52 (1·7%)	45 (1·5%)	0·54
Necrotising enterocolitis						
Suspected or proven	16 (1·0%)	12 (0·8%)	0·49	39 (1·2%)	31 (1·0%)	0·38
Proven	6 (0·4%)	4 (0·3%)	0·56	17 (0·5%)	13 (0·4%)	0·50
Abnormal cerebral ultrasonography	26 (1·6%)	29 (1·9%)	0·61	60 (1·9%)	56 (1·8%)	0·77
Death	43 (2·7%)	39 (2·5%)	0·75	90 (2·9%)	77 (2·5%)	0·37
Composite primary outcome	90 (5·6%)	78 (5·0%)	0·44	181 (5·7%)	154 (5·0%)	0·18

Abbreviations: NICU, Neonatal intensive care unit; *SCBU*, special care baby unit.

(Courtesy of Kenyon SL, for the ORACLE Collaborative Group: Broad-spectrum antibiotics for spontaneous preterm labour: The ORACLE II randomised trial. *Lancet* 357:989-994, 2001. Copyright The Lancet Ltd.)

lated; on more than 21% oxygen at 2, 7, 14, and 28 days; with respiratory distress syndrome; or treated with exogenous surfactant (Table 5).

Conclusion.—It appears that the role of subclinical infection as a cause of spontaneous preterm labor has been overestimated.

▶ This companion publication to the preceding results from the enrollment of 6295 women with the clinical diagnosis of threatened preterm labor with intact membranes and no clinical evidence of infection. The diagnosis was left to physician opinion and clearly exhibited a tendency toward overdiagnosis of preterm labor. In 54.9% of cases, the cervix was 0 to 1 cm dilated, and only 15.4% of women enrolled delivered within 7 days of entry. Antenatal corticosteroids were used in the 80.5% of cases and β-adrenergic agonists in 41.3%. There was no evidence that antimicrobial effect of a β-lactam or macrolide had any affect on prolongation of pregnancy or improvement of neonatal life in this study, which is the largest single trial of this undertaking yet reported. The rate of maternal infection during and after labor was decreased by antibiotic and co-amoxiclav and was once again associated with an increased risk of neonatal necrotizing enterocolitis. This is not a surprising result, and it should make clear the futility of antibiotic use for threatened preterm labor.

T. H. Kirschbaum, MD

Vaginal Clindamycin in Preventing Preterm Birth and Peripartal Infections in Asymptomatic Women With Bacterial Vaginosis: A Randomized, Controlled Trial

Kekki M, Kurki T, Pelkonen J, et al (Helsinki Univ; Oulu Univ, Finland; Vihti Health Ctr, Finland)
Obstet Gynecol 97:643-648, 2001   2–3

Objective.—There may be a link between preterm birth and ascending infection of the maternal genital tract. Bacterial vaginosis (BV) is a risk factor for preterm delivery, but it is unclear if BV is a cause of preterm delivery. This multicenter study evaluated whether clindamycin given intravaginally decreases the rates of preterm birth and peripartum infection in a low-risk population.

Methods.—Gram's stains were performed on 5432 pregnant women at 10 to 17 weeks' gestation between November 1994 and August 1998 at the first antenatal visit. Gram's stains were positive in 565 (10.4%) women. Women with BV who participated were treated for 7 days with either 2% vaginal clindamycin cream (n = 187) or placebo (n = 188). Repeat Gram's stains were done 1 week after treatment and during the third trimester. The outcome measures were peripartum infections and preterm birth.

Results.—The prevalence of BV was 10.4% (565 of 5432). The cure rate was 66% in the treated group and 62 in the placebo group (66% vs 34%). The preterm delivery rate was 4% (n = 16), 5% in the clindamycin group and 4% in the placebo group. The peripartum infection rate was 11% in the clindamycin group and 18% in the placebo group. The rate of preterm deliveries and peripartum infections were almost 3 times higher in women with persistent (31%) or recurrent (7%) BV than in women who were cured (28% vs 10%). There was no signifcant difference between the treatment and placebo groups. The preterm delivery rate was 15% in women with recurrent BV but only 2% in women cured of BV.

Conclusion.—Vaginal clindamycin did not decrease the rate of preterm delivery or peripartum infection. Recurrent BV significantly increased the rate of both.

▶ It is reasonably clear there is a relation between BV and preterm birth, but not at all clear that it is a causal one and not simply an associative relationship. Recently a large prospective NIH supported randomized trial of metronidazole failed to support evidence of prevention of preterm births (see 2001 YEAR BOOK OF OBSTETRICS, GYNECOLOGY, AND WOMEN'S HEALTH, pp 29-31), and a smaller study using 2% vaginal clindamycin in a prospective trial yielded very questionable evidence of benefit (see 2001 YEAR BOOK, pp 31-32). This prospective, randomized trial of predominantly white Finnish women at relatively low risk of preterm birth originated from 20 antenatal clinics, most of them operating in and around Helsinki. The diagnosis of BV was made by Gram's stain and enzyme linked immunoassays, and patients were randomly assigned to 2% clindamycin daily for 7 days or a placebo vaginal medication. Gonorrhea was excluded by culture. With randomization at 12 to 19 weeks, women were reexamined twice more during pregnancy to collect evidence of possible cure. Those reading smear results were blinded to therapy. The overall incidence of BV was 10.4%. Among women receiving antibiotics two thirds were smear negative in 1 week and one third of untreated controls. There was no difference in preterm delivery rates between patients treated (4.5%) and controls (3.7%). Among women with persistent BV (31%) or recurrent BV (7%), the preterm delivery rate was significantly higher than among those antibiotic treated and "cured." This is one more prospective, randomized trial that calls into question the value of routine prophylactic antenatal therapy for BV in pregnancy.

T. H. Kirschbaum, MD

Vaginal Indicators of Amniotic Fluid Infection in Preterm Labor

Hitti J, Hillier SL, Agnew KJ, et al (Univ of Washington, Seattle; Univ of Pittsburgh, Pa)
Obstet Gynecol 97:211-219, 2001   2–4

Background.—Amniotic fluid (AF) infection affects 10% to 15% of pregnancies complicated by preterm labor. Whether AF infection in such women can be predicted by vaginal interleukin-6 (IL-6), IL-8, neutrophils, bacterial vaginosis (BV), and selected vaginal bacteria was investigated.

TABLE 1.—Demographic and Reproductive Characteristics and Pregnancy Outcome, Stratified by Amniotic Fluid Culture and IL-6 Concentration

		Negative Culture		
	Positive Culture ($n = 18$) (%)	Interleukin-6 >2 ng/mL ($n = 21$) (%)	Interleukin-6 ≤2 ng/mL ($n = 158$) (%)	Total ($n = 179$) (%)
Median maternal age (y)	26	23	23	23
Maternal ethnicity, n (%)				
White	16 (89)	13 (62)	90 (57)	103 (58)*
Black	2 (11)	6 (29)	29 (18)	35 (20)
Other	0	2 (9)	39 (25)	41 (23)
Cigarette smoker	4 (22)	4 (19)	29 (19)	33 (19)
Nulliparity	11 (61)	10 (48)	71 (45)	81 (46)
Previous preterm delivery (parous women)	2/7 (28)	2/11 (18)	34/86 (39)	36/97 (37)
Enrollment findings				
Weeks' gestation	28†	29†	31	31
Cervical dilatation (cm)	3.75†	3.5†	2.5	2.5
Effacement (cm)	0.5	0.5	1.5	1.5
Contraction frequency (min)	4.5	2	3	3
Days from enrollment to delivery	2‡	3‡	22	20
Weeks' gestation at delivery	28‡	30‡	36	35
Infant birth weight (g)	1203‡	1296‡	2708	2580

*X^2 test P less than .05 for difference in ethnicity between positive culture and total negative culture group.

†Distributions differed from the negative culture, low IL-6 group (Mann-Whitney P less than .05 with Bonferroni correction); the positive culture group also differed from the total negative culture group (Mann-Whitney $P < .05$).

‡Distributions differ from the negative culture plus low IL-6 group (Mann-Whitney $P < .01$ with Bonferroni correction); the positive culture group also differed from the total negative culture group (Mann-Whitney $P < .001$).

(Courtesy of Hitti J, Hillier SL, Agnew KJ, et al: Vaginal indicators of amniotic fluid infection in preterm labor. *Obstet Gynecol* 97:211-219, 2001. Reprinted with permission from The American College of Obstetricians and Gynecologists.)

TABLE 2.—Vaginal Cytokines, Neutrophils, and Flora Stratified by Amniotic Fluid Culture and Interleukin-6 Concentration

	Positive Culture ($n = 18$) (%)	Negative Culture		Total ($n = 179$) (%)
		Interleukin-6 >2 ng/mL ($n = 21$) (%)	Interleukin-6 $\leq$2 ng/mL ($n = 158$) (%)	
Interleukin-6 (median, ng/mL)	3.3	0.9	1.0	1.0
Interleukin-8 (median, ng/mL)	140.2*	94.2*	15.3	17.3
Neutrophils per 400× field (mean)	12	5†	1.5	2
Vaginal Gram stain, n (%)				
Normal	6 (33)	3 (14)	93 (59)	96 (54)
Intermediate	7 (39)	11 (53)	45 (28)	56 (31)
Bacterial vaginosis	5 (28)	7 (33)	20 (13)	27 (15)
Vaginal culture, n (%)				
Lactobacillus >10^7 cfu/g	7 (39)	4 (19)	69 (44)	73 (41)
H$_2$O$_2$-producing *Lactobacillus*	5 (28)	3 (14)†	71 (48)	74 (44)
Group B *streptococcus*	3 (16)	2 (10)	12 (8)	14 (8)
Escherichia coli	5 (28)	6 (29)	43 (27)	49 (27)
Mycoplasma hominis	4/15 (27)	3/19 (16)	22/141 (16)	25/160 (16)
Ureaplasma urealyticum	8/15 (53)	12/19 (63)	76/139 (52)	85/158 (54)
Gardnerella vaginalis >10^6 cfu/g	6 (33)	6 (29)	41 (26)	47 (26)
Prevotella bivia/disiens >10^4 cfu/g	5 (28)	6 (29)	33 (21)	39 (22)
Black *Prevotella* >10^4 cfu/g	4 (22)	4 (19)	19 (12)	23 (13)
Bacteroides ureolyticus	3 (17)	4 (19)	8 (5)	12 (7)
Fusobacterium	1 (6)	4 (19)†	5 (3)	9 (5)
Peptostreptococcus >10^4 cfu/g	9 (50)	6 (29)	39 (25)	45 (25)

*Distributions differed from the negative culture low IL-6 group (Mann-Whitney P < .01 with Bonferroni correction): the positive culture group also differed from the total negative culture group (Mann-Whitney P < .001).

†Distributions differed from the negative culture, low IL-6 group (Mann-Whitney P < .05 with Bonferroni correction).

(Courtesy of Hitti J, Hillier SL, Agnew KJ, et al: Vaginal indicators of amniotic fluid infection in preterm labor. *Obstet Gynecol* 97:211-219, 2001. Reprinted with permission from The American College of Obstetricians and Gynecologists.)

TABLE 5.—Sensitivity, Specificity, and Positive and Negative Predictive Values of Vaginal Indicators to Detect Amniotic Fluid Infection or Interleukin-6 Levels Above 2 ng/mL

	No. Positive/ No. Tested (%)	Sensitivity (%)	Specificity (%)	Positive Predictive Value (%)	Negative Predictive Value (%)
Interleukin-8 >30 ng/mL	81/180 (45)	80	64	35	93
Neutrophils >5 per 400× field	70/197 (36)	54	69	30	86
Bacterial vaginosis or intermediate flora	95/197 (48)	31	87	38	84
Bacterial vaginosis or intermediate flora or neutrophils >5 per 400× field	129/197 (66)	90	41	27	94

(Courtesy of Hitti J, Hillier SL, Agnew KJ, et al: Vaginal indicators of amniotic fluid infection in preterm labor. *Obstet Gynecol* 97:211-219, 2001. Reprinted with permission from The American College of Obstetricians and Gynecologists.)

Methods.—The study included 197 afebrile women in preterm labor with intact membranes. Vaginal and AF samples were obtained for Gram's stain, culture, and IL-8 and IL-6 assessment.

Findings.—Vaginal IL-8 levels and neutrophil counts were significantly greater in the presence of AF infection as well as increased concentrations of AF IL-6 and IL-8 (Table 1). Vaginal IL-6 levels were unassociated with AF infection or high levels of AF cytokines. In addition, AF infection was correlated with BV or intermediate vaginal flora by Gram's stain, absence of hydrogen peroxide-producing *Lactobacillus*, and the presence of vaginal *Bacteroides ureolyticus* and *Fusobacterium* (Table 2). Vaginal IL-8 concentrations exceeding 30 ng/mL had a sensitivity of 80% and a positive predictive value of 35% for detecting AF infection or increased AF IL-6. An abnormal vaginal Gram's stain had a sensitivity of 90% and a positive predictive value of 27% for detecting AF infection or increased AF IL-6 (Table 5).

Conclusions.—In women with preterm labor, AF infection was strongly correlated with a high vaginal IL-8 level, abnormal vaginal Gram's stain, absent hydrogen peroxide-producing *Lactobacillus*, and anaerobic vaginal flora. An increased vaginal IL-8 level may be a useful, noninvasive marker for AF infection and proinflammatory cytokine production in women in preterm labor.

▶ There is no question that a relationship exists among latent chorioamnionitis, the presence of cervical vaginal proinflammatory cytokines (IL-6 and IL-8, in this case), and preterm labor, and that there is value in the ability to make the diagnosis of amnionitis without employing amniocentesis. Although these authors can reconfirm those relationships, one may reasonably argue with their view that these findings are "strongly associated with AF infection among women in preterm labor."

A group of 197 women in presumed preterm labor between 20 and 34 weeks underwent vaginal smears and amniocentesis. Gram's stains and neutrophil counts were performed on the vaginal smears; culture and enzyme-linked immunosorbent assay for IL-6 and IL-8 were done on both vaginal smears and amniotic fluid. The diagnosis of preterm labor was based on relatively loose criteria, and although the authors do not provide records of the number of women in false labor, it appears that slightly less than 80% of patients entered into this study delivered at term. Eighteen of the women were amniotic fluid culture positive, 21 were culture negative but had elevated IL-6 concentrations, and 158 were culture negative with normal IL-6 concentrations. The authors argue that because both the culture-positive women and those showing only elevated IL-6 delivered prematurely, the latter had low level infection even though their median IL-6 concentration was not greater than the mean value for the culture-negative women. Assuming low level infection without proof, but acknowledging that two thirds of such women were probably not infected, the authors calculated indices of predictability of vaginal findings against the likelihood of positive amniotic fluid culture or of amniotic fluid IL-6 concentrations greater than 2 ng/mL as evidence of infection.

Even with these questionable assumptions, their predictability was poor. Although vaginal cytokines and neutrophil counts were not different than those with BV and women with intermediate vaginal flora, those findings were said to have a sensitivity of 90% but a false-positive rate of 73% against their chosen criteria of infection. As Table 5 shows, other vaginal findings have lower sensitivities and lower specificity, with false-positive rates bearing from 62% to 70%. Adding findings of elevated cervical white cells seen in 17 women to those 95 women with BV or intermediate flora yields 112 cases, not the 129 they indicate in Table 5. In my view, more work and more proof for implicit assumptions are necessary before one can take this work seriously as an indirect means of diagnosing chorioamnionitis.

T. H. Kirschbaum, MD

Will Cervicovaginal Interleukin-6 Combined With Fetal Fibronectin Testing Improve the Prediction of Preterm Delivery?
LaShay N, Gilson G, Joffe G, et al (Univ of New Mexico, Albuquerque; Lovelace Med Ctr, Albuquerque, NM)
J Matern Fetal Med 9:336-341, 2000
2–5

Objective.—Although 10% to 12% of all deliveries are preterm, only 9% to 28% of women with preterm labor and intact membranes have positive amniotic fluid cultures and only a small fraction of those women have clinical signs and symptoms. Although the presence of cervicovaginal fetal fibronectin (fFN) is a potential useful marker for preterm birth, the positive predictive value was only 18% and 12% within 7 and 14 days before preterm birth. Interleukin (IL)-6 levels are significantly elevated in the amniotic fluid of women with preterm labor who deliver a preterm infant. Adding cervicovaginal IL-6 determinations to fFN to improve the positive predictive value of fFN testing for preterm birth was tested in a prospective cohort observational study.

Methods.—Cervicovaginal secretions were obtained from 118 women with intact membranes with suspected preterm labor between 24 and 34 weeks' gestation. IL-6 levels were determined by using an immunoassay with specific monoclonal antibodies. fFN concentrations were determined by using a solid phase enzyme-linked immunosorbent assay. Outcome measures included preterm delivery in less than 48 hours, in 7 days, and before 36 weeks.

Results.—Women were divided into 2 groups: those who delivered preterm and those who delivered after 37 weeks. Women became symptomatic at an average of 30.5 weeks, and all had a median cervical dilation of 1 cm. Ten (29%) women who delivered preterm and 24 (28%) women who delivered at term had pathogenic infections. Four (3%) women had deliveries in 48 hours or less, 5 (4%) within 7 days, and 34 (29%) before 37 weeks. Although both IL-6 and fFN concentrations were elevated in cervicovaginal secretions, the addition of IL-6 levels did not add any additional information (Table 1).

TABLE 1.—Cervicovaginal Fetal Fibronectin and Interleukin-6 as Predictors of Delivery at Less Than 37 Weeks' Gestation

	Sens (%)	Spec (%)	PPV (%)	NPV (%)	Odds Ratio	CI	P Value
fFN (+) (≥50 ng/mL)	29	91	59	77	4.58	1.54-13.35	<.003
IL-6 (+) (≥100 pg/mL)	62	30	37	79	1.57	.89-2.75	.11
fFN (+) and IL-6 (+)	26	94	58	75	4.00	1.31-12.17	.015

(Courtesy of LaShay N, Gilson G, Joffe G, et al: Will cervicovaginal interleukin-6 combined with fetal fibronectin testing improve the prediction of preterm delivery? *J Matern Fetal Med* 9:336-341, 2000. Reprinted by permission of Wiley-Liss, Inc., a subsidiary of John Wiley & Sons, Inc.)

Conclusion.—fFN testing is a reliable predictor of preterm birth. Adding IL-6 cervicovaginal levels does not enhance the predictive value of fFN alone.

▶ Because cervical-vaginal fFN is a clear correlate of preterm delivery, at least in women with threatened preterm labor, its use both as a predictor and indicator for therapy has been reviewed very extensively (see 1995 YEAR BOOK OF OBSTETRICS, GYNECOLOGY, AND WOMEN'S HEALTH, pp 69-70, 1996 YEAR BOOK, pp 129-130, 1997 YEAR BOOK, pp 29-31, and 145-148, 1998 YEAR BOOK, pp 53-54, 1999 YEAR BOOK, pp 11-13, and 35-37, 2000 YEAR BOOK, pp 47-49, and 2001 YEAR BOOK, pp 45-47, and 167-168). A minority of women with threatened preterm labor do not, anterorespectively, show evidence of chorioamnionitis, approximately 50% continue their pregnancies to term—the incidence of actual preterm delivery in such patients varies with the population studied from 10% to 30%. Accurate predictive characteristics would allow therapy to be focused more clearly on those at risk and avoid diluting the positive results of therapy by the preponderance of women who, without treatment, do not deliver preterm. The persistent problem with fetal fibronectin is the 50% to 80% false-positive rate which keeps it from being a clinically useful predictor.

Here, the authors hope to improve predictability by measuring a proinflammatory cytokine, IL-6, known to be increased in amniotic fluid in instances of chorioamnionitis and which can be detected in amniotic fluid with a predictive sensitivity of 64%. With amniotic fluid concentrations of IL-6 greater than 75 to 86 pg/mL, it can be used to predict delivery with 48 hours of testing in 92% of cases of threatened preterm labor. Such cases are infrequent, however.

The authors report cervical smears for IL-6 assayed by monoclonal immunoassay and fetal fibronectin by enzyme-linked immunosorbent assay in 118 gravidas seen with threatened preterm labor at a mean of 30.5 weeks. As Table 1 shows, vaginal IL-6 detects two thirds of cases of women who deliver at less than 37 weeks' gestation, but with a false-positive rate of 63%. Combined with fetal fibronectin assay, it adds nothing to the flawed capacity associated with that assay. These results should be borne in mind, as similar studies linking cervical length and other cytokines and leukotrienes to preterm delivery prediction continue to be reported.

T. H. Kirschbaum, MD

Vaginal Fetal Fibronectin Measurements From 8 to 22 Weeks' Gestation and Subsequent Spontaneous Preterm Birth

Goldenberg RL, Klebanoff M, Carey JC, et al (Natl Inst of Child Health and Human Development, Bethesda, Md)
Am J Obstet Gynecol 183:469-475, 2000   2–6

Background.—The presence of fetal fibronectin (fFN) in the cervix or vagina in women during the late second trimester who are not in labor increases the risk of spontaneous preterm birth by 60-fold. Whether measurements of vaginal fFN levels earlier in pregnancy would also be useful in predicting the risk of preterm birth was evaluated. Some of the factors that might affect vaginal fFN levels were also examined.

Methods.—The subjects were 13,360 pregnant women who were tested between 8 and 22 weeks' gestation to determine their eligibility for a bacterial vaginosis (*Trichomonas vaginalis*) treatment trial. Vaginal fFN levels were measured and correlated with the presence of *T vaginalis* infection, gestational age at screening and at delivery, and race.

Results.—At each gestational age between 8 and 22 weeks, vaginal fFN levels in individual subjects ranged from undetectable (in approximately one third of women) to 1000 ng/mL or more; in most subjects, the median value was less than 10 ng/mL (Fig 1). When data at each gestational age

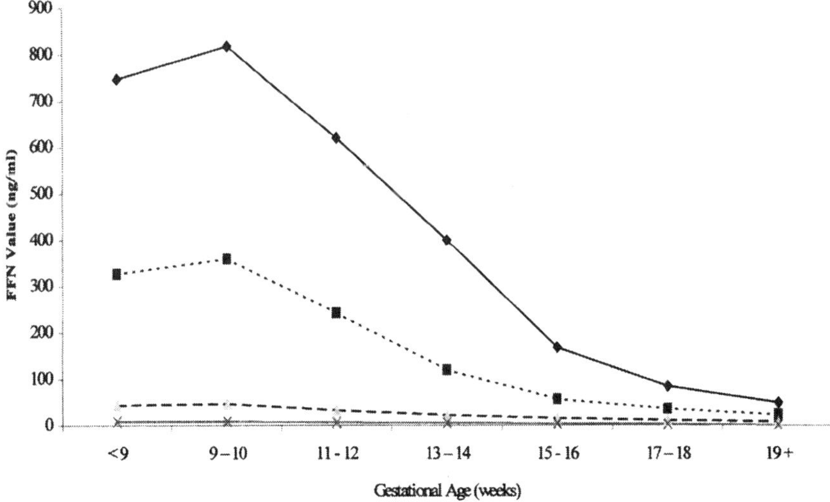

FIGURE 1.—Fetal fibronectin median (*times signs*) and 75th (*triangles*), 90th (*squares*), and 95th (*diamonds*) percentile values at various gestational ages. (Courtesy of Goldenberg RL, Klebanoff M, Carey JC, et al: Vaginal fetal fibronectin measurements from 8 to 22 weeks' gestation and subsequent spontaneous preterm birth. *Am J Obstet Gynecol* 183:469-475, 2000.)

TABLE II.—Relation Between Vaginal Fetal Fibronectin Value of ≥90th Percentile and Fetal Loss—Spontaneous Preterm Birth at <35 Weeks Gestation by Gestational Age at Sampling

Gestational Age at Sampling (wk)	Spontaneous Preterm Birth at <35 wk Gestation		Relative Risk and 95% Confidence Interval
	Fetal Fibronectin ≥90th Percentile	Fetal Fibronectin <90th Percentile	
<9 (n=1071)	12.6%	7.3%	1.73 (1.01-2.97)
9-10 (n=1423)	9.0%	6.3%	1.44 (0.82-2.53)
11-12 (n=1473)	6.3%	5.2%	1.22 (0.62-2.40)
13-14 (n=1206)	12.1%	5.5%	2.19 (1.27-3.80)
15-16 (n=1508)	13.5%	4.4%	3.06 (1.73-5.41)
17-18 (n=1441)	5.9%	3.8%	1.54 (0.74-3.17)
≥19 (n=2784)	9.7%	3.7%	2.63 (1.75-3.94)

(Courtesy of Goldenberg RL, Klebanoff M, Carey JC, et al: Vaginal fetal fibronectin measurements from 8 to 22 weeks' gestation and subsequent spontaneous preterm birth. *Am J Obstet Gynecol* 183:469-475, 2000.)

were pooled, median values ranged from 1 to 8 ng/mL and declined progressively and significantly as gestational age at sampling increased. Median values were significantly higher in black subjects and subjects with bacterial vaginosis and were significantly lower in nulliparous subjects and subjects with *T vaginalis* infection. Vaginal fFN levels at or above the 90th percentile for each gestational age at sampling were defined as abnormal. Between 13 and 16 weeks' gestation and after 19 weeks' gestation, abnormal vaginal fFN levels were associated with a significantly increased risk of spontaneous preterm birth (by 2- to 3-fold) (Table II). Furthermore, increasing fFN levels were significantly associated with earlier spontaneous preterm birth. The percentage of births at less than 28 weeks' gestation at a fFN level of 0 ng/mL (1.2%) doubled as the level increased from 0 to 24 ng/mL (2.3%), doubled again as levels increased to 49 ng/mL (4.8%), and almost doubled again at levels 50 ng/mL or greater (7.8% of births occurred at ≥28 weeks' gestation).

Conclusions.—Abnormal vaginal fFN levels detected as early as 13 weeks' gestation are a significant predictor of the risk of spontaneous preterm birth. Levels at or above the 90th percentile of normal for a particular gestational age increase the risk of spontaneous preterm birth by 2- to 3-fold. Additionally, as the fFN level increases, so does the risk of very early preterm birth and fetal loss. Thus, vaginal fFN screening late in the first trimester or early in the second trimester may help identify women at increased risk of spontaneous preterm birth earlier than screening is currently performed (late in the second trimester) and thus allow for specific interventions.

▶ The promise that fFN found in the vagina in early pregnancy might be a reliable indicator of disruption of the connective tissue matrixes connecting mother, placenta, and fetus with predictive strength in identifying women destined for preterm labor has not been fulfilled in numerous attempts (see 1996 YEAR BOOK OF OBSTETRICS, GYNECOLOGY, AND WOMEN'S HEALTH, pp 61-63, 1997 YEAR BOOK, pp 146-148, 1998 YEAR BOOK, pp 53-54, 1999 YEAR BOOK, pp 35-37, and 2000 YEAR BOOK, pp 47-48). The data used here by the Maternal Fetal Medicine Network of the NICHD were collected in an unsuccessful effort to demonstrate the use of metronidazole administered from 23 to 30 weeks' gestation in preventing preterm birth associated with bacterial vaginosis (see 2001 YEAR BOOK, pp 29-31). In an editorial comment in that issue, Dr R. F. Lamont pointed to the need to focus on antimicrobial use before 26 weeks' gestational age when the risk ratio for the coincidence of preterm birth and vaginal inflammatory changes is large. That comment has stimulated just such a controlled trial of antibiotic use in women with cervical vaginal fibronectin at 22 to 26 weeks, now in progress. Here the effort is to explore the possible usefulness of fFN activity in the interval from 8 to 22 weeks' gestation in a large population of women being screened for asymptomatic bacterial vaginosis. What is measured are risk ratios for the occurrence of spontaneous birth from 13 to 35 weeks' gestational age in women positive for fFN compared with those negative at the same age. The task is complicated by the absence of fFN or its presence in very low concentrations in the majority of the 13,360 women studied. During this pregnancy interval, concentration range for vaginal fibronectin declined sharply in women who were positive for fFN. Using the value of fFN equal to or greater than the 90th percentile of normal as a criterion for a positive finding, despite the fact that level represents less than the amount customarily used, the authors found a significant increase in risk ratio for preterm birth associated with fFN at 13 to 16 weeks' gestational age and at greater than 19 weeks, but not during the 17 to 18 weeks of gestation.

Significantly positive risk ratios suggest only an association between the presence of fFN and preterm birth but fail to deal with the predictive strength of that association. The authors calculate the incidence of positive tests among women with preterm birth (sensitivity) at 19% to 21% and the incidence of negative fFN normal women normals at 90.6% to 92.3% but do not publish data that would allow calculation of false-positive or false-negative rates. The authors are correct that measurements of predictability need to be coupled with prevalence and treatability estimates for fFN positivity to evaluate the utility of early second trimester fFN measurements. However, to date, no means of treating fFN positivity exists to allow therapy to be applied. The authors' data provide some but not much hope for a useful approach to identifying and preventing preterm birth. More observations in a study structured to evaluate predictability are needed in this area.

T. H. Kirschbaum, MD

Cervicovaginal Fibronectin and Cervical Length at 23 Weeks of Gestation: Relative Risk of Early Preterm Delivery
Heath VCF, Daskalakis G, Zagaliki A, et al (King's College Hosp, London)
Br J Obstet Gynaecol 107:1276-1281, 2000   2–7

Introduction.—The presence of fetal fibronectin (fFN) in cervicovaginal sections and the US finding of a short cervix as possible predictors of early preterm delivery have been the subject of recent interest. The prevalence of a positive fFN finding at 23 weeks' gestation in a routine population of 5146 singleton pregnancies in relation to cervical length and other maternal characteristics were assessed in a prospective clinical trial. The relative risks of spontaneous delivery at less than 33 weeks were also assessed with respect to maternal characteristics, fibronectin positivity and cervical length.

Methods.—The 5146 females with singleton pregnancies underwent measurement of cervicovaginal fFN and cervical length at 23 weeks' gestation. The distribution of fibronectin positivity within subgroups according to maternal characteristics was determined, and the relative risk (RR) of spontaneous delivery before 33 weeks was estimated. Patients were observed for prevalence of a fibronectin positive finding and its relation to cervical length measurement and spontaneous preterm delivery before 33 weeks.

TABLE 3.—The Predictive Properties of Fibronectin Positivity, a Cervical Length of Less Than or Equal to 15 mm, Cigarette Smoking, a Previous Delivery at 24 to 32 Weeks of Gestation, and Being of Afro-Caribbean Origin in the Calculation of Risk of Delivery Before 33 Weeks. Values are Given as %

			Predictive Value	
	Sensitivity	Specificity	Positive	Negative
Fibronectin positive	32·6	96·9	8·1	99·4
Cervical length ≤ 15 mm	27·9	99·5	30·8	99·4
Smoking	32·6	85·4	1·9	99·3
Previous delivery at 24-32^{-6} wks	9·3	98·6	5·5	99·2
Afro-Caribbean	60·5	58·9	1·2	99·4

(Courtesy of Heath VCF, Daskalakis G, Zagaliki A, et al: Cervicovaginal fibronectin and cervical length at 23 weeks of gestation: Relative risk of early preterm delivery. *Br J Obstet Gynaecol* 107:1276-1281, 2000, published by Elsevier Science Ltd.)

Results.—Of 5146 females, 182 (3.5%) had a fibronectin positive finding, and 76 (1.5%) had a cervical length of 15 mm or less. Females who were fibronectin positive were more likely to be Afro-Caribbean, to have had a previous second trimester miscarriage, and to have a short cervix (Table 3). For the 5068 women who were managed expectantly, the significantly independent RR of spontaneous delivery at before 33 weeks was 46.2 for a cervical length of 15 mm or less, 8.1 for a fibronectin positive finding, and 4.4 for cigarette smoking.

Conclusion.—Fibronectin positivity at 23 weeks' gestation is useful as a predictor of pregnancies at risk of spontaneous preterm delivery before 33 weeks. The RR of fibronectin positivity at 23 weeks is twice as high as cigarette smoking and one sixth that of cervical length.

▶ In yet another effort to explore the usefulness of cervical morphology and biochemistry in defining those at high risk of preterm birth to evaluate prophylaxis, these authors provide retrospective data from a cohort of 5000 gravid women. The women were seeking prenatal care and underwent vaginal ultrasonic determination of cervical length and determination of fFN from vaginal fluid at 22 to 24 weeks of gestational age. fFN concentration of 50 ng/mL or more and cervical length of 1.5 cm or less were deemed to have potentially positive values; their prevalence was 0.8% of the entire population. As others have, the authors demonstrate a correlative relationship among shortened cervical length, significant cervical vaginal fFN and the risk of delivery at less than 33 weeks' gestational age through the calculation of risk ratios (see 1997 YEAR BOOK OF OBSTETRICS, GYNECOLOGY, AND WOMEN'S HEALTH, pp 27-28, 2000 YEAR BOOK, pp 39-45, and 2001 YEAR BOOK, pp 45-47). Given the 39 women with shortened cervical length at 22 to 24 weeks, preterm birth occurred in one third, but the incidence of false positive predictions from the independent variables was 70%. Of 172 women with positive fFN, only 8% delivered prior to 33 weeks with a 67% false-positive rate. In both cases, the low prevalence of positive findings guaranteed a near 99% specificity. The correlative relationship is, as others have found before them, insufficiently strong for reliable clinical utility. These investigators also found that bacterial vaginosis leaves the risk of birth at less than 33 weeks unaltered from that of normal control subjects (see 2001 YEAR BOOK, pp 147-148).

T. H. Kirschbaum, MD

A Randomized Trial of Cerclage Versus No Cerclage Among Patients With Ultrasonographically Detected Second-Trimester Preterm Dilatation of the Internal Os

Rust OA, Atlas RO, Jones KJ, et al (Lehigh Valley Hosp, Allentown, Pa)
Am J Obstet Gynecol 183:830-835, 2000   2–8

Background.—For women with clinical indications of cervical incompetence, prophylactic transvaginal cerclage placement has been used for subsequent pregnancies, but the previous criteria have proved to be unreliable. On US examination, findings associated with cervical incompetence can be detected during the second trimester. The benefit associated with using transvaginal cerclage for patients with preterm dilatation of the internal os detected on second-trimester US evaluation was studied.

Methods.—Over a 1-year period, patients whose US findings at 16 to 24 weeks' gestation indicated preterm dilatation of the internal os were randomly assigned to have either no cerclage or a McDonald cerclage placed. All underwent amniocentesis and urogenital cultures as well as 48 hours of indomethacin and antibiotic therapy before randomization. Follow-up included bed rest and weekly US evaluations.

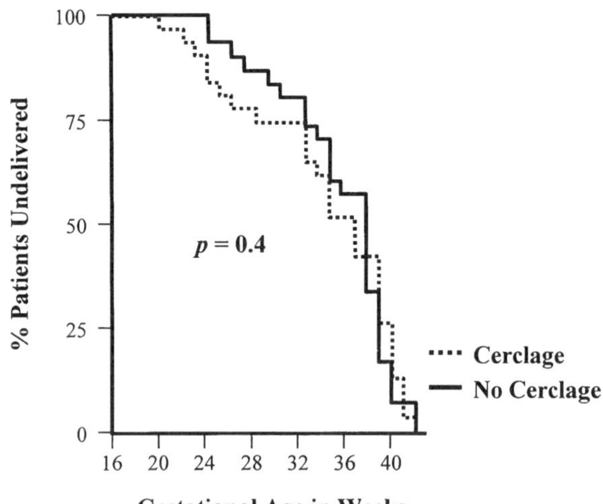

FIGURE 2.—Survival curve analysis with respect to gestational age at delivery. *Broken line*, cerclage group; *solid line*, no-cerclage group. (Courtesy of Rust OA, Atlas RO, Jones KJ, et al: A randomized trial of cerclage versus no cerclage among patients with ultrasonographically detected second-trimester preterm dilatation of the internal os. *Am J Obstet Gynecol* 183:830-835, 2000.)

Results.—Thirty-one patients received cerclage and 30 did not. The 2 groups had no significant differences in maternal demographics, risk factors for preterm birth, cervical dimensions, rescue procedures, readmission data, chorioamnionitis, or abruptio placentae. At delivery, the mean gestational ages and perinatal death rates were similar between the groups, with the cerclage group having children at a mean gestational age of 33.5 weeks versus 34.7 for those without cerclage, and respective death rates of 12.9% and 10.0% (Fig 2).

Conclusions.—No improvement in perinatal outcome was associated with use of the McDonald cerclage procedure in these women whose preterm dilatation of the cervix was detected by US.

▶ Though cervical shortening occurs throughout pregnancy and is related to preterm birth, whether and under what circumstances prophylactic cerclage is warranted remains controversial (see 1995 YEAR BOOK OF OBSTETRICS, GYNECOLOGY, AND WOMEN'S HEALTH, pp 52-54, 1999 YEAR BOOK, pp 70-71, and 2001 YEAR BOOK, pp 157-158). Resolution probably rests with a multicenter, prospective, randomized study of women at high risk with or without cervical findings. Meanwhile, smaller institutionally based studies are useful, and this is 1 of the best of recent efforts.

Women at risk of preterm birth by virtue of prior history, cervical surgery, uterine anomaly, and, in 7 cases here, multiple pregnancy were candidates for study. Those who were found on US examination to have cervical canals less than 2.5 cm long and/or to show membrane prolapse past the upper fourth of the length of the cervical canal without chorioamnionitis or membrane prolapse beyond the cervix or other structural or placental implantation abnormalities were accepted for randomization. Power analysis indicated that 60 patients would be required to detect a 20% reduction in the preterm birth rate. Before randomization, amniocentesis was used to detect chorioamnionitis, an exclusion criterion. Vaginal pooled fetal fibronectin, maternal white blood cell count, and hypercoagulation appraisal were followed by 48 to 72 hours of bed rest and treatment with indomethacin and clindamycin. Patients were discharged 24 hours after McDonald cerclage. Cerclage was offered at less than 24 weeks' gestation to 1 woman in the control group who showed continued dilatation of the internal os and membrane prolapse. No cases of chorioamnionitis were detected before cerclage, and though chorioamnionitis proved more common in women undergoing cerclage than in those who did not, there was no significant difference overall. In this sample of women, pregnancy survival analysis showed no positive effect of prophylactic cerclage in the selected candidates. Like any test of a negative hypothesis, that is, a test of no benefit, the strength of the conclusion rests on the efforts taken to demonstrate a possible difference. In this case, those efforts were considerable.

T. H. Kirschbaum, MD

Does Cervical Cerclage Prevent Preterm Delivery in Patients With a Short Cervix?

Hassan SS, Romero R, Maymon E, et al (Wayne State Univ, Detroit; Ben Gurion Univ, Beer-Sheva, Israel)

Am J Obstet Gynecol 184:1325-1331, 2001

Introduction.—Placement of a cerclage may reduce the rate of spontaneous preterm birth in women with a short cervix, but studies of the effectiveness of cervical cerclage have yielded contradictory conclusions. The outcome in patients with a short cervix ($\leq$15 mm) who were managed with cerclage placement was studied.

Methods.—Patients included in the analysis underwent transvaginal US at 14 weeks' gestation between April 1994 and September 1999. Excluded were patients with a multiple gestation, fetal congenital anomalies, or elective cerclage placement. Seventy patients with a short cervix met entry criteria. Logistic regression was used to examine factors that contributed to the risk of preterm delivery at less than 32 weeks' gestation.

Results.—Twenty-five of the 70 patients with a short cervix underwent cerclage placement (McDonald procedure). The cerclage and no-cerclage groups did not differ significantly in median cervical length, presence of a funnel, previous cervical surgery, or previous spontaneous abortion. A short cervix was detected at an earlier gestational age in patients managed with cervical cerclage (median, 19.6 weeks vs 21.3 weeks for patients with no cerclage). Patients with and without cervical cerclage did not differ in

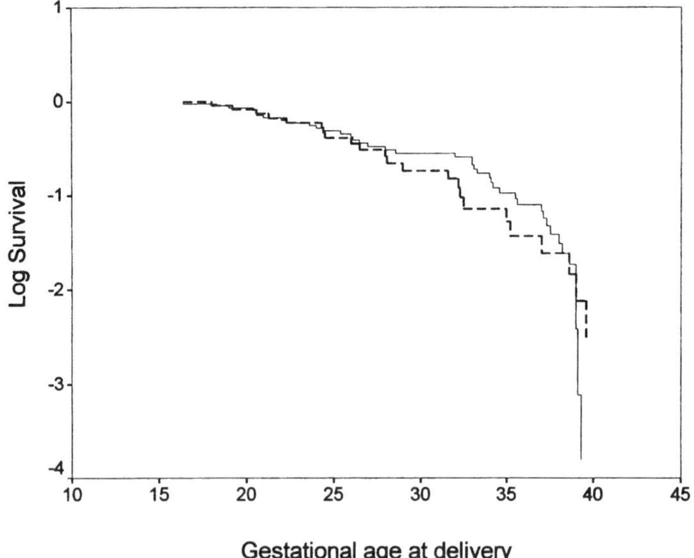

FIGURE 1.—Survival analysis of cerclage group (*dashed line*) and no-cerclage group (*solid line*). (Courtesy of Hassan SS, Romero R, Maymon E, et al: Does cervical cerclage prevent preterm delivery in patients with a short cervix? *Am J Obstet Gynecol* 184:1325-1331, 2001.)

TABLE 3.—Pregnancy Outcome

	Study Population (n = 70)	Cerclage Group (n = 25)	No Cerclage Group (n = 45)	Statistical Significance*
Rate of preterm delivery (No.)				
At <28 wk	27 (38.6%)	10 (40%)	17 (37.8%)	$P = .9$
At <32 wk	33 (47.1%)	14 (56%)	19 (42.2%)	$P = .3$
At <34 wk	41 (58.6%)	17 (68%)	24 (53%)	$P = .2$
At <37 wk	49 (70%)	19 (76%)	30 (66.7%)	$P = .4$
Interval between ultrasonography and delivery (wk, mean ± SD, range)	10.2 ± 6.8 (0-22.8)	10.6 ± 7.2 (0.3-22.7)	10.0 ± 6.7 (0-22.8)	$P = .7$
Gestional age at delivery (wk, median and range)	32.3 (16.4-40.3)	29.0 (18-40.3)	33.1 (16.4-40.3)	$P = .6$
Birth weight (g, median and range)	1740 (220-4310)	1320 (220-3390)	1900 (230-4310)	$P = .5$
Rate of preterm premature rupture of membranes (No.)	31/67 (46.3%)	15/23 (65.2%)	16/44 (36.4%)	$P < .05$†

*Cerclage group versus no-cerclage group.
†Statistically significant.
(Courtesy of Hassan SS, Romero R, Maymon E, et al: Does cervical cerclage prevent preterm delivery in patients with a short cervix? *Am J Obstet Gynecol* 184:1325-1331, 2001.)

pregnancy outcome. The 2 groups were similar in rate of preterm delivery, US-to-delivery interval, gestational age at delivery (Fig 1), and birth weight. Preterm premature rupture of membranes occurred at a higher rate in patients who underwent cerclage placement (Table 3). In logistic regression, the only factor significantly associated with spontaneous preterm delivery at less than 32 weeks' gestation was a history of voluntary termination of pregnancy.

Conclusion.—A short cervix is a risk factor for spontaneous preterm delivery, but the optimal management of patients with an US-detected short cervix has not been determined. In this series of patients, cervical cerclage failed to reduce the rate of spontaneous delivery and increased the risk of premature rupture of membranes.

▶ Indications for cervical cerclage have undergone a dramatic series of changes since the procedure was first described by Shiradkar[1] in 1955. As originally described, candidates for the procedure met the historic requisites for habitual abortion and, in the nonpregnant state, showed structural evidence of increased cervical compliance by means of uterine sounding, catheters, and x-ray examinations. When those selected women were treated with cerclage either in the non-pregnant state[2] or early in the next pregnancy, results were very favorable. Evidence that shortening of the cervix in early pregnancy is associated with preterm delivery for uncertain reasons and mechanisms has led to application of cerclage to such patients, and the results have been generally unsatisfactory (see 1994 YEAR BOOK OF OBSTETRICS, GYNECOLOGY, AND WOMEN'S HEALTH, pp 67-69, 1995 YEAR BOOK, pp 52-54, 1999 YEAR BOOK, pp 70-71, and 2000 YEAR BOOK, pp 41-44). This is another small but well-reported retrospective cohort study concerning 25 women who underwent cerclage compared with 45 who did not, all of whom had cervical lengths equal to or less than 15 mm as determined by transvaginal US at 14 to 24 weeks. These authors had previously shown that such women had a 48% likelihood of delivery before 32 weeks' gestation age, indeed, these 70 women exhibited a delivery rate of 47.1% before 32 weeks and 70% before 37 weeks. The criteria for surgery are not specified, but women of older age and earlier mean gestational age (19.6 weeks vs 21.3 weeks) were disproportionately represented among those operated upon. There was no significant difference in preterm delivery rates calculated at 2-week intervals from 28 weeks to term, and the incidence of preterm rupture of membranes in women who had undergone cerclage was significantly higher than those who had not; this was certainly the result of the inflammatory impact of surgery.

The problem, of course, is that the minority of women selected who might have met Lash's and Shirdakar's criteria for cervical incompetence were mixed with a vast majority of women who might well not but were engaged in the largely unknown process leading to preterm labor and delivery. As larger and larger prospective studies have been reported on this subject, that conclusion is becoming clear.

T. H. Kirschbaum, MD

References

1. Shiradkar VN: A new method of operative treatment for habitual abortions in the second trimester of pregnancy. *Antiseptic* 52:299, 1955.
2. Lash AF: Habitual abortion: The incompetent internal os of the cervix. *Am J Obstet Gynecol* 59:68, 1950.

Effectiveness and Safety of the Oxytocin Antagonist Atosiban Versus Beta-Adrenergic Agonists in the Treatment of Preterm Labour

Moutquin JM, for the Worldwide Atosiban Versus Beta-Agonists Study Group (CUSE, Site Fleurimont, Quebec)
Br J Obstet Gynaecol 108:133-142, 2001   2–10

Background.—Preterm birth is associated with an adverse neonatal outcome and is estimated to account for more than two thirds of all singleton neonatal deaths, excluding congenital malformations. The incidence of severe neonatal morbidity is increased with decreasing neonatal age at delivery; 10% of infants born at less than 28 weeks' gestation will be severely handicapped and will require lifelong care. In very preterm gestations, the prolonging of pregnancy by even a few days may result in improved neonatal survival, which increases by 3% per day before 26 gestational weeks. Among the strategies to prevent preterm birth in women in early preterm labor is the inhibition of uterine contractility through tocolysis. The effectiveness and safety of the oxytocin antagonist atosiban were compared with those of conventional β-adrenergic agonist therapy in women with preterm labor at 23 to 33 weeks of gestation.

Methods.—Three multinational, multicenter, double-blind, randomized controlled trials were conducted. Of the total of 742 women, 733 were randomly assigned to either atosiban (363 patients) or a β-agonist (379

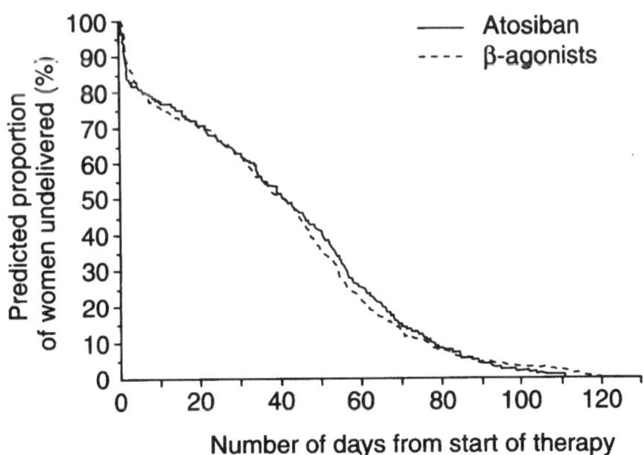

FIGURE 2.—Delivery rate and time to delivery for women administered atosiban or β-agonists. (Courtesy of Moutquin JM, for the Worldwide Atosiban Versus Beta-Agonists Study Group: Effectiveness and safety of the oxytocin antagonist atosiban versus beta-adrenergic agonists in the treatment of preterm labour. *Br J Obstet Gynaecol* 108:133-142. Copyright 2001 by Elsevier Science, publisher.)

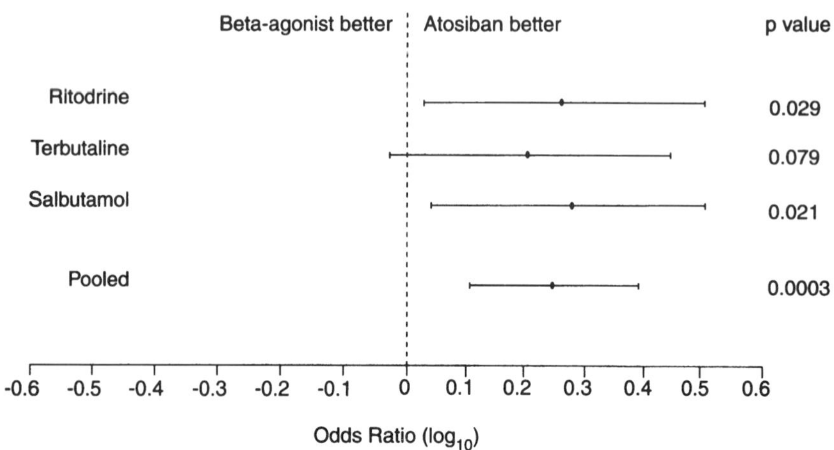

FIGURE 3.—Centre-stratified $\log_{10}$ odds ratio (with 95% CI) for the proportion of women undelivered and not requiring alternative tocolysis after 7 days of starting treatment in the three β-agonist trials and the pooled analysis. (Courtesy of Moutquin JM, for the Worldwide Atosiban Versus Beta-Agonists Study Group: Effectiveness and safety of the oxytocin antagonist atosiban versus beta-adrenergic agonists in the treatment of preterm labour. *Br J Obstet Gynaecol* 108:133-142. Copyright 2001 by Elsevier Science, publisher.)

patients) for at least 18 hours and for as many as 48 hours. The progression of labor was assessed by monitoring of the uterine contraction rate, cervical dilatation, and effacement. The Cochran-Mantel-Haenzel test was performed on all patients. The main outcome measures were tocolytic effectiveness in terms of the number of women undelivered after 48 hours and 7 days. The relationship between delivery rate and time to delivery for atosiban and beta-antagonists is shown in the Kaplan-Meier curve (Fig 2). Safety was assessed in terms of maternal side effects and neonatal morbidity.

Results.—No significant differences were noted between atosiban and β-agonists in delaying delivery for 48 hours (88.1% vs 88.9%) or 7 days (79.7% vs 77.6%). The 2 groups also had similar results for tocolytic effectiveness in terms of mean gestational age at delivery (35.8 weeks vs 35.5 weeks) and mean birth weight (2491 g vs 2461 g). However, maternal side effects, particularly adverse cardiovascular events, were reported more frequently in women who received β-agonists (8.3% vs 81.2%). These side effects resulted in a discontinuation of treatment in 1.1% of the atosiban group and in 15.4% of the β-agonist group. There were no statistical differences in neonatal/infant outcomes with either study medication.

Conclusions.—The findings of the largest study of tocolytic therapy to date were reported. Atosiban was found to be comparable in clinical effectiveness with β-agonist therapy, but had significantly fewer maternal cardiovascular side effects. Atosiban thus appeared to have clinical advantages over current tocolytic therapy (Fig 3).

▶ It has become conventional in evaluating tocolytics to make comparisons with β-adrenergic agents, the only class of tocolytics that has been compared in a randomized controlled study with placebo administered to controls. The bulk of that experience is contained in 2 articles.[1,2] The former is a meta-analysis of 16 controlled randomized trials, reporting the results from 851 case reports. The latter reports a Canadian collaborative trial of ritrodrine versus placebo in 708 patients. Both studies showed a significant effect of the β-agonist in preventing birth within 24 hours of administration, and the Canadian study extended the period of preventive effect to 48 hours. No significant difference was seen in the prevention of birth before 32 or 37 weeks' gestational age, in fetal or perinatal death, or the incidence of RDS in either study. Forty-two percent of women in the meta-analysis and 32% in the Canadian study delivered at term.

Here a consortium of 75 centers from 8 countries and 4 continents provides results in 742 cases to add to the 498 previously reported from a Michigan-Florida base study (see the 2001 YEAR BOOK OF OBSTETRICS, GYNECOLOGY, AND WOMEN'S HEALTH, pp 33-35). A complicated double-dose administration was employed to allow blinding because drug dosage schedules were different among the selected agents. Three different β-agonists were employed among the study centers. Regrettably, crossover medication was allowed as alternative tocolytics and at least 1 or more of 7 possible agents was given to 37.1% of atosiban subjects and 46.5% β-adrenergic controls. Since crossovers make it difficult to evaluate the use of either of the primary therapeutics alone, these cloud the results. Further, the criteria for designating atosiban failure were less than rigorous. The pattern, however, of the lack of difference between tocolytic efficacy of atosiban and β-adrenergic agents as judged 48 hours and 7 days after the beginning of therapy is clearly exhibited. Attesting to the difficulty in detecting preterm labor, 10% to 12% of women delivered within 48 hours after entry and only 18% to 22% delivered 7 days after the diagnosis of presumed premature labor. Part of the reason is that criteria for labor were less stringent here than in other studies cited. Patients' responses demonstrated the sometimes alarming symptoms of β-agonist use, undoubtedly reflected in the greater use of alternative agents among designated β-agonist users. Figure 3 is misleading because there are no differences in effectiveness between the 2 agents depicted, and using "need for an alternative tocolytic" simply seems to express the differences in symptomatic frequencies already demonstrated. In that sense, it is misleading to use in the header of Table 3 the words *Atosiban better* as applied only to those women undelivered after 7 days when its effectiveness in blocking labor is, in fact, no better than that of β-agonists. No benefit in fetal or infant death rates were seen.

What emerges is the same small benefit seen with other tocolytics without impact on shorter- or longer-term fetal and newborn outcome. Many of us have found magnesium sulfate a simpler and a less costly way to avoid the cardiovascular consequences of β-agonists.

T. H. Kirschbaum, MD

References

1. King JF, Grant A, Keirse MJNC, et al: Beta-mimetics in preterm labour: An overview of the randomized controlled trials. *Br J Obstet Gynaecol* 95:211-222, 1998.
2. Canadian Preterm Labor Investigators Group: Treatment of preterm labor with the beta-adrenergic agonist ritodrine. *N Engl J Med* 327:308-312, 1992.

A Randomized Trial of Augmented Prenatal Care for Multiple-Risk, Medicaid-Eligible African American Women

Klerman LV, Ramey SL, Goldenberg RL, et al (Univ of Alabama, Birmingham)
Am J Public Health 91:105-111, 2001   2–11

Background.—Low birth weight and preterm delivery have been correlated with increased rates of infant mortality and childhood illness and disability. Whether augmented prenatal care for high-risk African American women would improve pregnancy outcomes and patient knowledge of risks, satisfaction with care, and behavior was determined.

Methods.—Six hundred nineteen pregnant African American women were randomly assigned to receive augmented care or usual care. All women were eligible for Medicaid, had scored 10 or greater on a risk assessment scale, were 16 years of age or older, and had no major medical complications. More than half (58%) were multiparous. Augmented care consisted of educational peer groups, additional appointments, extended time with clinicians, and other supports.

Findings.—Women receiving augmented care rated their care as more helpful, knew more about their risk conditions, and spent more time with their nurse-providers than did those receiving usual care. A greater percentage of smokers in the augmented care group quit smoking compared with the usual care group. The 2 groups did not differ significantly in pregnancy outcomes. However, in the augmented care group, rates of preterm births were lower. In addition, cesarean deliveries and stays in neonatal intensive care units were less frequent. The rates of low birth weight were lower than predicted in both groups.

Conclusions.—High-quality prenatal care that stresses education, health promotion, and social support can significantly increase pregnant African American women's satisfaction with care, knowledge of risk conditions, and perceived mastery in their lives. However, it did not appear to decrease the rate of low birth weight deliveries in this study.

▶ Designed in part to explore means of dealing with the surplus of preterm delivery and births and growth retardation among African American women compared with white and Latino gravidas, this well-designed prospective randomized controlled study of 656 African American Medicaid recipients was implemented. Patients were at least 16 years of age and all had significant findings placing them at high risk for growth retardation and preterm birth. The study took place during slightly longer than 2 years and took place at a maternal and family specialty center financed by the Federal

Agency for Health Care Policy and Research. Selected women were exposed to care from specially trained and experienced prenatal care and research nurses as well as educators trained to explore and treat individual patient risk behaviors (including smoking, alcohol, obesity, and environmental stress) in private and group settings. The outcomes of these women were compared with women receiving nonaugmented, ongoing Medicaid-sponsored prenatal care. Studies aimed at evaluating the effect of prenatal care on premature birth and growth retardation have previously been reported from 5 states (see references 2-6 in the original article) and have failed to demonstrate significant improvement from either extended or early prenatal care. However, those studies were generally non-randomized, and the content and quality of prenatal care was uncertain and imperfectly controlled. Here, the experimental design includes a power calculation indicating an 80% likelihood of demonstrating a 50% reduction in the predicted 20% to 25% low birth weight incidence of women receiving standard care, if such an effect existed. The test group was offered prenatal visits every 2 weeks until the 36th week of gestational age, when they were seen weekly in facilities that were welcoming both in terms of comfort and decor. The results showed, largely on the basis of questionnaire responses, improved patient satisfaction, self and health knowledge, and some reduction in health-threatening behaviors as a result of the expanded care. No change in the incidence of low birth weight or preterm births was seen.

Although a negative result does not exclude the possibility that improvement in low birth weight rates might have been seen had larger numbers of patients been studied with an altered experimental design, the result does add 1 more well-designed and conducted experience that fails to demonstrate improvement in growth retardation and premature birth as a result of augmented prenatal care.

T. H. Kirschbaum, MD

Color Flow Mapping for Myometrial Invasion in Women With a Prior Cesarean Delivery

Twickler DM, Lucas MJ, Balis AB, et al (Univ of Texas, Dallas)
J Matern Fetal Med 9:330-335, 2000
2–12

Purpose.—Women who have previously undergone cesarean section are at increased risk of abnormal placental invasion into the myometrium. The ability to diagnose this problem before delivery could help in planning for surgery and possible transfusion. Previous studies have evaluated the use of US in assessing placental invasion, but the role of Doppler color flow mapping for this purpose remains unclear. The efficacy of color flow mapping in recognizing placental myometrial invasion in women with a history of cesarean delivery was evaluated.

Methods.—The study included 215 pregnant women with a history of previous cesarean delivery. Based on transvesical pelvic real-time imaging, all had placental implantations in proximity to the hysterotomy scar. Each patient underwent color Doppler mapping. In this examination, myometrial attenuation was evaluated by measuring the smallest myometrial thickness (SMT) under the placenta. The examiner also noted any unusual vascular lakes.

Findings.—Myometrial invasion was observed only in patients with marginal, partial, or complete placenta previa. Fifteen of the 20 women with placenta previa and cesarean delivery underwent cesarean hysterectomy because of bleeding complications. In 9 of these, the diagnosis of placental invasion was made. All of these had an SMT value of less than 1 mm and had vascular lakes. These variables predicted all cases of myometrial invasion, with a sensitivity of 100%, specificity of 72%, and positive and negative predictive value of 72% and 100%, respectively.

Conclusions.—Doppler color flow mapping can aid in predicting myometrial invasion in women with a history of previous cesarean delivery and US evidence of placenta previa. This information can aid in preparing for surgical management, including potential bleeding complications. Women who show an SMT of less than 1 mm and large intraplacental lakes on color flow mapping are highly likely to have myometrial invasion.

▶ This is the latest contribution to the important matter of preoperative diagnosis of placenta accreta in women pregnant following a prior cesarean section—an ever growing group (see 1993 YEAR BOOK OF OBSTETRICS, GYNECOLOGY, AND WOMEN'S HEALTH, pp 71-72, 1994 YEAR BOOK, pp 51-54, and 1996 YEAR BOOK, pp 154-156). In a group of 653 gravidas with prior cesarean section treated at Dallas Southwestern Medical Center, evaluation was by color-flow Doppler in 3 parallel vertical planes, focusing on the anterior uterine wall in relation to the bladder, and on Doppler velocimetry. The latter was used to demonstrate relatively slow flow in retroplacental vascular lakes, a sign of abnormal uterine venous return of an invasive placental implant. Among those examined, 195 proved to have anterior or low-lying placentas and 20 had placenta previa. Of those, 15 had section hysterectomies for excessive bleeding, and 9 (60%) had a confirmed diagnosis of placenta accreta. The remaining 5 scheduled for repeat cesarean section had uneventful deliveries. None of the patients characterized as having an anterior placenta implant area over a prior cesarean section's scar or those with low-lying anterior placentas had previa or hemorrhagic complications of delivery. The results are roughly the same as those reviewed here in 1994. The authors confuse the issue a bit by drawing a distinction between women without accreta with "no pathology" and "no invasion." Nonetheless, their conclusion that a minimal myometrial thickness in the anterior uterine wall less than 1 mm reflects the strong likelihood of accreta, given a prior cesarean section and an anterior placenta previa, is valuable. The chance of being wrong about such a prediction on this basis is roughly 50%.

T. H. Kirschbaum, MD

Prophylactic Amnioinfusion for Intrapartum Oligohydramnios: A Meta-Analysis of Randomized Controlled Trials

Pitt C, Sanchez-Ramos L, Kaunitz AM, et al (Univ of Florida, Jacksonville)
Obstet Gynecol 96:861-866, 2000   2–13

Introduction.—In animal models, the loss of amniotic fluid has been associated with variable decelerations in fetal heart rate (FHR) that resolve by fluid replacement with saline infusion. Oligohydramnios is commonly associated with cord compression during labor. The effectiveness of intrapartum prophylactic amnioinfusion in pregnancies complicated by oligohydramnios was assessed in a systematic review of grouped multiple randomized controlled trials.

Methods.—Computerized databases, index reviews, references cited in original trials, and review articles were used to identify randomized controlled trials of prophylactic amnioinfusion in women with oligohydramnios.

Results.—Of 35 trials identified, 14 met inclusion criteria. They included 1533 patients: 793 in the amnioinfusion group and 740 control subjects. An estimate of the odds ratio (OR) (with 95% CIs) and risk difference for dichotomous outcomes were performed using random and fixed-effects models. A test of homogeneity was performed across the trials. Females with oligohydramnios who received intrapartum amnioinfusion had lower rates of cesarean delivery for FHR abnormalities (OR, 0.23). Intrapartum amnioinfusion was also correlated with lower overall rates of cesarean deliveries (OR, 0.52), FHR abnormalities during labor (OR, .24), and Apgar scores under 7 at 5 min (OR, 0.52). All groups had similar postpartum endometritis rates.

Conclusion.—Prophylactic intrapartum amnioinfusion significantly improves neonatal outcome and reduces the rate of cesarean delivery without increasing the rate of postpartum endometritis in females with oligohydramnios.

▶ The suggestion in 1983 by Miyazaki and Taylor that saline intra-amniotic infusion is useful in ameliorating variable FHR patterns has readily been confirmed and is now a common obstetrical practice.[1] Though effective in reducing cesarean section rates largely attributable to concerns about FHR abnormality, it has had little effect on reducing the incidence of respiratory distress syndrome related to meconium-stained amniotic fluid (sec 1996 YEAR BOOK of OBSTETRICS, GYNECOLOGY and WOMEN'S HEALTH, pp 121-122). or newborn lung functioning (see 1996 YEAR BOOK, p 239). Further, attempts to prove reduction in perinatal morbidity and mortality rates through this modality have failed, except in emerging nations where neonatal care facilities are in short supply (see 1999 YEAR BOOK, pp 119-121). This meta-analysis of randomized unblinded trials of amnioinfusion in laboring women with oligohydramnios makes no claim to reducing perinatal morbidity, but it does, as others have, show a significantly decreased rate of cesarean section for FHR abnormality for women so treated. Since concerns regarding FHR included

83% of the indications for all cesarean sections here, the overall section rate was reduced as well. Data is aggregated for evidence of umbilical artery, blood pH less than 7.20 at birth is so heterogeneous as to preclude meta-analysis, and only 3 of 11 studies selected show independent significant relationships of amnioinfusion to maternal newborn acidosis. Although the authors claim evidence for significant reduction in incidence of Apgar scores of less than 7 at 5 minutes, the purported significance rests with only 1 study.[2] It seems reasonable to conclude that amnioinfusion, by diminishing the number and severity of variable decelerations, reduces obstetrician anxiety and the inclination to perform a cesarean section on that basis without improvement in perinatal outcome. In that limited sense, it is, however, a clinically useful procedure.

T. H. Kirschbaum, MD

References

1. Miyazaki FS, Taylor NA: Saline amnioinfusion for variable or prolonged decelerations. A preliminary report. *Am J Obstet Gynecol* 146:670-678, 1983.
2. Macri CJ, Schrimmer DB, Leung A, et al: Prophylactic amnioinfusion improves outcome of pregnancy complicated by thick meconium and oligohydramnios. *Am J Obstet Gynecol* 167:117-121, 1992.

Do Antenatal Corticosteroids Help in the Setting of Preterm Rupture of Membranes?
Harding JE, Pang J-M, Knight DB, et al (Natl Women's Hosp, Auckland, New Zealand)
Am J Obstet Gynecol 184:131-139, 2001   2–14

Introduction.—The administration of corticosteroids before preterm delivery is correlated with a marked decrease in the risks of neonatal death and respiratory distress syndrome. Corticosteroid use for patients with ruptured membranes continues to be controversial. A meta-analysis of the available randomized trials was conducted to settle the debate about the use of antenatal corticosteroids for the preterm rupture of membranes.

Methods.—A literature search for all randomized and appropriately controlled trials, including the 1972 Auckland, New Zealand Trial of females allocated to receive antenatal betamethasone or dexamethasone before anticipated preterm delivery was performed using the electronic databases MEDLINE, EMBASE, and the Cochrane Library.

Results.—Data from the Auckland Trial of 318 females with ruptured membranes disclosed a nonsignificant trend toward a decreased risk of respiratory distress syndrome with corticosteroids. Ruptured membranes had little effect on the risks of neonatal death, intraventricular hemorrhage, and fetal, neonatal, or maternal infection. Combined data from controlled trials including more than 1400 females with ruptured membranes verified that corticosteroids decrease the risks of respiratory distress syndrome (relative risk (RR), 0.56), intraventricular hemorrhage (RR,

0.47), and necrotizing enterocolitis (RR, 0.21). They also may diminish the risk of neonatal death (RR, 0.68). They do not seem to increase the risk of infection in either mother (RR, 0.86) or infant (RR, 1.05). The duration of rupture of membranes does not modify these outcomes.

Conclusion.—Corticosteroid administration is beneficial in the setting of a rupture of membranes. Future trials addressing this situation are not justified.

▶ Dr G.C. Liggins, exploring the mechanisms underlying the onset of labor in gravid sheep found, among other things, that he could induce labor at will by administering glucocorticoids to mother or fetus. He astonished the experienced veterinarians at UC Davis with the striking capacity of the prematurely delivered lambs to breathe and survive, and in a series of subsequent animal experiments, he demonstrated the role of maternal steroids in speeding development of the enzymatic capacity to produce fetal pulmonary surface active material in premature animals. With this background, he undertook a controlled prospective randomized study of 1142 women with 1218 infants at 24 to 37 weeks of pregnancy, which demonstrated a significant decrease in the risk of neonatal death and respiratory distress syndrome in pregnancies exposed to maternal glucocorticoids.[1] Subsequently, his findings were confirmed by more than 20 independent trials involving approximately 4000 pregnant women.

However, some questions remained regarding the impact of ruptured membranes prior to term (PROM) or premature labor (PPROM). Also concern for a possible increased risk of maternal and newborn infection arose from a study of 42 women, where prophylactic antibiotics were not given to women with PPROM who lacked clinical evidence of amnionitis.[2]

To deal with these uncertainties, records from more than 2000 women, half control subjects, from the 1972 study from Auckland were abstracted, categorizing ruptured membranes occurring before or at the time of study entry or exhibiting more than 24 or 48 hours after membrane rupture but before administering steroid. Since these categories divided the data into 4 subsets, acceptable data from 14 subsequent studies were added to attain statistical significance via meta-analysis. The results demonstrated clear evidence of a decreased risk of respiratory distress syndrome after maternal glucocorticoids, exempting the 2 studies with duration of ruptured membranes greater than 48 hours (see Figure 3 in the original article). Similarly, the incidence of intraventricular hemorrhage and necrotizing enterocolitis were significantly decreased, and risk ratios for neonatal death also exhibited a reduction with marginal statistical significance (see Figure 4 in the original article). No increase in the risk of fetal, neonatal, or maternal infection for women with ruptured membranes before entering the trial were seen, but again, 2 available studies did not suffice to provide adequate assurance of the absence of increased maternal infection risks after more than 24 hours of ruptured membranes had transpired before steroid treatment. These data stemmed from the Boston trial.[2]

With justifiable pride, the authors point to their 1972 experience as sufficient so that "further trials to address this [rupture of membranes] question cannot be justified."

T. H. Kirschbaum, MD

References

1. Liggins FC, Howie RN: A controlled trial of antepartum glucocorticoid treatment for prevention of the respiratory distress syndrome in premature infants. *Pediatrics* 50:515-525, 1972.
2. Taeusch HW Jr, Frigoletto F, Kitzmiller J, et al: Risk of respiratory distress syndrome after prenatal dexamethasone therapy. *Pediatrics* 63:64-72, 1979.

Serial Salivary Estriol to Detect an Increased Risk of Preterm Birth
Heine RP, McGregor JA, Goodwin TM, et al (Univ of Pittsburgh, Pa; Univ of Colorado, Denver; Univ of Southern California, Los Angeles; et al)
Obstet Gynecol 96:490-497, 2000   2–15

Background.—In human beings, the placenta and fetus are the primary sources for 90% or more of the estriol (E3) produced during late pregnancy. E3 levels can be directly measured in saliva, and a large increase in the salivary E_3-to-progesterone ratio occurs 3 to 4 weeks before birth. In a previous study, these authors used receiver operating characteristic (ROC) analysis to show that an increase in the salivary E3 level 2.1 ng/mL or greater was an accurate predictor of preterm labor. In this prospective study, whether weekly measurements of the salivary E3 level would identify women at increased risk of spontaneous premature labor and birth was examined.

Methods.—The subjects were 956 women with singleton pregnancies who were enrolled at 1 of 8 US medical centers. Based on the Creasy scoring system, 31.6% were considered at high risk of preterm birth (≤ 37 weeks' gestation). Subjects with symptoms of preterm labor, placenta previa, cervical changes requiring cerclage, ruptured membranes, preeclampsia, or planned cesarean delivery; subjects who used illicit drugs or drugs known to affect hormone levels; and subjects whose fetus had a major congenital abnormality, fetal growth restriction, or erythroblastosis fetalis or died in utero were excluded from analysis. Additionally, patients taking betamethasone, dexamethasone, or tocolytic agents were excluded because of the known or possible suppressive effects of these drugs on salivary E3. Beginning at gestational week 22, saliva samples were collected each week until birth and analyzed by enzyme-linked immunosorbent assay to determine unconjugated E3 levels. Fisher exact test (2-tailed; $\alpha = 0.05$) was used to examine differences in the incidence of preterm labor followed by preterm delivery based on a salivary E3 level less than 2.1 ng/mL or 2.1 ng/mL or greater. Additionally, ROC curves were developed to identify the salivary E3 level that best estimated the risk of preterm birth within 2 weeks of its measurement.

TABLE 3.—Predictive Accuracy of Salivary Estriol

	Sensitivity	Specificity	Positive Predictive Value	Negative Predictive Value	Relative Risk
Combined population					
Single positive test*	57 (34.5, 76.8)	78 (74.1, −81.0)	9 (5.0, 15.2)	98 (96.0, 99.0)	4.2 (1.9, 9.4)
Second positive test*	44 (23.2, 65.5)	92 (89.9, 94.4)	19 (9.3, 31.4)	98 (96.0, 98.7)	7.8 (3.6, 16.9)
Low-risk population					
Single positive test†	50 (21.1, 78.9)	81 (76.8, 84.4)	7 (2.5, 14.0)	98 (96.4, 99.4)	4.0 (1.3, 12.1)
Second positive test*	42 (15.2, 72.3)	93 (90.0, 95.3)	14 (4.8, 30.3)	98 (96.6, 99.3)	8.5 (2.8, 25.2)
High risk population					
Single positive test†	64 (30.8, 89.1)	68 (59.7, 75.7)	14 (5.6, 25.8)	96 (90.1, 98.9)	3.4 (1.0, 11.0)
Second positive test*	46 (16.8, 76.7)	90 (83.9, 94.5)	26 (9.2, 51.2)	96 (90.4, 98.3)	5.8 (2.0, 17.3)

Data are given as % (95% confidence interval).
*$P \leq .05$.
†$P \leq .005$.
(Courtesy of Heine RP, McGregor JA, Goodwin TM, et al: Serial salivary estriol to detect an increased risk of preterm birth. *Obstet Gynecol* 96:490-497, 2000. Reprinted with permission of The American College of Obstetricians and Gynecologists.)

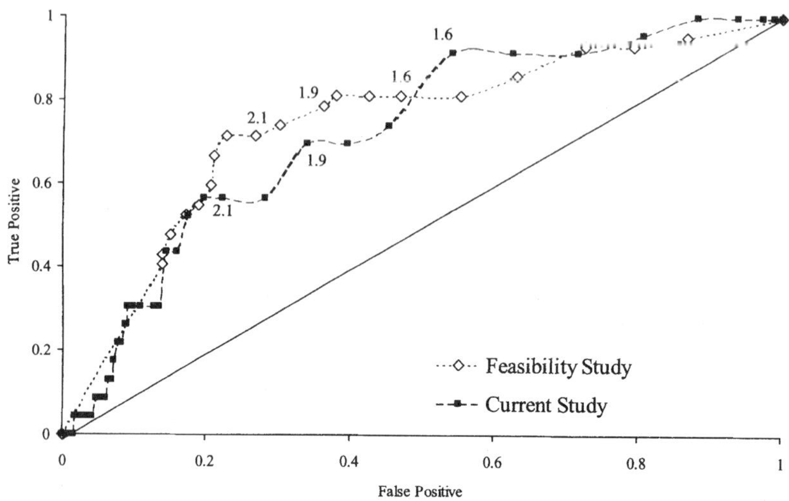

FIGURE 2.—ROC analysis: maximum intrapatient salivary E3 value and its ability to predict preterm birth, considering values collected at 24-36 weeks' gestation (n = 601) in our feasibility study and the current study. (Courtesy of Heine RP, McGregor JA, Goodwin TM, et al: Serial salivary estriol to detect an increased risk of preterm birth. *Obstet Gynecol* 96:490-497, 2000. Reprinted with permission of The American College of Obstetricians and Gynecologists.)

Results.—Of the 956 subjects enrolled, 247 were excluded from analysis because of noncompliance, the development of exclusion criteria after enrollment, and loss to follow-up. Of the remaining 714 subjects, 113 were excluded because of subsequent treatment with betamethasone, dexamethasone, or tocolytic agents, preterm premature rupture of membranes, medically indicated preterm birth, or a term birth despite preterm labor. Thus, primary analyses were based on 601 women, 152 (25.3%) of whom were at high risk of preterm birth. There were 578 term deliveries and 23 preterm deliveries (11 in the high-risk group) at a median gestational age of 36 weeks. A single, positive salivary E3 level 2.1 ng/mL or greater was associated with a significantly increased risk of spontaneous preterm labor and delivery not only in the group as a whole (relative risk [RR], 4.2), but within the high-risk (RR, 3.4) and low-risk (RR, 4.0) groups as well (Table 3). Having 2 or more positive salivary E3 tests significantly increased the positive predictive value in all 3 groups (RRs of 7.8, 5.8, and 8.5, respectively). ROC analysis confirmed that a cutoff of 2.1 ng/mL provided optimal sensitivity and specificity in predicting preterm birth (Fig 2). Among subjects who had 1 or more positive salivary E3 tests, the median time between the positive test and preterm birth was 2.3 weeks, and 86% delivered within 3 weeks. Furthermore, 158 (22%) of the 714 subjects presented with signs or symptoms of preterm labor, a salivary E3 level 1.4 ng/mL or greater identified 61% of subjects who delivered within 2 weeks.

Conclusions.—The risk of spontaneous preterm labor and birth was significantly associated with a salivary E3 test 2.1 ng/mL or greater. A lower threshold (1.4 ng/mL) effectively predicted the risk of preterm birth in almost two thirds of the symptomatic subjects. Thus, serial measurement of salivary E3 levels appears to be an effective, noninvasive means of assessing the risk of spontaneous preterm labor and delivery in both asymptomatic and symptomatic women.

▶ For several years, the possible use of salivary E3 measurements in predicting preterm labor has been an item of hopeful interest. The correspondence between salivary and serum E3 concentration is relatively good during pregnancy, and salivary E3 concentrations have been shown to be significantly greater in women delivering between 24 to 34 weeks' gestational age in comparison to women delivering at term.[1] Maternal E3 concentrations have been shown to increase a few weeks before the onset of normal human labor and clearly reflect fetal-placental production and release. Preliminary evidence established the presence of an association between salivary E3 and preterm birth, and this prospective masked multicenter study enables evaluation of the predictive utility of the noninvasive salivary E3 test. A population of 956 women enrolled was reduced to 601 women by virtue of noncompliance, failed follow-up and exclusions based on a wide range of pregnancy abnormalities, many of them risk factors for preterm birth. Perhaps this latter step, necessary to evaluate the use of the technique in patients with normal pregnancies, accounts for the low 3.8% preterm birth rate noted in this group of women, 25% of whom were believed to be at high risk for preterm birth. ROC analysis based on a feasibility study was used to define the optimal maximum normal E3 concentration that yielded a sensitivity figure of 55% with an approximately 22% false-positive rate. The derived criterion is based on the ability to predict preterm delivery within 2 weeks of the salivary E3 value equal to or greater than 2.1 ng/mL. When data from all 601 women were pooled, sensitivity was at most 57%, with a false-positive rate of 98% and 81% with 2 weekly consecutive abnormal salivary values, respectively. Limiting the study to higher risk women with 2 consecutive positive salivary values, sensitivity was 46% with a false-positive rate of 74%. This approach to predicting preterm birth falls into a familiar pattern, with demonstration of an association with premature birth insufficiently rigorous to serve as a useful predictor or an indication for special therapy.

T. H. Kirschbaum, MD

Reference

1. McGregor JA, Jackson GW, Lochelin GCO, et al: Salivary estriol as a risk assessment for preterm labor. *Am J Obstet Gynecol* 173:1337-1342, 1995.

Indomethacin Tocolysis and Intraventricular Hemorrhage

Suarez RD, Grobman WA, Parilla BV (Northwestern Univ, Chicago)
Obstet Gynecol 97:921-925, 2000

2–16

Background.—Indomethacin's tocolytic effect is equivalent to that of alternative regimens, and it has fewer side effects. However, most studies have concentrated on multiple tocolytic regimens, of which indomethacin is just a part, that may be associated with intraventricular hemorrhage (IVH). The independent association of indomethacin with neonatal IVH was the focus of this case control study.

Methods.—The study population consisted of 56 preterm neonates who had IVH and 224 gestational age–matched controls who did not have IVH. Each of the mothers' and infants' charts were evaluated to determine which tocolytic regimen the neonate had experienced. Analytic tools included the Student *t* test, chi-square analysis, and multivariate logistic regression.

Results.—No differences in maternal age, parity, betamethasone exposure, or gender were noted between the control and the affected infants (Table 1). Vaginal birth at an earlier gestational age and lower birth weight were characteristics found more often among the infants who experienced IVH, as was a greater tendency to have come from a pregnancy complicated by chorioamnionitis. It was more likely that affected infants would have sepsis, experience respiratory distress syndrome (RDS), and die than infants in the control group (Table 2). Exposure to indomethacin alone or combined with magnesium sulfate carried a higher risk of IVH according to univariate analysis (Table 3). According to multivariate analysis, exposure to indomethacin tocolysis alone or combined with magnesium sulfate introduced no higher risk of IVH. Variables that did correlate with IVH were earlier gestational age at delivery, chorioamnionitis during pregnancy, vaginal delivery, and RDS.

TABLE 1.—Pregnancy Characteristics of the Study Population

	IVH ($n = 56$)	Controls ($n = 224$)	P
Maternal age (y)	30.0 ± 6.5	30.0 ± 6.3	NS
Nulliparity	38 (68%)	151 (67%)	NS
Gestational age (wk)	28.0 ± 2.1	30.0 ± 2.2	<.001
Male	34 (61%)	22 (55%)	NS
Birth weight (g)	1070 ± 320	1392 ± 430	<.001
Vaginal delivery	40 (71%)	125 (56%)	<.05
Betamethasone exposure	51 (91%)	187 (84%)	NS
Chorioamnionitis	22 (39%)	30 (13%)	<.001

Note: Data are presented as mean ± standard deviation of *n* (%).
Abbreviations: IVH, Intraventricular hemorrhage; *NS,* not significant.
(Reprinted with permission of The American College of Obstetrics and Gynecology from Suarez RD, Grobman WA, Parilla BV: Indomethacin tocolysis and intraventricular hemorrhage. *Obstet Gynecol* 97:921-925, 2000.)

TABLE 2.—Neonatal Outcomes for the Study Population

Outcome	IVH ($n = 56$)	Controls ($n = 224$)	P
Sepsis	29 (52%)	50 (22%)	<.001
NEC	5 (9%)	22 (10%)	NS
RDS	53 (95%)	137 (61%)	<.001
Death	7 (13%)	7 (3%)	<.05
Umbilical artery pH	7.30 ± 0.10 ($n = 28$)	7.30 ± 0.10 ($n = 135$)	NS
Umbilical vein pH	7.25 ± 0.20 ($n = 36$)	7.27 ± 0.10 ($n = 150$)	NS

Note: Data are presented as mean ± standard deviation of n (%).
Abbreviations: As in Table 1; *NEC*, necrotizing enterocolitis; *RDS*, respiratory distress syndrome.
(Reprinted with permission of The American College of Obstetrics and Gynecology from Suarez RD, Grobman WA, Parilla BV: Indomethacin tocolysis and intraventricular hemorrhage. *Obstet Gynecol* 97:921-925, 2000.)

Conclusions.—No independent significance can be attached to the use of indomethacin for tocolysis leading to IVH. Because of its better tolerance, ease of administration, lower cost, and equivalent efficacy when compared with other tocolytics, indomethacin appears to be a good first-line choice for tocolysis.

▶ This is another example of the role of multivariate analysis, employed this time with questionable validity. In this cohort study, conducted over a 2-year period, 56 infants admitted because of IVH to a neonatal ICU (NICU) during the first 2 years of life represented 6.9% of total NICU admissions. They were matched with 224 NICU admissions in which infants failed to show IVH, and risk ratios were drawn between IVH group victims and controls. The index and control groups were grossly dissimilar because the IVH group, not unexpectedly, showed a lesser gestational age and birth weight and 3 times greater incidence of chorioamnionitis. The IVH group had a 2.4 times greater incidence of sepsis, a 1.5 times greater incidence of RDS, and a 4.3 times greater perinatal death rate. Since 1977, indomethacin was used in this center as primary tocolytic, and if the cervix changed within 7 days of use of that agent, magnesium sulfate was used either alone or in combination. Use of combinations of tocolytics complicates analysis, indeed, the authors use that point to question the results of others who claim a relationship between indomethacin use and IVH. Univariant analysis shows an increased risk of IVH in comparison with controls for pregnancies treated with indomethacin,

TABLE 3.—Univariate Analysis of Tocolytic Regimens*

	IVH ($n = 56$)	Controls ($n = 224$)	OR	95% CI
Indomethacin only	12 (21%)	27 (12%)	2.5	1.1, 5.6
Magnesium only	5 (9%)	26 (12%)	1.1	0.4, 3.1
Combination tocolysis	14 (25%)	29 (13%)	2.7	1.3, 5.9

Note: Data are presented as n (%).
*Reference group = No tocolysis.
Abbreviations: IVH, Intraventricular hemorrhage; *OR*, odds ratio; *CI*, confidence interval.
(Reprinted with permission of The American College of Obstetrics and Gynecology from Suarez RD, Grobman WA, Parilla BV: Indomethacin tocolysis and intraventricular hemorrhage. *Obstet Gynecol* 97:921-925, 2000.)

either alone or in combination with magnesium sulfate, but not with magnesium sulfate alone.

Multivariate analysis was then applied to a list of variables that failed to meet the test of the confounding variables, that is, those that are mutually related both to indomethacin use and to IVH. Multivariate analysis can't be used to correct for discordances between test and control groups which do not affect the independent variable, that is, the decision to use indomethacin. RDS occurrence, vaginal birth, chorioamnionitis, and prematurity have known relationships to IVH but not to a decision to use indomethacin. The use of combination tocolytics cannot say anything about indomethacin alone and has best been deleted from the analysis, which then confirms a relationship between indomethacin and IVH.

An equally important issue here is one that the authors avoid by stating, correctly, that indomethacin has been found to be clinically equivalent to alternative tocolytics. Those tocolytics, only 1 of which has been compared with untreated controls or placebos, failed to disclose any benefit from any tocolytic (see 1993 YEAR BOOK OF OBSTETRICS, GYNECOLOGY, AND WOMEN'S HEALTH, pp 44-45, 1997 YEAR BOOK, pp 113-114, 1999 YEAR BOOK, pp 115-117, and 2000 YEAR BOOK, pp 63-64). There is no basis for concluding that indomethacin is superior in any way to other tocolytics or that it affords any more advantage than the opportunity to give effective corticosteroid therapy to prevent RDS. Evidence that its use effects ductus arteriosus closure, reduced fetal cardiac output, oligohydramnios, and IVH continues to mean to me that indomethacin should not be used as a tocolytic.

T. H. Kirschbaum, MD

3 Fetal Complications of Pregnancy

Placental Insufficiency and Fetal Growth Restriction Lead to Postnatal Hypotension and Altered Postnatal Growth in Sheep
Louey S, Cock ML, Stevenson KM, et al (Monash Univ, Victoria, Australia)
Pediatr Res 48:808-814, 2000   3–1

Introduction.—An inverse relationship has been observed between arterial pressure and birth weight in both adults and children. In adults, this finding has been independent of current body size and lifestyle factors. Several investigations of fetal growth restriction in animals have demonstrated an association between a suboptimal intrauterine environment and arterial pressure. The effects of low birth weight resulting from intrauterine growth restriction (IUGR) on fetal and postnatal arterial pressure and the potential roles of circulating cortisol and renin were investigated in fetal sheep.

Methods.—Umbilico-placental embolization (UPE) was used to induce IUGR in fetal sheep from 120 days' gestation until birth (about 147 days). Eight IUGR and 8 control postnatal lambs were observed for 8 weeks. Both fetal and postnatal arterial pressures were measured, and blood samples were obtained for measurement of gas tensions, cortisol concentrations, and renin activity.

Results.—In IUGR fetuses, the mean arterial pressure (MAP) initially rose with UPE. Near term, it was similar to values in control fetuses (Fig 2). The IUGR sheep weighed 35% less than the control sheep at birth and remained lighter than the control sheep throughout the 8 weeks of follow-up. The IUGR growth pattern was different from that of the control group. The IUGR sheep had lower MAP than the control group; this relative hypotension (−4 mm Hg) persisted throughout the 8 weeks of postnatal follow-up. Covariate analysis revealed that the relative hypotension of IUGR sheep could have resulted from their smaller size. Plasma cortisol concentrations were similar in IUGR and control animals before and after birth. Compared to control sheep, plasma renin activity was similar in IUGR postnatal animals.

Conclusion.—Late gestational IUGR in sheep results in relative hypotension in the early postnatal period, probably because of decreased

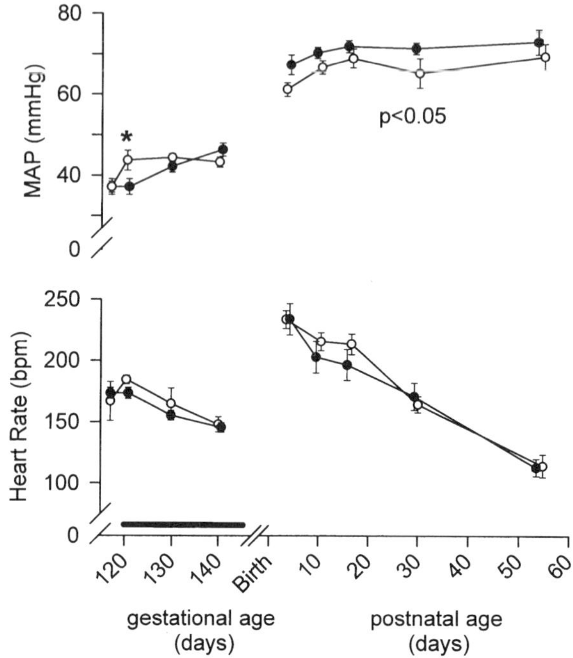

FIGURE 2.—Mean arterial pressure (MAP) and heart rate in IUGR (*open circle*) and control (*filled circle*) fetuses and postnatal lambs up to 8 weeks of age. The *bar* indicates the period of umbilico-placental embolization. *P*-values refer to a significant effect of treatment. Asterisk (*) indicates value that differs between groups (*P* < .05). (Courtesy of Louey S, Cock ML, Stevenson KM, et al: Placental insufficiency and fetal growth restriction lead to postnatal hypotension and altered postnatal growth in sheep. *Pediatr Res* 48:808-814, 2000.)

body size. Postnatal cortisol and renin levels were not associated with the development of either hypotension or hypertension.

▶ Starting with the observations of an inverse relationship between low birthweight and hypertension in later life, Barter and associates have generated a complex hypothesis based largely on epidemiologic evidence (see Abstract 1–4). What is posited is that, during states of nutrient deficiency in utero, as expressed by growth retardation at term birth, there are fetal metabolic adjustments that may predispose the infant, in later life, to hypertension, insulin resistance, dysfunctional carbohydrate and lipid metabolism, and atherosclerosis.[1] Some data analysis has led to the conclusion that hypertension can be discerned in infancy as well, though the evidence is tenuous.[2] The data compare systolic blood pressures done on 1895 term infants annually to age 10 years and at ages 4 days, 6 weeks, and 6 months of life. Their data were adjusted for variable blood pressure cuff sizes and body weight, and significant differences were reported only for low birth weight infants at 4 years of age; no significant differences existed in 1 year.

It is to this unsettled issue that these authors employ animal investigation, producing growth retardation in fetal sheep using umbilical placental embolization in utero with Sephadex microspheres, a technique with which they are experienced and successful (see 1999 YEAR BOOK OF OBSTETRICS, GYNE-COLOGY, AND WOMEN'S HEALTH, pp 18-19). Embolization was carried out from day 120 to approximately day 146 (term) with a resulting 33% reduction in mean birthweight together with hypoxemia, hypercarbia, and acidosis in growth-retarded lambs. Followed up through 55 days of postnatal life, growth-retarded lambs showed mean arterial blood pressures significantly lower than did normal control animals beginning at the fourth day of life.

Certainly the possibility of species differences from humans exist, and long term follow-up of these newborns will be important. However, these acute objective observations failed to confirm the data evaluation done by CM Low et al, which found epidemiologic evidence of early neonatal hypertension in growth-retarded infants.

T. H. Kirschbaum, MD

References

1. Barker BS: Fetal origins of coronary heart disease. *BMJ* 311:171, 1995.
2. Low CM, de Swiet M, Osmond C, et al: Initiation of hypertension in utero and its amplification throughout life. *BMJ* 306:24, 1993.

Early Nutrition in Preterm Infants and Later Blood Pressure: Two Cohorts After Randomised Trials
Singhal A, Cole TJ, Lucas A (Inst of Child Health, London)
Lancet 357:413-419, 2001   3–2

Background.—Evidence suggests that body size early in life is associated with cardiovascular events later in life. However, the effects of nutrition on such outcomes have not been established. The hypothesis that diet early in life can program blood pressure in later life was tested.

Methods.—A cohort of 926 children born prematurely were included in 2 parallel randomized studies in 5 neonatal units in England. In 1 study, children received donated banked breastmilk or preterm formula, in a second parallel study, they received standard term formula or preterm formula. Of the original cohort 216 (23%) had blood pressure measured at the age of 13 to 16 years.

Findings.—The mean arterial blood pressure of the children aged 13 to 16 years was lower in the 66 children given banked breastmilk than in the 64 given preterm formula (Table 3). In nonrandomized analyses, the proportion of enteral intake as human milk in the neonatal period was correlated inversely to later mean arterial presure (Fig 2). The groups given term formula and preterm formula did not differ.

Conclusions.—In these children born prematurely, breastmilk consumption was associated with lower blood pressure at the age of 13 to 16 years.

TABLE 3.—Blood Pressure in Relation to Early Diet

Variable	Mean (SD) Blood Pressure (mm Hg)		Mean (95% CI) Difference	p	Mean (SD) Blood Pressure (mm Hg)		Mean (95% CI) Difference	p
	Banked Breastmilk (n=66)	Preterm Formula (n=64)			Term Formula (n=44)	Preterm Formula (n=42)		
Diastolic	61·9 (8·1)	65·0 (6·7)	−3·2 (−5·8 to −0·6)	0·016	64·1 (7·7)	64·3 (6·8)	−0·2 (−3·4 to 2·9)	0·88
Systolic	113·6 (9·0)	116·3 (8·0)	−2·7 (−5·7 to 0·3)	0·075	117·9 (8·0)	116·4 (7·8)	−1·0 (−1·9 to 4·9)	0·37
Mean arterial	81·9 (7·8)	86·1 (6·5)	−4·1 (−6·6 to −1·6)	0·001	85·5 (7·3)	84·5 (6·4)	1·5 (−2·0 to 3·9)	0·51

(Courtesy of Singhal A, Cole TJ, Lucas A: Early nutrition in preterm infants and later blood pressure: Two cohorts after randomised trials. *Lancet* 357:413-419, 2001. Copyright by The Lancet Ltd., 2001.)

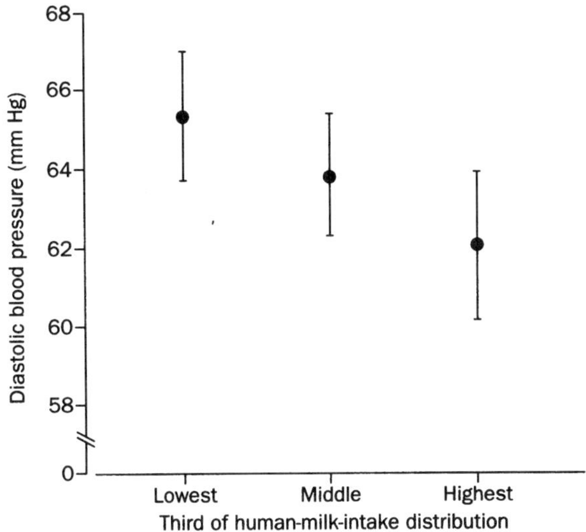

FIGURE 2.—Diastolic blood pressure in thirds of proportional intake of human milk. *Error bars =* 95% confidence interval. (Courtesy of Singhal A, Cole TJ, Lucas A: Early nutrition in preterm infants and later blood pressure: Two cohorts after randomised trials. *Lancet* 357:413-419, 2001. Copyright by The Lancet Ltd., 2001.)

The current findings suggest that early diet can program a cardiovascular risk factor.

▶ This work provides some support for the Barker hypothesis that fetal undernutrition and low birth weight increases the risk for diabetes mellitus, hypertension, dyslipidemia, and insulin resistance in later life. Some dispute over that definition has arisen, but more of that later. This study is unique among all others on this subject, including random assignment of nutrient availabilities in humans.

In 1980, human milk banks were available in London and, in the period from 1980 to 1985, 926 infants were randomly assigned to 2 study protocols involving breast milk availability. In the one of primary interest, 502 infants with birth weight less than 1.85 kg were randomized between banked breast milk feeding and preterm formula. Each of those 2 groups was additionally subdivided into women who used only the assigned feeding and those who supplemented their own breast milk with the assigned feeding product. Roughly, two thirds of women elected the latter regimen. Outcome measurements reported were confined to blood pressure measurements in all 4 subsets at a mean age between 7½ and 8 years and between the ages of 13 and 16 years. Note the experimental design assumes without proof that fetal and neonatal nutritional impacts are the same, though what is presented to the fetus via maternal feeding is likely different than direct infant nutritional intake. Note also, follow-up blood pressures were obtained in only 23% of subjects enrolled, and continuation in the follow-up may have been an uncontrolled variable, impacting on the blood pressure reported. No significant difference was noted in blood pressures as a result of feeding differences at the age of 7½-8 years. In the period from 13 to 16 years, no significant difference was noted in blood pressures between the third of infants receiving only breast milk and those receiving only preterm formula. In the two thirds of cases where breast milk was chosen to supplement the assigned diet, the mean diastolic blood pressure was 2.9 mm Hg and mean arterial blood pressures 4.8 mm Hg lower in those supplementing with breast milk than any of those using formula. No significant differences in arterial blood pressure were noted. The apparent effect in lowering blood pressure by breast milk appeared inversely related to a semi-quantitative estimate of the size of breast milk supplement. In a parallel study, no differences were noted when term formula was compared with preterm formula. The authors cite evidence in adults that a population-wide reduction of blood pressure of this magnitude has substantial public health benefits; there is no such evidence in infants, and no apparent health consequences at the age of 13 to 16 years are reported.

In correspondence from LH Lumey published on pages 472-473 of this journal issue, he claims that the original research support provided in 1994 by the Medical Research Council in London was for a study of nutrient impacts in early and mid fetal life, whereas the publication of data from that study[1] dealt with decreased fetal nutritional impacts in mid to late gestation. Assuming premature newborn and fetal nutritional impacts are the same, this study also fails to deal with early fetal conditioning, in the sense that it might take place in the first and second trimesters of pregnancy. Barker responds that he changed the hypothesis in 1995.[2] Lancet's editors confirm Lumey's charge and support some of his complaints of unethical publication practices when his direct participation in MRC-funded research was not properly described in the 1998 publication.

On page 405 of Reference 2, there is an editorial comment to the point that though the Barker hypothesis is an attractive, important, productive and well-funded one, it suffers from a lack of direct proof characterized by internal controls, randomization, and any solid evidence of mechanism underlying the epidemiologic data that supports it. Since the purported effects of impaired fetal growth take 30 to 40 years to become manifest in adult life, all data is retrospective, consisting of information collected years ago with uncertain precision and from natural experiments, such as the Dutch famine of 1944 to 1945, in which LH Lumey is particularly expert. Despite these uncertainties, the Barker hypothesis has spawned a First World Conference and The International Council for Research in 2001, and the hypothesis has broadened to include fetal nutritional impacts on the incidence of stroke, atopy, cancer, osteoporosis, depression, and aging. The editor urges research in cellular and metabolic processes underlying the purported effects of diminished birth weight and to "those research designs that seek to refute the 'Barker hypothesis' via the severest of challenges." It is a wise comment, for a concept that, with uncertain foundation, shows signs of encompassing a major share of all human pathophysiology without the presence of rigorous, objective, direct scientific support.

T. H. Kirschbaum, MD

References

1. Ravelli ACJ, van der Meulen, Michels RPJ, et al: Glucose tolerance in infants after prenatal exposure to famine. *Lancet* 351:173-177, 1998.
2. Barker DJB: Fetal origins of coronary heart disease. *BMJ* 311:171-174, 1995.

Antenatal Dexamethasone and Decreased Birth Weight

Bloom SL, Sheffield JS, McIntire DD, et al (Univ of Texas, Dallas)
Obstet Gynecol 97:485-490, 2001

3–3

Background.—Corticosteroids are routinely administered to women at risk for preterm delivery to promote fetal lung maturation. However, recent findings in animals suggest that these drugs may cause impaired fetal growth. The correlation between antenatal dexamethasone treatment and low birth weight in humans, corrected for gestational age, was analyzed.

Methods.—Birth weights for singleton, live-born infants given antenatal dexamethasone were compared with those for (1) a frequency matched (3:1) control group (maternal race, infant sex, gestational age at delivery; (2) a cohort group of infants who were delivered in the 12 months before Parkland Hospital in Dallas, Tex, began use of dexamethasone in 1994; and (3) a reference obstetric population.

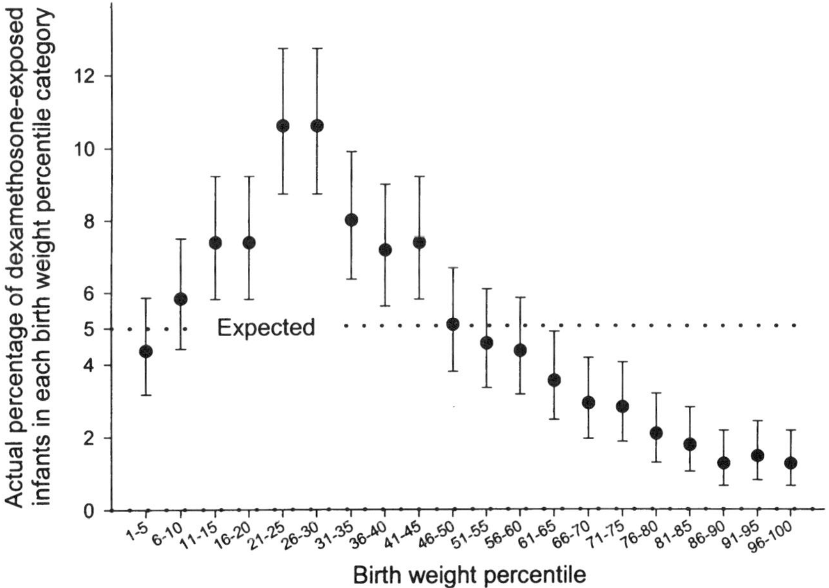

FIGURE 2.—Birth weight distribution of dexamethasone-treated infants compared with the distribution of the reference obstetric population of untreated infants. (Courtesy of Bloom SL, Sheffield JS, McIntire DD, et al: Antenatal dexamethasone and decreased birth weight. *Obstet Gynecol* 97:485-490, 2001. Reprinted with permission from The American College of Obstetricians and Gynecologists.)

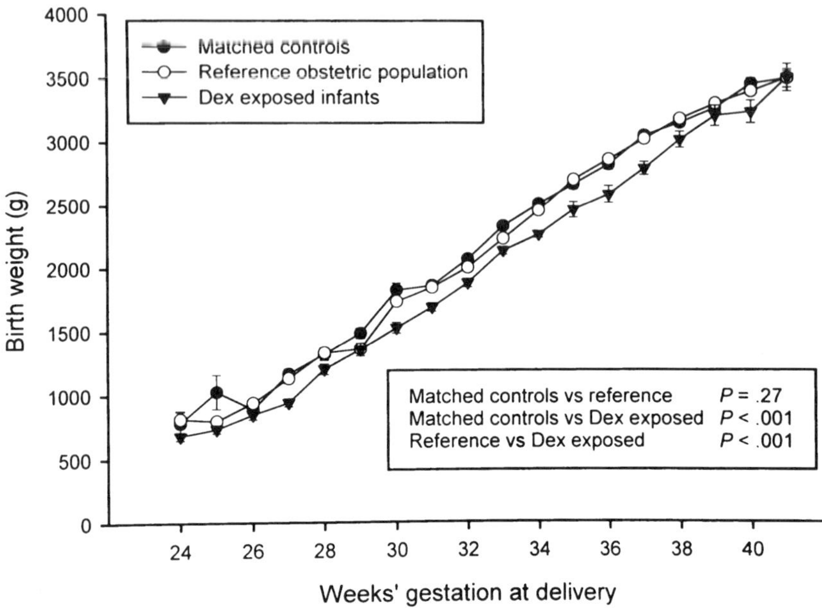

FIGURE 3.—Mean birth weights ± standard error of the mean for infants treated with dexamethasone compared with a matched control group and the reference obstetric population comprised of those infants unexposed to dexamethasone. *Abbreviations*: *DEX*, Dexamethasome. (Courtesy of Bloom SL, Sheffield JS, McIntire DD, et al: Antenatal dexamethasone and decreased birth weight. *Obstet Gynecol* 97:485-490, 2001. Reprinted with permission from the American College of Obstetricians and Gynecologists.)

Results.—After adjustment for week of gestation, the study group of dexamethasone infants (n = 961) showed lower birth weights when compared with the overall population (n = 122,629) or with the matched comparison group (n = 2808) (P < 0.001). However, the matched controls and reference population did not show significant difference when compared with each other. In comparison with the historical cohort infants, dexamethasone-treated infants had a birth weight that was smaller by 12 g at 24 to 26 weeks (gestational age), 63 g at 27 to 29 weeks, 161 g at 30 to 32 weeks, and 80 g at 33 to 34 weeks (Figs 2 and 3).

Conclusions.—The administration of antenatal dexamethasone to help with fetal maturation is associated with smaller birth weights.

▶ In his original test of the efficacy of maternal corticosteroids, Liggins et al[1] demonstrated a reduction in the incidence of respiratory distress syndrome and neonatal ICU admission of preterm infants exposed to a single maternal steroid dose. Assuming the active half life of the 25-mg betamethasone administration used, many groups, the Parkland Hospital included, opted for more frequent weekly maternal injection protocol. From 1994 to 1998, those 961 women deemed worthy of steroid treatment because of the risk of preterm birth, received 20 mg of dexamethasone administered over 48 hours weekly, to 34 weeks of gestational age, exempting for purposes of this study, women with multiple pregnancies, diabetes mellitus, hypertension, or temperature elevation. Looking for the impairment in birth weights associated with such administration in a variety of experimental animals, the authors compared birth weight at gestational age and resulting newborns in 3 ways.

The first was to plot the percentage of dexamethasone-treated infants corresponding to 20 5-percentile intervals derived from a reference population of more than 122,000 deliveries, all deliveries at Parkland during an unspecified period. It is not clear why the authors, expecting a 5% fraction in each such interval on the abcissa based on the 20 intervals they chose, elected to draw the expected value of the ordinate at the 6th percentile level in Figure 2. There does, however, seem to be a surplus of dexamethasone-treated infants in the birthweight percentile at stated gestational age from the 6th to the 50th percentile. A more straightforward comparison of dexamethasone-treated infants with 2:1 controls matched for race, gender, and gestational age derived both from the same historical reference population and from matched controls not receiving dexamethasone was then employed (see Figure 3). There were no surplus neonatal deaths among the dexamethasone-treated infants, and it was not possible to show any difference in mean birth weight among the 25% of gravidas who received 2 or more courses of steroids compared with those who received only 1. For me, this reaffirms an interpretation of the original work by Liggins et al that 1 course of therapy is enough for fetal protection against respiratory distress syndrome, and this renders concern for birth-weight reduction moot. With threatened preterm labor of 8 to 10 weeks duration, a second course close to the 34th week of gestational age may make sense.

T. H. Kirschbaum, MD

Reference

1. Liggins GC, Howie RN: A controlled trial of antepartum glucocorticoid therapy for prevention of the respiratory distress syndrome in premature infants. *Pediatrics* 50:515-525, 1972.

Expression of Vascular Endothelial Growth Factor in Third-Trimester Placentas Is Not Increased in Growth-Restricted Fetuses

Tse JYM, Lao TT, Chan CCW, et al (Univ of Hong Kong, People's Republic of China)

J Soc Gynecol Investig 8:77-82, 2001   3–4

Objective.—Vascular endothelial growth factor (VEGF) may initiate and coordinate early vascularization in the decidua and placenta and may regulate placental growth and invasion. VEGF in pathologic human pregnancies has not been well studied, although hypoxia is known to enhance its production. How the expression of VEGF in infants with intrauterine growth restriction (IUGR) and maintenance of umbilical artery diastolic flow compare with those in normal infants were prospectively investigated.

Methods.—Placentas from 17 pregnancies complicated by IUGR only were examined immunohistochemically for VEGF and cytokeratin con tents. Results were compared with those from 17 placentas from normal birth weight infants.

Results.—Birth weights and placental weights were significantly correlated in both groups. VEGF expression in normal and IUGR placentas was similar and was concentrated in the villous synctiotrophoblasts and intermediate trophoblasts. One-minute Apgar scores were significantly correlated with VEGF staining intensity, percentage of immunoreacive cells, and total score in synctiotrophoblasts and in intermediate trophoblasts. Placental weight was not correlated with VEGF staining in synctiotrophoblast and in intermediate trophoblast, and birth weight was not correlated with degree of VEGF staining. Hemoglobin levels and percentage of immunoreactive cells were correlated. Cord hematocrit was correlated with VEGF staining intensity, percentage of immunoreactive cells, and total score in villous synctiotrophoblasts. Neither cord hemoglobin nor hematocrit was correlated with intermediate trophoblasts.

Conclusion.—Although VEGF might play a role in local and focal control of angiogenesis by autocrine and paracrine mechanisms, its variability might not lend itself to an overall assessment of abnormal uteroplacental or fetal placental perfusion.

▶ As a series of protein growth factors have been identified in trophoblastic epithelium during the development and decidual anchoring of the placenta, they have come to constitute legitimate suspects for the development of fetal growth retardation unassociated with fetal maldevelopment, malnutrition infectious disease, and hypoxemia. Foremost among such candidates are placental growth factor and especially VEGF, the latter readily found in endometrium and cytotrophoblast in early pregnancy. VEGF is concentrated largely in syncytial trophoblast and wandering extravillous trophoblast embedded in the decidua in term placentas. It is important to exclude known causes of IUGR to evaluate the role of VEGF, one of the most important member of this class of proteins, as a cause of idiopathic IUGR.

Seventeen placentas from growth-retarded newborns at or below the 10th percentile for weight at gestational age were subjected to immunohistochemical analysis of VEGF with a rabbit-based polyclonal antibody and an anticytokeratin antibody to identify epithelial and extravillous trophoblast cells. A visual scoring system was used to show that no significant difference in the concentration and distribution of VEGF between placentas of normal and growth retarded infants existed. The investigative process will surely continue in this important matter of identifying the cause, currently unknown, of pathologic placenta development leading to fetal growth retardation.

T. H. Kirschbaum, MD

Planned Caesarean Section Versus Planned Vaginal Birth for Breech Presentation at Term: A Randomised Mulitcentre Trial
Hannah ME, for the Term Breech Trial Collaborative Group (Univ of Toronto)
Lancet 356:1375-1386, 2000   3–5

Introduction.—For most women with breech presentation at term, the approach to delivery is controversial. The Term Breech Trial was a prospective, randomized, multicenter trial (121 centers in 26 countries) that compared a policy of planned cesarean section with a policy of planned vaginal birth for selected breech-presentation pregnancies. Results of the trial are discussed.

Methods.—A total of 2088 women with a singleton fetus in a frank or complete breech presentation were randomized to planned cesarean section or planned vaginal birth. An experienced clinician was present at birth for women having a vaginal breech delivery (Table 3). Mothers and infants were followed for 6 weeks postpartum. The major outcomes were perinatal mortality, neonatal mortality or serious neonatal morbidity, and maternal morbidity or serious maternal morbidity. Intention-to-treat analyses were performed.

TABLE 3.—Characteristics of Labor and Delivery for Women Who Had a Vaginal Breech Delivery

Characteristic	Planned Caesarean Section (n=88)	Planned Vaginal Birth (n=558)
Induced labour	4 (4·6%)	83 (14·9%)
Induced labour with oxytocin or prostaglandins	3 (3·4%)	82 (14·7%)
Augmented labour	24 (27·3%)	278 (49·8%)
Augmented labour with oxytocin or prostaglandins	21 (23·9%)	266 (47·7%)
Epidural analgesia	23 (26·1%)	140 (25·1%)
Prolonged labour*	6 (6·8%)	20 (3·6%)
First stage ≥18 h	2 (2·3%)	1 (0·2%)
Second stage (no pushing) >2 h	1 (1·1%)	4 (0·7%)
Second stage (pushing) ≥1·5 h	3 (3·4%)	15 (2·7%)
Presentation at delivery		
Frank	55 (62·5%)	371 (66·5%)
Complete	29 (33·0%)	179 (32·1%)
Footing or uncertain	4 (4·5%)	8 (1·4%)
Type of vaginal delivery		
Spontaneous or assisted without forceps	67 (76·1%)	435 (78·0%)
Assisted with forceps	21 (23·9%)	123 (22·0%)
Experienced clinician at delivery*	82 (93·2%)	543 (97·3%)
Licensed obstetrician at delivery*	71 (80·7%)	436 (78·4%)
Clinician at delivery with >10 years vaginal breech-delivery experience*	50 (56·8%)	332 (60·0%)
Clinician at delivery with <20 years vaginal breech-delivery experience*	18 (20·5%)	133 (24·1%)

*For these variables there were a few missing values.
(Courtesy of Hannah ME, for the Term Breech Trial Collaborative Group: Planned caesarean section versus planned vaginal birth for breech presentation at term: A randomised multicentre trial. *Lancet* 356:1375-1386, 2000. Copyright by The Lancet Ltd, 2000.)

TABLE 5.—Perinatal or Neonatal Mortality at <28 Days of Age and Serious Neonatal Morbidity

Outcome	Planned Caesarean Section	Planned Vaginal Birth	Relative Risk (95% CI)	p
Perinatal/neonatal mortality or serious neonatal morbidity*	17/1039 (1·6%)	52/1039 (5·0%)	0·33 (0·19-0·56)	<0·0001
Low national PMR	2/514 (0·4%)	29/511 (5·7%)		
High national PMR	15/525 (2·9%)	23/528 (4·4%)		
Perinatal/neonatal mortality†	3/1039 (0·3%)	13/1039 (1·3%)	0·23 (0·07-0·81)	0·01
Low national PMR	0/514	3/511 (0·6%)		
High national PMR	3/525 (0·6%)	10/528 (1·9%)		
Serious neonatal morbidity‡	14/1036 (1·4%)	39/1026 (3·8%)	0·36 (0·19-0·65)	0·0003
Low national PMR	2/514 (0·4%)	26/508 (5·1%)		
High national PMR	12/522 (2·3%)	13/518 (2·5%)		

*P = .005 for interaction between treatment and national PMR for combined outcome of perinatal/neonatal mortality or serious neonatal morbidity.

†P = .96 for interaction between treatment and national PMR for outcome of perinatal/neonatal mortality.

‡P = .003 for interaction between treatment and national PMR for outcome of serious neonatal morbidity.

Abbreviation: PMR, Perinatal mortality rate.

(Courtesy of Hannah ME, for the Term Breech Trial Collaborative Group: Planned caesarean section versus planned vaginal birth for breech presentation at term: A randomised multicentre trial. *Lancet* 356:1375-1386, 2000. Copyright by The Lancet Ltd, 2000.)

TABLE 6.—Details of Neonatal Morbidity

	Planned Caesarean Section	Planned Vaginal Delivery	p
Birth trauma	6 (0·6%)	14 (1·4%)	0·05
Intracerebral or intraventricular haemorrhage*	0	2 (0·2%)	
Spinal-cord injury*	1 (0·1%)	0	
Basal skull fracture*	1 (0·1%)	0	
Fracture of long bone or clavicle	1 (0·1%)	6 (0·6%)	
Brachial plexus injury*†	2 (0·2%)	5 (0·5%)	
Significant genital injury*	1 (0·1%)	2 (0·2%)	
Seizures	1 (0·1%)	7 (0·7%)	0·03
During first 24 hr*	0	6 (0·6%)	
Needing ≥2 drugs*	1 (0·1%)	3 (0·3%)	
Hypotonia	2 (0·2%)	18 (1·8%)	0·0002
≥2 h*	2 (0·2%)	11 (1·1%)	
Abnormal level of consciousness	6 (0·6%)	16 (1·6%)	0·02
Hyperalert, drowsy, or lethargic	6 (0·6%)	13 (1·3%)	
Stupor/decreased response to pain*	0	1 (0·1%)	
Coma*	0	2 (0·2%)	
Apgar <7 at 5 min‡	8 (0·8%)	31 (3·0%)	0·0001
Apgar <4 at 5 min‡	1 (0·1%)	9 (0·9%)	0·01
Cord-blood base deficit ≥15*§	4/453 (0·9%)	13/446 (2·8%)	0·02
Cord-blood pH <7·00§	2/510 (0·4%)	13/503 (2·6%)	0·003
Intubation and ventilation	3 (0·3%)	13 (1·3%)	0·01
>24 h*	1 (0·1%)	4 (0·4%)	
Tube feeding	12 (1·2%)	32 (3·1%)	0·002
≥4 days*	2 (0·2%)	6 (0·6%)	
Care in neonatal ICU	16 (1·5%)	31 (3·0%)	0·02
>4 days*	4 (0·4%)	6 (0·6%)	
Birthweight >4000 g‡	32 (3·1%)	59 (5·8%)	0·002
Birthweight <2500 g‡	48 (4·6%)	49 (4·8%)	0·48

*Denotes measures of serious neonatal morbidity included in primary outcome (there were no cases of subdural hematoma).

†All were present at discharge from hospital and five were improving.

‡There were a few missing values for Apgar score and birthweight.

§Cord blood (arterial if available, otherwise venous) was not taken for some infants.

Abbreviations: ICU, Intensive care unit.

(Courtesy of Hannah ME, for the Term Breech Trial Collaborative Group: Planned caesarean section versus planned vaginal birth for breech presentation at term: A randomised multicentre trial. *Lancet* 356:1375-1386, 2000. Copyright by The Lancet Ltd., 2000.)

Results.—Data was available for 2083 women. Of the 1041 females assigned to planned cesarean section, 941 (90.4%) had cesarean section. Of the 1042 females assigned planned vaginal birth, 591 (56.7%) delivered vaginally. Perinatal mortality and neonatal mortality or serious neonatal morbidity were significantly lower for the planned cesarean group than for the planned vaginal delivery group (17/1039 [1.6%] vs 52/1039; [5.0%]; relative risk [RR], 0.33; *P* < .0001) (Tables 5 and 6). Maternal mortality and serious maternal morbidity were similar for the cesarean and planned vaginal delivery groups (41/1041 [3.9%] vs 33/1042 [3.2%]; [RR], 1.24; *P* = .35).

Conclusion.—Planned cesarean section was safer than planned vaginal delivery for the fetus in the breech presentation. Both groups had similar rates of maternal morbidity and mortality.

▶ This is an important account of the activities of the Term Breech Trial Collaborative Group organized at the University of Toronto from 1997 through April 2000. It involves 121 obstetrical centers in 36 countries, encompassing every continent except Antarctica. Its purpose is to evaluate the relative results of randomization of abdominal birth versus vaginal labor in delivery of women bearing singleton fetuses in frank or full breech presentation with an estimated fetal weight of 4 kilograms or less. Several nonrandomized case control studies, many reported here earlier, have failed to show benefit of cesarean section but they suffered by their experimental design and relatively small case numbers (see 1997 YEAR BOOK OF OBSTETRICS, GYNECOLOGY, AND WOMEN'S HEALTH, pp 189-190; 1998 YEAR BOOK, pp 195-196; 1999 YEAR BOOK, pp 179-180, and 2000 YEAR BOOK, pp 83-84). It is important that vaginal births in this study were conducted by physicians certified by their colleagues as experienced in vaginal breech deliveries. It's a concern that the quality of physician attendants may vary between third-world nations and other sites of origin of data. Women were excluded if their pregnancies exhibited fetal anomalies, hyperextended fetal heads, or maternal conditions precluding vaginal births, such as placenta previa. Data was segregated by perinatal mortality in the reporting county, using WHO data demonstrating national perinatal mortality equal to or less than 20 per thousand livebirths (low PNM) or greater than 20 per thousand live births (high PNM).

Included in this study were 1041 women randomized to planned abdominal delivery and 1042 scheduled for expectant management and vaginal birth. Ninety percent of women scheduled for cesarean section were delivered as planned, but 100 women were admitted in advanced labor or ultimately opted for vaginal birth instead. Among women scheduled for vaginal birth, 451 or 43.3% were delivered by cesarean section because of dystocia, fetal heart rate abnormalities, or medical or obstetrical complications. Clinical research data must be reported on the basis of intent-to-treat, but when such a large fraction of allocated vaginal birth required cesarean section as the result of complication of labor, it mitigates against the evaluable safety of vaginal breech birth.

The vaginal breech birth group contains data from 43% of pregnancies where breech presentation coexisted with sufficient intrapartum abnormality to merit emergency cesarean section. As Table 5 discloses, actual or intended vaginal birth is associated with greater perinatal morbidity and mortality than is elective abdominal birth. The finding was independent of the presence or absence of an experienced attendant; when cases without experienced attendants were excluded from the analysis, the apparent benefit of abdominal births still persisted. Similarly, the results did not change when cases marked by labor dystocia, oxytocin supplementation, footling breech deliveries or epidural anesthesia/analgesia were excluded. Reduction in fetal and neonatal risks associated with cesarean section was greater in countries with low perinatal mortality than those with high perinatal mortality, though the converse was true for serious neonatal morbidity. No statistically significant difference in maternal morbidity or mortality rates was seen between women scheduled for abdominal and vaginal births.

This study provides support for anyone who opts to deliver all breech-presenting fetuses by elective cesarean section. For those who have delivered breeches in any of their various presentations for years without birth trauma, that conclusion is troubling, and the loss of the skills derived from vaginal breech delivery, as teaching opportunities progressively decline with time, is regrettable. When, for instance, bilateral nuchal arms appear in course of delivery of a breech-presenting infant at cesarean section, it is helpful to have experience with vaginal birth. This study should at least motivate an obstetrical unit to look closely at its experience with vaginal breech delivery compared with abdominal birth, justify the continued practice if they wish. I would hope there are sufficient numbers of obstetricians who were content with their skills at vaginal breech delivery that they will be able, by teaching young obstetricians, to prevent the already somewhat marginal practice of those skills from disappearing from American obstetrics entirely.

T. H. Kirschbaum, MD

Magnesium Sulfate for Tocolysis and Risk of Spastic Cerebral Palsy in Premature Children Born to Women Without Preeclampsia

Grether JK, Hoogstrate J, Walsh-Greene E, et al (March of Dimes Birth Defects Found, Oakland, Calif; Natl Inst of Neurological Disorders and Stroke, Bethesda, Md)
Am J Obstet Gynecol 183:717-725, 2000   3–6

Background.—Disabling spastic cerebral palsy is relatively common among very low birth weight premature infants. Previous studies have found that magnesium sulfate protected against spastic cerebral palsy in these children. However, other studies have reported no or only weak evidence for a neuroprotective effect. The association between magnesium sulfate tocolysis and the risk of spastic cerebral palsy in very low birth weight premature infants was examined in this retrospective case-controlled study.

Methods.—Medical records were reviewed to identify all singleton infants with birth weights less than 2000 g who were born prematurely (gestational age <33 weeks) from 1998 through 1994 at a level 2 or 3 hospital in the San Francisco Bay area or the San Joaquin Valley of California. All infants had been delivered within 3 hours of the mother's admission to the hospital and had lived to 2 or more years of age. None of the infants had a prenatal diagnosis of major fetal malformation or disorder. Additionally, none of the mothers had preeclampsia, renal failure, myasthenia gravis, or a severe systemic illness, structural abnormality, or surgery that would affect management. Demographics and clinical char-

TABLE III.—Magnesium Sulfate Tocolytic Exposure in Children With Spastic Cerebral Palsy and Control Children, Born 1988-1994, Birth Weight <1500 g or 1500-1999 g, and Gestational Age <33 Weeks, to Women Without Preeclampsia

	Children With Cerebral Palsy (n = 170)	Control Subjects (n = 288)	Statistical Significance	Odds Ratio and 95% Confidence Interval
Any tocolytic treatment (No.)	126 (74%)	233 (81%)		0.68 (0.43-1.1)
Any tocolytic treatment with magnesium sulfate (No.)				
Proportion of total	98 (58%)	178 (62%)		0.84 (0.56-1.2)
Proportion of those treated with tocolytic agent	98 (78%)	178 (76%)		1.1 (0.65-1.8)
For magnesium sulfate, total duration of use (h)			NS*	
Mean ± SD	51 ± 78	53 ± 72		
Median	29	29		
For magnesium sulfate, time from first treatment to delivery (h)			NS*	
Mean ± SD	104 ± 162	97 ± 153		
Median	50	56		
For magnesium sulfate, time from last treatment to delivery (h)			NS*	
Mean ± SD	34 ± 92	31 ± 121		
Median	3.4	2.6		

*Multiple logistic regression model.

(Courtesy of Grether JK, Hoogstrate J, Walsh-Greene E, et al: Magnesium sulfate for tocolysis and risk of spastic cerebral palsy in premature children born to women without preeclampsia. *Am J Obstet Gynecol* 183:717-725, 2000.)

acteristics were compared between the children with cerebral palsy and those without.

Results.—Complete medical records were available for 170 children with cerebral palsy and 288 control subjects without cerebral palsy who met the inclusion criteria. Children with cerebral palsy were slightly but significantly younger than the controls (mean gestational ages, 27.1 vs 27.6 weeks) and were significantly more likely to receive surfactant (43% vs 31%). Mothers of children with cerebral palsy were significantly more likely to be white (47% vs 33%) and significantly less likely to have received antenatal corticosteroids for fetal lung maturity (52% vs 60%). Otherwise, clinical and treatment characteristics were similar between the cases and the controls, including the proportion of mothers who received magnesium sulfate alone or in combination with another tocolytic agent (58% and 62%, respectively) (Table III). Similarly, the total duration of magnesium sulfate therapy and the intervals from the beginning or the end of therapy to delivery were similar in the 2 groups. Multifactorial analysis of possible confounding factors (gestational age, birth weight, maternal race, year of birth, chorioamnionitis, histologically diagnosed intrauterine inflammation, corticosteroid use, mode of delivery, duration of labor, and neonatal surfactant treatment) did not significantly change the association between magnesium sulfate therapy and cerebral palsy. The authors also compared a subset of these children (146 cases, 244 controls) with 27 cases and 43 controls studied between 1983 and 1985; similar inclusion criteria were used in these subgroup analyses. Whereas the current data failed to show any protective effect of magnesium sulfate therapy on the risk of cerebral palsy (odds ratio, 0.80 for entire group), the previous data showed a significant neuroprotective effect (odds ratio, 0.16 for entire group) (Table IV).

Conclusions.—This study found no evidence that magnesium sulfate therapy protects against the risk of spastic cerebral palsy in very low birth weight premature infants born to women without preeclampsia. These data are in contrast to previous data indicating a significant neuroprotective effect for magnesium sulfate. Although the discrepant findings in these 2 studies cannot be easily explained, changes in medical practice between the 2 studies (1983-1985 and 1988-1994) may account for some of these differences.

▶ The initial comprehensive NIH-supported prospective study of obstetric care conducted from 1959 to 1966 yielded a group of 189 infants ultimately identified as having cerebral palsy. An analysis of the detailed datasets derived from their prenatal care, labor and delivery, and postnatal care yielded important observations regarding the uncommon relation of the obstetric events to the occurrence of cerebral palsy (see 1987 YEAR BOOK OF OBSTETRICS, GYNECOLOGY, AND WOMEN'S HEALTH, pp 243-245, 1988 YEAR BOOK pp 116-118). A subsequent retrospective case-control study mounted in northern California under the auspices of the California Department of Health Services dealt with 192 infants with cerebral palsy born in California in the interval from 1983 to 1985. The authors' intent was to explore the possibility

TABLE IV.—Selected Characteristics of Children With Moderate or Severe Spastic Cerebral Palsy and Control Subjects, Born 1988-1994, Birth Weight <1500 g, to Women Without Preeclampsia, in Comparison With Children Born 1983-1985, Birth Weight <1500 g, to Women Without Preeclampsia

	1983-1985*		1988-1994	
	Children With Cerebral Palsy (n = 27)	Control Subjects (n = 43)	Children With Cerebral Palsy (n = 146)	Control Subjects (n = 244)
Gestational age				
Mean ± SD (wk)	27.7 ± 2.9	28 ± 2.5	26.5 ± 2.1	27 ± 2.4
Median (wk)	28	28	26	27
Born at <26 wk (No.)	7 (26%)	8 (19%)	53 (36%)	73 (30%)
Birth weight				
Mean ± SD (g)	1002 ± 255	1112 ± 227	984 ± 258	1009 ± 267
Median (g)	1000	1100	960	980
Born at <1000 g (No.)	13 (48%)	12 (28%)	83 (57%)	128 (52%)
Any tocolytic treatment (No.)	15 (56%)	30 (70%)	110 (75%)	204 (84%)
Magnesium sulfate tocolysis (No.)	2 (7%)	13 (30%)	85 (58%)	159 (65%)
Antenatal corticosteroid use (No.)	14 (52%)	28 (65%)	77 (53%)	148 (61%)
Cesarean delivery (No.)	14 (52%)	18 (42%)	48 (33%)	92 (38%)
Placental histologic study done (No.)	18 (67%)	27 (63%)	114 (78%)	185 (76%)
Chorioamnionitis (No.)				
Definite or suspected clinical diagnosis only				
All subjects	20 (74%)	31 (72%)	52 (36%)	81 (33%)
Tocolysis subjects only	12 (80%)	21 (70%)	39 (35%)	66 (32%)
Histologic diagnosis only				
All subjects	2 (7.4%)	1 (2.3%)	49 (34%)	78 (32%)
Tocolysis subjects only	1 (6.7%)	0 (0%)	38 (35%)	69 (34%)
Clinical or histologic diagnosis, or both				
All subjects	22 (81%)	32 (74%)	101 (69%)	159 (65%)
Tocolysis subjects only	13 (87%)	21 (70%)	77 (70%)	135 (66%)
Neonatal surfactant (No.)	—	—	64 (44%)	79 (33%)

*For correspondence with later cohort, the following were excluded: women with preeclampsia, cases with <3 hours from admission to delivery, and cases with delivery in level 1 hospital.
(Courtesy of Grether JK, Hoogstrate J, Walsh-Greene E, et al: Magnesium sulfate for tocolysis and risk of spastic cerebral palsy in premature children born to women without preeclampsia. *Am J Obstet Gynecol* 183:717-725, 2000.)

that electronic fetal monitoring, not commonly used in the 1960s, might have resulted in different correlates of cerebral palsy occurrence in a study conducted 20 years later. No striking differences were seen (see 1995 YEAR BOOK, pp 135-138), but an apparently protective effect of magnesium sulfate administration, whether for tocolysis or seizure prevention in pregnancy hypertension, on the incidence of cerebral palsy was noted (see 1996 YEAR BOOK, pp 126-128, 1998 YEAR BOOK, pp 235-237, and 1999 YEAR BOOK, pp 56-57).

Here the authors have constructed a retrospective case-control study in 22 hospitals in the San Francisco Bay and Northern San Joaquin Valley areas, examining 170 infants with cerebral palsy with a control group of 288 matched for birth weight and gestational age, born in the interval from 1988 to 1994. Study entry was restricted to infants weighing less than 2 kg at birth, with particular attention to those weighing 1.5 kg because of the high prevalence of cerebral palsy in that group. Data were obtained from the California Birth Defects Monitoring Program and the records reviewed under those auspices. Pregnant women with preeclampsia were excluded to eliminate the diminished prevalence of cerebral palsy among their offspring as a complicating issue in the analysis. Cases where infants' central nervous system lesions were uncertain in nature or resulted from postnatal factors or congenital infection were also excluded.

The incidence of tocolytic use was 74% of the cases that resulted in cerebral palsy and 81% in normal controls. Similarly, no significant differences between groups were seen on the basis of unfulfilled intent to treat, use of magnesium sulfate alone or in combination with other tocolytics, and time from first or last magnesium exposure to delivery. Logistic regression was used to exclude gestational age, birth weight, race, year of birth, chorioamnionitis, antenatal steroids, route of birth, duration of labor, or use of surfactant as significant independent confounding variables. It is tempting to contribute the lack of evidence for protective effects in the latest study from the exclusion of pregnant hypertensive women, but when those women were removed from the 1983 to 1985 data, the apparent protective effect of magnesium is still seen (see Table IV).

Although the reasons for these observations are obscure, they may represent differences in obstetric or neonatal care in the 10 or so years bridging the 2 case studies. In any event, these results make the search for a protective role for magnesium sulfate tocolysis against cerebral palsy less compelling.

T. H. Kirschbaum, MD

Perinatal Death and Tocolytic Magnesium Sulfate
Scudiero R, Khoshnood B, Pryde PG, et al (Univ of Chicago; Univ of Wisconsin, Madison)
Obstet Gynecol 96:178-182, 2000   3–7

Introduction.—Magnesium sulfate is the first-line tocolytic agent used most often by obstetricians in the United States. Its safety and efficacy for this indication have not undergone rigorous examination. Retrospective data were used to determine whether there is a significant correlation between perinatal mortality and exposure to total doses of tocolytic magnesium sulfate larger than 48 grams.

Methods.—A case-control trial was conducted in which cases were defined as neonates or fetuses who died after exposure to tocolytic magnesium sulfate. The fetuses and neonates weighed 700 to 1249 grams. Their mothers received tocolytic magnesium sulfate from January 1, 1986 to March 31, 1999. Women who received prophylactic magnesium sulfate for pre-eclampsia or pre-eclampsia superimposed on chronic hypertension were excluded, as were fetuses or neonates with major congenital anomalies.

Results.—Using a multivariate model that controlled for birth weight or gestational age, year of delivery, receipt of betamethasone, acute maternal disease, and maternal race, it was found that exposure to total doses of tocolytic magnesium sulfate exceeding 48 grams was significantly correlated with increased perinatal mortality (adjusted odds ratio 4.7; $P = .035$). A significant dose response was present ($P = .03$) and was most consistent with a threshold effect.

Conclusion.—High doses of tocolytic magnesium sulfate were correlated with increased potential mortality among fetuses and neonates weighing 700 to 1249 grams.

▶ Motivated in part by an earlier report of unexpected perinatal death associated with tocolytic magnesium sulfate (see 1999 YEAR BOOK OF OB-STETRICS, GYNECOLOGY, AND WOMEN'S HEALTH, pp 56), these authors focus on very low birth weight infants in the range of 700 to 1250 grams, chosen for their high mortality rates. Patients receiving magnesium sulfate as an anticonvulsant during pregnancy hypertension were excluded, and a case control study was structured to compare perinatal death rates between women given at least 48 grams of magnesium sulfate, a critical value derived from the authors' earlier experience, and those receiving less than that dose, designated as control subjects. Univariate comparisons showed a surplus of white women with acute maternal disease among the large magnesium sulfate dose recipients as well as a greater incidence of fetuses at birth weight less than 1 kilogram. The test subset was also more likely to have been exposed to other tocolytic agents, specifically indomethacin and terbutaline. When multivariate techniques were applied to control for confounding relationships among these and other variables associated with perinatal death, multiple tocolytic agents and acute maternal disease failed to demonstrate significance. However, low birth weight and tocolytic magnesium sulfate in doses greater than 48 grams proved to have independent associations with perinatal mortality.

The authors feel their data suffice to motivate prudence in the use of magnesium sulfate as a tocolytic in this very low birth weight range. Results of their analysis are inconclusive, however, because of the significant independent impact of low birth weight, with 72% of infants weighing less than 1 kilogram in the high magnesium dose group compared with 44% in the low magnesium dose group. This uncontrolled variable could explain part or all of the results. What seems most important here is the failure to demonstrate benefit in outcome as a result of magnesium tocolysis in return for even this uncertain possibility of incremental risk of perinatal death. Regrettably, this study does not settle the issue.

T. H. Kirschbaum, MD

ORP150 Protects Against Hypoxia/Ischemia-Induced Neuronal Death
Tamatani M, Matsuyama T, Yamaguchi A, et al (Osaka Univ, Japan; Hyogo College of Medicine, Japan; Natl Ctr for Cardiac Disease and Circulation Research, Osaka, Japan)
Nat Med 7:317-323, 2001   3–8

Introduction.—The authors have previously identified a new, 150 kd protein, designated oxygen-regulated protein (ORP) 150, that is synthesized by astrocytes in response to hypoxia. This endoplasmic reticulum-associated chaperone appears to play an important role in cell viability in culture under conditions of oxygen deprivation. The effects of further studies of ORP150 on cell survival during hypoxic/ischemic stress are discussed.

Methods and Results.—Immunohistochemical studies of autopsy specimens of human brains indicated that neurons expressed ORP150 in response to ischemia during the acute phase after stroke. In the subacute or chronic phase, ORP150 expression was induced in astrocytes. Cultured cortical neurons expressed low levels of ORP150 antigen. These levels increased significantly after 4 to 8 hours of hypoxia, decreasing to control levels at 12 to 24 hours. In cultured astrocytes, the increase in ORP150 antigen increased up to 48 hours after hypoxia. Resistance to hypoxemic stress was greater in cultured neurons overexpressing ORP150, lesser in astrocytes with inhibited ORP150 expression.

In further studies, transgenic mice were generated using the platelet-derived growth factor (PDGF) B-chain promoter to drive ORP150 expression. When subjected to cerebral ischemia, mice with targeted neuronal ORP150 overexpression had smaller stroke volumes, suggesting that ORP150 overexpression protects neurons against ischemic stress. These neurons also showed suppression of caspase-3-like activity and enhancement of brain-derived neurotrophic factor in the presence of hypoxic signaling.

Conclusions.—The new findings suggest that ORP150 has an important impact on cell survival under hypoxic/ischemic stress. The mechanisms of its induction suggest that ORP150 can coordinate the response to ischemic stress, in the form of enhancing the processing of various elements involved in the cytoprotective response to stress. The findings raise the possibility that upregulation of ORP150 could provide a new approach to enhancing cell survival during ischemia.

▶ When investigators studying the mechanics of hypoxic-ischemic fetal brain injury used experimental animals so that the timing of the vascular injury produced is precisely known, they were able to demonstrate a biphasic brain response, only the second of which, beginning 24 to 48 hours after the insult, resulted in significant neural destruction and irreversible functional loss (see 1992 YEAR BOOK OF OBSTETRICS, GYNECOLOGY, AND WOMEN'S HEALTH, pp 189-191). The same pattern was confirmed in humans using magnetic resonance spectroscopy (see 1990 YEAR BOOK, pp 206-207, and 1993 YEAR BOOK, pp 123-124). This means that a window of several hours of opportunity is present between an hypoxic ischemic brain insult and neuronal loss, during which preventive therapy might be useful. Thereafter, a search for such agents began. Included have been GM1 ganglioside, IGF-1, glutamate antagonists, and brain cooling (see 1996 YEAR BOOK, pp 20-21). The use of nitric oxide synthase inhibitors was found to aggravate brain injury (see 1998 YEAR BOOK, pp 241-242). These authors explore the possible value of a 150 kilodalton oxygen-regulated protein ORP (150) released by astrocytes exposed to significant hypoxia in vitro and in vivo.

The protein, associated with cytoplasmic endoplasmic reticulum, was found localized in the ischemic focus of a human brain infarct in a patient who died 6 hours after a stroke. Using an antigen extracted from nerve tissue an antibody proven specific by cytohistochemistry, the authors were able to prove the presence of ORP150 of neuronal origin within the 6 hours that preceded death. In contrast, in a human patient who lived 3 days after brain infarction, with ORP150 antibody localized to the periphery of the infarct and, using co-labeling, they were able to show its localization in astrocytes. Using cell culture techniques, the authors were able to show neurons expressed increased ORP150 for 4 to 8 hours after hypoxia, returning to control values at 12 to 24 hours. In contrast, astrocyte production reached maximum augmentation at 8 to 12 hours after hypoxia, at which time neuronal apoptosis was prominent. Astrocyte ORP150 remained hyperexpressed for more than 48 hours. When transfection with an adenovirus vector (A_xCAORP150s) proved to increase cellular ORP150 production, the result provided a 50% to 60% production of neurons exposed to hypoxia over 24 hours but showed no protection against cellular toxins that do not result in hypoxia. When transgenic mice containing a promoter sequence for PDGF expression, a protein that stimulates ORP150 production, were exposed to a hypoxic-ischemic insult, they proved to be significantly resistant to hypoxic brain injury.

These authors have therefore provided us one more potential candidate for the prevention of neuronal loss when given soon after hypoxic ischemic injury has occurred. In this journal issue, other investigators[1] explored the role of plasma fibronectin produced by hepatic cells as a possible deterrent to hypoxic neuronal injury. The search for agents that prevent neuronal loss soon after brain injury is very important to obstetricians and perinatologists; it will continue and merits our close attention.

T. H. Kirschbaum, MD

Reference

1. Sakai CT, Johnson JJ, Murozono M, et al: Plasma fibronectin supports neuronal survival and reduced brain injury following transient focal cerebral ischemia but is not essential for skin wound healing and hemostasis. *Nat Med* 7:324-330, 2001.

Early Prediction of Severe Twin-to-Twin Transfusion Syndrome
Sebire NJ, Souka A, Skentou H, et al (Kings College Hosp, London)
Hum Reprod 15:2008-2010, 2000   3–9

Background.—Fetal loss rates are much higher in monochorionic twins than in dichorionic twins. Part of this increase in mortality rate in monochorionic twins is likely from severe early onset twin-to-twin transfusion syndrome (TTS). Some data suggest that an increase in nuchal translucency (NT) as seen on US may predict the subsequent development of TTS. The possible association between increased NT and risk for TTS in monochorionic diamniotic twin pregnancies between 10 and 14 weeks' gestation was examined prospectively.

Methods.—The subjects were 303 pregnant women with monochorionic diamniotic twin pregnancies in which both fetuses were alive at 10 to 14 weeks' gestation. At this time, all women underwent US evaluation of the fetuses; 153 women (50%) also underwent US at 15 to 17 weeks' gestation. US results were correlated with the development of TTS, defined as either US evidence of anhydramnios and nonvisible bladder in the donor fetus with polyhydramnios and a dilated bladder in the recipient fetus that resulted in miscarriage, fetal death, or the need for intrauterine treatment, or postmortem evidence that the cause of death was TTS.

Results.—In 16 of the 303 monochorionic diamniotic twin pregnancies (5%), either 1 or both fetuses had structural or chromosomal abnormalities. Among the remaining 287 pregnancies, either 1 or both of the fetuses died in 40 pregnancies (13.9%), for a total fetal loss rate of 11.5% (66 of 574). Most of the fetal deaths occurred before 24 weeks' gestation (Fig 1). Severe TTS developed in 43 of these 287 pregnancies (15%); in 19 cases both fetuses died, in 10 cases 1 fetus died and 1 survived, and in 14 cases both fetuses survived. The median fetal NT was 1.0 multiples of the mean, and NT thickness was increased (above 95th percentile) in 47 fetuses (8.2%) and 37 pregnancies (12.9%). Increased NT was significantly more common in the pregnancies with TTS (15 fetuses [17.4%] and 12 pregnancies [28%]) than in the pregnancies that did not have TTS (32 fetuses [6.6%] and 25 pregnancies [10.2%]). The likelihood ratio of increased fetal NT thickness at 10 to 14 weeks' gestation for the subsequent development of severe TTS was 3.5. Among the 153 pregnancies examined by US at 15 to 17 weeks' gestation, intertwin membrane folding was noted in

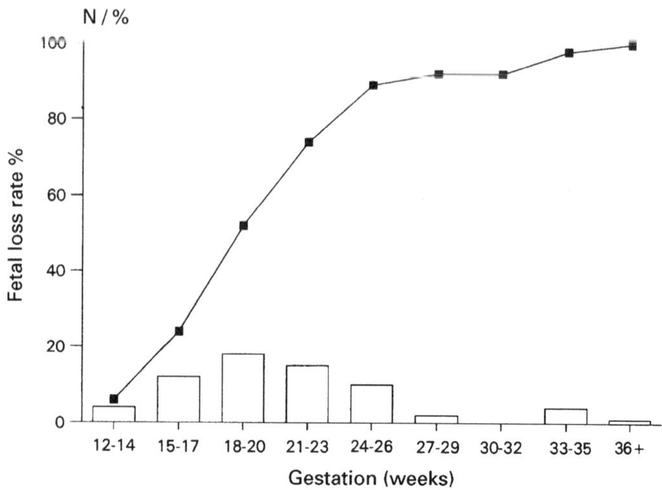

FIGURE 1.—Fetal loss rate by weeks of gestation (*bars*) and cumulative (%) fetal loss rate (*line*) in monochorionic twin pregnancies examined at 10 to 14 weeks' gestation. (Courtesy of Sebire NJ, Souka A, Skentou H, et al: Early prediction of severe twin-to-twin transfusion syndrome. *Hum Reprod* 15:2008-2010, 2000. Copyright European Society for Human Reproduction and Embryology, by permission of Oxford University Press.)

49 (32%). Almost half of these pregnancies (21, or 43%) subsequently had TTS develop, compared with only 2 (2%) of 104 pregnancies in which intertwin membrane folding was absent (*P* < .001). The likelihood ratio of the presence of intertwin membrane folding at 15 to 17 weeks' gestation for the subsequent development of severe TTS was 4.2.

Conclusions.—The loss of 1 or both infants occurred in about 15% of monochorionic diamniotic twin pregnancies in which both fetuses were alive at 10 to 14 weeks' gestation. More than 75% of these losses occurred before 24 weeks' gestation. Additionally, about 15% of these pregnancies were complicated by severe TTS. Increased NT at 10 to 14 weeks' gestation was significantly associated with the subsequent development of severe TTS, as was the presence of intertwin membrane folding at 15 to 17 weeks' gestation.

▶ Although the intent of this study, to determine whether NT is a useful predictor of TTS in monochorionic twins is not conclusive, there is a related observation of interest here. Of 287 cases of monochorionic twins without apparent developmental anomalies, 43, or 15%, had TTS develop at some time after their entry into this cohort study at 10 to 14 weeks. In 15 cases, or roughly a third of diagnosable TTS, increased NT was noted. Among monochorionic twins without TTS, the incidence of NT was 13%. With NT as a predictor of TTS, the predictive value of a positive finding is 40.5%, the predictive value of a negative finding 88%, and the false-positive rate is approximately 60%. The presence of fetal congestive heart failure is a confounding variable in the relation between TTS and NT, and because it is difficult to evaluate the presence or degree of congestive heart failure, little predictive capacity for NT is apparent. But what is useful is the author's demonstration that fetal death in TTS occurs predominantly before 26 weeks of gestational age, and fetal loss thereafter is relatively uncommon, occurring in fewer than 10% of cases here. That observation is useful in counseling and guiding antenatal testing in third-trimester cases of TTS.

T. H. Kirschbaum, MD

Long-Term Outcome in Twin-Twin Transfusion Syndrome Treated With Serial Aggressive Amnioreduction

Mari G, Detti L, Oz U, et al (Yale Univ, New Haven, Conn; Eastern Virginia Med School, Norfolk)

Am J Obstet Gynecol 183:211-217, 2000   3–10

Introduction.—The prognosis for untreated twin-twin transfusion syndrome is extremely poor, and the optimal treatment for this complication of pregnancy remains controversial. At the study institution, serial aggressive amnioreduction has been used in cases of twin-twin transfusion syndrome since 1990. Perinatal outcome and long-term outcome were reported for 33 pregnancies managed between 1990 and 1997.

Methods.—Five criteria were used for the prenatal diagnosis of twin-twin transfusion syndrome: (1) monochorionic-diamniotic twin pregnancies with discordance in size, (2) polyhydramnios in the gestational sac of the recipient twin, (3) oligohydramnios in the gestational sac of the donor twin, (4) polyuria of the recipient (diagnosed by finding of a distended bladder), and (5) oliguria of the donor (diagnosed by finding of a collapsed bladder). A US diagnosis of monochorionic twin pregnancy was based upon the presence of concordant fetal gender, single placenta, and thin separating membranes. Fifteen parameters were used to assess perinatal outcome; the main outcome at 2 years or greater was the absence of cerebral palsy.

Results.—Twin-twin transfusion syndrome was diagnosed at a median of 20.6 weeks' gestation; the median gestational age at delivery was 30.5 weeks. The median number of therapeutic amnioreductions per pregnancy was 2, and the median amniotic fluid volume withdrawn per amniocentesis was 1420 mL. Fifty-one (77%) twins were born alive. At 24 months, at least 1 infant was alive from 70% of pregnancies, and both infants were alive from 57% of pregnancies. At the last follow-up, 78% of survivors were older than 36 months. One of the twins died after amnioreduction in 8 pregnancies. In these cases, only 1 co-twin survived with a clinically normal outcome (Table 2).

Conclusion.—No available data indicate that other forms of therapy offer a better outcome than therapeutic amniocentesis in twin-twin transfusion syndrome. In the cases reported here, no major neurologic handicaps developed when both twins were delivered alive after 27 weeks' gestation without congenital malformations and survived the neonatal

TABLE 2.—Management and Pregnancy Outcomes Among Patients With a Single Intrauterine Fetal Death

Case	Gestational Age at Diagnosis (Wk)	Amnioreductions (No.)	Gestational Age at Death (Wk)	Gestational Age at Delivery (Wk)	Mode of Delivery	Outcome of Cotwin
1	14.5	1	18	18.5	Therapeutic abortion	Ventriculomegaly (recipient)
2	16.5	2	18	19	Spontaneous abortion	Fetal death at 19 wk
3	26.5	1	27.1	27.2	Cesarean	Neonatal death of severe respiratory distress syndrome; necrotizing enterocolitis (recipient)
4	17.9	8	27	27	Cesarean	Neonatal death of respiratory distress syndrome, disseminated intravascular coagulation, brain infarction (recipient)
5	25	2	27-29	29	Vaginal	Multicystic encephalomacia (recipient)
6	23	5	29	29	Vaginal	Fetal death at 29 wk
7	19.5	10	32	32	Cesarean	Clinically normal at 37 mo of age (recipient)
8	21.5	4	35	35	Cesarean	Cerebral palsy, spastic quadriplegia (recipient)

Note: In case 3, the amnioreduction was discontinued after the removal of 170 mL because the patient reported discomfort.
(Courtesy of Mari G, Detti L, Oz U, et al: Long-term outcome in twin-twin transfusion syndrome treated with serial aggressive amnioreduction. *Am J Obstet Gynecol* 183:211-217, 2000.)

period. Poor prognostic signs were hydrops of the recipient and the absence of end-diastolic waveforms of the umbilical artery in 1 twin.

▶ The optimal management for this complication of monochorionic twin pregnancy is uncertain because of its relative rarity, the uncertain role of laser or bipolar cautery of umbilical vessels, the lack of a uniform approach to therapy, and the lack of sufficiently long follow-up to allow accurate newborn evaluation. This account of 30 patients treated with amnioreduction meets many of those concerns and serves as a good basis for comparing future reports of management. Case reports date to the interval from 1990 to 1997, and surviving infants were followed to at least 24 months of age, 78% of them for at least 36 months. The median gestational age at diagnosis was 20.6 weeks and at delivery, it was 30.5 weeks. The experience included 25 cases of "stuck twins" and 12 cases of hydrops in 1 of the twin pairs. A median of 2 amnioreductions to normal or reduced amniotic fluid volume were done, and patients were examined twice a week until delivery.

Fifty-one (77%) twins were born alive and 43 survived to 1 month of age, a neonatal death rate of 130/1000 live births. Both twins survived in 57% of cases and at least 1 of the twin pairs survived in 70%. There were 2 infants with cerebral palsy and 1 infant likely to attain that diagnosis with further evaluation, an incidence of 5%. In 8 cases of death in 1 of the fetal pairs, the outcome for the surviving twin was unfavorable in 7 cases, including 2 instances of cerebral palsy. The presence of fetal hydrops and of absent end-stage diastolic flow velocity in umbilical arteries were unfavorable signs but not necessarily insurmountable. This relatively large, well-recorded experience should serve as a benchmark for comparisons in the future.

T. H. Kirschbaum, MD

Triplets: Outcomes of Expectant Management Versus Multifetal Reduction for 127 Pregnancies
Leondires MP, Ernst SD, Miller BT, et al (NIH, Bethesda, Md)
Am J Obstct Gynecol 183:454-459, 2000   3–11

Background.—Assisted reproductive technologies have greatly increased the number of multifetal pregnancies. These pregnancies carry certain risks to both the mother (eg, preeclampsia) and the infants (eg, fetal growth restriction), and thus many centers offer multifetal pregnancy reduction. But does multifetal pregnancy reduction significantly improve outcomes? Fetal outcomes between triplet pregnancies managed expectantly and triplet pregnancies managed by embryo reduction were compared retrospectively.

Methods.—Between August 1995 and July 1997, 127 women initiated an assisted reproductive technology cycle that resulted in an ultrasonographically confirmed viable triplet pregnancy at 9 weeks' gestation and in whom the triplet pregnancy continued beyond 9 weeks' gestation. All

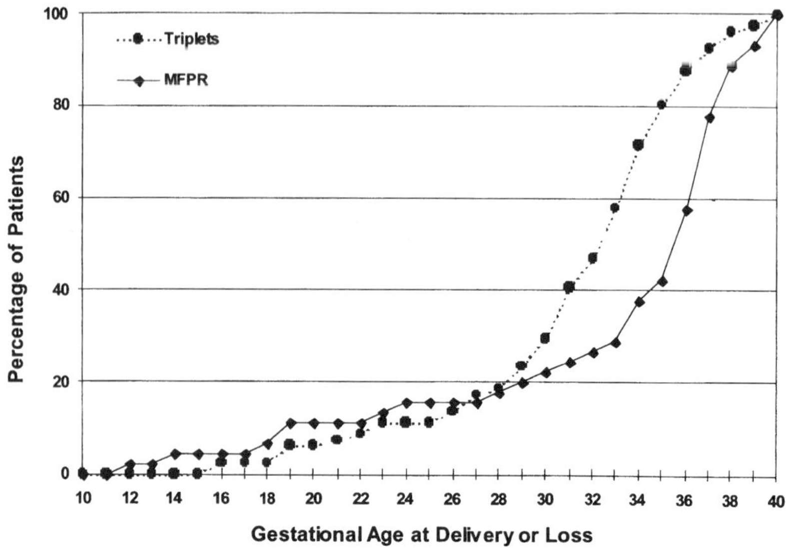

FIGURE 1.—Percentage of patients delivered versus gestational age at delivery for 81 expectantly managed triplet pregnancies and 46 triplet pregnancies managed by multifetal pregnancy reduction (*MFPR*). (Courtesy of Leondires MP, Ernst SD, Miller BT, et al: Triplets: Outcomes of expectant management versus multifetal reduction for 127 pregnancies. *Am J Obstet Gynecol* 183:454-459, 2000.)

patients were referred to a maternal-fetal medicine specialist and to 1 of 3 centers experienced in multifetal pregnancy reduction. After counseling, 81 patients (64%; mean age, 34.0 years) chose to continue the triplet pregnancy, whereas 46 (36%; mean age, 34.9 years) opted for transabdominal embryo reduction (to twins in all but 2 cases) between 11 and 13 weeks' gestation. Fetal outcomes were compared between the 2 groups.

Results.—Of the 81 patients in the expectant management group, 11 (13.5%) had spontaneous reductions after 9 weeks' gestation (to twins in 8 cases, to a singleton in 3 cases). The rates of complete fetal loss before 24 weeks' gestation did not differ significantly in the expectant management and the multifetal pregnancy reduction groups (9.9% [8 of 81] vs 13.0% [6 of 46]) (Fig 1). After 24 weeks' gestation, 3 fetuses (3.7%) in the expectant management group were lost, but none in the multifetal pregnancy reduction group were lost. The perinatal mortality rate (stillbirths and live births after 20 weeks' gestation with neonatal loss before 29 days of life) per birth did not differ significantly between the expectant management and the multifetal pregnancy reduction groups (5.5% vs 2.6%), nor did the "take home" infant per delivery rate (90.1% vs 87%). Mean gestational age at delivery was 33.25 weeks in the expectant management group and 32.04 weeks in the multifetal pregnancy reduction group. However, among the infants delivered at 24 weeks' or more gestation, the mean birth weight was significantly higher in the multifetal pregnancy reduction group (2226 vs 1796 g).

Conclusions.—Perinatal mortality rate, gestational age at delivery, and the "take home" infant per delivery rate did not differ significantly between women with triplet pregnancies who were managed expectantly and those who underwent multifetal pregnancy reduction. The only significantly different fetal outcome between the 2 groups was that birth weights were significantly higher in the multifetal pregnancy reduction group. Thus, patients with triplet pregnancies as a result of assisted reproductive technologies should be counseled to make their decisions regarding pregnancy reduction based on personal choice rather than on expectations of improved fetal outcomes.

▶ Among the implicit tenets of fetal reduction in multiple pregnancies are that the procedure results in decreased risks of preterm delivery, operative birth, fetal growth retardation, preeclampsia, and fetal malformations. It is difficult to evaluate the impact of the procedure because of the wide range in number of prereduction fetuses reported and the variable number of fetuses injected per pregnancy. This converts the number of reported cases into a large number of subsets each consisting of relatively few cases. These authors wisely confine themselves to a comparison of triplets (no longer a rarity because of assisted reproductive technology) subjected to reduction to twins treated by expectant management. Because randomization of patient choice is not feasible, this is an uncontrolled experience with respect to parent attitudes toward reproduction and the geographically separated nature of facilities where pregnancy and newborn care were carried out. Further, rates of occurrence are based on various denominators, each chosen to express the odds appropriate to couples undergoing the stepwise sequence of decisions as they encounter them.

Entry criteria consisted of ultrasonic proof of triplet pregnancies with fetal heart rate activity at 9 weeks' gestation. Roughly one third of couples opted for fetal reduction carried out in 3 regional centers between 11 and 13 weeks' gestational age. Of the 81 women opting for expectant care for triplets, 13.5% underwent spontaneous reduction to twin pregnancies or a singlet on pregnancy between 9 and 24 weeks. There was a small surplus of pregnancy losses between 9 and 16 weeks among those undergoing reduction. Total loss of pregnancy occurred spontaneously before 24 weeks in 9.9% of triplet pregnancies unreduced and 13% of reduced twin pregnancies. Three triplet pregnancies lost 4 fetuses in the interval from 26 weeks to term. Perinatal mortality rate for pregnancies delivered from 20 weeks gestational age to 29 days of neonatal life was 5.5% among triplets and 2.6% among twins, a nonsignificant difference. No differences were noted in the duration of pregnancy, but birth weight among triplet pregnancies averaged 1796 g compared with 2226 g for twins.

Because of differences between groups based on their counseling decisions, prenatal and pregnancy care, and sites of reduction procedures, it is difficult to define the outcome of pregnancy reduction beyond increases in mean fetal weight at delivery. There appeared to be no impact on perinatal survival. The reader may wish to review the 1999 YEAR BOOK OF OBSTETRICS, GYNECOLOGY, AND WOMEN'S HEALTH, pp 67 to 70 for a recent literature review in this area. This study suggests little was accomplished by fetal reduction beyond decreasing the number of live births that eventually ensued.

T. H. Kirschbaum, MD

Intrauterine Transmission of Cytomegalovirus to Infants of Women With Preconceptional Immunity

Boppana SB, Rivera LB, Fowler KB, et al (Univ of Alabama, Birmingham; Univ of Erlangen-Nürnberg, Germany)
N Engl J Med 344:1366-1371, 2001   3–12

Objective.—Preconceptional immunity against cytomegalovirus (CMV) provides only partial protection from intrauterine transmission of the virus. Factors associated with intrauterine transmission have not been defined. Whether acquisition of 1 strain of CMV in women with preexisting immunity against another strain resulted in intrauterine transmission of CMV was investigated in women who delivered infants with congenital CMV infection.

Methods.—Serum samples were obtained from 46 women who were seropositive at a previous delivery and at subsequent deliveries and analyzed for antibodies against CMV. IgG antibodies were measured against CMV and the envelope glycoprotein B with gradient purified AD169 virions and glycoprotein B recombinant protein. Virus-neutralizing activity was analyzed by a microneutralization assay. CMV isolates, obtained from 7 of 16 infected infants, were sequenced with amplified products from polymerase chain reaction.

Results.—Of the 16 infected infants, 7 had clinical abnormalities during the neonatal period and 5 had permanent neurodevelopmental abnormalities. Fourteen (88%) of 16 mothers with infected infants and 22 of 30 women without infected infants had antibodies reactive with at least 1 of 2 antigens (AP86 and TO86). Significantly more women with infected infants had antibodies against both antigens. Ten mothers of infected

TABLE 3.—Comparison of Strain-Specific Antibody Responses Against Glycoprotein H in Serial Samples From Mothers With Preconceptional Immunity Against CMV, According to Whether Their Infants Had Congenital CMV Infection

Acquisition of New Antibody Specificities Between Pregnancies	Mothers of Infected Infants (N = 16)	Mothers of Uninfected Infants (N = 30)
	no. (%)	
Yes	10 (62)	4 (13)*
No	6 (38)	26 (87)

*$P < .001$ for the comparison with the mothers of infected infants.
(Courtesy of Boppana SB, Rivera LB, Fowler KB, et al: Intrauterine transmission of cytomegalovirus to infants of women with preconceptional immunity. *N Engl J Med* 344:1366-1371. Copyright 2001, Massachusetts Medical Society. All rights reserved.)

infants and 4 mothers of uninfected infants had new antibodies specificities at the time of the current delivery (Table 3). The difference was significant. The sera of 4 of the 7 mothers of uninfected infants contained twice as much neutralizing antibody against CMV isolated from their infants in the subsequent delivery than in the previous delivery. The predicted nucleotide sequence of the region of the glycoprotein H gene encoding the aminoterminal region of the protein obtained from 4 of 7 infected infants correlated with the newly acquired antibody specificities of the mothers. Three of these 4 children had symptomatic congenital infection and permanent neurodevelopmental deficits.

Conclusion.—Intrauterine transmission of reactivated CMV was probably responsible for congenital CMV infection in women who were seropositive after the previous delivery.

▶ Maternal antibody to CMV increases progressively in incidence with maternal age and appears at an earlier age of onset in women from lower socioeconomic strata. The presence of maternal IgG for CMV does not protect against fetal infection during pregnancy but is usually associated with lesser rates of occurrence of severe signs of infection such as jaundice, purpura, chorioretinitis, seizures, and deafness than in infants born to women who convert from IgG antibody–negative to–positive status during pregnancy. There are exceptions to this generality and those exceptions are important in the counseling of women about this, the most common of human fetal infections, involving roughly 1% to 2% of all births.

In this cohort study, 46 women known to be seropositive for CMV before pregnancy delivered in 1993 to 1995 were characterized as having 2 of 3 infected and 1 of 3 uninfected infants and compared. Among the 16 infected infants 7 (44%) had significant neonatal symptoms and 5 suffered permanent sensorineural abnormalities. Using antibodies specific to envelope glycoproteins of 2 known strains of CMV, it was possible to show that 10 of 16 infected newborns had been infected by a CMV strain different from that for which preconceptional antibody was identified before conception. Because more examples of infection by a new strain might have been noted if more than 2 strains were used for interrogation, this is almost certainly an underestimate. In addition to the reactivation of virus responsible for preconceptional CMV infection, CMV seropositive women should be warned of the occasional occurrence of symptomatic fetal infection that might stem from a new viral strain and new maternal infection. This work does not enable an estimate of the frequency of such an event.

T. H. Kirschbaum, MD

4 Medical Complications of Pregnancy

A Comparison of Glyburide and Insulin in Women With Gestational Diabetes Mellitus

Langer O, Conway DL, Berkus MD, et al (St Luke's-Roosevelt Hosp Ctr, New York; Univ of Texas, San Antonio)

N Engl J Med 343:1134-1138, 2000   4–1

Background.—Many authors advise against the use of sulfonylurea drugs in women with gestational diabetes because these drugs can cause neonatal hypoglycemia and fetal anomalies. However, many of these recommendations are made based on studies performed before newer sulfonylurea drugs, such as glyburide and glipizide, became available. Laboratory studies have shown that, in contrast to the older drugs of its class, glyburide does not cross the human placenta in appreciable quantities. Whether glyburide would be a safe and effective alternative to insulin therapy in women with mild gestational diabetes was evaluated.

Methods.—The subjects were 440 women between 11 and 33 weeks' gestation with a singleton pregnancy who had gestational diabetes requiring treatment develop (failed oral glucose tolerance test and fasting plasma glucose level 95-140 mg/dL). Patients were randomly assigned to receive either glyburide (n = 201; initial dose 2.5 mg orally, increasing by 5 mg/wk up to a total of 20 mg) or insulin (n = 203; initial dose 0.7 U/kg subcutaneously 3 times a day, increasing each week as necessary) for glycemic control. The targets for glycemic control were a mean blood glucose level of 90 to 105 mg/dL, a fasting blood glucose level of 60 to 90 mg/dL, a preprandial blood glucose level of 80 to 95 mg/dL, and a postprandial blood glucose level less than 120 mg/dL. Maternal and neonatal outcomes were evaluated and compared between the groups.

Results.—The glyburide and insulin groups were similar at baseline in age (mean, 29 vs 30 years, respectively) and other demographic and

TABLE 3. —Blood Glucose Concentrations Measured at Home and Glycosylated Hemoglobin Values During Treatment in Women With Gestational Diabetes

Variable	Glyburide (N = 201)	Insulin (N = 203)	P Value*
Week of gestation when blood glucose testing started	28±6	27±8	0.22
No. of weeks of testing	10±6.	11±7	0.12
Blood glucose (mg/dl)†			
Fasting	98±13	96±16	0.17
Preprandial	95±15	97±14	0.17
Postprandial	113±22	112±15	0.60
Mean	105±16	105±18	0.99
Glycosylated hemoglobin (%)‡	5.5±0.7	5.4±0.6	0.12

Values are mean ± SD.

*P values were calculated by a 2-tailed t test.

†Blood glucose values are means of measurements obtained throughout pregnancy. To convert values for glucose to millimoles per liter, multiply by 0.056.

‡The test was performed late in the third trimester.

(Courtesy of Langer O, Conway DL, Berkus MD, et al. A comparison of glyburide and insulin in women with gestational diabetes mellitus. *N Engl J Med* 343:1134-1138, 2000. Copyright 2000 by the Massachusetts Medical Society. All rights reserved.)

clinical variables. Both treatments caused significant reductions in blood glucose levels compared with levels measured at home for 1 week before treatment (Table 3): Mean blood glucose levels in the glyburide group decreased from 114 to 105 mg/dL, whereas those in the insulin group decreased from 116 to 105 mg/dL. Eight patients in the glyburide group (4%) did not achieve glycemic control with the maximum dose; these patients were switched to insulin therapy. None of the patients had severe symptoms develop, and the glyburide and insulin groups had a similar incidence of preeclampsia (6%) and cesarean section (23%-24%). Neonatal outcomes did not differ significantly between the 2 groups (Table 4). Specifically, the glyburide and insulin groups had a similar incidence of large-for-gestational-age infants (12% and 13%, respectively), macrosomia (birth weight ≥4000 g; 7% and 4%), lung complications (8% and 6%), hypoglycemia (9% and 6%), admission to a neonatal intensive care unit (6% and 7%), and fetal anomalies (2% and 2%). The mean cord-serum insulin concentration was 15 µU/mL in each group, and no glyburide was detected in the cord serum of any infant in the glyburide group.

Conclusions.—Glyburide appears to be a safe and effective alternative to insulin therapy in women with mild gestational diabetes. The extent of glycemic control was similar with glyburide and insulin, and maternal and fetal outcomes were similar as well. Concerns of teratogenicity with glyburide appear to be unfounded, given that no drug was found in the cord serum of infants in the glyburide group and that patients began therapy only after 11 weeks of gestation (ie, after organogenesis was completed).

TABLE 4.—Neonatal Outcomes

Outcome	Glyburide (N = 201)	Insulin (N = 203)	P Value
Neonatal features			
Large size for gestational age —no. (%)	24 (12)	26 (13)	0.76
Birth weight—g	3256 ± 543	3194 ± 598	0.28
Ponderal index >2.85 —no. (%)*	18 (9)	24 (12)	0.33
Macrosomia—no. (%)	14 (7)	9 (4)	0.26
Metabolic outcomes			
Cord-serum insulin—µU/ml†	15 ± 13	15 ± 21	0.84
Intravenous glucose therapy —no. (%)	28 (14)	22 (11)	0.36
Hypoglycemia—no. (%)	18 (9)	12 (6)	0.25
Hypocalcemia—no. (%)	2 (1)	2 (1)	0.99
Hyperbilirubinemia—no. (%)	12 (6)	8 (4)	0.36
Polycythemia—no. (%)	4 (2)	6 (3)	0.52
Lung complications—no. (%)	16 (8)	12 (6)	0.43
Respiratory support—no. (%)	4 (2)	6 (3)	0.52
Admission to neonatal intensive care unit—no. (%)	12 (6)	14 (7)	0.68
Congenital anomaly	5 (2)	4 (2)	0.74
Perinatal mortality—no. (%)‡			
Stillbirth	1 (0.5)	1 (0.5)	0.99
Neonatal death	1 (0.5)	1 (0.5)	0.99

Plus-minus values are mean ± SD.

*The ponderal index was calculated as 100 times the weight in grams divided by the cube of the length in centimeters.

†To convert values for insulin to picomoles per liter, multiply by 6.0.

‡Numbers include infants with congenital anomalies.

(Courtesy of Langer O, Conway DL, Berkus MD, et al. A comparison of glyburide and insulin in women with gestational diabetes mellitus. *N Engl J Med* 343:1134-1138, 2000. Copyright 2000 by the Massachusetts Medical Society. All rights reserved.)

▶ As concerns about the possible fetal effects of metformin have arisen (see Abstract 4–3), it has become appropriate to look again to the value of some of the newer sulfonylurea compounds now in renewed use in treating late-onset diabetes. Use of this class of agents arose with the observation that sulfonamides used in treating infectious disease were sometimes associated with hypoglycemic episodes. By the 1960s it became clear that sulfonylurea compounds stimulate pancreatic beta cells to increased insulin production and release. Beta cell surface receptors to sulfonylurea alter adenosine triphosphate–dependent potassium channels, decreasing cellular efflux of potassium. This change tends to open voltage regulated calcium channels, allowing beta cells the influx of calcium and activation of protein kinase C and myosin light chain kinase, which in turn stimulates insulin secretion. Perhaps more interesting, long-term use of the drug increases insulin receptor site density and, through a mechanism not entirely clear, decreases insulin resistance just as metformin does. Metformin is a chemically simple biguanide whereas glyburide and other sulfonylureas are larger, more complex molecules. It is no surprise that some of these authors using isolated perfused human cotyledons demonstrated only 1.5% of maternal-to-fetal transfer at a maternal glyburide concentration of 1000 ng/mL over a 3-h period and 2.11% of transfer at a maternal concentration of 20,000 ng/mL.[1] In this prospective, randomized but unblinded clinical trial of gestational diabetics with abnormal oral glucose tolerance tests and fasting blood sugars greater than 95 mL/dL, treated either with insulin or glyburide, criteria for control were based on 7 blood samples per day demonstrating normal fasting blood sugars and 2-h postcibum blood sugars less than 120 mg/dL. Glyburide was not found in cord blood samples. Only 4% of women receiving glyburide failed to achieve adequate control and had less hypoglycemia than those taking insulin. There were no significant maternal side effects from glyburide, and neonatal outcomes were indistinguishable between the 2 treatment groups. Those receiving glyburide had 7% incidence of large-for-gestational-age newborns and 4% macrosomia; corresponding rates for insulin recipients were 10% and 3%. The incidences of cesarean section (23%-24%) and preeclampsia (6%) were virtually identical between the 2 groups. Glyburide has a half-time of elimination of 10 hours, and a single daily oral dose suffices for management.

These authors have demonstrated a viable option to the use of insulin in gestational diabetics who have not responded to fasting blood sugar control on diet alone. Still to be evaluated in diabetic pregnancy are the merits of combining insulin with sulfonylurea agents in view of the evidence for both insulin deficiency and insulin resistance in type 2 diabetics.[2]

T. H. Kirschbaum, MD

References

1. Elliott BD, Langer O, Schenken S, et al: Insignificant transfer of glyburide occurs across the placenta. *Am J Obstet Gynecol* 165:807-812, 1991.
2. Riddle M (ed): The two defects of type 2 diabetes mellitus. *Am J Med* 108:6A, 2000.

Impact of Prenatal Glucose Screening on the Diagnosis of Gestational Diabetes and on Pregnancy Outcomes
Wen SW, Liu S, Kramer MS, et al (Bureau of Reproductive and Child Health, Ottawa, Ont, Canada; McGill Univ, Montreal; Dalhousie Univ, Halifax, Nova Scotia, Canada; et al)
Am J Epidemiol 152:1009-1014, 2000   4–2

Introduction.—Routine screening for gestational diabetes with an oral glucose challenge test late in the second trimester was recommended in 1985 at the Second International Workshop-Conference on Gestational Diabetes Mellitus; it was reaffirmed by the American Diabetes Association in 1986. No trial has evaluated whether these guidelines have influenced the rate of gestational diabetes or diabetes-related adverse pregnancy outcomes in the general population. The impact of these guidelines was examined by reviewing temporal and geographic trends in gestational diabetes and diabetes-related pregnancy outcomes in Canada from 1984 to 1996.

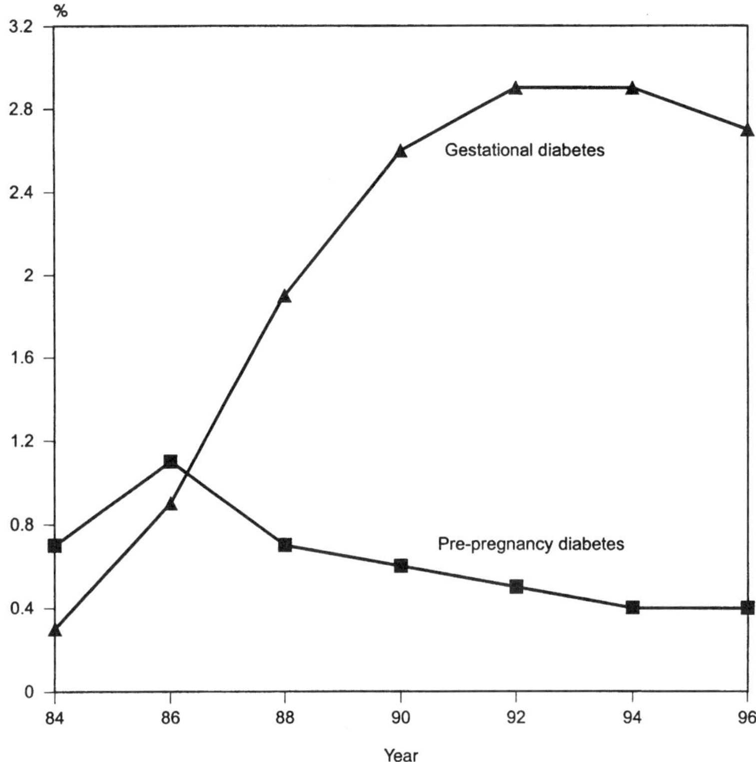

FIGURE 1.—Age-adjusted rates of gestational and prepregnancy diabetes in Canada, 1984-1996. (Courtesy of Wen SW, Liu S, Kramer MS, et al: Impact of prenatal glucose screening on the diagnosis of gestational diabetes and on pregnancy outcomes. *Am J Epidemiol* 152:1009-1014, 2000, by permission of Oxford University Press.)

Findings.—The proportion of females with gestational diabetes increased 9-fold (from 0.3% to 2.7%) and the proportion of females with prepregnancy diabetes decreased from 0.7% to 0.4% (Fig 1). As rates of gestational diabetes increased, a corresponding decrease in the risks of complications (polyhydramnios, amniotic cavity infection, cesarean delivery, and precclampsia) occurred for females with gestational diabetes (Fig 2). The ratc of gestational diabetes decreased in Metro-Hamilton (where screening was discontinued in 1989) but remained high in the rest of Ontario (where screening continued in most areas). No related temporal trends for fetal macrosomia, cesarean delivery, or other diabetes-related complications were seen, regardless of screening policy. Rates of polyhydramnios and amniotic infection increascd and rates of cesarean delivery decreased during the evaluation period in both regions; rates of fetal macrosomia and pre-eclampsia fluctuated (Fig 5).

Conclusion.—The marked increase in gestational diabetes in Canada is an artifact resulting from universal screening with no evidence of beneficial effects on pregnancy outcomes.

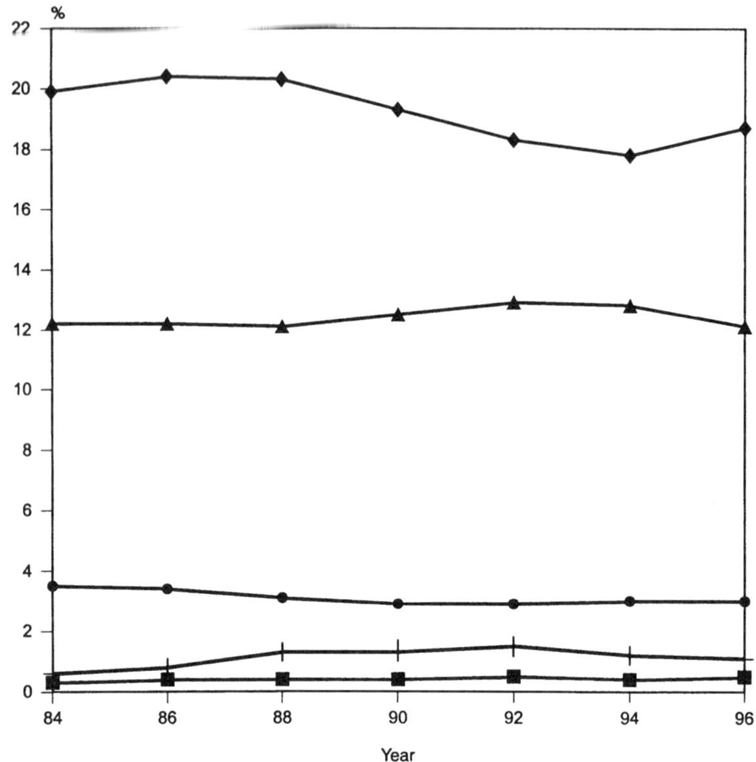

FIGURE 2.—Rates of diabetes-related pregnancy complications in Canada, 1984-1996. All rates (except those for fetal macrosomia) were adjusted for maternal age. (*Diamond*), cesarean delivery; (*triangle*), fetal macrosomia; (*circle*), preeclampsia; (*vertical lines*), amniotic infection; (*square*), polyhydramnios. (Courtesy of Wen SW, Liu S, Kramer MS, et al: Impact of prenatal glucose screening of the diagnosis of gestational diabetes and on pregnancy outcomes. *Am J Epidemiol* 152:1009-1014, 2000, by permission of Oxford University Press.)

▶ In an effort to explore the impact of routine antenatal diabetic screening, these investigators collected data filed with the Canadian Institute for Health Information for more than 1.7 million births, representing 78% of all Canadian births during the interval from April 1984 to March 1997. That interval was chosen to bridge the time before and after the recommendations for routine glucose testing in pregnancy made by an International Workshop Conference in 1985 and the American Diabetic Association in 1986. A complicating feature was the withdrawal from routine glucose testing begun in 1989 in the Hamilton, Ontario metropolitan area as the result of the urging of faculty at the McMaster University School of Medicine. Comparisons were made between the incidence of ICD coding for diabetic complications of pregnancy, between those with an associated diagnosis of gestational diabetes, and those with prepregnancy diabetes across the provinces and, after 1989, between the Hamilton metropolitan area and the rest of Ontario.

In both sets of comparisons, those with gestational diabetes showed a reduction of cesarean section incidence, of preeclampsia, polyhydramnios,

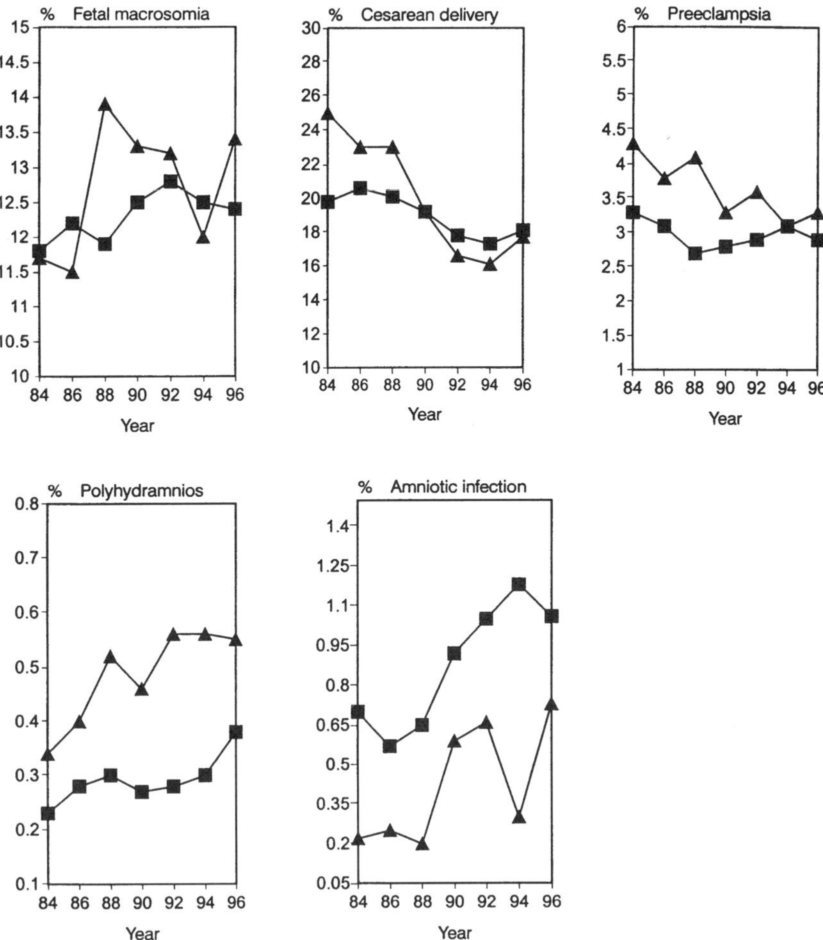

FIGURE 5.—Age-adjusted (except fetal macrosomia) rates of fetal macrosomia, cesarean delivery, preeclampsia, polyhydramnios, and amniotic infection in Metro-Hamilton (*triangle*) versus the rest of Ontario (*square*), Canada, 1984-1996. (Courtesy of Wen SW, Liu S, Kramer MS, et al: Impact of prenatal glucose screening on the diagnosis of gestational diabetes and on pregnancy outcomes. *Am J Epidemiol* 152:1009-1014, 2000, by permission of Oxford University Press.)

and amnionitis. However, a decline in cesarean section incidence was present in all Canadian regions (see Figure 2) regardless of glucose testing, and no trends, other than an increase in the diagnosis of hydramnios, probably an impact of the introduction of ultrasonic antenatal monitoring, were seen after the institution of routine glucose testing. No clear decreases in the rate of diabetic complications were seen in Ontario data, excluding the Hamilton experience, where routine testing was in operation. The authors conclude that screening detects gestational diabetes, which accrues some benefit through diabetic management. However, since general indices of diabetic morbidity were not affected in the 2.7% of women found to have gestational diabetes, complications like macrosomia, preeclampsia and am-nionitis noted and treated in screened women were very likely mild-to-moderate problems, not sensitively related to indices of poor pregnancy outcome. This is a view that assumes that associative events are also causal, and that is an uncertain assumption. However, these investigators introduce a new view of the nature of the conflict about routine glucose testing between those who have seen the benefits in the short term for the treatment of gestational diabetes mellitus and those who fail to find general improvement in morbidity and mortality rates as a result of those efforts over the longer time scale.

T. H. Kirschbaum, MD

A Randomised Controlled Pilot Study of the Management of Gestational Impaired Glucose Tolerance

Bancroft K, Tuffnell DJ, Mason GC, et al (Univ of Leeds, England)
Br J Obstet Gynaecol 107:959-963, 2000   4–3

Background.—Many clinicians advocate intensive management of women with impaired glucose tolerance in pregnancy even though there is no clear evidence that this approach improves maternal or fetal outcomes. Large randomized trials to determine whether intensive management regimens truly benefit women with impaired glucose tolerance in pregnancy and/or their infants are sorely needed. But would patients be willing to be randomized and to comply with an intensive blood glucose monitoring regimen? This prospective, randomized, controlled pilot study addresses that question.

Methods.—Eligible subjects were 70 pregnant women with impaired glucose tolerance (fasting blood glucose level <7.0 mmol/L and a blood glucose level 2 hours after a 75-g oral glucose dose of 7.8 to 11 mmol/L). Two subjects declined to participate, leaving a total of 68 women to be randomly assigned to the monitored or unmonitored groups. The patient's diabetologist knew whether she was in the monitored or unmonitored group, but the patient's obstetrician did not to avoid influencing decisions related to obstetric management. Both groups were given standard dietary advice and underwent monthly determinations of glycosylated hemoglobin (HbA1c) levels. Antenatal care was also the same in each group and consisted of routine serial US, amniotic fluid analyses, and Doppler umbilical artery velocity profiling. Additionally, patients in the monitored group performed capillary glucose sampling 1 to 2 hours after a meal 5 times per week. Patients with ≥5 samples that were >7.0 mmol/L in 1 week were switched to insulin therapy.

Results.—The monitored (n = 32) and unmonitored (n = 36) groups did not differ significantly in age at delivery (mean, 29.7 vs 31.9 years), body mass index at booking (mean, 31.2 vs 27.5 kg/m²), or other demographic variables. Mean HbA1c levels at 32 weeks were significantly higher in the unmonitored group than in the monitored group (5.9% vs

TABLE 4.—Neonatal Outcome Measures

	Monitored Group (*n* = 32)	Unmonitored Group (*n* = 36)
Frequency of admission to SCBU	2 (6)	6 (17)
Frequency of hypoglycaemia	2 (6)	6 (17)
Gestation at delivery (weeks)	39 {36–41}	39 {34–41}
Birthweight (kg)	3·58 [0·55]	3·62 [0·55]
Birthweight ratio	1·07 [0·16]	1·10 [0·15]
Birthweight > 90th centile for gestation	8 [25]	7 [19]

Values are given as n (%), mean [SD], or median {range}.
Abbreviations: SCBU, Special care baby unit.
(Courtesy of Bancroft K, Tuffnell DJ, Mason GC, et al: A randomised controlled pilot study of the management of gestational impaired glucose tolerance. *Br J Obstet Gynaecol* 107:959-963, 2000. Copyright Elsevier Science Ltd.)

5.2%), but not at 28, 36, or 38 weeks or at term. At admission, patients in the unmonitored group had significantly higher 2-hour plasma glucose levels than patients in the monitored group (8.9 vs 8.5 mmol/L). Nonetheless, neonatal outcomes did not differ significantly between the 2 groups (Table 4). Patients in the monitored group performed between 0 and 500 plasma glucose measurements (median, 118), and 6 (19%) were switched to insulin therapy on the basis of serially elevated levels. Yet again, maternal outcomes did not differ significantly between the 2 groups (Table 5).

Conclusions.—This small pilot study shows that women with gestational impaired glucose tolerance will comply with randomization to intensive glucose monitoring. Such a program involves substantial inconvenience; some of the patients in the monitored group obtained as many as

TABLE 5.—Maternal Outcome Measures

	Monitored Group (*n* = 32)	Unmonitored Group (*n* = 36)
No. of capillary specimens performed*	118 (0–520)	0 (0)
Frequency of insulin use†	6 [19]	0 [0]
No. of antenatal visits	17 (2–28)	14 (6–33)
No. of hospital admissions	1 (0–6)	0 (0–8)
Delivery type		
Vaginal	22 [69]	25 [69]
LSCS	10 [31]	11 [31]

Values are given as median (range) and n [%].
Abbreviations: LSCS, Lower segment caesarean section.
*P < .005.
†P < .008.
(Courtesy of Bancroft K, Tuffnell DJ, Mason GC, et al: A randomised controlled pilot study of the management of gestational impaired glucose tolerance. *Br J Obstet Gynaecol* 107:959-963, 2000. Copyright Elsevier Science Ltd.)

500 capillary glucose samples, and 19% underwent insulin therapy. Nonetheless, despite intensive monitoring of blood glucose levels, neither maternal nor fetal outcomes were significantly improved in the monitored group compared with the unmonitored group.

▶ Doubts about the efficacy of routine antenatal glucose tolerance testing and treatment of gestational diabetes have largely been expressed as opinions, unaccompanied by data. This pilot study suffers from small numbers of cases but is an item of support for a large-scale international randomized controlled trial of gestational diabetes therapy that is now underway. Gestational diabetics were randomly divided into monitored and unmonitored subsets. Both received dietary consultation and prescription and monthly determinations of hemoglobin A1C. The monitored women also performed capillary blood glucose determinations 5 times weekly. Both groups were exposed to serial ultrasound and Doppler umbilical artery velocity profiles. Diabetic management status was blinded to obstetricians who determined delivery time and route.

The unmonitored group had significantly higher 2-hour post-cibum blood sugar levels and higher concentrations of hemoglobin A1C at 32 weeks of gestation, suggesting their carbohydrate abnormality might be more severe than in the monitored group. Neonatal outcomes, including birth weight and gestational age at birth, were not different between monitored and non-monitored groups; there were no fetal or neonatal deaths. Nearly 20% of the monitored groups of patients were placed on insulin therapy, a product of the median number of 118 capillary blood samples in a frequency distribution that ranged as high as 500 samples per pregnancy. Despite the effort, cost, and anxiety associated with glucose monitoring, no benefit was discernable in the pilot study. Clearly an important issue, a broader study with more numerous subjects is therefore certainly desirable.

T. H. Kirschbaum, MD

Oral Hypoglycaemic Agents in 118 Diabetic Pregnancies
Hellmuth E, Damm P, Mølsted-Pedersen L (Univ of Copenhagen)
Diabet Med 17:507-511, 2000   4–4

Background.—Oral hypoglycemic agents would appear to be an attractive alternative to insulin therapy in pregnant women who have gestational diabetes mellitus (GDM) develop or with type 2 diabetes mellitus (DM) who cannot achieve glycemic control by diet alone. But are these agents safe for use in pregnancy? The maternal and neonatal side effects of metformin, sulfonylurea, and insulin in pregnant women with GDM or type 2 DM were evaluated.

Methods.—Three groups of diabetic pregnant patients and their infants who were treated at the same hospital were studied. The first 2 groups were treated between 1966 and 1984 with either metformin or sulfonylurea; the third group was treated after 1984 with insulin and served as a

TABLE 2.—Characteristics of Infants of Diabetic Women With GDM or Type 2 Diabetes Treated With Oral Hypoglycemic Agents or Insulin During Pregnancy

Infant Data	Metformin (n = 50)	Sulphonylurea (n = 69)	Insulin (n = 43)
Gestational age (weeks)	38 (33-39)	37 (29-39)	37 (31-39)
Gestatioial age < 37 completed weeks	11 (22%)	14 (20%)	11 (26%)
Birthweight (g)	3700 (1700-5470)	3437 (1710-4460)	3400 (1440-4600)
Birthweight > 90th percentile	19 (38%)	20 (29%)	19 (44%)
Birthweight < 10th percentile	2 (4%)	0	2 (5%)
Stillborn infants	4 (8.0%)	0	1 (2.3%)*

Data are median (range) or n (%).
*P = .042.
(Courtesy of Hellmuth E, Damm P, Mølsted-Pedersen L: Ora. Hypoglycaemic agents in 118 diabetic pregnancies. *Diabet Med* 17:507-511, 2000. Reprinted by permission of Blackwell Science, Inc.)

reference group. The 50 patients who received metformin (mean age at delivery, 32 years; 76% white; 30% nulliparous) included 31 patients with GDM who received metformin for a median of 3 weeks and 19 patients with type 2 DM who received metformin for a median of 9 weeks. The 68 patients who received sulfonylurea (mean age at delivery, 28 years; 83% white; 37% nulliparous) included 39 patients with GDM who received sulfonylurea for a median of 4 weeks and 29 patients with type 2 DM who received sulfonylurea for a median of 9 weeks. The 42 patients in the insulin group (mean age at delivery, 29 years; 71% white; 26% nulliparous) included 35 patients with GDM who received insulin beginning in week 26 (median) and 7 patients with type 2 DM who received insulin beginning in week 15 (median). Maternal, perinatal, and neonatal complications were recorded and compared among the 3 groups.

Results.—Insulin therapy was required in 4 patients with GDM and 7 patients with type 2 DM in the metformin group and in 11 patients with GDM and 20 patients with type 2 DM in the sulfonylurea group. The 3 groups were similar at baseline, except that the prepregnancy body mass index was significantly higher in the metformin group than in the sulfonylurea or insulin groups (median, 31.2 vs 22.8 and 24.8 kg/m^2, respectively). The incidence of pregnancy-induced hypertension, intrauterine growth retardation, polyhydramnios, placenta abruptio, or cesarean section did not differ significantly among the 3 groups. However, the incidence of preeclampsia was significantly greater in the metformin group than in the sulfonylurea or insulin groups (31% vs 7% and 10%). The incidence of a stillborn infant was also significantly greater in the metformin group (8.0% vs 0% and 2.3%), respectively) (Table 2). However, neonatal mortality and morbidity rates (including preterm birth, asphyxia, severe hypoglycemia, jaundice, and respiratory problems) were similar in the 3 groups.

Conclusions.—Pregnant women with GDM or type 2 DM who took metformin during their pregnancy were significantly more likely to have preeclampsia and to have a stillborn child than diabetic women who took sulfonylurea or insulin. The current study cannot determine whether these associations are causal or merely coincidental. Nonetheless, the authors recommend against the use of metformin in pregnant diabetic women until more data are available.

▶ Metformin has been shown to be effective in increasing insulin sensitivity in men and nonpregnant women with type 2 DM when insulin resistance appears to be the principal problem. Additionally, the drug increases fibrinolysis in nonpregnant women, a possible benefit to women with hypercoagulable states unrelated to DM. Because the drug was initially thought not to cross the placenta, it was believed to be a potential value in treating type 2 diabetics in pregnancy, though the effects on the fetus were uncertain (see 1998 YEAR BOOK OF OBSTETRICS, GYNECOLOGY, AND WOMEN'S HEALTH, pp 99-100).

This study compares 118 women treated for diabetic pregnancy at the famed Rigshospital in Copenhagen from 1966 to 1991. Subjects were either gestational diabetics or type 2 diabetics who could not satisfactorily be controlled by diet alone and received oral hypoglycemic agents in order to avoid insulin therapy. Oral hypoglycemic agents were used routinely for these indications from 1966 to 1984, but the practice was discontinued in favor of insulin thereafter because of unproven concerns for the fetus. From 1984 to 1991, only occasional cases qualified for entry into the study and were identified from the records of care at the hospital. Fifty such women had received only metformin and 68 received either tolbutamide or another sulfonylurea compound. Forty-two randomly selected women who received insulin therapy instead of oral hypoglycemic agents were enrolled as controls in this retrospective cohort study.

Metformin-treated women had significantly greater body mass indexes than the other 2 groups and, perhaps related, a higher prevalence of pregnancy-induced hypertension than did the others. The women were predominantly multiparous (65% to 75%). Most significantly, the incidence of fetal death was higher in metformin-treated women than in the other 2 groups, especially when treatment occupied the third trimester. Incidences of neonatal pathology or death were not affected. The increased incidence of fetal death would seem to render metformin contraindicated in type 2 diabetic pregnancies until evidence to refute this study and prove metformin's safety to the fetus is generated.

T. H. Kirschbaum, MD

Decreased Insulin Receptor Tyrosine Kinase Activity and Plasma Cell Membrane Glycoprotein-1 Overexpression in Skeletal Muscle From Obese Women With Gestational Diabetes Mellitus (GDM): Evidence for Increased Serine/Threonine Phosphorylation in Pregnancy and GDM
Shao J, Catalano PM, Yamashita H, et al (Case Western Reserve Univ, Cleveland, Ohio; Louisiana State Univ, Baton Rouge; Univ of San Francisco)
Diabetes 49:603-610, 2000   4–5

Background.—Insulin-mediated glucose disposal decreases by up to 60% from early to late pregnancy to provide glucose for the developing fetus. Women who cannot compensate by increasing their secretion of insulin develop gestational diabetes mellitus (GDM). At a cellular level, insulin receptor binding capacity is not changed in GDM, which implies that postreceptor mechanisms are responsible for insulin resistance. Insulin binds to the α-subunit of its transmembrane receptor, which triggers its β-subunit to undergo autophosphorylation of various tyrosine residues. This phosphorylation activates insulin receptor tyrosine kinase (IRTK), which catalyzes other cellular signaling proteins to undergo tyrosine phosphorylation. IRTK activity is inhibited by the phosphorylation of serine/threonine residues on the insulin receptor. Studies have also shown that plasma cell membrane glycoprotein-1 (PC-1) inhibits IRTK activity in human skeletal muscle and thus may also influence postreceptor insulin activity. The roles of increased insulin receptor serine/threonine phosphorylation and PC-1 expression on IRTK function in GDM were examined.

Methods.—Rectus abdominus muscle samples were obtained from 6 nonpregnant women without diabetes mellitus, 6 pregnant women without GDM, and 6 pregnant women with GDM. All women were obese (body mass index $\geq$30 kg/m²) and were similar in age (group means ranged from 34.2 to 37.0 years). Basal insulin receptor content was measured by enzyme-linked immunosorbent assay. IRTK phosphorylation was measured by liquid scintillation counting of the extent of uptake of ³²P-labeled poly(Glu,Tyr) in immunocaptured insulin receptors. Insulin receptors were then dephosphorylated by the addition of alkaline phosphatase, and IRTK activity was measured by enzyme-linked immunosorbent assay. PC-1 content was measured by Western blotting.

Results.—Basal insulin receptor tyrosine phosphorylation and IRTK activity did not differ significantly in the 3 groups. Maximal insulin stimulation (10⁻⁷ mol/L) caused a significant increase in IRTK activity in all 3 groups (Fig 1). However, the increase in insulin-stimulated IRTK activity was significantly lower in the patients with GDM compared with the nonpregnant controls (39% lower) and the pregnant controls without GDM (21% lower). After dephosphorylation of serine/threonine residues

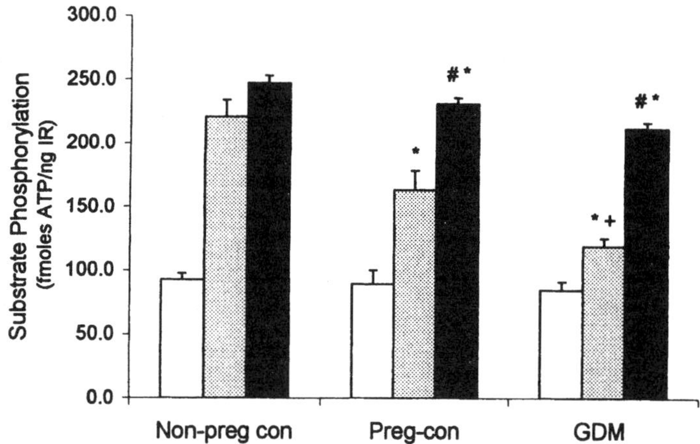

FIGURE 1.—Effect of prior alkaline phosphatase treatment on IRTK activity in skeletal muscle from nonpregnant control (*Non-preg con*), pregnant control (*Preg-con*), and GDM subjects. Rectus abdominus muscle biopsies were obtained during gynecological surgery or at the time of scheduled cesarean section delivery and were stored at–70°C. The muscle tissues were homogenized under denaturing conditions at 4°C, and the same amount of insulin receptors (determined previously) were immunocaptured on a 96-well plate precoated with anti-insulin receptor antibody. One aliquot of insulin receptors was treated with 20 U alkaline phosphatase before assaying the IRTK activity. Before assaying the kinase activity, the receptors were incubated with [γ³²P]-labeled adenosine trisphosphate. Substrate phosphorylation was determined by adsorbing peptide substrate poly(Glu,Tyr) 1:4 per nanogram of insulin receptor. The data are means ± SE for nonpregnant control (n = 6), pregnant control (n = 6), and GDM (n = 6) subjects. *, Significantly lower than nonpregnant control subjects (*P* < .05); +, significantly lower than pregnant control subjects (*P* < .05); #, significantly greater than the corresponding kinase activity in the same group without alkaline phosphatase treatment (*P* < .05); *open bars*, insulin (–) and alkaline phosphatase (–); *gray bars*, insulin (+) and alkaline phosphatase (–); *solid bars*, insulin (+) and alkaline phosphatase (+). (Courtesy of Shao J, Catalano PM, Yamashita H, et al: Decreased insulin receptor tyrosine kinase activity and plasma cell membrane glycoprotein-1 overexpression in skeletal muscle from obese women with gestational diabetes mellitus (GDM): Evidence for increased serine/threonine phosphorylation in pregnancy and GDM. *Diabetes* 49:603-610. Copyright 2000, by the American Diabetes Association.)

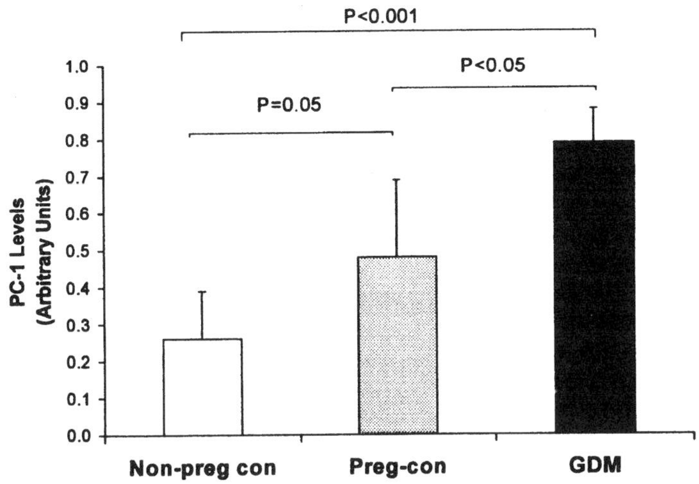

FIGURE 2.—PC-1 content in the skeletal muscle of nonpregnant control (*Non-preg con*), pregnant control (*Preg-con*), and GDM subjects. Frozen muscle tissues were homogenized, and the protein samples were run on a denatured gel system. After transfer to the membrane, the PC-1 was probed by polyclonal anti PC-1 antibody. Quantification of the 110-kDa band was performed with a Bio-Rad imaging densitometer with 8 µg of whole cell lysate of the human hepatoma cell line HepG2 to control for gel-to-gel variation. Results are expressed as a ratio to the HepG2 control. Data are expressed in arbitrary units and as means ± SE for 6 to 8 patients per group. (Courtesy of Shao J, Catalano PM, Yamashita H, et al: Decreased insulin receptor tyrosine kinase activity and plasma cell membrane glycoprotein-1 overexpression in skeletal muscle from obese women with gestational diabetes mellitus (GDM): Evidence for increased serine/threonine phosphorylation in pregnancy and GDM. *Diabetes* 49:603-610. Copyright 2000, by the American Diabetes Association.)

by alkaline phosphatase, insulin-stimulated IRTK activity increased significantly compared with basal values in the pregnant controls without GDM (by 48%) and the patients with GDM (by 80%); yet these increases were still significantly less than values in the nonpregnant controls. PC-1 levels in the patients with GDM were significantly greater than those in pregnant controls without GDM (by 63%) and nonpregnant controls (by 206%) (Fig 2). PC-1 levels were significantly and negatively correlated with insulin receptor phosphorylation, IRTK activity, and IRTK activity after dephosphorylation.

Conclusions.—Compared with the nonpregnant controls without diabetes mellitus, both the pregnant controls without GDM and the patients with GDM had significantly higher PC-1 levels and excessive phosphorylation of serine/threonine residues in skeletal muscle insulin receptors. The extent of these changes was significantly greater in the pregnant women with GDM than in the pregnant women without GDM. PC-1 overexpression and excessive serine/threonine phosphorylation were each associated with decreased IRTK activity. Thus, these postreceptor alterations in insulin signaling likely contribute to the pathogenesis of GDM.

► Pregnancies associated with insulin resistance, measured in normal gravidas maintained artificially at a normal blood glucose concentration, require as much as a 50% to 60% increase in insulin administration to obtain normal rates of glucose utilization and storage. Because no changes in insulin receptor density or affinity are noted in normal pregnancy, it seems likely that events after insulin-receptor coupling operate in reducing insulin sensitivity and ensuring periodic·maternal hyperglycemia, important during pregnancy in maintaining a positive concentration gradient between mother and fetus. This helps ensure adequate fetal blood glucose concentration and metabolism. Maternal inability to maintain the requisite increased insulin release results in GDM, a precursor to chemical diabetes in later life. These authors explore the changes in postreceptor mechanisms responsible for those attenuations in insulin resistance. Evidence that insulin resistance in nonpregnant women and in men is associated with hypertension, dyslipidemia atherosclerosis, and arteriosclerotic heart disease in later life adds urgency to understanding these mechanisms. The insulin receptor is a transmembrane protein complex. When insulin combines with its external alpha subunit, structural alterations of the intracellular beta subunit follow and initiate autophosphorylation of several of its tyrosine components, in turn activating tyrosine-specific protein kinase (IRTK). This enzyme catalyzes the production of a number of second messengers, among them insulin receptor substrate 1, which conducts the glucose transport, utilization, and carbohydrate storage that results from insulin administration. The kinase can be inhibited by other agents, among them PC-1, which inhibits the activity of tyrosine kinase and is therefore a potential source of insulin resistance.

Using 3 groups of women, all obese to control for this variable, some nonpregnant, 6 pregnant with normal glucose tolerance tests, and 6 pregnant with GDM at 36 to 40 weeks, the investigators used tissue preparations from rectus abdominus biopsies taken during surgery to explore changes in IRTK and its inhibitor PC-1 in a basal state and in response to insulin and an inhibitor of receptor phosphorylation (alkaline phosphatase). They showed constant IRTK at basal conditions and progressively less IRTK response to insulin in normal glycemic pregnancies and gestational diabetics. Dephosphorylation with alkaline phosphatase demonstrated a small decrease in maximum possible IRTK in pregnancy, but no observations directly bearing on this change were made. Simultaneously, the authors measured progressive increases in the tyrosine kinase inhibitor PC-1 in pregnancy compared with nonpregnancy and in GDM.

This is impressive evidence of postreceptor changes marked by increases in PC-1 and decreases in IRTK responsible for both insulin resistance of normal pregnancy and in GDM, different only in magnitude. It opens new questions but is a step in our understanding of the mechanisms responsible for insulin resistance, a matter of vital interest to obstetricians and internists alike.

T. H. Kirschbaum, MD

Complications According to Mode of Delivery Among Human Immuno-deficiency Virus–Infected Women With CD4 Lymphocyte Counts of ≤ 500/µL
Watts DH, for the Pediatric AIDS Clinical Trials Group 185 Study Team (Natl Inst of Child Health and Human Development, Bethesda, Md; et al)
Am J Obstet Gynecol 183:100-107, 2000   4–6

Introduction.—Although the risk of HIV transmission is lower with planned cesarean delivery than with vaginal delivery, cesarean delivery is associated with an increased risk of maternal morbidity and mortality. Further information on the risk of complications is needed, however, to adequately counsel HIV-infected pregnant women on mode of delivery.

Methods.—The study cohort consisted of women in the Pediatric AIDS Clinical Trials Group Protocol 185. Those enrolled were HIV-seropositive, had a CD4 lymphocyte count of ≤500 cells/µL, were between 20 and 30 weeks' gestation, and received zidovudine for treatment of HIV infection. Excluded were women treated with protease inhibitors. Delivery was categorized as planned cesarean (before onset of labor and rupture of membranes), other cesarean (after onset of labor or rupture of membranes), and vaginal (spontaneous or forceps- or vacuum-assisted). Risk factors for complications were calculated for each mode of delivery.

Results.—Planned cesarean delivery was carried out in 37 women and other cesarean delivery in 95; 365 women delivered vaginally. Major complications occurred more often in cesarean groups than in the vaginal delivery group. The rate of amnionitis or endometritis was 16%, 27%, and 7%, respectively, in the planned cesarean, other cesarean, and vaginal delivery groups. Rates of wound infection were 5%, 8%, and 1%, and transfusion rates were 8%, 6%, and 3%, respectively. Factors associated with amnionitis/endometritis in multivariate analyses were cesarean deliv-

---

TABLE 3.—Patient Characteristics Associated With Selected Outcomes in Univariate and Multivariate Analyses

Factor	Univariate Odds Ratio and 95% Confidence Interval	Adjusted Odds Ratio and 95% Confidence Interval
Amnionitis or postpartum endometritis		
Cesarean delivery	4.4 (2.5-7.7)	4.8 (2.5-9.3)
African American race	2.3 (1.3-4.2)	3.0 (1.6-5.7)
Delivery <37 weeks' gestation	1.9 (1.0-3.6)	1.4 (0.7-2.9)
Peripartum antibiotic prophylaxis	2.2 (1.3-3.8)	1.3 (0.6-2.5)
Red blood cell transfusion		
Cesarean delivery	2.4 (1.0-5.8)	2.8 (1.0-8.4)
African American race	5.5 (1.6-18.9)	3.3 (0.9-12.5)
Hematocrit level at 32-38 wk	0.8 (0.7-0.9)	0.8 (0.7-0.9)*
Sexually transmitted disease anytime		
during pregnancy	3.5 (1.4-8.6)	2.6 (0.9-7.5)

*Odds ratio indicates decrease in risk for transfusion with each percentage point increase in hematocrit level at 32 to 38 weeks.

(Courtesy of Watts DH, for the Pediatrics AIDS Clinical Trials Group 185 Study Team: Complications according to mode of delivery among human immunodeficiency virus–infected women with CD4 lymphocyte counts of ≤500/µL. *Am J Obstet Gynecol* 183:100-107, 2000.)

ery and African-American race; a factor associated with transfusion was third trimester anemia (Table 3). Neither entry nor third-trimester CD4 lymphocyte counts or HIV plasma viral loads was associated with increased risk of these complications.

Conclusion.—Cesarean delivery before onset of labor or rupture of membranes can reduce the risk of perinatal HIV transmission. The findings of this study suggest that the increased risk for complications after cesarean delivery is not specifically related to HIV status.

▶ This account of postdelivery complications of HIV-positive women is a byproduct of the AIDS Clinical Trials Group Protocol 185 (see 2001 YEAR BOOK OF OBSTETRICS, GYNECOLOGY, AND WOMEN'S HEALTH, pp 92-94). In that study, the effects of HIV hyperimmune globulin passive immunization in reducing maternal to fetal transmission of HIV in infected gravidas receiving azidothymidine (AZT) but not protease inhibitors was studied. In this uncontrolled cohort study, the incidence and pattern of complications of delivery of 497 HIV-positive women delivered in 1993 to 1997 were compared with normals. Mode of delivery was determined by individual obstetricians, and 26% of the women were delivered abdominally, 37 of them by elective procedures prior to labor.

Entry into this study required the presence of maternal HIV-1 antibody, CD4 counts less than 500/mm^3 at a gestational age between 20 and 30 weeks, and use of AZT and other antiviral agents, excluding protease inhibitors, during pregnancy. The investigators were concerned primarily with the role of increasing abdominal delivery in reducing vertical transmission of HIV-1. The contribution of this study is to explore the possibility that increasing the incidence of cesarean section in such women might increase anticipated maternal morbidity.

The results confirm the finding of a recent meta-analysis demonstrating that, in the developed nations, HIV-positive women appear to have the same perinatal outcomes as noninfected gravidas (see 2000 YEAR BOOK, pp 125-127). The impact of cesarean section, not unexpectedly, was to increase rates of amnionitis and endometritis, wound infection, pneumonia, and the need for platelet transfusions. Multivariate analysis demonstrated a corelationship between endometritis and cesarean section, Afro-American race, low presurgical hematocrit, the need for transfusion, and wound infection, as well as CD4 counts of less than 200/mm^2. These associations had been established earlier. All other complication rates were within their usual range in normal gravidas. At least one part of the primary question is clear: Increasing the cesarean section rate in HIV-positive women taking AZT should result in no significant increase in the rate of anticipated postpartum complications.

T. H. Kirschbaum, MD

Probability of HIV-1 Transmission per Coital Act in Monogamous, Heterosexual, HIV-1-Discordant Couples in Rakai, Uganda

Gray RH, and the Rakai Project Team (Johns Hopkins Univ, Baltimore, Md; et al)
Lancet 357:1149-1153, 2001   4–7

Background.—While estimates of transmission probabilities for HIV-1 per coital act have been published based on studies in Europe and the United States, the probability of HIV-1 transmission per coital act in representative African populations has not been determined. The overall probability of HIV-1 transmission per coital act in an African cohort was calculated, and how such transmission is affected by a variety of factors that are thought to influence infectivity was estimated.

Methods.—The study group consisted of 174 monogamous couples retrospectively identified from a population cohort in Rakai, Uganda. In each couple, 1 partner was HIV-1 positive. The frequency of intercourse and the reliability of reporting by couples were prospectively assessed. HIV-1 viral load was determined for the infected partners, and HIV-1 seroconversion was determined in the uninfected partners. Poisson regression was used to determine the adjusted rate ratios of transmission per coital act. The probabilities of transmission per act were estimated by means of log-log binomial regression.

Results.—There was a mean frequency of intercourse of 8.9 times per month, with declines in frequency with age and HIV-1 viral load. Similar frequencies of intercourse were reported by members of couples. The overall unadjusted probability of HIV-1 transmission per coital act was determined to be 0.0011, and transmission probabilities increased from 0.0001 per coital act at viral loads of less than 1700 copies/mL to 0.0023

TABLE 2.—Probabilities of HIV-1 Transmission per Coital Act*

			Viral Load (Copies/mL)		
		<1700	1700 −12 499	12 500 −38 500	>38 500
Age (years)	Age†		Age and viral load§		
15-24	0·0013	0·0001	0·0020	0·0019	0·0032
25-29	0·0017	0·0001	0·0018	0·0026	0·0048
30-34	0·0006	0·00003	0·0005	0·0005	0·0014
35-59	0·0009	0·00004	0·0007	0·0008	0·0020
Viral load‡		0·0001	0·0013	0·0014	0·0023
Genital ulcer disease¶					
No	0·0041	0·0002	0·0033	0·0039	0·0049
Yes	0·0011	0·0001	0·0012	0·0014	0·0018

*Calculated from $(1-\exp[-\exp](k)])$, where $k = b_0+b_1X$ and X is the vector of regression coefficients.
†Model for age alone.
‡Model for viral load alone.
§Model for age and viral load.
¶Model for genital ulcer disease and viral load.
(Courtesy of Gray RH, and the Rakai Project Team: Probability of HIV-1 transmission per coital act in monogamous, heterosexual, HIV-1–discordant couples in Rakai, Uganda. *Lancet* 357;1149-1153, 2001, copyright by The Lancet Ltd.)

per coital act at 38,500 copies/mL or more. Transmission probability in the presence of genital ulceration was 0.0041 compared with 0.0011 when genital ulceration was not present (Table 2). There was no difference in transmission probability per act by HIV-1 subtypes A and D, gender, sexually transmitted diseases, or symptoms of discharge or dysuria in the HIV-1-positive partner.

Conclusions.—In the Ugandan population studied, the primary determinants of HIV-1 transmission were higher viral load and genital ulceration.

▶ The probability of HIV-1 transmission by vaginal coitus among partners discordant for HIV-1 positivity in Europe and the United States has been well studied and ranges from 0.0001 to 0.0014. The purpose of this study was to explore the possibility that the explosive spread of the disease in sub-Saharan Africa might be caused by differences in transmission rates or to differences in HIV-1 strains, identified by serotyping of the V3 loop of the virus, a relatively exposed segment of its structure amenable to antibody formation and subtyping. US and European infection involves type B; types A and D are seen dominantly in Africa.

A hundred seventy-four monogamous heterosexual couples using vaginal but not anal intercourse, a route of greater infectivity, were seen at 10-month intervals with blood samples for HIV-1 tested by enzyme-linked immunosorbent assay and Western blots performed for HIV-1 diagnosis. Serologic tests for syphilis, herpes simplex virus type 2, chlamydia, trichomoniasis and bacterial vaginosis (BV) were determined immunologically and by culture. Interviews were used to establish coital frequency per month, and estimates by partners were compared to assure agreement. Statistical analysis was by multiple regression techniques using sex of the HIV-positive partner, age, viral load of HIV-RNA, and the presence or absence of genital ulcerative lesions as covariants. No antiviral agents or condoms were used.

The overall rate of transmission was 0.0011 and varied inversely with age when controlled for coital frequency and directly with viral load. Reported genital ulceration increased the risk of transmission by a factor of 2.58, a statistically significant increase. The transmission rate by HIV-positive women to men was 0.0013; from HIV-positive men to women, it was 0.0009, not a statistically significant difference. Coinfection with syphilis, gonorrhea, chlamydia, BV, or trichmoniasis did not influence transmission rates, though case numbers are small.

Since the transmission rates noted here are within the range reported for US and European populations, the study supports the premise that neither viral subtype nor greater propensity for transmission independent of viral load and age accounts for the remarkably rapid spread of the disease in the African continent.

T. H. Kirschbaum, MD

A Trial of Shortened Zidovudine Regimens to Prevent Mother-to-Child Transmission of Human Immunodeficiency Virus Type 1

Lallemant M, for the Perinatal HIV Prevention Trial (Thailand) Investigators (Institut de Recherche pour le Développement, Paris; et al)
N Engl J Med 343:982-991, 2000   4–8

Background.—In much of the Western world, standard therapy for preventing the vertical transmission of HIV type 1 involves maternal administration of zidovudine beginning at 28 weeks' gestation, intravenous zidovudine during labor, and fetal administration of zidovudine for 6 weeks after birth. However, this intensive regimen may not be feasible in areas where resources are limited. The efficacy of 4 different zidovudine regimens in preventing mother-to-child transmission of HIV was prospectively evaluated in Thailand.

Methods.—The subjects were 1437 pregnant women with HIV (median age, 24 years) who were randomly assigned at 28 weeks' gestation to 1 of 4 zidovudine treatment groups. The "long-long" regimen involved treating the mother with oral zidovudine (300 mg twice a day) beginning at 28 weeks' gestation and treating the infant with oral zidovudine (2 mg/kg every 6 hours) for 6 weeks after birth. The "long-short" regimen involved treating the mother beginning at 28 weeks' gestation and treating the infant for 3 days. The "short-long" regimen involved treating the mother beginning at 35 weeks' gestation and treating the infant for 6 weeks. The "short-short" regimen involved treating the mother beginning at 35 weeks' gestation and treating the infant for 3 days. All women received 300 mg zidovudine orally at the onset of labor and every 3 hours thereafter until delivery, and all infants were fed formula. Infants were evaluated for HIV DNA at 2, 4, and 6 weeks and 4 and 6 months after birth.

Results.—At baseline, the groups were similar in demographics, clinical characteristics, and delivery characteristics. At the first interim analysis, HIV vertical transmission rates in the short-short group (n = 230) were significantly higher than those in the long-long group (n = 221; 10.5% vs 4.1%), and thus the short-short regimen was discontinued. Thus, the final analysis includes 403 subjects in the long-long group, 343 in the long-short group, and 338 in the short-long group. For the entire study period, HIV vertical transmission rates for the long-long, long-short, and short-long regimens were 6.5%, 4.7%, and 8.6%, respectively, and did not differ significantly from one another. In pooled analyses, the vertical transmission rate was significantly lower when the mother was treated beginning at 28 weeks' gestation rather than at 35 weeks' gestation (1.6% vs 5.1%). The incidence of serious adverse events in the mothers was similar regardless of when zidovudine therapy was started (Table III). Similarly, the incidence of serious adverse events in the infants was similar in all 4 treatment groups.

Conclusions.—The short-short regimen clearly led to an increased rate of mother-to-child HIV transmission. However, the other 3 regimens had similar efficacy and safety in preventing vertical HIV transmission. Vertical

TABLE III.—Serious Adverse Events*

Event	Long Maternal Regimen (N = 769)	Short Maternal Regimen (N = 668)	Total (N = 1437)
	no. of women (%)		
Women			
Death†	3	8	11
Stillbirth	8	4	12
Severe anemia	7	4	11
Neutropenia	0	1	1
Infection or other HIV-related event	20	17	37
Event related to pregnancy or delivery	24	17	41
Other	6	13	19
≥1 Event	48 (6)	45 (7)	93 (6)

Infants	Long–Long (N = 403)	Long–Short (N = 343)	Short–Long (N = 338)	Short–Short (N = 315)	Total (N = 1399)
	no. of infants (%)				
Infants					
Death‡	5	7	5	4	21
Severe anemia (requiring hospitalization and transfusion)	4	0	1	4	9
Congenital abnormalities§	7	7	6	1	21
Neutropenia or leukopenia¶	7	3	5	2	17
Infection or other HIV-related event	43	43	40	33	159
Neonatal or obstetrical event	22	12	9	14	57
Other	6	4	5	20	
≥1 Event	71 (18)	63 (18)	55 (16)	52 (17)	241 (17)

*Serious adverse events, defined according to the Good Clinical Practice Guidelines, were reported immediately to the Thai Ministry of Public Health and the Department of International Product Safety and Pharmacovigilance at Glaxo Wellcome. Events were reported during pregnancy and for the first 6 months postpartum for the mothers and during the first 6 months of life for the infants. In the case of twins, only the first twin was included in the analysis.

†All 11 maternal deaths occurred after delivery. Five women died from pneumonia, 2 from sepsis, 1 from cryptococcal meningitis, and 1 from an AIDS-defining event; 2 deaths were suicides.

‡Seven infants died from recurrent infections, 4 from severe prematurity, 3 from neonatal events, 2 from AIDS, 1 from anemia and pneumonia at 10 weeks, 1 from tuberculosis, 1 from congenital diaphragmatic hernia and patent ductus arteriosus, 1 from an accidental injury, and 1 from neonatal asphyxia from a cleft palate.

§There were 24 congenital abnormalities in 21 infants; 5 infants had a ventricular septal defect, 4 had polydactyly, 3 had a cleft lip or cleft palate or both, 3 had congenital heart disease, 2 had Down's syndrome, 2 had monorchidism, 1 had a diaphragmatic hernia, 1 had omphalocele, 1 had hydrocephalus, 1 had microcephaly, and 1 had a microcornea.

¶All episodes of neutropenia and leukopenia resolved spontaneously without complications.

(Courtesy of Lallemant M, for the Perinatal HIV Prevention Trial (Thailand) Investigator: A trial of shortened zidovudine regimens to prevent mother-to-child transmission of human immunodeficiency virus type 1. *N Engl J Med* 343:982-991, 2000. Copyright 2000 by the Massachusetts Medical Society. All rights reserved.)

transmission rates were significantly higher when treatment of the mother was delayed from 28 to 35 weeks' gestation, regardless of whether the infant received 3 days or 6 weeks of treatment. Thus, the long-short zidovudine regimen is recommended for women who can be treated earlier in their pregnancy. If zidovudine treatment can only be instituted late in therapy, however, treatment of the infant for 6 weeks according to the short-long regimen appears prudent.

▶ Use of the results of the pediatric AIDS Clinical Trial Group Protocol 076 involving 12 weeks of intrapartum maternal zidovudine dosage, 300 mg of zidovudine every 3 h during labor, and 6 weeks of newborn therapy at 2 mg/kg per day dosage has become part of standard care for HIV infected gravidas in much of the Western world (see 1996 YEAR BOOK OF OBSTETRICS, GYNECOLOGY, AND WOMEN'S HEALTH, pp 84-85). The regimen is too expensive and too demanding of systematized health care services to be effective in most of Subsaharan Africa and Asia, where the epidemic rages most furiously. To this point, a variety of shortened zidovudine protocols have been reported (see 2000 YEAR BOOK, pp 121-125, 2001 YEAR BOOK, pp 90-92) as have abbreviated exposure to a new agent, Nevirapine (see 2000 YEAR BOOK, pp 46-47) in an attempt to reduce costs with minimal loss of effectiveness. This account of a 2.5-year systematic Thai trial exploring 4 zidovudine protocols varying in length of maternal and infant zidovudine exposure explores the effects of shortening either or both maternal and infant drug therapy on the risk of maternal fetal HIV transmission. Maternal trials tested therapy beginning at 28 weeks' gestational age, comparing them with those beginning at 35 weeks' gestational age (long and short maternal trials) with oral zidovudine during labor; infant trials varied between 3 days and 6 weeks of zidovudine exposure (short and long infant exposure) involving 1437 HIV-positive gravidas. Only those with contraindications to zidovudine, significant anemia, or abnormality in amniotic fluid volume were excluded from this study. Infants were seen at 2-week intervals for the first 6 weeks of life and at 4 and 6 months of age for ultimate HIV diagnosis. Vertical infection was based on 2 positive assays for HIV-RNA on PCR done after 1 month of life.

The initial 1.5 years compared standard therapy (long-long) with shortening of both maternal and fetal drug exposure (short-short). As noted before, standard dosage resulted in fetal transmission of 4.1%, whereas the short-short regimen resulted in a 10.5% transmission rate. For women delivering prematurely, presumably because of more extensive disease, transmission rates were increased roughly 3- to 4-fold. When results with standard care were compared with shortened maternal or infant dosage, maintenance of the 12-week maternal drug exposure was found essential to maintain infant transfer rates less than 5%; the shortened infant drug exposure from 6 weeks to 3 days produced no increase in infant transmission rates.

The authors provide strong evidence against the value of reducing maternal zidovudine exposure but find reduction in infant therapy to be an acceptable option in the interest of economy of time and effort. In managing maternal HIV infection, a vital issue in the third world, these observations support the premise that zidovudine reduces vertical transmission of maternal HIV by reducing cervical vaginal HIV-RNA copy numbers thereby reducing fetal infection in transit through the lower birth canal (see 2001 YEAR BOOK, pp 90-92).

T. H. Kirschbaum, MD

Effect of Breastfeeding on Mortality Among HIV-1 Infected Women: A Randomised Trial

Nduati R, Richardson BA, John G, et al (Univ of Nairobi, Kenya; Univ of Washington, Seattle)
Lancet 357:1651-1655, 2001

4–9

Background.—From 1992 to 1998, a randomized clinical trial was conducted regarding breast-feeding and formula feeding among the infants of a group of Kenyan women who were infected with HIV-1. The goal of the study was the identification of the frequency of breast milk transmission of HIV-1. In addition, the authors analyzed data from the study to determine the effects of breast-feeding on maternal death rates during the first 2 years after delivery. The findings of this secondary analysis are reported.

Methods.—HIV tests were offered to pregnant women who attended 4 Nairobi city council clinics. At about 32 weeks' gestation, a group of 425 HIV-1 seropositive women were randomly selected to either breast-feed their infants or feed them with formula. The mother-infant pairs were followed monthly in the first year after delivery and quarterly during the second year until death or the end of the study.

Results.—Mortality was found to be higher among mothers in the breast-feeding group (18 deaths) than among those in the formula group (6 deaths) (Fig 2). In the breast-feeding group the cumulative probability of maternal death at 24 months after delivery was 10.5%, compared with 3.8% in the formula group. Compared with formula-feeding mothers, the relative risk of death for breast-feeding mothers was 3.2. The attributable

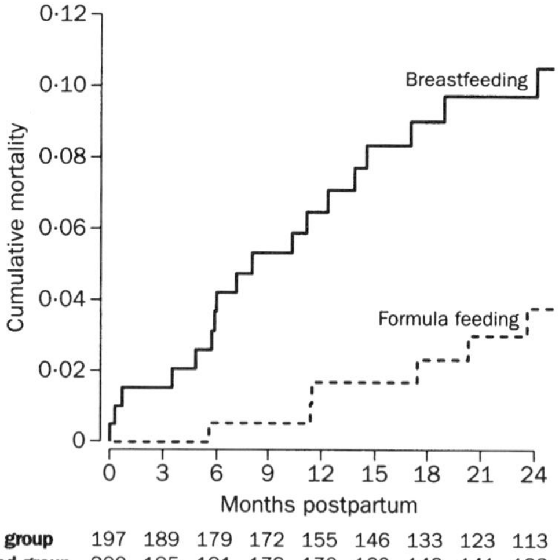

Breastfeed group	197	189	179	172	155	146	133	123	113
Formula feed group	200	195	191	179	170	160	149	141	123

FIGURE 2.—Mortality of mothers in breastfeeding and formula-feeding groups. Breastfeeding was associated with a higher risk of death in mothers than formula feeding. *P* = .009. (Courtesy of Nduati R, Richardson BA, John G, et al: Effect of breastfeeding on mortality among HIV-1 infected women: A randomised trial. *Lancet* 357:1651-1655, 2001, copyright by The Lancet Ltd.)

risk of maternal death because of breast-feeding was 69%. An association between maternal death and subsequent infant death was evident even after controlling for infant HIV-1 infection status.

Conclusions.—The findings suggest the possibility of adverse outcomes for both mother and infant from breast-feeding by HIV-1-infected women.

▶ These authors present a secondary analysis of a randomized, prospective controlled trial, previously published, that was originally designed to estimate the risk of infant and fetal transmission associated with breast-feeding in HIV-positive gravidas not on active HIV drug therapy.[1] They were able to establish that nursing adds a risk of 16.2% to the underlying risk of infant infection and accounted for 44% of all transmitted HIV infection to newborns. The authors were moved to analyze maternal deaths in the population of 397 women with complete follow-up to 2 years postpartum by the reports of others who found that infant death rates increased 3 to 4 times when death claimed the infants' mothers in comparison with those with intact parentage. One possibility is that the considerable energy costs of lactation which might decrease maternal host resistance to the HIV infection might be ameliorated by formula feeding. A further possibility is that endocrine or other physiologic factors associated with nursing might influence viral replications rates.

During the period from 1992 to 1998, aggregate maternal mortality in the study population was 6%, 9% occurring in breast-feeding mothers (18 of 197), and 3% in formula feeders (6 of 200). No significant difference was noted in infant death rates between the groups, and AIDS was identified as the cause of death in two thirds of the cases, complicated by opportunistic infections in 20%. The laboratory data are insufficient for the firm establishment of the cause of death in many cases, but many decedents showed CD4 counts of less than 200 per milliliter and HIV-RNA copy numbers greater than 100,000 per milliliter. In many cases, the clinical diagnosis was affirmed by evidence of Kaposi sarcoma, tuberculosis, cryptococosis, and marasmus. Though the number of cases of maternal death are few and compliance with formula feeding only 71%, it's likely some breast-feeding occurred in those assigned formula based on issues of cost, cultural norms, and inadequate clean water for formula preparation. All of these would serve to diminish the apparent savings in maternal life. Nonetheless, a 2-year mortality rate of 3% among HIV-infected Nairobi gravidas is a statistically significant decrease and warrants a therapeutic trial aimed at the role of maternal nutrient support and infant formula feeding in HIV-1-positive gravidas to reduce maternal and infant mortality.

T. H. Kirschbaum, MD

Reference

1. See Nduati R, John G, Mbori-Ngacha D, et al: Effect of breastfeeding and formula feeding on transmission of HIV-1: A randomized clinical trial. *JAMA* 283:1167-1174, 2000.

Preeclampsia: Evidence for Impaired Shear Stress–Mediated Nitric Oxide Release in Uterine Circulation

Kublickiene KR, Lindblom B, Krüger K, et al (Huddinge Univ, Sweden; Uppsala Univ, Sweden)
Am J Obstet Gynecol 183:160-166, 2000   4–10

Introduction.—Endothelial dysfunction has been linked to impaired nitric oxide activity in preeclampsia, but published data on the levels of stable nitric oxide metabolites in preeclampsia have varied. It is increasingly accepted, however, that shear stress generated by blood flow is the predominant physiologic stimulus for endothelial nitric oxide synthesis. Arteries from women with preeclampsia and from healthy pregnant women were studied for shear stress–mediated vasodilatation and for the role of nitric oxide in the modulation of pressure-induced myogenic and norepinephrine-induced tone.

Methods.—Study participants were 6 nulliparous women with preeclampsia who were undergoing cesarean delivery because of worsening of the preeclamptic state. Their median age was 27 years; the median gestational age was 36 weeks. Controls were 9 healthy pregnant women (median age, 27 years; median gestational age, 39 weeks). Five were scheduled for cesarean delivery because of breech presentation and 4 because of

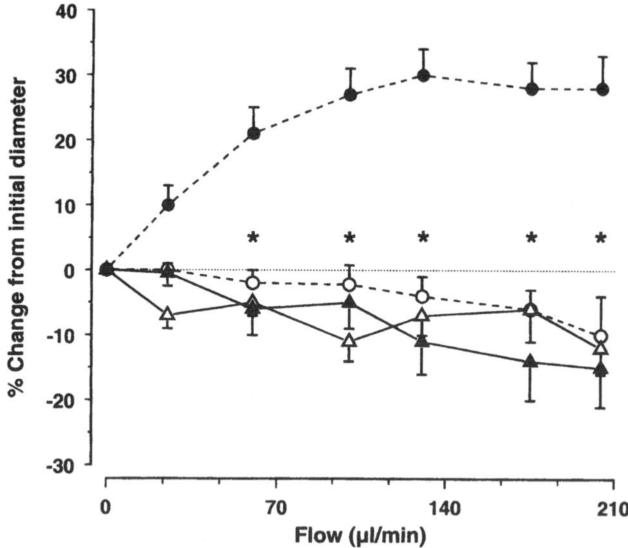

FIGURE 1.—Percentage of flow-mediated vasodilatation in myometrial arteries from women with preeclampsia *solid line* and normal pregnant women (*dashed line*) in physiologic sodium chloride solution (*filled circles* and *triangles*, respectively) and in Nω-nitro-L-arginine (*open circles* and *triangles*, respectively). Data were analyzed by multivariate analysis of variance for repeated measurements and presented as mean ± SEM. *Asterisks indicate* post hoc comparisons between 2 groups in physiologic sodium chloride solution at different flow steps (P < .001). (Courtesy of Kublickiene KR, Lindblom B, Krüger K, et al: Preeclampsia: Evidence for impaired shear stress–mediated nitric oxide release in uterine circulation. *Am J Obstet Gynecol* 183:160-166, 2000.)

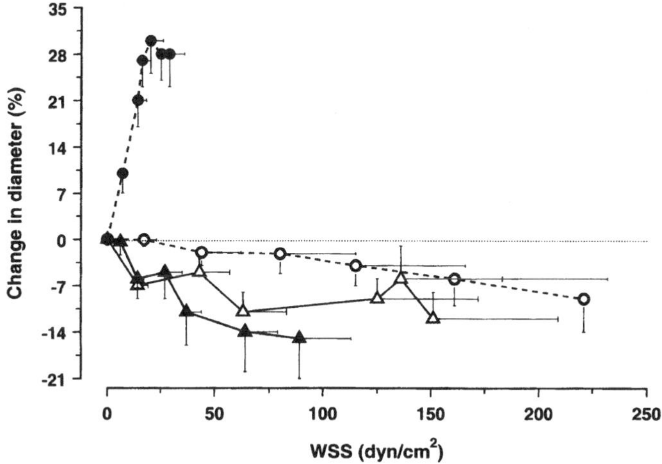

FIGURE 2.—Relationship between wall shear stress (*WSS*) and percentage of dilation (*change in diameter*) in myometrial arteries from women with preeclampsia (*solid line*) and normal pregnant women (*dashed line*), in physiologic sodium chloride solution (*filled circles* and *triangles*, respectively) and in Nω-nitro-L-arginine (*open circles* and *triangles*, respectively). (Courtesy of Kublickiene KR, Lindblom B, Krüger K, et al: Preeclampsia: Evidence for impaired shear stress–mediated nitric oxide release in uterine circulation. *Am J Obstet Gynecol* 183:160-166, 2000.)

previous cesarean delivery. Arteries were dissected from myometrial biopsy specimens and mounted on a pressure arteriograph. Responses to intraluminal flow, pressure, and a constrictor agonist (norepinephrine) were examined in the presence and absence of the nitric oxide synthase inhibitor Nω-nitro-L-arginine.

Results.—In healthy controls, but not in patients with preeclampsia, an increase in intraluminal flow led to dilation of isolated myometrial arteries (Fig 1). Addition of Nω-nitro-L-arginine failed to significantly affect flow-mediated responses in arteries from women with preeclampsia. In arteries from healthy controls, flow-mediated dilation was abolished by Nω-nitro-L-arginine. The range of shear stress values achieved was considerably greater in the arteries from women with preeclampsia, implying that their arteries were less sensitive to shear stress than were the healthy women's arteries because no vasodilatation was observed (Fig 2). After incubation with Nω-nitro-L-arginine, myogenic tone increased in arteries from both groups. Norepinephrine-induced tone did not differ significantly between control and preeclampsia groups.

Conclusion.—Preeclampsia was found to be associated with a failure of shear stress–mediated nitric oxide release in vitro, despite a lack of change in basal production. The failure of shear stress–mediated dilation in myometrial arteries might contribute to impaired uteroplacental blood flow in preeclampsia.

▶ This complex study makes fairly clear one of the principal barriers to evaluating the possible role of altered endothelial nitric oxide production in the increased vascular resistance of preeclampsia. The original observation by Furchgott and associates[1] that the vasodilating properties of acetylcholine are lost as vascular endothelium, a source of nitric oxide, was experimentally removed or damaged, as in preeclampsia, has led many investigators to look to blood concentrations of nitric oxide metabolites and simple pressure-driven models of vasoconstriction for answers. Vascular physiologists have established that the dominant stimulus to endothelial nitric oxide production results from blood flow in the form of transmitted shear stress directed at the endothelial surface and the subepithelial layer of the intima.[2]

As this report shows, study protocols for investigating shear stress in maternal vessels are demanding. These investigators worked with intramyometrial arteries dissected from uteri with segments with an internal diameter of 0.2 mm and lengths of less than one third of a centimeter. Vessel segments are mounted in a perfusion system allowing fluid perfusion at a measured rate and pressure, as well as the ability to measure small changes in vessel segment diameter with changing pressure as a measure of myogenic tone. These observations enable the calculation of the magnitude of shear stress. In this way, the investigators evaluated differences between vessels of 6 preeclamptics and 9 pregnant controls with respect to the effects of flow-mediated shear stress of hydrodynamic and vasoconstrictor (norepinephrine) increases in myogenic tone. They studied the role of nitric oxide in endothelial cells through the addition of an arginine antagonist to the perfusate which blocked the conversion of arginine to nitric oxide.

The results showed that normal gravidas exhibit considerable vasodilatation with increased blood flow, an effect that was lost and resulted in vasoconstriction with nitric oxide inhibition. In contrast, vessels from preeclamptics showed vasoconstriction in response to increased blood flow, a result that was independent of pharmacologic inhibition of nitric oxide synthesis (Fig 1). Where vessel dilatation was displayed as a function of calculated shear stress, the differences imposed on preeclamptic arterioles was marked (Fig 2). On the other hand, alteration of myogenic tone by changes in pressure at constant flow or the use of norepinephrine showed increased sensitivity in preeclamptic vessels unmediated by nitric oxide inhibition. This means that the effects of nitric oxide production by vascular endothelium in preeclamptics is a reflection of the loss of response to vascular shear stress and that we should not expect to see decreases in nitric oxide metabolic products in preeclampsia for that reason.

Although nitric oxide plays no role in the enhanced sensitivity to the pressure amines and vasoconstriction that results in peripheral vascular resistance in preeclampsia, the endothelial lesions more likely exist in endothelial receptor sites or subendothelial cytoskeleton, integrin adhesion sites, or some similar region. It may be that increased shear stress and pregnancy hypertension caused by the increased flow velocity in constricted blood vessels, a consequence of the Bernoulli principal, accounts for the increased nitric oxide metabolites seen in women with pregnancy-induced hypertension (see 1998 YEAR BOOK OF OBSTETRICS, GYNECOLOGY, AND WOMEN'S HEALTH, pp 23-25, and 1997 YEAR BOOK, pp 24-25). This is an important contribution to our knowledge of vasoregulation in normal and hypertensive pregnancy.

T. H. Kirschbaum, MD

References

1. Furchgott RF, Carvalho MH, Kahn MT, et al: Evidence for endothelial dependent vaso-dilatation of resistance vessels by acetylcholine. *Blood Vessel* 24:145, 1987.
2. Novis CM, Morigi M, Dondadelli R, et al: Nitric oxide synthesis by cultured endothelial cells is modulated by flow conditions. *Circ Res* 76:536, 1995.

Increased Fetal Erythroblasts in Women Who Subsequently Develop Pre-Eclampsia
Al-Mufti R, Hambley H, Albaiges G, et al (King's College Hosp, London)
Hum Reprod 15:1624-1628, 2000   4–11

Introduction.—Some fetal blood cells escape into the maternal circulation during pregnancy. Approximately 1 in 10^3 to 10^7 of nucleated cells in maternal blood are fetal. Recent studies have shown that in pregnancies complicated by preeclamptic toxemia (PET) and/or intrauterine growth restriction (IUGR), the number of fetal erythroblasts in maternal blood is higher. It is not known whether this rise in feto-maternal cell traffic precedes or is the result of placental damage related to these pregnancy complications. Uterine artery Doppler findings were reviewed to determine whether the number of fetal cells in maternal blood is increased before the onset of these complications.

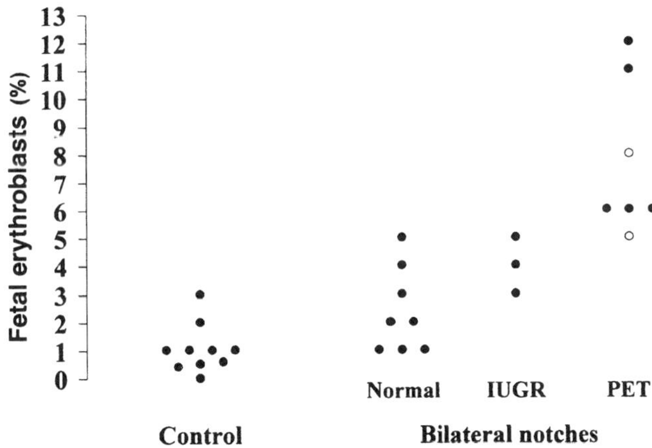

FIGURE 3.—Percentage of fetal erythroblasts in the enriched maternal blood sample (Kleihauer-Giemsa staining) from the control with normal waveforms, and the abnormal Doppler group with bilateral notches, which is subdivided into those with normal outcome, those delivering growth-restricted babies (IUGR), and those that developed pre-eclampsia (PET). In the latter group, *open circles* represent those patients with IUGR. (Courtesy of Al-Mufti R, Hambley H, Albaiges G et al: Increased fetal erythroblasts in women who subsequently develop pre-eclampsia. *Hum Reprod* 15:1624-1628, 2000. Copyright European Society for Human Reproduction and Embryology, by permission of Oxford University Press.)

Methods.—Maternal blood was collected from 18 pregnancies with abnormal Doppler findings at 22 to 24 weeks gestation and from 10 normal control subjects. Fetal erythroblasts were enriched from maternal blood via triple-density gradient centrifugation and magnet cell sorting with CD71 antibody. The percentages of these erythroblasts were calculated.

Results.—The median proportion of fetal erythroblasts in the group with abnormal Doppler findings was 4.5% (range, 1%-12%). This was significantly higher, compared with control subjects (median 1%; range, 0-3%; *P* < .001). The median proportion of fetal erythroblasts was higher among the 10 patients with an abnormal Doppler test who subsequently developed PET and/or IUGR (median, 5.5%; range, 3%-12%), compared with those with normal pregnancy outcome (median 2%; range, 1%-5%; *P* < .01) (Fig 3).

Conclusion.—Impaired placental perfusion is probably related to an increase in feto-maternal cell traffic, which precedes the onset of PET and/or IUGR by several weeks.

▶ The relatively poor ability to predict the presence of preeclampsia and intrauterine growth retardation based on second trimester uterine artery ultrasonic velocity patterns constitutes a serious problem in this study. The work does however comprise a small step in exploring the increase in mean normoblast numbers in the blood of women with preeclampsia compared to normotensives. Eighteen women, all but 1 primigravid, were found to have diastolic notching in their uterine artery Doppler velocity patterns at 22 to 26 weeks gestational age. Of this group, 7 proved to develop preeclampsia based on a blood pressure greater than 140/90 mm Hg and the presence of albuminuria measured quantitatively. A false-positive rate of 60%, using the Doppler finding, is not unexpected. Five women were said to develop infants with birthweight less than the 5th percentile, yielding a false-positive rate of 72% for second trimester ultrasonic prediction of intrauterine growth retardation. As Figure 3 illustrates, median maternal normoblast count established both by Kleihauer-Betke staining and FISH using a gammaglobin probe was greater in women developing preeclampsia than in 10 normal controls. The data is insufficient to calculate a useful mean value. No significant difference was noted in the comparison of pregnancies yielding growth-retarded infants compared to controls with respect to normoblast count. The authors' contention rests on the unproven assumption that ultrasonic diastolic notching of the uterine arteries at 22 to 26 weeks denotes high uterine artery impedance. They further hypothesize that elevated normoblast counts are a result of abnormal implantation of the placenta in preeclampsia. Whether this is true or not, they at least demonstrate that increased numbers of normoblasts appear as early as the middle of the second trimester in the course and development of preeclampsia in some women.

T. H. Kirschbaum, MD

Antiphospholipid Antibodies in Women at Risk for Preeclampsia
Branch DW, for the National Institute of Child Health and Human Development Maternal-Fetal Medicine Units Network (Univ of Utah, Salt Lake City; et al)
Am J Obstet Gynecol 184:825-834, 2001   4–12

Objective.—Antiphospholipid antibodies are associated with miscarriage and preeclampsia. Whether detection of antiphospholipid antibodies signals risk for preeclampsia was tested in women with a history of preeclampsia.

Methods.—Between July 1992 and January 1996, serum samples were obtained at 13 and 26 weeks of pregnancy from 317 women, average age 24.4 years, with a history of preeclampsia and from 100 nonpregnant, healthy, fertile women. Immunoglobulins G (IgG) and M (IgM) phospholipid binding assays were performed. The outcome variables were recurrent preeclampsia, miscarriage, stillbirth, neonatal death, intrauterine growth restriction (IUGR), and preterm birth.

Results.—Recurrent preelampsia developed in 62 (19.6%) women. Nineteen women had severe preeclampsia and 4 had delivery at less than 34 weeks' gestation. Eighteen (5.8%) of 309 women had infants with IUGR, and 3 of these had preeclampsia. Antiphospholipid antibody was not associated with an increased risk for preeclampsia. Two of 9 women with IgG antiphosphatidylserine antibody at more than 99th percentile had severe preeclampsia. This result was significant. IgM antiphosphatidylglycerol and IgM antiphosphatidylethanolamine antibodies were associated at the 95th percentile with preterm delivery. At least 1 of the 5 IgG antiphospholipid antibodies was associated with IUGR. Positive predictive values ranged from 22% to 50%.

Conclusion.—IUGR is modestly associated with IgG antiphospholipid antibodies. Screening women at risk for preeclampsia is of little value.

▶ This study, an extension of a previous study to evaluate the prophylactic use of aspirin in preventing preeclampsia (see 1999 YEAR BOOK OF OBSTETRICS, GYNECOLOGY, AND WOMEN'S HEALTH, pp 81-83), explores the usefulness of 5 assays of antiphospholipid antibody in predicting recurrent pregnancy-induced hypertension among those women who become preeclamptic. Here, 317 of the 508 women, 75% of them black, who had preeclampsia develop, were followed up through a subsequent pregnancy. The incidence of recurrent hypertensive disease was 19.6% and severe disease was 6%. None of the 5 anticardiolipin assays proved to have sufficient predictive strength to be clinically useful. Although risk ratios for recurrence were increased with those antibody positive, and 5.3% of women with recurrent hypertension were positive for IgG anticardiolipin, these cases were not associated with an increased rate of preterm birth. Findings were judged to be of no clinical significance.

The authors err, I believe, in ignoring the conclusive evidence produced by Leon Chesley years ago that preeclampsia is overwhelmingly a disease of primigravidas delivering at term.[1] Parous women with recurrent PIH are those with latent or unrecognized chronic cardiovascular renal disease, brought to clinical recognition by the cardiovascular changes of normal pregnancy and/or increased medical access. The question here is one of the relation of IgG or IgM antiphospholipid antibody to those chronic hypertensive syndromes. It is not clinically significant.

A further problem, which Dr Branch makes clear, is the technical problems associated with the antibody assays that yield coefficients of variation of 14.8% to 16.8% for IgG and 8.4% to 14.3% for IgM in their laboratory, the most experienced in the nation in those determinations. He cites a 1999 College of American Pathology study showing coefficents of variation up to 32% among laboratories performing anticardiolipin assays on the same samples. This adds a great deal of noise to results from the single lab and makes comparisons among separate labs even more hazardous.

T. H. Kirschbaum, MD

Reference

1. Chesley CL: Recognition of long term sequela of eclampsia. *Am J Obstet Gynecol* 189:249, 2000.

Umbilical Cord Serum Levels of Thromboxane B2 in Term Infants of Women Who Participated in a Placebo-Controlled Trial of Low-Dose Aspirin

Parker CR Jr, Hauth JC, Goldenberg RL, et al (Univ of Alabama, Birmingham)
J Matern Fetal Med 9:209-215, 2000
4–13

Introduction.—The effects of cyclooxygenase inhibitors, including aspirin (ASA), on platelet production of thromboxane A2 in males and nonpregnant females are well documented. Few trials have addressed this relationship for pregnant females and newborn infants of females exposed to ASA during gestation. Thromboxane B2 (TXB2), the stable metabolite of thromboxane A2, was measured in the umbilical cord serum of term infants of nulliparous, low-risk women, who were randomized to placebo or low-dose (60 mg) ASA on a daily basis from 24 weeks' gestation through delivery as part of a randomized clinical trial for prevention of preeclampsia.

Methods.—Umbilical cord sera from 230 singleton, term infants whose mothers were involved in the low-dose ASA trial were examined for TXB2 by investigators blinded to maternal treatment or maternal TXB2 levels. The data was analyzed in relation to assigned treatment group, longitudinal pattern of maternal serum TXB2 levels, and other maternal and newborn characteristics. The data were also assessed according to whether maternal serum levels of TXB2 were decreased 50% or more at 29 to 31 weeks, 34 to 36 weeks, and at delivery, compared with levels before trial initiation (Fig 1).

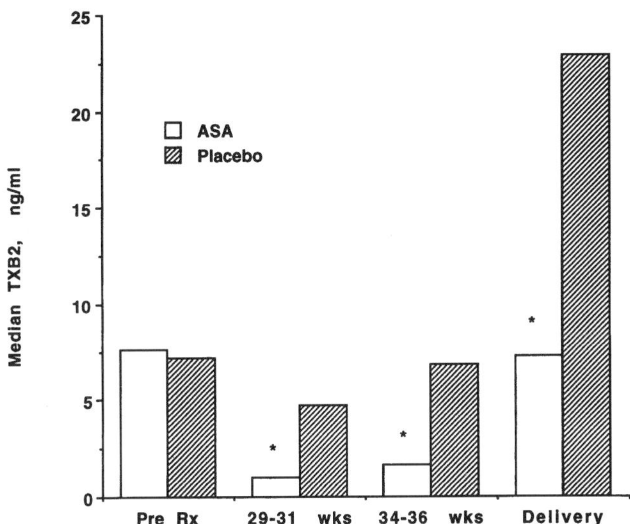

FIGURE 1.—Maternal serum TXB2 levels in women assigned to receive low-dose aspirin or placebo: intent to treat analysis. *P < .01 vs the placebo group. (Courtesy of Parker CR Jr, Hauth JC, Goldenberg RL, et al: Umbilical cord serum levels of thromboxane B2 in term infants of women who participated in a placebo-controlled trial of low-dose aspirin. *J Matern Fetal Med* 9:209-215, 2000. Reprinted by permission of Wiley-Liss, Inc., a subsidiary of John Wiley & Sons, Inc.)

Results.—In each treatment group, about 75% of females had serum TXB2 levels corresponding to that expected on the basis of their assigned treatment group (Fig 3). Umbilical cord TXB2 levels (ng/mL, mean ± SE) were significantly lower at term in the ASA group, compared with control subjects (56.6 ng/mL vs 119 ng/mL; P = .002). Umbilical cord TXB2 levels were correlated with those in the maternal serum at delivery in the ASA group (r = .24; P = .0005). This correlation was not observed in the placebo group (r = .06; P = .53). Despite their assigned treatment group, the 114 infants whose mothers had a 50% or greater longitudinal reduction in serum TXB2 had lower umbilical cord TXB2 levels (39.2 ng/mL) compared with the 116 infants whose mothers had less than 50% decreases in TXB2 (54.6 ng/mL; P = .027). The birthweights of these infants were inversely correlated (r = .17; P = .017) with maternal serum TXB2 at delivery and not correlated to umbilical cord TXB2 levels (Table 2). The best correlation between birthweight and TXB2 levels in maternal serum was observed in pregnancies assigned to receive placebo (r = .26; P = .0009).

Conclusion.—The umbilical cord serum TXB2 levels are (1) decreased with long-term ingestion of ASA, (2) well correlated with maternal serum TXB2 levels at delivery when there is evidence for consistent maternal use of ASA, and (3) not correlated with maternal serum TXB2 levels when there is no evidence for frequent maternal ingestion of cyclooxygenase inhibitors. The capacity for platelet production of TXA2 in fetal and maternal compartments is apparently independently regulated. An inverse

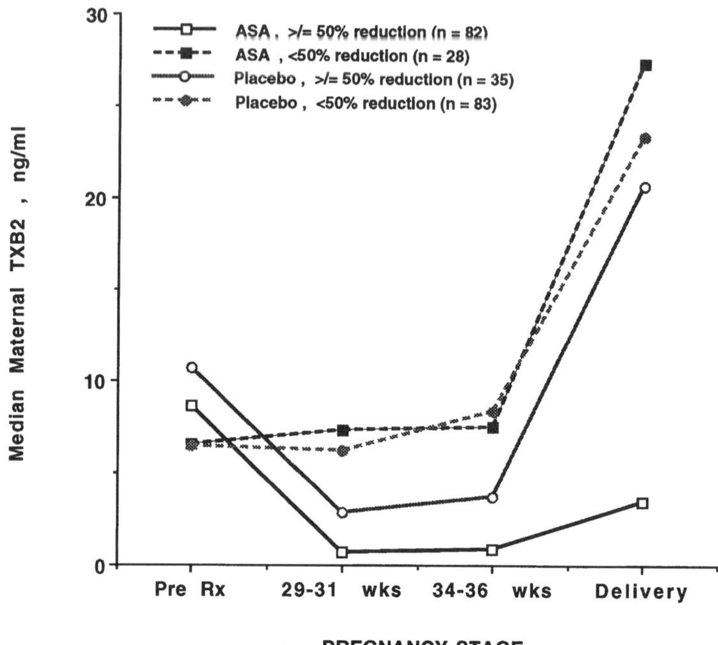

FIGURE 3.—Maternal serum TXB2 levels before and after treatment with low-dose aspirin or placebo: longitudinal pattern in women according to whether or not TXB2 levels were reduced ≥50% compared to pretreatment values. Serum TXB2 levels at the three sampling periods after initiation of the trial were compared to the pretreatment levels in each woman. The women were then subdivided according to whether or not there was a ≥50% reduction in two of the three posttreatment serum TXB2 levels compared to the pretreatment concentration. We excluded data for two women in whom insufficient serum samples were obtained to ascertain longitudinal TXB2 responses. (Courtesy of Parker CR Jr, Hauth JC, Goldenberg RL, et al: Umbilical cord serum levels of thromboxane B2 in term infants of women who participated in a placebo-controlled trial of low-dose aspirin. *J Matern Fetal Med* 9:209-215, 2000. Reprinted by permission of Wiley-Liss, Inc., a subsidiary of John Wiley & Sons, Inc.)

relationship was observed between maternal serum TXB2 levels at delivery and birthweight of newborn infants. This was most seen among pregnancies assigned to placebo and also among pregnancies in which little evidence was present to indicate a pattern of cyclooxygenase inhibitor use during pregnancy.

▶ It is clear that prophylactic use of 60 mg of aspirin daily in the prevention of preeclampsia has proven ineffective except in 1 1993 study conducted in part by this group of investigators (see 1994 YEAR BOOK OF OBSTETRICS, GYNECOLOGY, AND WOMEN'S HEALTH, pp 61-63). Subsequent work on that study population failed to show an effect in preventing preeclampsia, even in gravidas who showed a significant decrease in maternal serum thromboxane B2, the major stable metabolite of thromboxane A2, following aspirin therapy. Thromboxane A2 is a vasoconstrictive product largely of platelet but also of endothelial origin (see 1997 YEAR BOOK, pp 46-48 and 2000 YEAR BOOK, pp 133-134). Aspirin acts by inactivating platelet cyclooxygenase

TABLE 2.—Birthweights and Gestational Ages at Delivery of Infants of Women in ASA and Placebo Groups: Relation to Maternal TXB2 Levels

	Birthweight	Gestational Age
ASA		
Reduced ≥50%	3,441 ± 59 g*	39.5 ± 0.19 wks
Reduced <50%	3,150 ± 117 g	39.0 ± 0.41 wks
Placebo		
Reduced ≥50%	3,388 ± 74 g	39.1 ± 0.29 wks
Reduced <50%	3,176 ± 52 g	38.7 ± 0.21 wks

Note: Data expressed as mean ± SE.
*$P < .05$ vs values for infants of women in the same treatment group whose TXB2 levels were not reduced ≥ 50% compared to protreatment values.
Abbreviations: ASA, Aspirin; *TBX2*, thromboxane B2.
(Courtesy of Parker CR Jr, Hauth JC, Goldenberg RL, et al: Umbilical cord serum levels of thromboxane B2 in term infants of women who participated in a placebo-controlled trial of low-dose aspirin. *J Matern Fetal Med* 9:209-215, 2000. Reprinted by permission of Wiley-Liss, Inc., a subsidiary of John Wiley & Sons, Inc.)

which, in turn, reduces the production of thromboxane A2 and prostacyclin (PGI$_2$) differentially, depending on dosage. This new prospective double-blinded placebo-controlled study of 606 low-risk primigravidas conducted from 28 weeks to delivery was designed to study the relationship between maternal and fetal thromboxane B2 reduction by aspirin compared with controls. Further, the authors looked to the possibility of benefits other than the prevention of preeclampsia in those 228 women in whom both maternal and cord blood serum was available. Compliance in aspirin administration was judged by reduction in pretreatment maternal thromboxane B2 concentration.

Decreased umbilical cord blood thromboxane B2 occurred in instances of maternal aspirin administration and correlated well with those women with consistent aspirin intake, as judged by reduced serum thromboxane B2. The relationship between aspirin intake and reduced thromboxane B2 was complex, since it was seen not only in about 75% of pregnant women taking aspirin but also in nearly 30% of controls without aspirin intake. This phenomenon probably contributed to the failure to show clinical benefits of aspirin prophylaxis, since the reduction in thromboxane B2 in controls not taking aspirin diminished the likelihood of seeing a significant difference in those who received the drug. In those women receiving placebo who had reduced serum thromboxane concentrations, there was no correlated decrease in cord blood thromboxane B2. Interestingly, when infants of gravidas with reduced thromboxane B2 concentration, whether treated with aspirin or placebo, were identified, they proved to have a significant increase in birth weight at comparable gestational age, compared with those who had sustained less reduction in thromboxane B2 concentration. There was also a small but significant increase in mean pregnancy duration of approximately 4 days in those with reduced thromboxane B2 concentration. As the authors point out, the possible role of low-dose aspirin in influencing birth weight and duration of gestation warrants further study.

T. H. Kirschbaum, MD

Decreased Maternal Serum Leptin in Pregnancies Complicated by Preeclampsia

Laml T, Preyer O, Hartmann BW, et al (Univ of Vienna)
J Soc Gynecol Investig 8:89-93, 2001   4–14

Objective.—Leptin regulates appetite and body weight and may also regulate fetal growth and development during pregnancy. Whether leptin levels in maternal plasma and umbilical venous plasma differ between women with and without preeclampsia was investigated. The correlation between leptin levels and several clinical measures was also determined.

Methods.—All neonates born to 36 pairs of women, matched for prepregnancy body mass index (PPBMI) and gestational age, were healthy and delivered vaginally at term. Plasma leptin levels were compared with PPBMI, maternal and fetal hormone levels, and birth weight.

Results.—The preeclamptic and normal cohorts were well-matched except for systolic (155.7 vs 120.1 mm Hg) and diastolic (93.8 vs 75.1 mm Hg) blood pressures (Table 1). Median leptin concentration was significantly lower in the preeclamptic group than in the normal group (8.3 vs 20.2 ng/mL, OR 7.8). Maternal leptin levels were not correlated with PPBMI or fetal leptin levels in either group. Fetal leptin levels and birth weight were independently and significantly correlated in both groups.

Conclusion.—Leptin levels and birth weight were correlated in mothers with and without preeclampsia. Leptin levels were significantly lower in the preeclamptic group than in the normal group.

▶ There is little significant association between maternal leptin, which correlates with maternal weight, and umbilical blood leptin concentration, which appears strongly related to birth weight but not maternal weight or weight changes (see Abstract 1–2). This study attempts to clarify the uncertain status of maternal leptin in preeclampsia and in 36 pairs of preeclamptics and normal controls and to present data from both groups with similar body mass indexes. Maternal weight was therefore controlled as a confounding variable; maternal age has been shown by others to be unrelated to leptin concentration in women with similar body mass indexes. The

TABLE 1.—Composite Group Characteristics Between Women With Preeclampsia and Normal Controls

	Normal Pregnancy (n = 36)			Preeclampsia (n = 36)		
	Mean ± SD	Median	Range	Mean ± SD	Median	Range
Age at delivery (y)	28.0 ± 5.2	27.5	19.0-40.0	29.3 ± 6.0	31.0	15.0-39.0
Prepregnancy BMI (kg/m^2)	21.1 ± 2.1	20.9	17.6-25.3	21.1 ± 2.1	21.0	17.7-25.3
BMI at delivery (kg/m^2)	27.1 ± 2.3	27.1	23.0-32.0	26.2 ± 2.3	26.1	21.6-31.6
Leptin (ng/mL)	...	20.2	6.0-63.7	...	8.3	3.5-20.0*

Abbreviations: SD, Standard deviation; *BMI,* body mass index.
*P < .001, Mann-Whitney U test.
(Courtesy of Laml T, Preyer O, Hartmann BW, et al: Decreased maternal serum leptin in pregnancies complicated by preeclampsia. *J Soc Gynecol Investig* 8:89-93. Copyright 2001 by Elsevier Science.)

authors find leptin concentrations significantly lower in women with pre-eclampsia than in controls. As in the study referenced above, they show a relation between cord blood leptin and birth weight and none between maternal and cord blood leptin. This makes the problem clear. Preeclampsia in some way is associated with decreased maternal serum leptin. We will look forward to the reason.

T. H. Kirschbaum, MD

Should the Definition of Preeclampsia Include a Rise in Diastolic Blood Pressure of ≥15 mm Hg to a Level <90 mm Hg in Association With Proteinuria?
Levine RJ, Ewell MG, Hauth JC, et al (NIH, Bethesda, Md; Emmes Corp, Potomac, Md; Univ of Alabama, Birmingham; et al)
Am J Obstet Gynecol 183:787-792, 2000   4–15

Background.—While a rise in blood pressure is not considered technically to be included in the definition of preeclampsia, proteinuria concurrent with a rise in diastolic pressure of at least 15 mm Hg to less than 90 mm Hg may be associated with adverse outcome in pregnancy. Baseline characteristics and the outcomes of pregnancy were compared between a group of normotensive women whose diastolic blood pressure did not rise over 15 mm Hg along with proteinuria and a group of normotensive women who did have a rise in blood pressure and proteinuria.

Methods.—The study population was derived from the Calcium for Preeclampsia Prevention trial, which consisted of 4302 healthy nulliparous women who delivered at a minimum of 20 weeks' gestation. Baseline blood pressure was defined as the mean of measurements taken at 2 clinic visits before 22 weeks' gestation. Eighty-two women were normotensive but developed proteinuria within 7 days of having a rise in diastolic blood pressure of at least 15 mm Hg over baseline on 2 occasions separated by 4 to 168 hours. Comparison was made with normotensive women who had proteinuria but no rise in diastolic blood pressure and no gestational hypertension (Table 1).

Results.—The 82 women weighed more, had a higher body mass index, and had higher systolic blood pressure than the other normotensive women. Few data indicated any adverse effect on the pregnancy outcome, although these women gained weight at a greater rate, had larger babies, and had a twofold increase in abdominal delivery (Table 2).

Conclusions.—No clinical usefulness was attached to a rise in diastolic blood pressure of 15 mm Hg or greater in women who had proteinuria but were otherwise normotensive.

▶ This is an important study which attacks the utility of incremental increases in blood pressure during pregnancy (at least 15 mm Hg of diastolic or 30 mm Hg of systolic pressure above baseline values) in establishing the diagnosis of pregnancy hypertension. These criteria have been viewed as

TABLE 1.—Characteristics at Study Entry of Healthy Nulliparous Women During Normotensive Pregnancy With or Without a Rise in Diastolic Blood Pressure of ≥ 15 mm Hg in Association With Proteinuria

Characteristic	With Rise in Diastolic Blood Pressure Plus Proteinuria (n = 82)	Without Rise in Diastolic Blood Pressure Plus Proteinura (n = 3147)
Age (y)	21.0	21.0
Height (cm)	162.7	162.4
Weight (kg)	73.1*	66.8
Body mass index (kg/m²)	27.5*	25.3
Blood pressure (mm Hg)		
Systolic	107.5†	105.6
Diastolic	58.9	58.7
Previous abortion (%)	23.2	25.7
Current smoker (%)	13	13
Race (%)		
White non-Hispanic	42	37
White Hispanic	22	17
Black	33‡	44
Other	4	3

*$P < 0.001$.
†$P = 0.05$.
‡$P = 0.06$.
(Courtesy of Levine RJ, Ewell MG, Hauth JC, et al: Should the definition of preeclampsia include a rise in diastolic blood pressure of ≥ 15 mm Hg to a level < 90 mm Hg in association with proteinuria? *Am J Obstet Gynecol* 183:787-792, 2000.)

valuable in evaluating young gravidas who present in the first trimester with low normal blood pressures. For a teenage woman whose baseline blood pressure is 90/60, a blood pressure of 135/85 would be distinctively pathologic using incremental criteria. Such young women make up the bulk of those erroneously reported as showing normotensive eclampsia in our literature.

Data analysis here is based on 4302 nulliparous women collected from 5 maternal-fetal medicine centers and followed to at least 20 weeks' gestational age. The patients were admitted to the study at 13 to 21 weeks' gestational age (a mean of 17 weeks) and were required to have had screening blood pressures less than 135/85 without albuminuria on at least 2 prenatal visits. Women were judged to have gestational hypertension if their diastolic pressure exceeded 90 mm of mercury, to have albuminuria with greater than 300 mg with albumin excreted for 24 hours, and to be preeclamptic if both were present. Routine glucose tolerance testing was carried out in the second trimester. In this population, 92% of women had evidence of at least 1 incident in which an increase in diastolic blood pressure of 15 mm of mercury or more occurred, and 50% of women showed 2 such episodes. In this latter group, the subsequent likelihood of diagnosis of preeclampsia or gestational hypertension was 50%, that is, they made up half of all women entered into this retrospective study.

It's important that few, if any, first-trimester blood pressures were used here, and that nearly all entry blood pressures were done in the second

TABLE 2.—Selected Maternal and Perinatal Outcomes Among Healthy Nulliparous Women With Normotensive Pregnancies With or Without a Rise in Diastolic Blood Pressure of ≥ 15 mm Hg in Association With Proteinuria

Outcome	With Rise in Diastolic Blood Pressure Plus Proteinuria (n = 82)	Without Rise in Diastolic Blood Pressure Plus Proteinuria (n = 3147)
Maternal outcomes		
Plasma glucose concentration		
1 h after 50-g oral glucose	111	107
challenge (mg/dL)		
Gestational diabetes mellitus (%)	1.4	1.9
Weight gain in third trimester (lb/wk)	1.5*	1.2
Induced labor (%)	9.8	11.3
Cesarean delivery (%)	28.1†	13.0
Perinatal outcomes		
Gestational age at birth (d)	276	275
Gestational age at birth <34 wk (%)	2.4	3.2
Gestational age at birth >41 wk (%)	8.5‡	3.5
Birth weight (g)	3369‡	3201
Birth weight <2500 g (%)	6.1	8.3
Birth weight >4000 g (%)	12.2§	6.1
Intrauterine growth restriction‖ (%)	6.1	5.7
Neonatal intensive care unit		
admission (%)	14.6	12.9
Perinatal morbidity or death¶ (%)	4.9	5.7
Respiratory distress syndrome (%)	4.9	3.8
Mechanical ventilation (%)	0.0	2.2
Intraventricular hemorrhage grade		
III/IV (%)	0.0	0.2
Necrotizing enterocolitis (%)	0.0	0.2
Intrauterine death (%)	0.0	1.0
Death in neonatal intensive care unit (%)	0.0	0.5

Note: Outcomes were available for ≥ 97% of the women except for plasma glucose concentration (88%), gestational diabetes mellitus (86%), and third-trimester weight gain (85%). Perinatal outcomes are based on live births only.

*$P < 0.005$.

†$P = < 0.001$.

‡$P = ≤ 0.05$

§$P = 0.06$.

‖Intrauterine growth restriction considered to represent < 10th percentile for gestational age according to the standards of Brenner et al uncorrected for parity, race, and infant sex. According to the standards of Zhang and Bowes with adjustment for parity, race, and infant sex, intrauterine growth restriction prevalences were 13.4% in those with blood pressure elevation in association with proteinuria and 9.2% in those without, a difference that was not statistically significant.

¶This category included births with 1 or more of the following negative outcomes: respiratory distress syndrome, seizures, need for ventilatory support, grade III/IV intraventricular hemorrhage, necrotizing enterocolitis, intrauterine death, or death in the neonatal intensive care unit.

(Courtesy of Levine RJ, Ewell MG, Hauth JC, et al: Should the definition of preeclampsia include a rise in diastolic blood pressure of ≥ 15 mm Hg to a level < 90 mm Hg in association with proteinuria? *Am J Obstet Gynecol* 183:787-792, 2000.)

trimester. This means that women whose first-trimester blood pressures underwent a significant increase were not recognized, and the possible utility of recognizing incremental blood pressures values from first-trimester baselines was unrecognizable in principle among the study subjects. Further, women with screening diastolic blood pressures equal to or greater than 75 mm of mercury were operationally excluded, since if their diastolic blood pressure increased by greater than 15 mm of mercury to 90 mm Hg or more, they were labeled hypertensive and excluded from the study. This means that women with diastolic blood pressures in the upper range of normal were rejected from the study. Assuming that blood pressure changes were, in part, randomly distributed, this would tend among those women accepted to increase the number who showed a diastolic blood pressure increment of 15 mm or more during prenatal care.

Few clinicians make a diagnosis of hypertension in pregnancy based on a single elevated value, for good reasons as this study shows. The diagnosis should rather be based on a pattern of progressive increments with time during prenatal care, an approach that is unevaluable by the structure of this study. Preeclamptic or gestationally hypertensive women showed little or no perinatal morbidity as an apparent consequence of that diagnosis as previously reported (2001 YEAR BOOK OF OBSTETRICS, GYNECOLOGY, AND WOMEN'S HEALTH, pp 101-103). Among women with diastolic blood pressure increases of 15 mm of mercury or more and albuminuria, prominent weight gain, gestational diabetes, increased birth weight, and an increased likelihood of delivery past 41 weeks but not macrosomia were seen in comparison with those without hypertension. For uncertain reasons, those with hypertension and albuminuria had a cesarean section rate greater than 2-fold higher than those without. Failure to use first-trimester blood pressures in establishing baselines and the differential exclusion of normotensive women with screening blood pressures in the upper normal range make the authors' conclusions of questionable reliability.

T. H. Kirschbaum, MD

Elevated Circulating Homocyst(e)ine Levels in Placental Vascular Disease and Associated Pre-Eclampsia
Wang J, Trudinger BJ, Duarte N, et al (Univ of Sydney, Australia; Univ of New South Wales, Sydney)
Br J Obstet Gynaecol 107:935-938, 2000   4–16

Introduction.—Maternal preeclampsia and fetal intrauterine growth restriction are related to vascular disease in the maternal uteroplacental and fetal umbilical placental circulations. The fetal syndromes associated with this vascular lesion have been correlated with pathology in the maternal uteroplacental circulation similar to that observed with preeclampsia. Maternal and fetal plasma homocysteine levels were examined in pregnancies with preeclampsia and/or Doppler US-identified umbilical placental vascular disease.

Methods.—Twenty-six normal third-trimester pregnancies and 60 with clinical evidence of placental vascular disease were examined. Umbilical Doppler was used to confirm abnormal vascular findings. There were 19 pregnancies with preeclampsia, 17 with Doppler-identified umbilical placental vascular disease, and 24 with both preeclampsia and umbilical placental vascular disease. Maternal venous blood was obtained within 1 week before delivery and fetal blood was collected from the umbilical vein between delivery of the infant and delivery of the placenta. Total homocysteine levels were determined.

TABLE 1.—Clinical Characteristics and Plasma Homocysteine Levels. Values Are Given as [%] or mean (SEM)

	NP (n = 26)	PE (n = 19)	UPVD (n = 17)	PE with UPVD (n = 24)
Maternal age (year)	31·6 (0·9)	32·4 (1·4)	30·1 (1·7)	29·4 (1·3)
Parity (no. of primiparae)	4 [15·3]	8 [42·1]	11 [64·7]†	14 [58·3]†
GA at delivery (weeks)	39·3 (0·4)	35·8 (1·0)†	32·8 (0·9)‡	31·3 (0·6)‡
Infant birthweight (g)	3481·7 (121·9)	2304·8 (230·1)‡	1519·3 (157·8)‡	1296·2 (116·1)‡
Centile	50·5 (5·9)	20·2 (5·4)†	13·9 (6·6)‡	8·4 (4·2)‡
No. < 10th centile	0 [0]	10 [52·6]‡	12 [70·6]‡	21 [87·5]‡
Placenta weight (g)	689·8 (27·0)	567·9 (70·1)	323·6 (43·5)‡	311·8 (24·3)‡
Delivery method: caesarean section	26 [100]	13 [68·4]*	17 [100]	23 [95·8]
Homocyst(e)ine (μmol/L)				
Maternal	5·9 (0·3) (n = 22)	9·4 (0·6)‡ (n = 16)	8·8 (0·9)† (n = 12)	8·8 (0·5)‡ (n = 21)
Fetal	4·7 (0·3) (n = 26)	6·7 (0·6)† (n = 18)	5·5 (0·9) (n = 16)	6·0 (0·6) (n = 21)

*P < 0.05
†P < 0.01
‡P < 0.001

Abbreviations: NP, normal pregnancy; PE, pre-eclampsia; UPVD, umbilical placental vascular disease; GA, gestational age.

(Courtesy of Wang J, Trudinger BJ, Duarte N, et al: Elevated circulating homocyst(e)ine levels in placental vascular disease and associated pre-eclampsia. *Br J Obstet Gynaecol* 107:935-938, 2000, Elsevier Science, publisher.)

Results.—Mean gestational age at delivery was later, and birth weight was higher, in the normal than in the affected group. The homocysteine levels were higher for affected fetal and all 3 affected maternal groups compared with the normal fetal and maternal groups (Table 1). Fetal plasma homocysteine levels were significantly associated with maternal levels in the whole study population (P = .0001). Analyses of fetal and maternal concentrations showed significant correlations for normal pregnancy (r = .65, P = .001), preeclampsia (r = .68, P = .005), and preeclampsia and umbilical placental disease (r = .48; P = .042). No such correlation was observed for the subset of fetuses with umbilical placental vascular disease in the absence of maternal hypertension (r = .12; P = .73). Of interest, fetal plasma homocysteine was weakly associated with infant birth weight (r = .40; P = .043).

Conclusion.—Elevated circulating homocysteine may be involved in the pathogenesis of uteroplacental vascular disease related to preeclampsia, and may be a risk marker for this in the mother.

▶ The presence of elevated concentrations of blood homocysteine in patients with peripheral, coronary, and cerebral vascular disease has generated a hypothesis that this intermediate in the metabolism of methionine, vitamin B_{12}, and folic acid may serve as the origin of epithelial injury underlying atherosclerotic change (2001 YEAR BOOK OF OBSTETRICS, GYNECOLOGY, AND WOMEN'S HEALTH, pp 87-89.) It's also a candidate for the blood-borne basis for the pathologic changes in maternal endothelium in pregnancy hypertension. Such endothelial changes in the uteroplacental and systemic maternal vasculature result in arteriolar vasoconstriction, atherosclerosis in decidual vessels, and thrombotic ischemic lesions in kidney, liver, brain, and myocardium associated with severe pregnancy-induced hypertension. Homocysteine plasma concentrations from 26 women with normal pregnancies were compared with samples from 19 preeclamptics and 41 women with "uteroplacental vascular disease" with or without preeclampsia. The patient categorizations are regrettably unclear. Of the 19 women with preeclampsia, only 8 were primigravid, leaving the majority better described as multiparas with pregnancy-induced hypertension. Uteroplacental vascular disease was based on the diagnosis of fetal growth retardation with abnormal umbilical Doppler artery velocity profiles. The first of these findings is not pathognomonic for placental abnormality, and the second has proven to be an unreliable measure of placental function of any sort. Of the 24 women with "preeclampsia with uteroplacental vascular disease," only 14 were primigravid and likely preeclamptic. Most patients categorized as showing uteroplacental vascular disease had blood sampling performed significantly earlier in pregnancy than other subjects did, for uncertain reasons. However, plasma homocysteine was significantly elevated in all test subjects compared with control subjects, and fetal umbilical plasma homocysteine concentrations were elevated in fetuses from "preeclamptics." Without providing definitive answers, this work supports the hypothesis that altered homocysteine metabolism is in some way part of the mechanism of the pathophysiology of pregnancy-induced hypertension. This is a potentially important area which warrants better investigative efforts.

T. H. Kirschbaum, MD

Expectant Management of Early Onset, Severe Pre-Eclampsia: Perinatal Outcome
Hall DR, Odendaal HJ, Kirsten GF, et al (Univ of Stellenbosch, Tygerberg, South Africa)
Br J Obstet Gynaecol 107:1258-1264, 2000   4–17

Background.—While delivery is the only way to eliminate severe preeclampsia, high perinatal mortality and morbidity caused by prematurity result from this course. Expectant management may improve neonatal outcome. Perinatal outcomes with expectant management of severe preeclampsia were evaluated.

Methods.—The study population consisted of all 340 women with singleton pregnancies who came for treatment for early onset severe preeclampsia over a 5-year period. Mother and fetus were otherwise stable. The interventions included frequent clinical and biochemical monitoring of the mother's status, particularly blood pressure control. For the fetus, the heart rate was monitored at 6-hour intervals, weekly Doppler studies were done, and US was performed every 2 weeks. The interventions were planned to prolong gestation, reduce the perinatal mortality rate, and improve neonatal survival without major complications.

Results.—The number of days gained in gestation ranged from 1 to 47, with a mean of 11 days. Perinatal mortality was 24 per 1000, with fetal distress being the most common indication for delivery (44.4%). None of the mothers died, and only 3 required admission to the adult intensive care unit. Maternal factors were the chief indication for delivery in 25.9% of deliveries. The neonatal survival rate was 94%. Only gestational age at delivery was significantly linked to neonatal outcome. The factors contributing most to neonatal mortality and morbidity were pulmonary complications and sepsis. Two intrauterine deaths occurred, and 3 pregnancies were terminated before viability was achieved. Cesarean section was used for 81.5% of women whose pregnancy was threatened by fetal distress. Intensive care of the neonate was required in 40.7% of cases, with a median stay of 6 days.

Conclusions.—High perinatal and neonatal survival rates were achieved with expectant management of women with early onset severe preeclampsia as well as careful neonatal care. Judicious use of neonatal intensive care facilities was achieved.

▶ Because severe pregnancy hypertension can be associated with serious progressive impairment of maternal and fetal organ systems, it is usually treated with its only definitive remedy: delivery. This South African study explores the merits of temporary expectant nonoperative management in women with diastolic blood pressures ranging from 110 to 120 at 24 to 34 weeks. Candidates for immediate delivery with multiple maternal organ system disturbances including coagulopathy or gross fetal abnormalities were excluded from the study. Hypertensive women were treated with antihypertensive agents, and magnesium sulfate if in labor. Betamethasone was administered weekly to 33 weeks, and inpatient monitoring included fetal US, amniotic fluid index determination, and umbilical artery Doppler velocimetry. Expectant management lasted a mean of 11 days with wide variability in duration (SD 7 days). Elective delivery was carried out at 34 weeks in 16% of women (54 cases); delivery was selected on grounds of "fetal distress" in 44% of cases and maternal deterioration in 26%. Most deliveries were abdominal (81.5%), but 103 women had labor induction. Abruption was an important complication in 20.2% of cases, resulting in 2 fetal deaths. Perinatal mortality overall was 24 per 1000 live births, and neonatal survival was 94%. The authors' experience indicates that expectant management of this grave complication of pregnancy is at least feasible with careful monitoring and flexibility in management decisions. Sudden unanticipated abruption is a major problem which rapidly changes the treatment options, but with care and luck, immaturity, the major correlative of perinatal death in such pregnancies, may be partly ameliorated by this approach.

T. H. Kirschbaum, MD

Factor V Leiden Paradox: Risk of Deep-Vein Thrombosis but not of Pulmonary Embolism

Bounameaux H (Univ Hosp of Geneva)
Lancet 356:182-183, 2000

4-18

Introduction.—The Leiden mutation of blood coagulation factor V is seen in approximately 5% of white persons. This mutation confers coagulation inhibitor–activated protein C (APC) resistance. The risk of deep vein thrombosis (DVT) and pulmonary embolism (PE) in persons with this mutation is discussed.

Risk of DVT and PE.—Persons heterozygous for the Leiden mutation carry about a 5-fold increased risk of DVT. The relative risk of PE is lower than that of DVT in patients with APC resistance. Thrombosis occurs markedly less often in the iliofemoral veins in factor V Leiden. Since PE originates most commonly from large, proximal (iliofemoral) thrombi, this finding could explain why patients with factor V Leiden are less prone than those without to develop PE when they have DVT. The relationship of this phlebographic pattern with this common inherited hypercoagulable state may have implications for the treatment of carriers of the mutation who experience DVT. Since their propensity for PE appears to be lower than that of noncarriers, they do not require a lengthy period of anticoagulation treatment.

Conclusion.—The differing risk of DVT and PE among persons with factor Leiden Va is not consistent with the concept of DVT and PE being 2 clinical manifestations of a single disorder named venous thromboembolism. This factor V Leiden DVT/PE paradox does not jeopardize the venous thromboembolism concept. It merely highlights the range of this disease—from isolated calf DVT to massive PE. The question remains: Why does APC resistance decrease the likelihood of proximal and extensive DVT?

▶ The Leiden mutation is a replacement mutation in the gene for clotting factor V found on chromosome 1. It renders the factor V protein relatively resistant to the anticoagulant-activated β-protein-C and its cofactor protein S. Proteins C and S are normally activated in the presence of thrombin, thrombomodulin, and platelets, in turn activated at sites of epithelial injury. Inhibition of this anticoagulant effect has been associated with an increased risk of thromboembolus,[1,2] abortion,[3] fetal death,[4] and pregnancy-induced hypertension[5] (YEAR BOOK 2000, pp 115-121, 134-137). The carrier incidence for the mutation is 5% in Caucasians and its presence increases the risk of DVT 3-fold in pregnancy. The chance of a thrombotic episode among gravidas heterozygous for the mutation is about 10%.

The author summarizes the results of 7 publications to establish that the incidence of PE in women exhibiting factor V resistance to surplus activated protein C is much less than is the risk of DVT, albeit the rate of occurrence is larger than in normal controls. The cause of this differential phenomenon is uncertain but may reflect the increased thrombin generation by the mutated factor V protein, which tends to hold venous thombi in situ and prevent embolization. The finding should offer some comfort to women bearing the Leiden mutation and to their obstetric attendants.

T. H. Kirschbaum, MD

References

1. Dizon-Townson DS, Nelson LM, Easton K, et al: The factor V Leiden mutation may predispose women to severe preeclampsia. *Am J Obstet Gynecol* 175:902-905, 1996. (1998 YEAR BOOK OF OBSTETRICS, GYNECOLOGY, AND WOMEN'S HEALTH, p 210.)
2. McColl MD, Ramsay JE, Tait RC, et al: Risk factors for pregnancy associated venous thromboembolism. *Thromb Haemost* 78:1183-1188, 1997. (1999 YEAR BOOK OF OBSTETRICS, GYNECOLOGY, AND WOMEN'S HEALTH, p 71.)
3. Dizon-Townson DS, Meline L, Nelson LM, et al: Fetal carriers of the factor V Leiden mutation are prone to miscarriage and placental infarction. *Am J Obstet Gynecol* 177:402-405, 1997. (1999 YEAR BOOK OF OBSTETRICS, GYNECOLOGY, AND WOMEN'S HEALTH, p 63.)
4. Meinardi JR, Middeldorp S, de Kam PJ, et al: Increased risk for fetal loss in carriers of the factor V Leiden mutation. *Ann Intem Med* 130:736-739, 1999. (2000 YEAR BOOK OF OBSTETRICS, GYNECOLOGY, AND WOMEN'S HEALTH, p 136.)
5. van Pampus MG, Dekker GA, Wolf H, et al: High prevalence of hemostatic abnormalities in women with a history of severe preeclampsia. *Am J Obstet Gynecol* 180:1146-1150, 1999. (2000 YEAR BOOK OF OBSTETRICS, GYNECOLOGY, AND WOMEN'S HEALTH, p 119.)

Safety of Withholding Heparin in Pregnant Women With a History of Venous Thromboembolism

Brill-Edwards P, for the Recurrence of Clot in This Pregnancy Study Group (McMaster Univ, Hamilton, Ont, Canada; et al)
N Engl J Med 343:1439-1444, 2000   4–19

Background.—The risk of pregnancy-related venous thromboembolism appears to be increased among women with a past history of such events. There is ongoing debate over whether these women should continue to receive heparin during the antepartum period. The situation is complicated by the lack of accurate data on the risk of recurrent thromboembolism in women not receiving heparin. The safety of withholding heparin during the antepartum period for women with a history of venous thromboembolism was prospectively assessed.

Methods.—The multicenter prospective cohort study included 125 consecutive pregnant women with 1 previous episode of venous thromboembolism. During the antepartum period, heparin therapy was withheld. Anticoagulant therapy was then resumed, continuing through 4 to 6 weeks post partum. The rate of recurrent venous thromboembolism during the antepartum period was analyzed. In addition, 95 patients underwent laboratory studies to assess the incidence of thrombophilia.

Results.—Three women had recurrent venous thromboembolism during the antepartum period, an incidence of 2.4%. No recurrences developed in

TABLE 1.—Risk Factors and Rate of Recurrent Venous Thromboembolic Events in 95 Women With Previous Venous Thomboembolism

Variable	Idiopathic Condition and Abnormal Test Results	Temporary Risk Factor and Abnormal Test Results	Idiopathic Condition and Normal Test Results	Temporary Risk Factor and Normal Test Results
Recurrent events (no.)				
Total	2	2	2	0
Ante partum	1	1	1	
Post partum	1	1	1	
No recurrence (no.)	8	13	24	44
Recurrent rate				
Percent (95% CI)	20 (2.5-55.6)	13 (1.7-40.5)	7.7 (0.01-25.1)	0 (0.0-8.0)

Note: Temporary risk factors were pregnancy, use of oral contraceptives, surgery, trauma, immobility, and chemotherapy. Only women in whom laboratory studies were performed are included.

Abbreviation: CI, Confidence interval.

(Reprinted by permission of *The New England Journal of Medicine* courtesy of Brill-Edwards P, for the Recurrence of Clot in This Pregnancy Study Group: Safety of withholding heparin in pregnant women with a history of venous thromboembolism. *N Engl J Med* 343:1439-1444, 2000. Copyright 2000, Massachusetts Medical Society. All rights reserved.)

a subgroup of 44 patients who had no evidence of thrombophilia and whose previous thrombotic episode was related to a temporary risk factor (Table 1). Abnormal laboratory results or a previous episode of idiopathic thrombosis were present in 51 women. For this group, the incidence of antepartum recurrence of venous thromboembolism was 5.9%.

Conclusion.—Pregnant women with a single previous episode of venous thromboembolism are at low risk for recurrent episodes during the antepartum period. Antepartum heparin therapy does not appear to be indicated on a routine basis for such patients. Postpartum anticoagulant therapy is still recommended.

▶ Although pulmonary embolus is an uncommon event in pregnancy, occurring in roughly 0.3% or fewer of all pregnancies, it continues as the leading cause of maternal mortality. The prophylactic use of anticoagulants in women with a prior history of thromboembolus is an important consideration. The estimates of rates of recurrence range from 0% to 13%, and the majority of reports of relatively high prevalence occurred prior to the common employment of objective diagnostic measurements such as compression, venous US, or venography for the diagnosis of pulmonary embolus.

This observational study attempts a more rigorous estimate of risk, studying a 125 gravida with a single prior episode of thromboembolus proven by modern imaging techniques. Women were enrolled prior to 20 weeks' gestational age. Women with known congenital thrombophilia associated with protein C or S deficiency, antiphospholipid antibody, lupus anticoagulant, Leiden factor V mutation, or prothrombin G2021A mutation were excluded from entry. All enrolled women were screened by compression US of iliac veins bilaterally, and in 95 cases, procoagulant testing was carried out. The gravidas received postpartum anticoagulant both heparin and warfarin, within 24 hours after delivery. No antepartum anticoagulants were employed.

Antepartum thromboembolus occurred in 3 women; 2 had antepartum deep venous thrombosis and 1 woman experienced pulmonary embolus at 9 weeks' gestational age. Three women had deep vein thrombosis post partum, 1 at 11 weeks after a missed abortion and 2 at 3 and 8 weeks post partum. All 3 of these women received postpartum anticoagulants prior to the thrombosis. None of the 44 women who had temporary prior risk factors (pregnancy, oral contraceptive use, surgery, physical trauma, etc) and normal screens from thrombophilia experienced thromboembolus.

This is support for the premise that women with prior thomboembolus should first be screened for thrombophilic elements in plasma and prophy-lactic heparin confined largely to those with positive screens. This proposi-tion has been advanced in 2 recent comprehensive reviews of the subject.[1,2] As the authors indicate, the small number of cases here generate a wide range of rates of probable recurrence, and the exclusion of women with a pulmonary embolus within 3 months of the onset of pregnancy diminishes the generalizability of their results. This work supports prior claims that the risk for pregnancy thromboembolus decreases with time after the primary event, and fatal pulmonary embolus is a rare, singular recurrent event after a prior embolus.

T. H. Kirschbaum, MD

References

1. Green I: Thrombosis in pregnancy: Maternal and fetal issues. *Lancet* 353:1258, 1999.
2. McCall MD, Walker ID, Greer IA: The role of inherited thrombophilia in venous thromboembolus associated with pregnancy. *Br J Obstet Gynaecol* 106:756, 1999.

Percutaneous Balloon Mitral Valvuloplasty in Comparison With Open Mitral Valve Commissurotomy for Mitral Stenosis During Pregnancy
de Souza JAM, Martinez EE Jr, Ambrose JA, et al (Federal Univ of São Paulo, Brazil; Saint Vincent's Hosp, New York)
J Am Coll Cardiol 37:900-903, 2001   4–20

Background.—In developing countries, mitral stenosis and consequent heart failure are common during pregnancy. In 1984, percutaneous bal-loon mitral valvuloplasty (PBMV) was introduced and has since become an effective alternative to open heart surgery. Before then, mitral valve commissurotomy (MVC) was the only treatment available for symptoms of refractory heart failure. MVC was generally safe for pregnant women but often unsafe for their fetuses (fetal mortality rates, 6%-33%). No fetal loss has been reported for PBMV performed during pregnancy. Maternal and fetal outcomes from PBMV were compared with those from MVC.

Methods.—The study included 45 pregnant patients with severe heart failure caused by mitral stenosis who underwent PBMV (group I, n = 21; from 1990 to 1995) or open MVC (group II, n = 24, from 1985 to 1990).

TABLE 3.—Neonatal and Fetal Mortality

Mortality	PBMV n (%)	MVC n (%)
Yes	1 (4.8%)	8 (37.9%)*
No	20 (95.2%)	16 (62.1%)
Total	21 (100%)	24 (100%)

*$P = .025$ by the Fisher exact test.

Abbreviations: MCV, Mitral valve commissurotomy; *NYHA*, New York Heart Association; *PBMV*, percutaneous balloon mitral valvuloplasty.

(Courtesy of de Souza JAM, Martinez EE Jr, Ambrose JA, et al: Percutaneous balloon mitral valvuloplasty in comparison with open mitral valve commissurotomy for mitral stenosis during pregnancy. *J Am Coll Cardiol* 37:900-903, 2001. Reprinted with permission from the American College of Cardiology.)

The clinical and obstetric outcomes for group I were compared with group II.

Results.—Success of procedures was determined by the final mitral valve area achieved. PBMV had a success rate of 95%, as determined by the Gorlin formula. Using the echocardiographic "pressure half-time" method, 90.5% success rates were noted for PBMV. Although patients in both PBMV and MVC groups showed improved symptoms, the PBMV group had markedly fewer fetal complications. In the PBMV group, only 1 neonatal death occurred. This was in a premature child with an esophageal malformation. In contrast, the MVC group experienced 2 neonatal and 6 fetal deaths. The difference between the deaths in the PBMV and MVC group were significant (1 vs 8, $P = .025$) (Table 3).

Conclusions.—PBMV during pregnancy is effective and safe and promotes fetal survival better than MVC.

▶ This study provides demonstration of the benefit of balloon commissurotomy for mitral stenosis during pregnancy complicated only by persistent heart failure. Such patients are relatively rare in this country but this collaborative project of the cardiovascular surgical units in New York City's St. Vincent's Hospital and the Federal University of Sao Paulo, Brazil, provides a retrospective cohort study of 45 such women compared with historical control patients. In the interval from 1985 to 1990, the only therapy available to women with mitral stenosis functional Class III or IV, despite good medical inpatient management, was open mitral commissurotomy with extracorporeal circulatory support. Twenty-four such women are reported, and an additional 8 were treated by mitral valve replacement because of leaflet calcification and valve deformity, which makes commissurotomy less efficacious. Those women undergoing thoracotomy received general anesthesia, hypothermia, heparin, and appropriate cardiopulmonary support and pump output was guided by fetal heart rate monitoring. Beginning in 1990 to 1995, transseptal balloon commissurotomy after Inoue of functional Class III and IV pregnant patients was used in 21 women. Extracorporeal circulatory support was not necessary in such patients. Maternal results were good in both groups. There was 1 surgical death and 1 patient persisted at functional Class IV postoperatively in those patients treated by thoracotomy. Among those treated with percutaneous balloon commissurotomy, results were successful in reducing the patient's functional class to I or II, but 4 cases of mild mitral incompetence were noted. The major difference was improvement in perinatal mortality in the balloon valvulotomy group, apparently a result of the avoidance of extracorporeal support.

Historical controls always cloud data interpretation. With time, surgical groups acquired skill and experience, which is reflected partly on the results of the more recent endoscopic subset. It's unlikely that improvement in perinatal care accounted for the improved outcome for pediatric patients alone. This study offers support for balloon commissurotomy as the preferred approach to managing gravidas with refactory heart failure associated with mitral stenosis.

T. H. Kirschbaum, MD

The Effect of Valvular Heart Disease on Maternal and Fetal Outcome of Pregnancy

Hameed A, Karaalp IS, Tummala PP, et al (Univ of Southern Calif, Los Angeles)
J Am Coll Cardiol 37:893-899, 2001   4–21

Background.—The risks during pregnancy for patients with valvular heart disease (VHD) have been recognized, but have not been well defined. Most of the current research is based on a small number of patients in uncontrolled studies. The association between VHD and outcomes for mother and fetus in a fairly large group were compared with the same variables for a well-matched group of control subjects, the purpose being to aid physicians in designing therapeutic plans for patients and also to aid physicians in risk assessment.

Methods.—The study included 66 pregnancies in 64 women with VHD who attended a high-risk obstetrics/cardiology clinic at a tertiary-care center and were compared with 66 normal pregnant women matched for year of pregnancy, time of initial prenatal care, obstetrical and medical history, age, and ethnicity. The women with VHD were divided into 3 categories: (1) mitral stenosis (MS); (2) aortic stenosis (AS); or (3) mitral regurgitation (MR). Maternal outcomes were assessed as follows: (1) change in functional class as defined by the New York Heart Association (NYHA); (2) new cases of congestive heart failure (CHF); (3) hospitalization unrelated to child-birth; (4) arrhythmic exacerbation; (5) new cardiac medication or increased doses of old medications; and (6) delivery mode. Fetal outcomes assessed included birth weight, stillbirth, and preterm labor.

Results.—Higher rates of arrhythmia (15% vs 0%, $P = .002$), incidence of CHF (38% vs 0%; $P = .00001$), increased cardiac medications (41% vs 2%, $P < .0001$), and hospitalization (35% vs 2%, $P = .0001$) were found in women with VHD who were pregnant. Only 1 patient with aortic stenosis and coarctation died (2% vs 0%, P not significant). Fetal out-

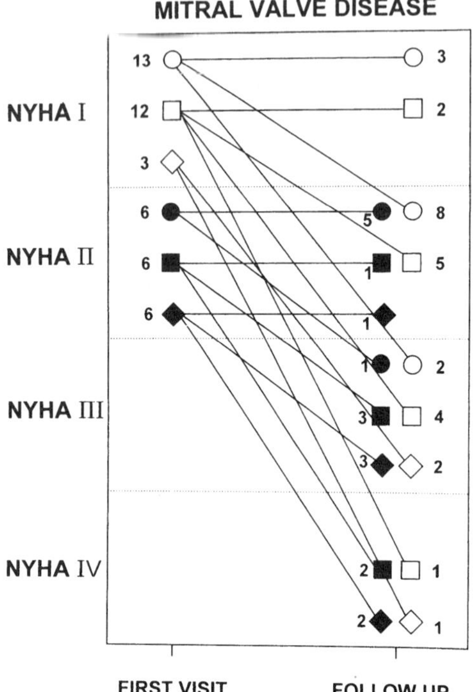

FIGURE 1.—Change in New York Heart Association functional class between first visit and follow-up during pregnancy in patients with predominant mitral valve disease. *Circles*, mild mitral stenosis; *squares*, moderate mitral stenosis; *diamonds*, severe mitral stenosis; *open symbols*, NYHA functional class I on presentation; *closed symbols*, NYHA functional class II on presentation. *Abbreviations*: *NYHA*, New York Heart Association. (Courtesy of Hameed A, Karaalp IS, Tummala PP, et al: The effect of valvular heart disease on maternal and fetal outcome of pregnancy. *J Am Coll Cardiol* 37: 893-899, 2001. Reprinted with permission from the American College of Cardiology [*Journal of the American College of Cardiology*, 2001, 37, 893-899.])

comes were also significantly more negative in women with VHDs. Fetal effects observed included intrauterine growth retardation (21% vs 0%, $P < .0001$), increased preterm delivery (23% vs 6%, $P = .03$), and reduced mean birth weight (2897 g vs 3366 g, $P = .0003$). Patients with moderate or severe MS and AS were most likely to have negative outcomes for both mother and fetus. Sixty-two percent of women deteriorated in at least 1 functional class during pregnancy (Figs 1 and 2).

Conclusions.—Women with AS and MS are much more likely to have maternal morbidity and negative fetal effects. Those with more severe VHD are more likely to show negative outcomes. However, even though maternal morbidity rates are high, death is rare.

▶ It is seldom that any program, even the Cardiology service run jointly by the Cardiology Division of Internal Medicine of the Department of OB GYN at USC, can provide definitive answers to comparisons among the varied levels of functional impairment of gravidas with mitral, aortic, and pulmonary

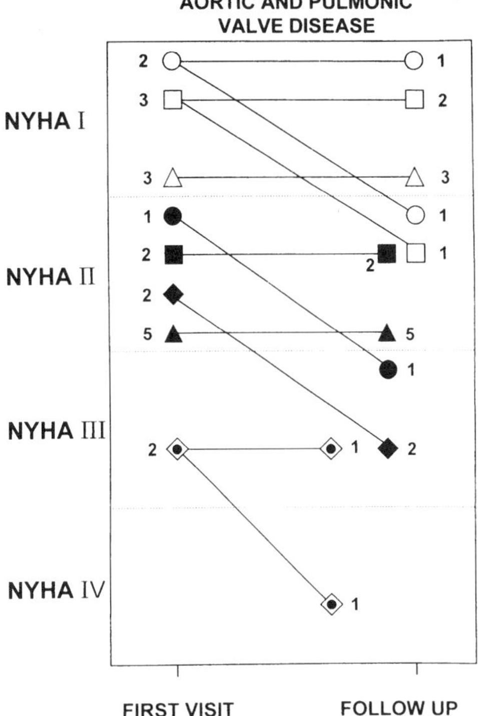

FIGURE 2.—Change in New York Heart Association functional class between first visit and follow-up during pregnancy in patients with predominant aortic and pulmonic valve disease. *Circles*, mild aortic stenosis; *squares*, moderate aortic stenosis; *diamonds*, severe aortic stenosis; *triangles*, pulmonic stenosis; *open symbols*, NYHA functional class I on presentation; *closed symbols*, NYHA class II on presentation; *dotted diamonds*, NYHA functional class III on presentation. *Abbreviations*: *NYHA*, New York Heart Association. (Courtesy of Hameed A, Karaalp IS, Tummala PP, et al: The effect of valvular heart disease on maternal and fetal outcome of pregnancy. *J Am Coll Cardiol* 37: 893-899, 2001. Reprinted with permission from the American College of Cardiology [*Journal of the American College of Cardiology*, 2001, 37, 893-899.])

valve disease. Here, they present an account of 66 pregnancies among 64 women seen during an uncertain interval in Boyle Heights. They report results of 46 pregnancies in women with mitral stenosis, 12 of whom also had mitral incompetence; 12 women with aortic stenosis; and 8 with pulmonary valve disease. Only 2 women with aortic or pulmonic valvular lesions were functional Class III on entry, all 44 others were functional Class I or II. In general, the deterioration of cardiac status was most common among women with mitral stenosis, occurring in 82% women originally functional Class I and 55 percent of those originally functional Class II prior to pregnancy. Comparable figures for progression in functional class for 20 pregnancies in women with aortic and pulmonary valve lesions were 25% and 30%, respectively. In addition to changes in functional class, those women with mitral stenosis showed an increased number of hospitalizations for cardiac evaluation and therapy, of a new onset of arrhythmia, and of a need for adjusted cardiac management. Following obstetrical department policy,

92% of the women delivered vaginally, but in 58%, operative vaginal delivery was employed. In a control group without heart disease selected for age, ethnicity, obstetrical and medical history, and time of pregnancy and delivery, 87% delivered vaginally, all spontaneously. There was 1 maternal death in a woman with aortic stenosis and coarctation of the aorta and 5 cases of postpartum pulmonary edema. Neonatal outcomes are not provided, a major barrier to evaluating adequacy of care, but as one would expect, growth retardation, preterm delivery, and low birth weight were noted among the newborns. None of the women with pulmonic stenosis, 3 of them functional Class I and 5 functional Class II, showed deterioration during pregnancy, a reflection of the good general condition of the women on entry. Granted that mitral sclerosis appeared to offer more opportunities for new evidence of dysfunction during pregnancy than to those with other valve lesions, it is generally true that this young population appeared to enter pregnancy with good clinical cardiac reserve.

T. H. Kirschbaum, MD

A Comparison of Echocardiography and Pulmonary Artery Catheterization for Evaluation of Pulmonary Artery Pressures in Pregnant Patients With Suspected Pulmonary Hypertension

Penning S, Robinson KD, Major CA, et al (Univ of California, Orange)
Am J Obstet Gynecol 184:1568-1570, 2001   4–22

Introduction.—The significant hemodynamic changes that occur in pregnancy may affect the ability of echocardiography to estimate pulmonary artery pressures in women with suspected pulmonary hypertension. Cardiac catheterization provides a reliable estimate but is an invasive procedure with a risk of complications. A retrospective chart review compared the accuracy of echocardiography and pulmonary artery catheterization in the setting of suspected pulmonary hypertension during pregnancy.

Methods.—Included in the review were all pregnant patients with a diagnosis of cardiac disease who were admitted to the University of California, Irvine Medical Center, between January 1990 and February 2000. The study subjects had documented pulmonary artery pressures by echocardiography and cardiac catheterization in the same pregnancy. Pulmonary hypertension was defined as pulmonary artery systolic pressure greater than 30 mm Hg.

Results.—Twenty-seven of the 159 patients whose charts were reviewed were eligible for analysis. These women had an average age of 28.6 years and a mean gravidity of 3.2. The mean gestational age at echocardiography was 27.4 weeks, compared with 31.7 weeks at catheterization. Mean pulmonary artery pressure was significantly overestimated with echocardiography compared with catheterization (55.4 vs 51.1 mm Hg). Eight women had pulmonary hypertension when estimated by echocardiography, but subsequent catheterization revealed normal pulmonary artery pressures. The 2 measurements did not differ significantly in the 7 patients who had no structural cardiac defects (mean, 43.4 mm Hg with echocardiography vs 40.7 mm Hg with catheterization). No complications were attributed to pulmonary artery catheterization.

Conclusion.—Because of the high risk of maternal death, it is essential to diagnose pulmonary hypertension in pregnancy. Echocardiography significantly overestimates the condition, and approximately one third of pregnant patients with normal pulmonary artery pressures may be misclassified if catheterization is not performed. Coexistent structural cardiac defects may affect the accuracy of echocardiography.

▶ With the advent of Doppler echocardiography, cardiologists have found it useful to estimate peak right atrial pressure based on the velocity of the regurgitation jet of blood passing during systole from right ventricle to right atrium through the partially incompetent tricuspid valve. In men and non-pregnant women, the results compare reasonably well with the results of pulmonary artery catheterization, the invasive standard for establishing the diagnosis of pulmonary artery hypertension. This is a first attempt at evaluation of the Doppler technique in pregnant women. The changes in endocardiac functions and structure make this an important consideration. During pregnancy there are changes in stroke volume, chamber dimensions, and cardiac output, and most echocardiographers report that some degree of tricuspid insufficiency is seen in nearly all women by mid pregnancy. Furthermore, the adverse consequences of the diagnosis based on reported complications of pulmonary hypertension in pregnancy sometimes lead to recommendation of abortion in early pregnancy or to extended inpatient care in later months.

This is a cohort study of gravidas treated for cardiac disease over a 10-year period. Among such women, there were 27 who had both echocardiography and pulmonary artery catheterization to allow comparison of the 2 techniques. When a value of 30 mm Hg peak was used as normal peak systolic pulmonary artery pressure, 25 women were judged hypertensive on echocardiography, but one third were normotensive on catheterization. Two patients judged to be normotensive on echocardiography were subsequently found to be hypertensive on catheterization. Although this is a small series, it probably would be prudent for obstetricians to insist on right heart catheterization before initiating the recommendations customary for this severe cardiac complication of pregnancy.

T. H. Kirschbaum, MD

Maternal and Fetal Outcomes of Subsequent Pregnancies in Women With Peripartum Cardiomyopathy

Elkayam U, Tummala PP, Rao K, et al (Univ of Southern California, Los Angeles)

N Engl J Med 344:1567-1571, 2001

4–23

Background.—The cause of peripartum cardiomyopathy is unknown, but its outcome includes partial or complete recovery in 80% of those affected and cardiac transplant or death in 20% of the cases. Becoming pregnant again may increase the risk of redevelopment of cardiomyopathy. Maternal and fetal outcomes of subsequent pregnancies in women who had a history of peripartum cardiomyopathy were evaluated.

Methods.—Members of the American College of Cardiology were surveyed and identified 44 women in whom peripartum cardiomyopathy had been diagnosed and who had 60 subsequent pregnancies. These women's medical records were analyzed, and either the women themselves or their physicians were interviewed. Two groups of women were identified: those in whom left ventricular function had returned to normal (group 1, 28 subsequent pregnancies) and those with persistent left ventricular dysfunction (group 2, 16 subsequent pregnancies).

Results.—Both groups and the entire cohort had reduced mean left ventricular ejection fraction, with values falling from 49% to 42% for the entire cohort, from 56% to 49% for group 1, and from 36% to 32% for group 2. Twenty-one percent of the women in group 1 experienced symptoms of heart failure in their subsequent pregnancies; 44% of those in group 2 did so (Table 1). The frequency of premature delivery in women with persistent dysfunction (group 2) was 37%, with a rate of therapeutic

TABLE 1.—Incidence of Maternal Complications During the First Subsequent Pregnancy in Women Who Had Had Peripartum Cardiomyopathy*

Group	No. of Women	Symptoms of Heart Failure	>20% Decrease in LVEF	Decreased LVEF at Follow-up	Death
		no. of women (%)			
All women	44				
Group 1	28	6 (21)	6 (21)	4 (14)	0
Group 2	16	7 (44)	4 (25)	5 (31)	3 (19)†
Women who did not have abortions	35				
Group 1	23	6 (26)	4 (17)	2 (9)	0
Group 2	12	6 (50)	4 (33)	5 (42)	3 (25)‡

*Group 1 consisted of women with recovered left ventricular function, defined as a left ventricular ejection fraction (LVEF) of 50% or higher, before the subsequent pregnancy; group 2 consisted of women with persistent left ventricular dysfunction (an LVEF of less than 50%).

†*P* .06 for the comparison with group 1.

‡*P* .05 for the comparison with group 1.

(Reprinted by permission of the New England Journal of Medicine, from Elkayam U, Tummala PP, Rao, K, et al: Maternal and fetal outcomes of subsequent pregnancies in women with peripartum cardiomyopathy. *N Engl J Med* 344:1567-1571. Copyright 2001, Massachusetts Medical Society. All rights reserved.)

abortion of 25%; these values were 11% and 4% in group 1. The mortality rate was 0% in group 1 and 19% in group 2.

Conclusions.—In women with a history of peripartum cardiomyopathy, especially those with persistent left ventricular dysfunction, subsequent pregnancy increases the risk of redevelopment of symptoms of heart failure in the mother and increases the rate of premature delivery or therapeutic abortion. Thus, both clinical deterioration and death may result from these subsequent pregnancies, a fact to be considered in any decision to become pregnant again.

▶ Peripartum cardiomyopathy is fortunately an infrequent disease that is usually but not always manifest after delivery and marked by dilated cardiomyopathy, decreased ventricular efficiency, and obscure etiology. One study employing ventricular biopsy suggested that viral myocarditis may be a cause in some cases (see 1988 YEAR BOOK OF OBSTETRICS, GYNECOLOGY, AND WOMEN'S HEALTH, pp 49-51). In others, abnormal myometrial development in infancy is suggested. It is not uncommon for cardiac transplant to be necessary to prevent maternal death during or after a pregnancy marked by this complication.

These authors have executed a detailed survey of members of the American College of Cardiology and a South African cardiology group to identify 44 women who had 1 or more pregnancies after surviving an earlier episode of peripartum cardiomyopathy. Records of these pregnancies sufficed to make the diagnosis of cardiomyopathy in the earlier pregnancy based on dilatation of left and right ventricles and the presence of a left ventricular ejection fraction less than 40%. Their results suggest that myocardial dysfunction tends to persist after delivery and alter the outcome of subsequent pregnancies. The ability normally to increase the left ventricular ejection fraction during a prior pregnancy by at least 50% was an important predictive finding, since congestive heart failure occurred in 21% of the women in that group versus 44% of those who failed the pregnancy-related increase in injection fraction in a prior pregnancy. The increase in ejection fraction, part of the ventricular remodeling that occurs during pregnancy, and the increases in both diastolic ventricular volume and stroke volume are essential parts of the normal cardiovascular adjustment to the demands of pregnancy. In addition, preterm delivery and maternal death in 3 cases also complicated subsequent pregnancies. Clearly, survival of an episode of peripartum cardiomyopathy leaves residual myocardial injury and suboptimal ventricular functional reserve in a subsequent pregnancy. Such women require careful counseling and contraceptive assistance by those who care for them.

T. H. Kirschbaum, MD

Relationship Between Parity and Clinical and Biological Features in Patients With Systemic Sclerosis

Launay D, Hebbar M, Hatron P-Y, et al (Hôpital Claude Huriez, Lille, France)
J Rheumatol 28:509-513, 2001   4–24

Objective.—Compared with healthy women, women with systemic sclerosis (SSc) more frequently and markedly carry fetal progenitor cells for decades after childbirth. Whether this microchimerism of fetal origin is involved in the pathogenesis of SSc was investigated retrospectively in a group of pregnant women with SSc.

Methods.—Between 1990 and 1999, 100 consecutive women with SSc were entered into the study. Age, duration of SSc before diagnosis, cutaneous extension of SSc, pulmonary involvement, antinuclear antibodies, and number, sex, and date of birth of children born before and after SSc onset were recorded.

Results.—SSc was limited in 72 patients and diffuse in 28%. SSc duration was longer in patients with limited disease (15.6 vs 11.6 years). Patients with diffuse disease were significantly more likely to have pulmonary involvement than were patients with limited disease (22 of 28 vs 17 of 72). Although anticentromere antibodies were more common in patients with limited SSc (47 of 72 vs 0 of 28), antiSc170 antibodies were more common in patients with diffuse disease (15 of 28 vs 7 of 72). Patients with limited SSc had significantly more children than patients with diffuse disease before disease onset. Although patients with limited SSc and pulmonary fibrosis had significantly more children than patients without pulmonary fibrosis, the difference was not significant for patients with diffuse disease. Although there were no significant differences for either group with respect to the interval between first pregnancy and SSc onset, the interval between the first birth and SSc onset was significantly shorter for patients with limited disease than for those with diffuse disease (11.0 vs 23.5 years). Although both groups of patients had the same number of girls, age of mother at first birth was significantly higher for girls than for boys (26.8 vs 22.9 years), and the interval between the first birth and SSc onset was significantly shorter when the first child was a girl rather than a boy (16.2 vs 25.4 years).

Conclusion.—Because multiparity appears to be associated with limited SSc and pulmonary fibrosis, it may be a subset of SSc in which microchimerism is involved or it may be a distinct disorder.

▶ The presence of maternal microchimerism arising from fetal to maternal transplantation of fetal cells during pregnancy has been demonstrated before in relation to this and other diseases (see 1999 YEAR BOOK OF OBSTETRICS, GYNECOLOGY, AND WOMEN'S HEALTH, pp 189-191, and 2001 YEAR BOOK, pp 219-220). This study of 100 consecutive French women bearing the diagnosis helps confirm that relationship and points to some differences in the pattern of the disease associated with increase in parity. Eight-three of the women were parous with a mean of 2.2 children at the time of the diagnosis of the disease at a mean of 52 years of age. With increasing parity, women had an increased likelihood of SSc limited to face and extremities and to pulmonary fibrosis based on pulmonary x-ray and function tests. Diffuse disease was limited to the trunk and acral regions. The mean interval between first delivery and the diagnosis of sclerosis was shorter for those with the limited form (1.1 years) than for those with the diffuse form (23.5 years), suggesting pregnancy is the more proximate cause of the former more limited pattern. No clear relation of parity or the presence of antinuclear or anticentromere maternal antibodies was seen. Finally, for the 17 women with SSc who were nulliparous, the hypothetical relation to microchimerism is impossible to support, and the origin of the disease in those cases remains unexplained.

T. H. Kirschbaum, MD

The Maternal Lifestyle Study: Drug Use by Meconium Toxicology and Maternal Self-Report

Lester BM, ElSohly M, Wright LL, et al (Brown Med School, Providence, RI; Elsohly Labs Inc, Oxford, Miss; Natl Inst of Child Health and Human Development, Bethesda, Md; et al)
Pediatrics 107:309-317, 2001   4–25

Background.—A thorough understanding of the nature and magnitude of the problem of prenatal cocaine exposure and the determination of appropriate interventions are dependent on the accurate identification of prenatal cocaine exposure. An effort was made to characterize drug use by pregnant women who participated in the 4-site Maternal Lifestyle Study of in utero cocaine or opiate exposure.

Methods.—At 4 sites, immunoassay with gas chromatography/mass spectrometry (GC/MS) confirmation was performed in the analysis of meconium specimens from 8527 newborns for metabolites of cocaine, opiates, cannabinoids, amphetamines, and phencyclidine. Hospital interviews were used to obtain maternal self-reports of drug use.

Results.—Overall, the prevalence of cocaine/opiate exposure at the 4 sites was 10.7%. Most of the exposure (9.5%) was to cocaine, according to the combination of meconium analysis and maternal self-report. However, exposure status varied by site and was found to be higher in low birth weight infants (18.6% for infants with very low birth weight and 21.1% for infants with low birth weight). The rate of GC/MS confirmation of presumptive positive cocaine screens was 75.5%. In the group exposed to cocaine/opiates, the mothers of 38% of the infants denied use, but the results of meconium tests were positive. Agreement between positive meconium results and positive maternal report was 66%. Only 2% of the mothers reported that they used only cocaine during pregnancy, and mothers who used cocaine were 49 times more likely to use another drug.

Conclusions.—GC/MS confirmation and the coupling of a maternal hospital interview with meconium assay were shown to improve the accurate identification of prenatal drug use. However, the use of GC/MS may have different implications for research than for public policy. It is recommended that caution be used in the application of quantitative analysis of drugs in meconium for the estimation of the degree of exposure. In addition, the polydrug nature of what was once considered only a cocaine problem is highlighted by these findings.

▶ With recognition that maternal cocaine and opiate use during pregnancy is a significant problem with serious implications for the maternal cardiovascular system, placental abruption, and fetal injury, its detection and definition of patterns of illicit use have become increasingly important (see 1998 YEAR BOOK OF OBSTETRICS, GYNECOLOGY, AND WOMEN'S HEALTH, pp 133-134). Traditionally, clinicians have employed urine analysis for cocaine metabolites for detection, but their presence in urine and blood is evanescent and disappears with discontinuance within 4 to 5 days.

Introduction of meconium analysis has revolutionized what we know about the natural history of illicit drug use in pregnancy (see 1993 YEAR BOOK, pp 203-204, 223-224). Cocaine is lipid soluble and readily crosses the placenta to be metabolized by the fetal liver. Metabolites are excreted via fetal bile into the fetal intestinal tract where, contained in meconium, they lie discoverable until birth. Meconium analysis gives a record of maternal drug use over weeks of fetal life. Metabolites tend to become concentrated with time compared with their decreasing concentration in urine and blood, and multiple drug metabolites may be sought by enzyme-linked immunoassays. Finally, confirmation for possible legal implications of such evidence can be carried out by GC-MS.

This is, to date, the definitive report of the application of these techniques in a study financed by the NICHD Neonatal Research Network and the NIDA's Federal Center for Drug Abuse and Treatment, reporting 11,811 analyses from 4 research sites operating from 1993 to 1995. Participants were offered NIDA certification of confidentiality, which rendered them immune from state mandatory reporting statutes, triggered by the collection of evidence of drug use, a step that facilitated patient participation considerably. Initial analytes included metabolites of cocaine, opiates, cannabinol (THC), and PCP, but cannabinol was dropped with evidence of an inadequate screening assay in the course of the study. Thereafter, several other reagents were added to the program when it became clear that only 2% of cocaine users employed that agent alone and that women who used cocaine were nearly 50 times more likely to use other illicit agents than were nonusers.

Cocaine use was found by screening examination in 9.5% of gravidas and confirmed by GC-MS in 7%. Opiates were found on screening examination in 2.3% and confirmed in 2.2%. In both cases, patient self-reports quite accurately reflected laboratory findings, once the threat of prosecution was removed. THC was found on screening in 7.2%, but only 2.4% could be confirmed by GC-MS. There is wide variability of incidence of illicit drug use among centers with high rates in Detroit, but lower in Miami and Providence. The incidence of metabolite positivity also varied with gestational age (Table 4 in the original article).

It is very clear that cocaine is only part of what is in reality a multidrug exposure problem. Clearly, the actual problem for us all is addiction among pregnant women to a large and growing number of agents affecting somewhere around 10% of pregnancies.

T. H. Kirschbaum, MD

Ursodeoxycholic Acid in Intrahepatic Cholestasis of Pregnancy: A Retrospective Study of 19 Cases
Berkane N, Cocheton J-J, Brehier D, et al (Hôpital Tenon, Paris)
Acta Obstet Gynecol Scand 79:941-946, 2000   4–26

Objective.—Cholestasis of pregnancy is characterized by an increase in circulating total bile acids resulting in pruritus and possibly cytolysis through their hepatic toxicity. Cholestasis can lead to prematurity, fetal distress, and death in utero. Ursodeoxycholic acid (UDCA) has been used to treat this condition. One institution's experience with UDCA in the treatment of severe and early-onset cholestasis of pregnancy is retrospectively reported.

Methods.—Files of 431 patients with cholestasis of pregnancy, 19 of whom received UDCA, between January 1991 to June 1997, were reviewed for maternal clinical and biologic effects of treatment, term and mode of delivery, fetal distress, birth weight, and malformations.

Results.—Thirteen of 19 pregnancies were singleton, 4 were twin, and 2 were triplet. Signs of cholestasis appeared at week 29.7 of pregnancy on average. Treatment with UDCA began at week 32 on average and continued for an average of 28.5 days. Fourteen (73%) had a favorable clinical outcome, and 11 had favorable changes in biologic parameters. Two patients deteriorated. Deliveries were spontaneous in 9 cases, induced in 7, and by cesarean section in 3. Ten of 27 neonates were low-birth-weight babies, with 9 of 10 from multiple pregnancies.

Conclusion.—Although UDCP appears to be effective in the treatment of cholestasis of pregnancy, its safety in pregnancy remains to be determined.

▶ Although this is an uncontrolled study of the use of UDCA in only 19 patients, it adds to the recorded experience in the use of the only agent demonstrating promise of clinical efficacy in this sometimes compelling clinical problem. Since use of the drug has last been reviewed here (see 2001 YEAR BOOK OF OBSTETRICS, GYNECOLOGY, AND WOMEN'S HEALTH, pp 36-38), more has been learned of the mechanism of action of this substituated bile acid. It appears to act not only by competitive inhibition of endogenous bile acids known to be hepatocytotoxic, but also to decrease intestinal absorption and increase biliary excretion of bile acids generally. The agent also appears to stabilize hepatocytes as measured by reduced elevation of serum alkaline phosphatase, perhaps by attenuation of expression of the HLA antigens of the major histocompatibility complex that serve as receptor sites for some cytotoxic effectors, at least in biliary cirrhosis.

Of the 19 recipients receiving UDCA for an average of 30 days beginning at 32 weeks' gestation, improvement was noted in 74%; 42% of the women showed full resolution of signs and symptoms of cholestasis. Improvement in laboratory evidence of cholestasis was seen in two thirds of cases. Seven inductions of labor were done primarily for cholestasis, but 3 cesarean sections were done solely for obstetrical indications. The authors cite 2 randomized controlled studies that purport to demonstrate a reduction in preterm birth in women using UDCA for cholestasis.

It seems time to mount a large prospective controlled study to prove the utility of this agent and to explore in detail the safety to fetuses exposed to the drug, which surely crosses the placenta with ease.

T. H. Kirschbaum, MD

Hepatitis C Virus Among High and Low Risk Pregnant Women in Dundee: Unlinked Anonymous Testing
Goldberg D, McIntyre PG, Smith R, et al (Scottish Centre for Infection and Environmental Health, Glasgow, Scotland; Ninewells Hosp, Dundee, Scotland)
Br J Obstet Gynaecol 108:365-370, 2001   4–27

Objective.—The prevalence of hepatitis C virus (HCV) transmitted by sexual intercourse was investigated in pregnant women (1) to determine what proportion of infected pregnant women would be detected if a selective screening strategy, targeted at women who injected drugs or who had partners who injected drugs, was used and (2) to estimate the number of babies being born with HCV infection.

Methods.—In 1997, 3548 pregnant women who attended Ninewells Hospital, Dundee, Scotland, for prenatal care or pregnancy termination were offered HIV testing. Anonymous testing for HCV was also performed on anonymous samples. Each woman was asked if she or her partner used injected drugs.

Results.—The overall prevalence of anti-HCV was 0.6% and 41% among those who used injected drugs (relative risk [RR], 131), 15% among those whose partners used injected drugs (RR, 48), and 0.3% of those who had neither risk. Eighteen women were estimated to have given birth to an infected baby.

Conclusion.—Women with partners who inject drugs are at substantially increased risk for hepatitis C infection. Use of condoms should be promoted in this high-risk population. About half the cases would not have been detected by screening.

▶ This report attacks the common presumption that HCV is infrequently transmitted by sexual contact (see 2001 YEAR BOOK OF OBSTETRICS, GYNECOLOGY, AND WOMEN'S HEALTH, pp 138-139). What makes this hypothesis difficult to prove is the need to differentiate the risk of sexual transmission from the serious risk of transmission through common use of illicit drug products and/or paraphernalia. This interview study coupled with HCV serologic examination together with an offer of HIV antibody testing to 3548 Scottish gravidas suggests, but does not prove, a definable independent sexual transmission route exists. Among those tested, the HCV positive antibody rate was 41% among 7 women who admitted to drug use. For those 98.5% of women who indicated neither drug use nor cohabitation with a user, the HCV antibody positivity rate was 0.3%. For 33 women who denied drug use but cohabitated with a drug user, the HCV positivity rate was 15% or 58 times the incidence rate for those who denied both possible exposures. The problem is with the interpretation of the interview data which presumes candor, honesty, and good recall capacity. To avoid those problems is not easy, and we are left with the likelihood that there is a small risk of sexually transmitted HCV infection until better data become available.

T. H. Kirschbaum, MD

Pregnancy in Cystic Fibrosis: Fetal and Maternal Outcome
Gilljam M, Antoniou M, Shin J, et al (Göteborg Univ, Sweden; Univ of Toronto)
Chest 118:85-91, 2000   4–28

Background.—In the past few decades, there has been a dramatic improvement in the survival of patients with cystic fibrosis (CF). The adult population of patients with CF has been increasing to the point that issues such as fertility, family planning, and pregnancy have become important topics for these patients and their caregivers. The initial reports of pregnancy in patients with CF were discouraging, but studies have demonstrated the safety of pregnancy in women with good lung function. However, there have also been reports of premature delivery. It has been suggested that impairment of pulmonary function may be the most important predictor of maternal and fetal outcome. Other factors that may be an influence on long-term survival are nutritional status, the presence of diabetes mellitus, the presence of *Burkholderia cepacia*, and frequent infectious exacerbation. The effects of pregnancy on pulmonary function and survival in women with CF were evaluated, and fetal outcome was assessed.

Methods.—The cohort of patients comprised all women with CF who attended the Toronto Cystic Fibrosis Clinics at the time of diagnosis or pregnancy, between 1961 and 1998. The data were collected from the Toronto CF database, from chart review, and from a patient questionnaire.

Results.—In the period 1961 to 1998, there were 92 pregnancies in 54 women. Among this group, there were 11 miscarriages and 7 therapeutic abortions. A total of 74 children were born to 49 women. The mean follow-up was 11 ± 8 years. One patient was lost to follow-up soon after delivery, and another was lost to follow-up after 12 years. Nine of 48

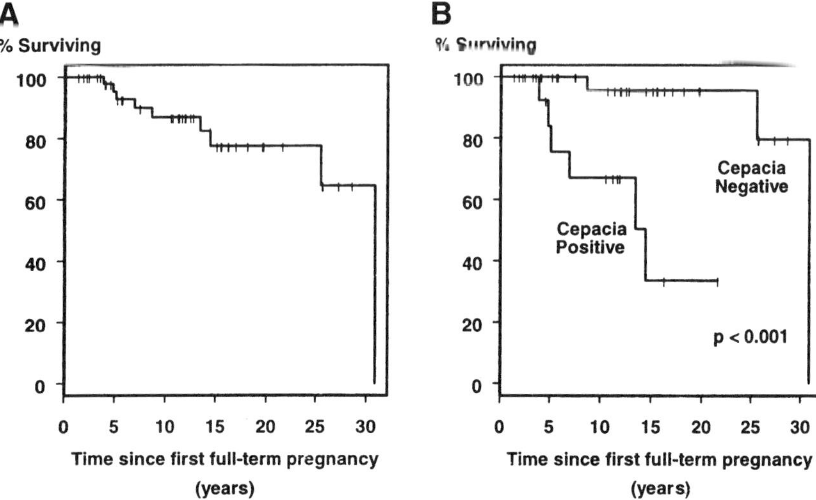

FIGURE 1.—Kaplan-Meier survival curves for 49 women with cystic fibrosis after their first completed pregnancy. Overall survival (**A**) and survival (**B**) for *Burkholderia cepacia*–negative versus *Burkholderia cepacia*–positive women ($P < .001$ [log rank test]). *Vertical lines* indicate censored observations, ie, those patients still alive on December 31, 1998. (Courtesy of Gilljam M, Antoniou M, Shin J, et al: Pregnancy in cystic fibrosis: Fetal and maternal outcome. *Chest* 118:85-91, 2000.)

patients died, for an overall mortality rate of 19%. Better survival rates were found in association with the absence of *B cepacia*, pancreatic sufficiency, and prepregnancy forced expiratory volume in 1 second (FEV_1) of greater than 50% predicted (Fig 1). When adjusted for the same factors, pregnancy was shown not to affect survival when compared with the entire adult female CF population. The decline observed in FEV_1 was comparable to the decline in FEV_1 seen in the entire CF population. Diabetes mellitus was present in 3 of the women in the study, and gestational diabetes developed in 7 women. Six preterm infants were born, and there was 1 neonatal death. Two children were found to have CF.

Conclusion.—For most women with CF, maternal and fetal outcome is good; risk factors for mortality in these women are similar to the risk factors for the nonpregnant CF population. Planning of the pregnancy is important to allow an opportunity for counseling and optimization of the patient's medical condition. This necessitates good communication between the obstetrician and the CF team.

▶ At least in the program based in Toronto's Cystic Fibrosis Treatment Center, there has been significant improvement in the care of gravidas with CF, expressed in improved pregnancy results over the last 2 to 3 decades. The severity of pulmonary functional impairment has decreased with systematic antibiotic therapy, sputum liquefaction agents and efforts to reduce the incidence of chronic infection caused by *B cepacia*. Early diagnosis of pancreatic islet insufficiency has led to earlier and more effective treatment of diabetes mellitus. Efforts at maintaining adequate maternal nutrition have decreased the incidences of maternal and fetal malnutrition.

In this collection of 74 infants born of 49 women receiving care at this center, based on antepartum visits 1 to 4 times a year and delivering over the 3½ decades prior to 1998, mean birth weight was 3.2 kg and mean gestational age was 40 weeks. The incidence of preterm delivery was 8% and birth weight less than 2.5 kg occurred in only 6% of deliveries. There were no consistent differences in maternal and fetal outcome based on FEV$_1$ impaired to 50% of normal. There were no fetal deaths and 1 neonatal death caused by sepsis generated a neonatal death rate of 20 per 1000 live births. Of pregnancies for which adequate obstetric information was available, the cesarean section rate was 12.5%, based largely on obstetric indications, and 17.5% of women had labor inductions on maternal indications.

Long-term follow-up in 39 women, ranging from 7 months to 28 years, confirmed the underlying maternal hazard. Three of those women required bilateral lung transplants, and the maternal mortality rate was 10% after 5 years and 20% 10 years after delivery. Risk factors for increased maternal mortality proved to be the presence of pancreatic insufficiency, impaired ventilatory function, and chronic *B cepecia* infection. It is well to remember these good obstetric and neonatal results in women with CF benefitting by this type of systematic, experienced antepartum and prepartum care.

T. H. Kirschbaum, MD

Appendicitis in Pregnancy
Tracey M, Fletcher HS (Saint Barnabas Med Ctr, Livingston, NJ)
Am Surg 66:555-560, 2000   4–29

Introduction.—Although acute appendicitis continues to be the most common nonobstetric surgical diagnosis in pregnancy, there is little improvement in the success of accurate diagnosis of this problem. The physiologic and anatomical changes in pregnancy are believed to obscure, thereby delaying diagnosis of acute appendicitis and contributing to its increased risk in pregnancy. A retrospective contemporary evaluation of pregnant patients with diagnosis of acute appendicitis between 1991 and 1998 was performed to further evaluate its overall incidence, determine the factors contributing to its delay in diagnosis, and analyze the overall outcomes in appendicitis for pregnancy.

Methods.—Medical records were reviewed for data concerning age, parity, gestational age/trimester, symptoms and symptom duration, temperature on admission, physical findings, diagnostic (ultrasonography), deliveries, Apgar scores, and overall length of admission. Pathology reports were also reviewed.

Results.—Among 44,845 births in women aged 19 to 42 years, 22 (0.05%) pregnant women were taken to the operating room with a diagnosis of appendicitis. The gestational stage at diagnosis was first, second, and third trimester, in 5 (22%), 6 (27%), and 11 (50%) patients, respectively. Nineteen patients (86%) had pathologically confirmed acute appendicitis. Sixteen patients (73%) were seen within 24 hours of abdominal symptoms. Seventeen patients (77%) had findings of rebound and guarding on initial physical examination. Of 15 patients (68%) taken to the operating room within 24 hours of being seen, 10 (68%) had acute perforated appendixes. Overall, there were 12 patients (55%) with perforated appendices. This incidence is higher than that reported in the literature. There were no fetal deaths.

Conclusion.—This population paralleled the incidence (0.05%-0.07%) of gestational appendicitis. The most reliable diagnostic tool for appendicitis was physical examination at presentation. A higher rate of perforation was observed with increased gestational age, which was not associated with fetal mortality rate.

▶ Because appendicitis remains a management problem for obstetricians and their surgical colleagues, this current review of the subject from a hospital with a fine reputation in patient care warrants our consideration. The authors provide a retrospective cohort study of 22 gravidas with a preoperative diagnosis of appendicitis managed in the last decade. The incidence of the diagnosis, 0.05%, is likely an underestimate in view of the low incidence of normal appendices they report (4.5%) and the 50% incidence of women operated on in the third trimester, 9 of 11 of whom had perforated appendices. Only 14% of all gravidas presented with fever. Their leukocyte counts were, in 54% of cases, less than 12,000/mm^3 and right lower-quadrant pain localization was seen in only one third. It is likely that some women with appendicitis in the first and second trimesters in the authors' treatment area had insufficient findings to enable a clinical diagnosis and responded to temporization and antibiotic therapy. The most common symptom noted among these patients was nausea and vomiting in one third of women; half of all operated on in the third trimester had right upper-quadrant pain. Ultrasonic examination of the abdomen did not appear useful in the 10 women in whom it was used and the most valuable diagnostic sign appeared, in retrospect, to be abdominal rebound pain and guarding. The high incidence of appendiceal perforation (55%) did not reflect physician delay, since 72% of women had surgery within 24 hours of admission.

The failure of pregnant women to present with clear intense abdominal pain localization together with the customary relative leukocytosis of pregnancy, and coupled with the poor diagnostic efficacy of abdominal US, means that all obstetricians need to be aware of appendicitis as a possibility in their pregnant patients.

T. H. Kirschbaum, MD

5 Surveillance

The Preterm Prediction Study: Can Low-Risk Women Destined for Spontaneous Preterm Birth Be Identified?
Iams JD, for the National Institute of Child Health and Human Development Maternal-Fetal Medicine Units Network (Ohio State Univ, Columbus)
Am J Obstet Gynecol 184:652-655, 2001   5–1

Background.—It is difficult to determine those women without risk factors for preterm births who will deliver early. Further confounding this problem, half of preterm births occur in women without risk factors. Early indicators that could possibly predict preterm deliveries were assessed, even though successful interventions do not currently exist to prevent preterm deliveries.

Methods.—The study included 2929 women with no apparent risk factors for preterm birth who underwent screening, including digital examination, fetal fibronectin assays, and cervical US as part of the Preterm Prediction Study done by the National Institute of Child Health and the Human Development Maternal-Fetal Medicine Units Networks. Researchers performed a secondary analysis of data collected at 22 to 24 weeks' gestational age. Patient records included in the data analysis came from women with no history of preterm birth or loss of pregnancy before 20 weeks' gestation. Variables included in analysis were Bishop scores (≥ 4), cervical length (≤ 25 mm) at 24 weeks' gestation, and fetal fibronectin levels (≥ 50 ng/mL). These variables were analyzed both in isolation and in sequence to determine which might predict spontaneous delivery before 35 weeks' gestation.

Results.—Of the original candidates, 2197 were included in this secondary analysis. Of these, 1207 were pregnant for the first time and 900 were multiparous but low risk. Sixty-four births occurred spontaneously before 35 weeks' gestation (3.04%). The 3 tests all related significantly to preterm births (before 35 weeks); however, the sensitivities of the tests were low (high Bishop score, 23.4%; short cervix, 39.1%; fetal fibronectin detection, 23.4%). Sensitivity, specificity, and positive and negative predictive value for each of the 3 variables are shown in (Table I). Taken in sequence, the sensitivities of these tests were still low (Table II). Specifically, as related to birth before 35 weeks, high Bishop scores had a relative risk (RR) of 3.6; 95% confidence interval (CI), 2.1-6.3; short cervical

TABLE I.—Prediction of Spontaneous Preterm Birth Before 35 Weeks' Gestation Among 2107 Low-Risk Women

	Bishop Score	Cervical Length	Fetal Fibronectin Assay
Positive test result (No.)	165 (7.8%)	179 (8.5%)	76 (3.6%)
Spontaneous preterm birth before 35 wk (No.)	15	25	15
Sensitivity (No.)	15/64 (23.4%)	25/64 (39.1%)	15/64 (23.4%)
Specificity (No.)	1893/2043 (92.6%)	1889/2043 (92.5%)	1982/2043 (97.0%)
Positive predictive value (No.)	15/165 (9.1%)	25/179 (14.0%)	15/76 (19.7%)
Negative predictive value (No.)	1893/1942 (97.5%)	1889/1928 (98.0%)	1982/2031 (98.0%)
Relative risk of spontaneous preterm birth before 35 wk	3.6	6.9	8.2
95% Confidence interval for relative risk	2.1-6.3	4.3-11.1	4.8-13.9

Note: Sensitivity, specificity, and positive and negative predictive values were calculated for the population of 2107 women.
(Courtesy of Iams JD, for the National Institute of Child Health and Human Development Maternal-Fetal Medicine Units Network: *Am J Obstet Gynecol* 184:652-655, 2001.)

TABLE II.—Sequential Screening for Spontaneous Preterm Birth
Before 35 Weeks' Gestation

	Delivery at <35 Wk
Population (N = 2107)	64
Positive fetal fibronectin result (n = 76)	15
Positive fetal fibronectin result plus cervical length ≤25 mm (n = 20)	10
Sensitivity	15.6%
Specificity	99.5%
Positive predictive value	50.0%
Negative predictive value	94.4%
Relative risk	19.3
95% Confidence interval for relative risk	11.6-32.2
Bishop score ≥4 (n = 165)	15
Bishop score ≥4 plus cervical length ≤25 mm (n = 33)	9
Sensitivity	14.1%
Specificity	98.8%
Positive predictive value	27.3%
Negative predictive value	97.4%
Relative risk	10.3
95% Confidence interval for relative risk	5.6-19.1

(Courtesy of Iams JD, for the National Institute of Child Health and Human Development Maternal-Fetal Medicine Units Network: *Am J Obstet Gynecol* 184:652-655, 2001.)

length, RR, 6.9, 95% CI, 4.3-11.1; and fetal fibronectin detection, RR, 8.2, 95% CI, 4.8-13.9.

Conclusions.—The sensitivities of digital examination, fetal fibronectin assays, and cervical ultrasonography were all low when used in women with low-risk of preterm delivery. Sequential screening decreased the sensitivity of these tests to only 15% among low-risk women.

▶ This study is noteworthy primarily for the authoritativeness it lends to some generally well-known conclusions. In a search for the prediction of preterm birth in a primigravid population without symptoms, cervical vaginal fibronectin 15 ng/mL or more, cervical length on ultrasound 2.5 cm or less, and a Bishop score 4 or more have all been demonstrated to be independently associated with an increased risk of preterm birth. This study sponsored by NICHD's Maternal Fetal Medicine Network based in 10 national centers was designed solely to test the predictive strength of these findings, individually and combined, in reliably identifying a population subset sufficiently at risk of preterm birth, so that prophylactic therapy might be tested on it. In a population of 2017 women, 57% of them nulliparous and the remainder multiparas without prior history of preterm birth, examinations were carried out at 22 to 24 weeks, using all 3 modalities. The incidence of preterm birth was 4.3% of which from 23% to 39% of cases were predicted by each of the 3 modalities with false-positive rates that varied from 80% to 91%. Combining fetal fibronectin assays with cervical length yielded a sensitivity of 15.6%, with 50% false positives. Combining cervical length with Bishops score, sensitivity was 14%, with 73% false positives. This group concludes "at present no screening tests for preterm birth other than a thorough obstetric history can be recommended. . ." for care of an asymptomatic low-risk gravida. Keep that in mind as you continue to read reports of the employment of these techniques.

T. H. Kirschbaum, MD

A Multicenter Controlled Trial of Fetal Pulse Oximetry in the Intrapartum Management of Nonreassuring Fetal Heart Rate Patterns

Garite TJ, Dildy GA, McNamara H, et al (Univ of California Irvine Med Ctr, Orange; Utah Valley Regional Med Ctr, Provo; McGill Univ, Montreal)
Am J Obstet Gynecol 183:1049-1058, 2000   5–2

Introduction.—Electronic fetal heart rate (FHR) monitoring is associated with increased cesarean delivery rates, partly because nonreassuring FHR patterns are an inaccurate indicator of fetal hypoxia and acidosis. The question of whether fetal pulse oximetry (FPO) could be used to assess abnormal FHR patterns in labor and improve accuracy of fetal evaluation to allow the safe reduction of cesarean delivery performed because of nonreassuring fetal status was investigated.

Methods.—Patients with full term pregnancies who were in active labor when abnormal fetal heart patterns developed were randomized to either electronic FHR monitoring alone (control group) or to the combination of electronic FHR and FPO (study group) in a randomized, controlled trial conducted concurrently in 9 centers. The main outcome was a decrease in the number of cesarean deliveries for nonreassuring fetal status as a measure of improved accuracy of evaluation of fetal oxygenation.

Results.—Of 1010 patients evaluated, 502 were randomized to the control group and 508 to the study group. A decrease of more than 50% was noted in the number of cesarean deliveries performed because of nonreassuring fetal status in the study group compared with the number performed in the control group (4.5% vs 10.2%; $P = .007$). No net difference in overall cesarean delivery rates was observed between the 2 groups (147 [29%] in the study group vs 130 [26%] in the control group;

TABLE 4.—Delivery Route and Indication

Delivery Mode and Indication	FHR Alone ($n = 502$) (No.)	FHR Plus FSpo$_2$ ($n = 508$) (No.)	Statistical Significance by χ^2
Spontaneous vaginal delivery	255 (51%)	241 (47%)	NS
Assisted vaginal delivery	117 (23%)	120 (24%)	NS
For nonreassuring fetal status	57 (11%)	55 (11%)	
For all other indications	60 (12%)	65 (13%)	
Cesarean deliveries, all indications	130 (26%)	147 (29%)	NS ($P = .49$)
Nonreassuring fetal status, single indication	51 (10%)	23 (5%)	$P < .0001$
Fetal intolerance to labor with dystocia, mixed indication	35 (7%)	27 (5%)	NS
Dystocia, single indication	43 (9%)	94 (19%)	$P < .0001$
Other indication	1 (0%)	3 (1%)	NS

Abbreviations: FHR, Fetal heart rate; *FSpo$_2$,* fetal pulse oximetry
(Courtesy of Garite TJ, Dildy GA, McNamara H et al: A multicenter controlled trial of fetal pulse oximetry in the intrapartum management of nonreassuring fetal heart rate patterns. *Am J Obstet Gynecol* 183:1049-1058, 2000.)

TABLE 8.—Neonatal Outcomes

Variable	Control	Study	Statistical Significance
1-min Apgar score <4 (No.)	29	26	NS
5-min Apgar score <7 (No.)	19	8	$P = .05$
Apgar score (mean)			
1-min	7.6	7.5	NS
5-min	8.8	8.7	NS
Cord arterial pH			
Mean	7.24	7.24	NS
<7.15	56	62	NS
<7.10	26	28	NS
<7.05	11	8	NS
<7.0	4	3	NS
Cord arterial base excess (mean)	−3.4	−3.6	NS
Resuscitation (No.)			
Bag and mask	58	73	NS
Intubation	14	6	NS
Neonatal intensive care unit admissions (No.)	74	92	NS
Suspected sepsis (No.)	21	25	NS
Respiratory disease (No.)	41	39	NS
Jaundice (No.)	59	58	NS
Neonatal length of stay (d)	1.35	1.40	NS

(Courtesy of Garite TJ, Dildy GA, McNamara H et al: A multicenter controlled trial of fetal pulse oximetry in the intrapartum management of nonreassuring fetal heart rate patterns. *Am J Obstet Gynecol* 183:1049-1058, 2000.)

$P = .49$), because there was an increase in deliveries performed in the study group because of dystocia (Table 4). A blinded partogram analysis showed that 89% of study patients and 91% of control subjects who underwent cesarean delivery because of dystocia met defined criteria for actual dystocia. No between-group differences were noted in adverse maternal or neonatal outcomes (Table 8). With respect to the surgical intervention for nonreassuring fetal status, an improvement was noted in sensitivity and specificity for the study group compared with the control group for the end points of metabolic acidosis and the need for resuscitation (Table 7).

Conclusion.—Although FPO allowed a safe reduction in cesarean deliveries performed as a result of nonreassuring fetal status, the addition of FPO did not result in an overall decrease in cesarean deliveries. The rise in cesarean deliveries because of dystocia seemed to result from well-documented labor arrest. It is not known why this occurred. The use of FPO improved the obstetrician's ability to more appropriately intervene by cesarean or operative vaginal delivery for fetuses who were actually depressed or acidotic.

TABLE 7.—Accuracy of Fetal Assessment: Agreement Between Operative Intervention* for Nonreassuring Fetal Status and Index Values in Cases of Fetal Acidosis and Depression

Immediate Neonatal Condition	FHR ($n = 108$) (No.)	SpO_2 ($n = 78$) (No.)	Sensitivity (%)		Specificity (%)		Odds Ratio†
			FHR	SpO_2	FHR	SpO_2	
Arterial pH <7.05	11	8	27	75	78	86	$P = .001$
Arterial base excess ≤−10	32	29	34	52	79	87	$P = .001$
Apgar score <7 at 5 min	18	9	28	33	79	85	$P = .17$
Bag and mask ventilation	58	73	22	27	79	87	$P = .02$
Tracheal intubation	14	6	21	50	79	85	$P = .25$

Note: A comparison is presented between the study and control groups including only those patients in whom cesarean or operative vaginal delivery was performed because of nonreassuring fetal status.
Abbreviations: FHR, Fetal heart rate; *FSpO₂,* fetal pulse oximetry.
*Includes cesarean and operative vaginal delivery intervention because of nonreassuring fetal status.
†Cochran-Mantel-Haenszel test for homogeneity of odds ratio.
(Courtesy of Garite TJ, Dildy GA, McNamara H et al: A multicenter controlled trial of fetal pulse oximetry in the intrapartum management of nonreassuring fetal heart rate patterns. *Am J Obstet Gynecol* 183:1049-1058, 2000.)

▶ This is a large prospective randomized controlled study, a counterpart to the comparable French study (see 1999 YEAR BOOK OF OBSTETRICS, GYNECOLOGY, AND WOMEN'S HEALTH, pp 147-149) aimed at evaluating the role of FPO in antenatal surveillance. The French study compared FPO with fetal blood analyses in its ability to predict newborn acidosis and neonatal impairment at birth and found that both were equally characterized by 40% to 50% false-positive rates and predictive sensitivities in the range of 35% to 40%. Here the focus is on possible utility of FPO in decision making, given a nonreassuring fetal heart rate tracing. In a large well-conducted study of 1010 women, fetal acidosis was noted in 108 pregnancies subject to FHR evaluation alone, a prevalence of 21.5%, and to FHR analysis augmented by FPO, acidosis was noted in 78 cases with a prevalence of 15.4%. Both rates are relatively high, perhaps a reflection of the lack of observer blinding and certainly a function of the well-known observer ability in evaluation of FHR patterns and management decisions based on them. FPO values indicating fetal scalp blood oxyhemoglobin saturation less than 30% for 10 to 15 minutes were deemed abnormal, despite the uncertainty of that threshold value. An occurrence of oxyhemoglobin saturation values less than 30% in more than half of monitored normal fetuses in labor was largely derived from transient cord compromise and prolonged fetal oxygen extraction from umbilical blood as fetal blood transit time is prolonged (see 2000 YEAR BOOK, pp 167-168).

Use of FPO resulted in no decrease in the incidence of cesarean section in pregnancies with nonreassuring FHR tracings but resulted in a decrease in concerns for fetal status as indication for surgery—evidence that obstetricians were reassured about fetal well-being by the FPO data. However, in the cases employing FPO, the incidence of dystocia as indication for cesarean section was nearly doubled compared with those cases treated with FHR analysis alone. That is, the same likelihood of cesarean section among pregnancies with nonreassuring FHR tracings (26% and 29%) was evident with or without use of FPO; only a shift in the nature of the preoperative diagnosis prior to section was noted. No differences in fetal neonatal outcome were noted.

The authors' primary conclusion is that FPO increased the sensitivity of prediction of real fetal jeopardy, as measured by hypoxia, acidosis, and depression at birth after delivery by forceps or cesarean section for nonreassuring fetal status, as they indicate in Table 8. However, in the FHR subset, 11 fetuses with umbilical artery pH less than 7.05 of 143 forceps and abdominal deliveries, yields a sensitivity of 7.6% and a 90% false-positive rate, not the 27% sensitivity the authors report. Among the FPO subset, there were 8 acidotic fetuses among 105 forceps plus abdominal deliveries for a sensitivity of 7.6% and a false positive rate of 90%. My calculations are the same as the authors with respect to specificity values.

The certain conclusions here are that the use of FPO, as described, neither influences the chances of cesarean sections for fetuses with nonreassuring fetal heart rate tracings nor improves fetal or neonatal outcome. If it improves predictability of an unimpaired fetus, and I believe it does not on the basis of their data, it is hard to discrimate improvement in outcome based on that prediction.

I. H. Kirschbaum, MD

Screening With a Uterine Doppler in Low Risk Pregnant Women Followed by Low Dose Aspirin in Women With Abnormal Results: A Multicenter Randomised Controlled Trial
Goffinet F, Aboulker D, Paris-Llado J, et al (INSERM U 149, France; Gen Council of Seine-Saint-Denis, France; Jean Verdier Hosp, France; et al)
Br J Obstet Gynaecol 108:510-518, 2001   5–3

Background.—Preeclampsia and intrauterine growth restriction have been significant causes of perinatal and maternal morbidity and mortality. In very high-risk populations, low doses of aspirin have been shown to help reduce the incidence of both preeclampsia and intrauterine growth restriction. However, because aspirin therapy has not appeared to be effective in low- or moderate-risk populations, it is important to find a way to identify women who could benefit from aspirin therapy. The uterine artery Doppler examination has been found to have a good predictive value for intrauterine growth restriction and preeclampsia in a general population. Systematic screening by uterine artery Doppler examination in low-risk pregnant women followed by low-dose aspirin therapy in patients with abnormal results was assessed to determine whether this strategy could reduce the incidence of intrauterine growth restriction and pre-eclampsia.

Methods.—In a multicenter randomized trial, a group of 3317 low-risk pregnant women underwent uterine artery Doppler evaluation in the 20th to 24th week. The women were randomly divided into 2 groups: those women who had uterine artery Doppler evaluation on the day of the second-trimester abdominal US examination, and those who did not have a Doppler examination (control group). Aspirin (100 mg) was administered until the 35th week to women who had abnormal results on the Doppler examination. The primary outcome measure was restriction of intrauterine growth, which was defined as birth weight below the 10th and the third percentile according to gestational age. In this study, preeclampsia was defined as hypertension associated with proteinuria greater than 9.5 g/L.

Results.—There was no significant difference between the 2 groups in the degree of intrauterine growth restriction, whether defined by the third or 10th percentile. Uterine artery Doppler screening did not appear to have any effect on birthweight or any criteria of prenatal morbidity. Doppler screening also had no effect on the incidence of preeclampsia or hypertensive disorders. The results were identical for nulliparous and multiparous women.

Conclusions.—These findings offer no justification for the use of uterine artery Doppler screening in a low-risk population, even when abnormal results are followed by increased prenatal surveillance and the administration of aspirin therapy. In future studies, predictive tests that can be performed early in pregnancy and can identify populations at very high risk of preeclampsia and intrauterine growth restriction should be assessed.

▶ This is another prospective randomized trial of uterine artery Doppler evaluation in the second trimester that fails to support routine Doppler surveillance in identifying and predicting intrauterine growth retardation and preeclampsia. It also, somewhat less convincingly, demonstrates the lack of prophylactic benefit of 0.1 gm of aspirin each to women with abnormal Doppler studies (see 1996 YEAR BOOK OF OBSTETRICS, GYNECOLOGY, AND WOMEN'S HEALTH, pp 153-155 and 2001 YEAR BOOK, pp 165-167). The population studied originates in 17 French centers. Women with prior pregnancy hypertension, fetal death, growth retardation, or diabetes were excluded, and 90.4% of uterine artery Doppler exams were performed in the 20th to 24th week of gestation. Randomization yielded 1572 women for routine Doppler exam and 1561 control subjects given standard care. The combined incidence of growth retardation was 7.6% and of preeclampsia 1.5%, with a total incidence of pregnancy hypertension of 6.3%. Aspirin 0.1 gm/d was given to all 232 women with abnormal Doppler exams, of whom only 52% were compliant. The results showed no significant difference between the 2 groups in the incidence of growth retardation based on the 8th percentile of body weight at stated gestational age, preeclampsia, birth weight, prenatal death, or newborn care requirements. It is not necessary to emphasize this point much further—there is no reason for routine Doppler uterine artery surveillance in contemporary obstetrics.

T. H. Kirschbaum, MD

The Continuing Value of the Apgar Score for the Assessment of Newborn Infants

Casey BM, McIntire DD, Leveno KJ (Univ of Texas, Dallas)
N Engl J Med 344:467-471, 2001   5–4

Background.—Some investigators have suggested that measuring pH in umbilical-artery blood is a more objective method of assessing newborns than the Apgar score. This hypothesis was tested in a retrospective cohort analysis.

Methods.—Data on 151,891 live-born singleton newborns with no malformations who were born between 1988 and 1998 were reviewed. All had been delivered at 26 weeks' gestation or later at an inner-city public hospital. Paired Apgar scores and umbilical-artery blood pH values for 145,627 infants were analyzed to determine which data best predicted neonatal death in the first 28 days of life.

Findings.—Among 13,399 infants born preterm, the neonatal mortality was 315 per 1000 for those with 5-minute Apgar scores of 0 to 3 and 5 per

TABLE 1.—Incidence of Neonatal Death in 13,399 Singleton Infants Born Before Term (At 26 to 36 Weeks of Gestation) in Relation to Apgar Scores at 5 Minutes of Age*

Five-Minute Apgar Score	No. of Live Births	Neonatal Death	Relative Risk (95% CI)
		no. (rate per 1000 births)	
0-3	92	29 (315)	59 (40-87)
4-6	556	40 (72)	13 (9-20)
7-10	12,751	68 (5)	1

*Infants with 5-minute Apgar scores of 7 to 10 served as the reference group.
(Courtesy of Casey BM, McIntire DD, Leveno KJ: The continuing value of the Apgar score for assessment of newborn infants. N Engl J Med 344:467-471, 2001. Copyright 2001, Massachusetts Medical Society. All rights reserved.)

1000 for those with 5-minute Apgar scores of 7 to 10 (Table 1). Among the 132,228 infants born at term, mortality was 244 per 1000 for those with 5-minute Apgar scores of 0 to 3 and 0.2 per 1000 for those with 5-minute Apgar scores of 7 to 10 (Table 2 and Fig 1). The risk of neonatal death in term infants with a 5-minute Apgar score of 0 to 3 was 8 times that of term infants with umbilical-artery blood pH values of 7.0 or less.

Conclusions.—The value of the Apgar score is controversial because of attempts to use it to predict infant neurologic development. However, this measure was never intended for this purpose. For predicting neonatal outcome, the Apgar score is as relevant today as it was 50 years ago.

▶ In the early 1950s, Dr Virginia Apgar introduced her method of neonatal evaluation by using linear estimates of 5 items of newborn behavior at 1 and 5 minutes of age.[1] Intended to standardize and objectify newborn behavioral characteristics to facilitate evaluation of obstetrical, anesthetic, and resuscitative performance during the first 28 days of life, her method quickly gained popularity. Not only did it meet the intended goals mentioned above, it also reinforced the growing concern of obstetricians and pediatricians with fetal and neonatal welfare. Later, the Collaborative Perinatal Study sponsored by 2 of the National Institutes of Health demonstrated that the 5-minute Apgar score correlated better with perinatal injury than did the 1-minute score, and that Apgar scores of 0 to 3 at 5 minutes, particularly when they lasted as long as 10 to 15 minutes of age had some predictive

TABLE 2.—Incidence of Neonatal Death in 132,228 Singleton Infants Born at Term (37 Weeks of Gestation or Later) in Relation to Apgar Scores at 5 Minutes of Age*

Five-Minute Apgar Score	No. of Live Births	Neonatal Death	Relative Risk (95% CI)
		no. (rate per 1000 births)	
0-3	86	21 (244)	1460 (835-2555)
4-6	561	5 (9)	53 (20-140)
7-10	131,581	22 (0.2)	1

*Infants with 5-minute Apgar scores of 7 to 10 served as the reference group.
(Courtesy of Casey BM, McIntire DD, Leveno KJ: The continuing value of the Apgar score for assessment of newborn infants. N Engl J Med 344:467-471, 2001. Copyright 2001, Massachusetts Medical Society. All rights reserved.)

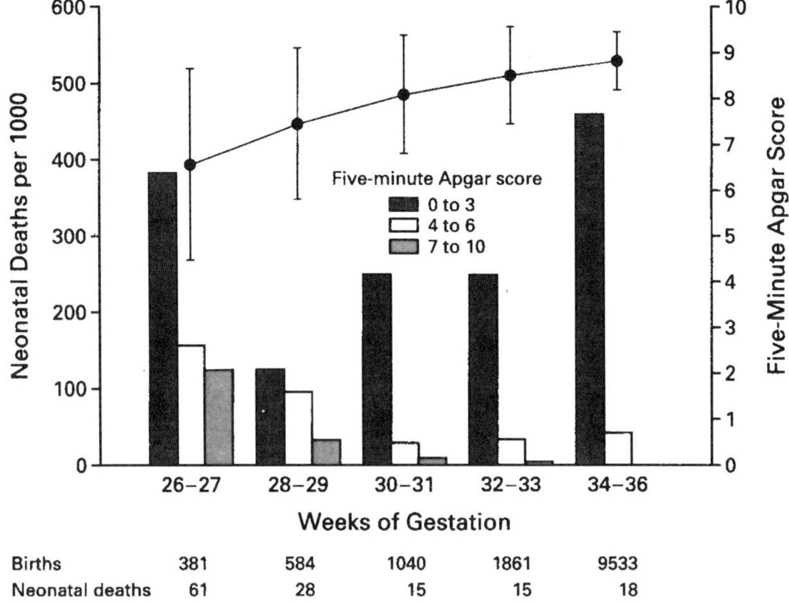

	26–27	28–29	30–31	32–33	34–36
Births	381	584	1040	1861	9533
Neonatal deaths	61	28	15	15	18

FIGURE 1.—Mean (±SD) 5-minute Apgar scores in preterm infants according to gestational age (*curve*) and neonatal death rates for infants with 5-minute Apgar scores of 0 to 3, 4 to 6, and 7 to 10 (*bars*). At 34 to 36 weeks of gestation, the neonatal death rate was 0.5 per 1000 for Apgar scores of 7 to 10. (Courtesy of Casey BM, McIntire DD, Leveno KJ: The continuing value of the Apgar score for assessment of newborn infants. *N Engl J Med* 344:467-471, 2001. Copyright 2001, Massachusetts Medical Society. All rights reserved.)

capacity for newborn CNS injury and cerebral palsy (see 1987 YEAR BOOK OF OBSTETRICS, GYNECOLOGY, AND WOMEN'S HEALTH, pp 243-245 and 1988 YEAR BOOK, pp 116-118). It also became clear that immature fetal development impeded the newborn's behavioral repertoire enough that the Apgar score was less useful in the gestational age range at greatest jeopardy for CNS injury. However, because episodes of fetal hypoxemia and respiratory acidosis may be evanescent, they are sometimes poorly reflected in the Apgar score and those often short-term events are better reflected in umbilical-artery blood analysis.

In this study of 145,627 births in which both Apgar scores and umbilical-artery blood analysis were conducted during 1988 to 1995 at the Parkland Hospital in Dallas, Tex, the relative merits of these 2 approaches to newborn evaluation are compared. For both term and premature births, the 5-minute Apgar score aggregated into 3- or 4-minute intervals significantly and inversely related to neonatal death rates. Further, the group of patients with 5-minute Apgar scores of 3 or less at 5 minutes reflected a significant increase in the prospect of neonatal death in both term and preterm infants, exempting infants with congenital malformations. Without providing the data in full, the authors indicate that umbilical-artery pH of 7 or less adds nothing to the predictability of neonatal morbidity inferred by the Apgar score alone, except that the addition of newborn acidosis to newborns with

Apgar scores of 3 or less to 5 minutes results in greater prospects for neonatal death than does either finding alone.

The study is hampered by the low prevalence of Apgar scores in the range of 0 to 3 at 5 minutes (0.12% of the total), and the omission of 4% of births where either Apgar score or umbilical artery pH was not available. This omitted group suffered a neonatal death rate 3 times higher than the cases reported here and may conceivably have altered some of the authors' conclusions. This study does, however, affirm the merits of newborn Apgar scoring, just as Virgina Apgar pointed out 50 years ago.

T. H. Kirschbaum, MD

Reference

1. Apgar V: Proposal for new method of evaluation of the human infant. *Curr Res Anesth Analg* 32:260, 1953.

6 Fetal Therapy

Differentiation of Embryonic Stem Cell Lines Generated From Adult Somatic Cells by Nuclear Transfer
Wakayama T, Tabar V, Rodriguez I, et al (Rockefeller Univ, New York; Sloan-Kettering, New York)
Science 27:740-743, 2001   6–1

Background.—Stem cells are pluripotent, undifferentiated cells that are able to differentiate into all cell types, including gametes. The potential use of such cells is limited by the ability to obtain stem cells for a given patient. A way to obtain stem cells is to take them from an embryo generated by cloning from the nuclei of the person's somatic cells. The ability to derive embryonic stem (ES) cells in vitro from the inner cell mass of blastocysts produced by cloning via nuclear transfer was evaluated.

Methods.—Nuclei obtained from adult-derived somatic donor cells of 5 mouse strains were used to produce cloned blastocysts, with each yielding at least 1 nuclear transfer ES (ntES) cell line. A total of 35 cryopreserved stable ntES cell lines were produced. Pluripotency was established by differentiating them in vitro to various ectodermal, mesodermal, and endodermal lines and by attempting to induce a highly differentiated cell type (dopaminergic neurons).

Results.—Each of the 7 lines tested was able to efficiently differentiate into the neural cell lines. The cells yielded were confirmed to be functional. Serotonergic neurons were found on histochemical testing, with the release of serotonin confirmed by reversed-phase HPLC. In reversal of the reprogramming that produced pluripotent ntES cells, a process involving re-derivation of the original nucleus donor cell types in cloned offspring, cells developed to the blastocyst stage were transferred to pseudopregnant surrogate mothers, and resulted in the births of 20 pups (all healthy with normal fertility) from 6 of the cell lines. Nine pups that died perinatally of unknown causes also contained genomic contribution from the hybrid, possibly reflecting a critical contribution made by the hybrid genetic background of that strain.

Conclusions.—Thirty-five ES cell lines were derived by nuclear transfer from adult mouse somatic cells of inbred, hybrid, and mutant strains. Various cell types were then demonstrated, including dopaminergic and serotonergic neurons (in vitro) and germ cells (in vivo). Cloning by transfer of ntES cell nuclei could be used to produce normally developed fertile

"

adults. This demonstration of the pluripotency of ntES cells is particularly applicable in providing a source of differentiated cells for human autologous transplant therapy.

▶ Embryonic stem cells are undifferentiated cells found in inner cell masses of embryos; they are capable of differentiation and replication into any cell type in the body. Their characterization and proof of totipotentiality in cells of human blastocysts by virtue of their cell surface markers was the most important event in cell biology of the decade (see 2000 YEAR BOOK OF OBSTETRICS, GYNECOLOGY, AND WOMEN'S HEALTH, pp 171-172). Initially, it was thought that embryonic stem cells existed in an undifferentiated state for a variable time period, after which they became pluripotential progenitor cells of limited developmental potential and later irreversibly became organ specific cells, where they functioned amid a few progenitor cells, which afforded some cell repair potential. Further research carried out in experimental animals because of state laws, federal research guidelines, and ethical and political considerations has revolutionized those earlier concepts.

Stem cells can be produced from nuclei of fully differentiated somatic cells by microinjecting the nucleus into an enucleated species-specific oocyte, using an electrical field to produce a reversible porelike opening in its plasma membrane-electroporesis. These ntES cells are then injected into host mouse embryonic donor blastocysts, where it has been possible to direct differentiation by nutrient and environmental manipulation into myocardial cells, neurons, CNS connective tissue cells, and hematologic and dopaminergic neurons, among other choices. The clonal colonies established in donor blastocysts serve as a source of embryonic stem cells for introduction into recipients suffering from such problems, to use human examples, as islet cell–deficiency diabetes mellitus, Parkinson's disease, hemophilia, muscular dystrophies, hepatic cirrhosis, and epithelial and connective tissue disorders.

Producing stem cells from adult somatic cells and clonal intermediates has many advantages. The clonal colonies provide a ready source of large numbers of stem cells in comparison to the very few that may be obtained from any embryonic inner cell mass. Direct use of fetal tissues is avoided. Such stem cells are autoregulated. That is, hematologic stem cells may be given in large numbers and will result in regulated hematopoesis, despite ignorance of the internal regulatory processes that prevail. Host toxicity for such transplantation has reduced the effects of drugs used to prepare the host for injection, and no long-standing immune suppression is necessary. Finally, when autoimmune rejection is minimized, only a single application of stem cells may be needed to establish an effective level of the new gene product. There are no immediate applications for fetal use here, but the potential for fetal repair is almost unlimited. Obstetricians should know about this exciting set of opportunities and lend our voices in support of stem cell research by federal sources. Readers might find "Stem Cells Branch Out" by Hines and Powell[1] a helpful reference in this regard.

T. H. Kirschbaum, MD

References

1. Hines PJ, Powell BA: Stem cells branch out. *Science* 287:1417-1446, 2000.

Fetal Immunization by a DNA Vaccine Delivered Into the Oral Cavity
Gerdts V, Babiuk LA, Van Drunen Littel-van den Hurk S, et al (Univ of Saskatchewan, Saskatoon, Canada)
Nature Med 6:929-932, 2000   6–2

Introduction.—Estimates provided by the World Health Organization indicate that infectious diseases caused the death of approximately 8 million infants in 1995. Among the important pathogens involved are herpes simplex virus, HIV, hepatitis B virus, and chlamydia. Prophylactic antibiotics and cesarean section are used in an attempt to reduce the risk of disease transmission, but these approaches are not always effective. A DNA vaccine, delivered into the amniotic fluid in the oral cavity of fetal lambs, induced high serum antibody titers and a cell-mediated immune response.

Methods.—Delivery of DNA into the amniotic fluid in the oral cavity was performed at day 123 or 124 of pregnancy (148-day gestation). Investigators used a plasmid encoding a truncated form of bovine herpes-virus 1 glycoprotein D with the transmembrane portion removed (tgD). Four fetuses were immunized with a single injection of 500 µg tgD plasmid and 4 more fetuses received PBS. Fetal sera were obtained and organ tissues were collected at day 143 or 144 of gestation.

Results.—There were no fetal deaths, and the fetal lambs were of normal size and had normal organ development. Histologic examination revealed no pathologic changes. All DNA-vaccinated fetuses responded with high titers of gD-specific serum antibodies, which were not found in any PBS-injected fetuses or in the ewes. The primary site of gD expression and antigen presentation was determined to be the oral cavity area. Effective mucosal immunity is a chief factor in preventing initial infec-tion of the infant, for most infectious agents enter the host through the mucosal surfaces. Analysis of gD-specific immune responses of lympho-cytes isolated from lymph nodes draining various mucosal surfaces indi-cated that mucosal immunity had been achieved with the DNA vaccine.

Conclusion.—In the fetal lamb, a single immunization with a DNA vaccine delivered into the amniotic fluid in the oral cavity induced local immunity. This method may minimize the hazards associated with intra-uterine injections and provide a safe and effective means of preventing or reducing the high risk of vertical disease transmission during pregnancy and after birth.

► These investigators, using DNA vaccination in an experimental animal, have demonstrated the possibility of introducing acquired specific cellular and humoral immunity in late pregnancy in utero. The experimental technique involved gene insertion of a viral DNA segment using a plasmid vector rendered nonpathogenic by truncating part of the DNA sequence yet leaving enough material to allow generation of specific antibody. That antibody has the capacity to recognize and combine with the complete viral antigen complex in vivo. The vector allows incorporation of the foreign DNA into the host genome, resulting in gene transformation and providing a template upon which antibody formation in the course of development in later life depends.

Here the chosen DNA segment was specific to a glycoprotein, gD, derived from the bovine herpes virus. Laparotomy was performed on gravid ewes and the DNA preparation injected through the uterine wall into the amniotic fluid–filled mouth of the fetus. Four animals were treated and compared with 4 controls. All treated fetuses showed normal development as marked by the increase in fetal cortisol appropriate to the onset of labor near term. There was no resultant maternal fetal or neonatal injury from the procedure. High serum titers to gD developed in all test fetal animals, and neither control nor maternal animals showed significant antibody development to this antigen. The presence of intact immune function in fetal animals was proven by their ability to perform conversion from immunoglobulin-M to immunoglobulin-G for gD with time. Further, the development of cellular immunity was proven by the ability of fetal mononuclear cells to undergo lymphoproliferation on exposure to antigen. Local mucosal immunity was proven by the demonstration of gD-specific antibody production from immune cells isolated from lymph nodes draining the oropharynx.

Clearly, there is work to be done to prove the capability of orally ingested DNA to evoke a general immune reaction through exposure in the human fetal gastrointestinal tract. The technique is applicable to bacterial organisms as well as viruses. The prospects of using this technique in late pregnancy to influence infection by HIV-1, cytomegalovirus, group B *Streptococcus*, and hepatitis B and C in cases of high fetal infectivity are exciting. US can be used to perform the fetal injections without laparotomy in the human. It will be interesting to watch for results of further work on this approach, which has the potential to produce acquired immunity in fetuses infected or at risk of infection in utero.

T. H. Kirschbaum, MD

Fetal Syphilis: Clinical and Laboratory Characteristics
Hollier LM, Harstad TW, Sanchez PJ, et al (Univ of Texas, Dallas)
Obstet Gynecol 97:947-953, 2001   6–3

Background.—Because of the increased incidence of HIV infection among pregnant women and the increased findings of gonorrhea, it is anticipated that syphilis will similarly increase. Detection of congenital disease in the fetus has been rare for various reasons, leading to a lack of information concerning the pathophysiology of fetal disease. Biochemical, immunologic, and sonographic means were used to detect intrauterine

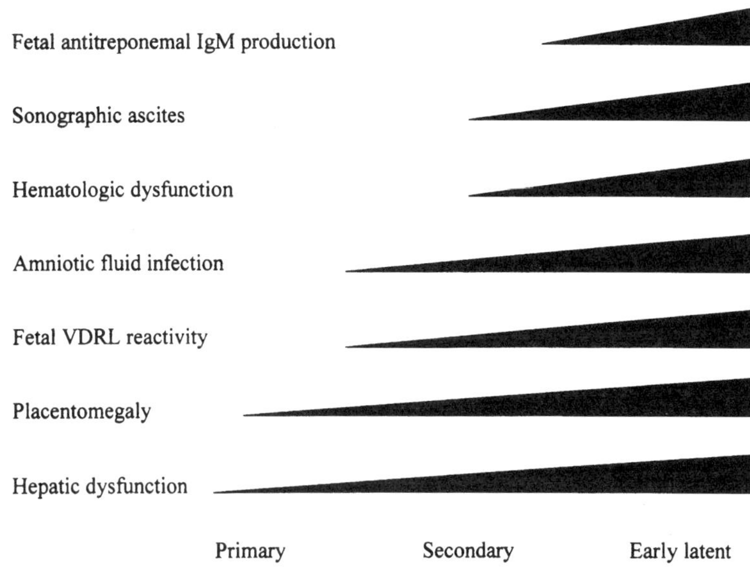

FIGURE 1.—Hypothesized continuum of fetal syphilis infection. (Reprinted with permission of The American College of Obstetrics and Gynecology from Hollier LM, Harstad TW, Sanchez PJ, et al: Fetal syphilis: Clinical and laboratory characteristics. *Obstet Gynecol* 97:947-953, 2001.)

infection by *Treponema pallidum*, and the results were correlated with treatment outcomes.

Methods.—Prospective identification was made of 24 pregnant women with untreated syphilis. All underwent sonography with amniocentesis and percutaneous umbilical blood sampling. Samples of amniotic fluid were subjected to dark-field examination, rabbit infectivity testing, and polymerase chain reaction to detect *T pallidum*. Fetal blood samples were used for hematologic and chemical tests, with fetal antitreponemal IgM detected with Western blot assay. Mothers were treated with 2.4 to 4.8 million units of benzathine penicillin G IM. The signs of congenital syphilis in the infants were noted, and outcomes were evaluated.

Results.—Six women had primary syphilis, 12 had secondary syphilis, and 6 had early latent disease. Abnormal US findings were noted in 16 fetuses; 13 had hepatomegaly, and 3 had hepatomegaly with ascites. Systolic/diastolic ratios were above normal for gestational age in 3 fetuses and 1 had hydrops; hydramnios was noted in 1 patient. Seventeen of the placentas had increased thickness for gestational age, which affected half of the fetuses of mothers with primary syphilis, 75% of those with secondary syphilis, and 83% of those with early latent disease. *T pallidum* was found in 14 of 22 amniotic fluid specimens, with positive dark-field testing in 6 cases and positive rabbit infectivity test results in 12 cases. Overall, 66% of the fetuses had either congenital syphilis or *T pallidum* in the amniotic fluid. Other fetal abnormalities included fetal antitreponemal

IgM (3 infants), abnormal liver transaminases (88% of cases), anemia (26% of cases), and thrombocytopenia (35% of cases). Treatment of the mother was successful in 83% of the cases. When both hepatomegaly and ascites were present, the risk of treatment failure rose.

Conclusions.—Fetal syphilis resembles neonatal syphilis. Projecting from the data discovered, elevated levels of fetal transaminase occur early in the infection, and then hematologic problems and hydrops develop (Fig 1). More severe infections are associated with greater chances that treatment will be ineffective.

▶ This is a first effort to define the pathophysiologic sequence of changes in fetal congenital syphilis with the use of contemporary imaging, amniocentesis, and cordocentesis. It suffers from the availability of only 24 cases of untreated early syphilis in pregnancy, but the authors are breaking a previously untrodden path. The study is important because of the likely future increase in congenital syphilis associated with the AIDS epidemic. Over a period of 3 years, it was possible to identify 24 women with untreated primary, secondary, or early latent syphilis past 24 weeks of pregnancy. Since fetuses lack discernible immune responses to syphilis before 24 weeks, women at less than 24 weeks of pregnancy were treated with standard antibiotic therapy and were not followed up for study purposes. The others received routine US together with estimates of liver size, umbilical artery, and vein Doppler S to D ratios and measurements of placental size and thickness. Amniotic fluid samples were used for rabbit injection and examined by dark-field and fluorescent *Treponema* antibody techniques for identification of *T pallidum*. Cord blood was submitted for VDRL, IgM for syphilis, and liver function assays were performed on fetal blood. From a small number of cases, the authors attempt to estimate the time sequence of changes observed in the fetus.

Two thirds of the cases of maternal infection past 24 weeks of pregnancy showed evidence of fetal infection. Placentomegaly was an early and progressive change in 70% of the cases, especially with primary syphilis. Cord blood VDRL was positive in 83% of the cases, and in two thirds of the cases, *T pallidum* could be found in amniotic fluid. Changes in fetal platelets and leukocyte count occurred relatively late in fetal infection and were seen in only about a third of the cases. Sonographic ascites was seen in 3 patients and, coupled with hepatomegaly, was associated in all cases of fetal infection. In only 3 infants was cord blood positive for IgM, and evidence of liver injury by virtue of elevated gamma glutamyl transpeptidase proved to be the most sensitive measure of fetal infection (positive in 94% of the subsequently confirmed cases). The authors' figure 1 serves as a crude means of estimating the presence and extent of changes in fetal infection when, despite the success rate of antibiotic therapy of 83% in such cases, evidence of fetal infection is seen.

T. H. Kirschbaum, MD

Histologic Chorioamnionitis, Antenatal Steroids, and Perinatal Outcomes

Elimian A, Verma U, Beneck D, et al (New York Med College, Valhalla)
Obstet Gynecol 96:333-336, 2000   6–4

Background.—The association between histologic chorioamnionitis and preterm neonatal morbidity and mortality has not been defined clearly. The perinatal effects of histologic chorioamnionitis on preterm neonates and the efficacy of antenatal steroids in the presence of histologic chorioamnionitis were investigated.

Methods.—Between 1990 and 1997, 1260 neonates weighing 1750 g or less were born at 1 center. This cohort was stratified primarily by the presence of histologic chorioamnionitis and secondarily by antenatal steroid exposure.

Findings.—The placentas of 527 neonates showed evidence of histologic chorioamnionitis, and those of 733 did not. The former group had a lower gestational age, a lower birth weight, and a higher rate of major neonatal morbidities than the latter group. After adjustment for confounding variables, histologic chorioamnionitis was correlated independently with lower gestational age, lower birth weight, and neonatal death. Neonates with histologic chorioamnionitis who were exposed to steroids antenatally had a significantly lower incidence of low Apgar scores, respiratory distress syndrome, intraventricular hemorrhage and periventricular leukomalacia, major brain lesions, patent ductus arteriosus, and neonatal death compared with neonates with histologic chorioamnionitis and no antenatal exposure to steroids (Table 4).

TABLE 4.—Antenatal Steroids in Presence of Histologic Chorioamnionitis

Characteristic	HCA + ANS ($n = 169$)	HCA − ANS ($n = 358$)	P
Maternal age (y)	29.1 ± 5.9	28.9 ± 5.7	.58
Gestational age (wk, mean ± SD)	27.8 ± 2.6	27.7 ± 3.4	.74
Birth weight (g, mean ± SD)	1125 ± 335	1078 ± 370	.16
Birth weight (%, ± SD)	49.0 ± 22	46.3 ± 22	.19
5-min Apgar score<7	31 (18%)	120 (33.5%)	<.001
Surfactant	107 (63.3%)	210 (58.7%)	.31
RDS	67 (39.6%)	200 (55.9%)	<.001
Total IVH/PVL	37 (21.9%)	132 (36.9%)	<.001
Major brain lesions*	13 (7.7%)	66 (18.4%)	<.001
Necrotizing enterocolitis	10 (5.9%)	22 (6.1%)	.91
Patent ductus arteriosus	25 (14.8%)	85 (23.7%)	.018
Proved neonatal sepsis	31 (18.3%)	50 (14%)	.24
Neonatal death	14 (8.3%)	58 (16.2%)	.01

*Major brain lesions include periventricular leukomalacia with or without associated intraventricular hemorrhage, or grades 3 and 4 intraventricular hemorrhage.

Abbreviations: +ANS, Antenatal steroids exposed; −ANS, antenatal steroids unexposed; RDS, respiratory distress syndrome; IVH/PVL, all abnormal neurosonograms, including all grades of intraventricular hemorrhage, periventricular leukomalacia, or both.

(Reprinted with permission from The American College of Obstetricians and Gynecologists from Elimian A, Verma U, Beneck D, et al: Histologic chorioamnionitis, antenatal steroids, and perinatal outcomes. *Obstet Gynecol* 96:333-336, 2000.)

Conclusion.—Through its association with preterm birth, histologic chorioamnionitis is correlated with an increase in major perinatal morbidity. This condition is independently associated with neonatal death. Antenatal steroid exposure in affected neonates significantly reduces the incidence of respiratory distress syndrome, intraventricular bleeding and periventricular leukomalacia, major brain lesions, and neonatal death, without increasing sepsis.

▶ Antenatal steroids are probably contraindicated for women in preterm labor with clinical evidence of chorioamnionitis because of the risk of decreased host resistance to infection. Further, they are probably unnecessary because those fetuses are likely to be undergoing maximum endogenous stress-related steroid production (see 2000 YEAR BOOK OF OBSTETRICS, GYNECOLOGY, AND WOMEN'S HEALTH, pp 66-71). In the absence of clinical evidence of chorioamnionitis, the value of improved very low birth weight pulmonary function appears to outweigh the risk of steroid administration to the subset of newborns with latent chorioamnionitis destined eventually without delivery to clinical infection.

There have been relatively few directly applicable data to support that contention, especially in the birth range from 0.5 to 1.75 kg where latent chorioamnionitis is relatively common and this analysis provides a clear answer. Of 1260 women in preterm labor without clinical evidence of chorioamnionitis, preterm premature rupture of membranes, or pregnancy-induced hypertension, 527, or 42%, proved to have histologic evidence of chorioamnionitis at delivery. That group, compared with women delivering without chorioamnionitis, was composed of women delivering at a lesser mean gestational age and birth weight as Dr. Hillier demonstrated years ago (see 1990 YEAR BOOK, pp 34-36).

On univariate analysis, those with positive cultures post partum expressed higher rates of immediate and delayed postpartum neonatal morbidity, including brain injury and neonatal death. On logistic regression analysis, those findings tended to be a reflection solely of the lesser gestational age and birth weight in the women delivering with positive cultures. Thirty-two percent of the 527 women whose placentas showed latent chorioamnionitis received appropriate antenatal steroids and showed no increase in the incidence of neonatal sepsis but benefitted in comparison with 358 culture-positive women with a gestational age and birth weight comparable to the others who did not receive steroids. Although it is certainly no favor for a fetus in the very low birth weight range to be exposed to latent chorioamnionitis, this study clearly shows that the value of exposing it to antenatal steroid administration clearly exceeds the hypothetical risk of augmented infection.

T. H. Kirschbaum, MD

7 Surgical Obstetrics, Anesthesia, and Delivery

Uterine Rupture During Induced Trial of Labor Among Women With Previous Cesarean Delivery
Ravasia DJ, Wood SL, Pollard JK (Univ of Calgary, Alta, Canada)
Am J Obstet Gynecol 183:1176-1179, 2000   7–1

Introduction.—Nonsignificant trends toward higher rupture rates have been reported with use of prostaglandin E_2 (PGE_2) for labor induction for patients with vaginal birth after cesarean delivery (VBAC). Some reports have indicated there is no increased risk. The rates of uterine rupture and vaginal delivery among women with previous cesarean delivery whose deliveries were induced were compared retrospectively with those of women with previous cesarean delivery who entered labor spontaneously.

Methods.—All deliveries between 1992 and 1998 of females with previous cesarean delivery were evaluated. The rates of uterine rupture were determined for spontaneous labor and various methods of induction.

Results.—Of 26,868 deliveries between 1992 and 1998, 2119 (87%) attempted VBAC, of which 575 (27%) were induced VBAC labors. The overall uterine rupture rate was 0.71% (15/2119) for women undergoing VBAC. Women who underwent induced VBAC labor had a significantly higher rate of uterine rupture than those who had spontaneous labor (1.4% vs 0.45%; $P = .004$). Compared with spontaneous labor, the uterine rupture rates associated with different methods of induction were PGE_2 gel, 2.9% (5/172; $P = .004$); intracervical Foley catheter, 0.76% (1/129; $P = .47$); and labor induction not necessitating cervical ripening, 0.74% (2/274; $P = .63$). The uterine rupture rate related to inductions other than PGE_2 was 0.74% (3/474; $P = .38$) (Table 2). The relative risk of uterine rupture with PGE_2 use was 6.41, compared with spontaneous trial of labor.

Conclusion.—Labor induction was correlated with increased risk of uterine rupture among women with a previous cesarean delivery; this corrclation was highest when PGE_2 gel was used.

TABLE 2.—Uterine Ruptures During Induced Trial of Labor According to
Method of Induction

Method	Ruptures (No.)	Trials of Labor (No.)	Rupture Rate (%)	Statistical Significance*
PGE$_2$ gel	5	172	2.9	$P = .004$
Intracervical Foley catheter	1	129	0.76	NS
Induction not requiring cervical ripening	2	274	0.73	NS
Spontaneous labor (baseline risk)	7	1544	0.45	Referent

Note: $\chi^2 = 13.26$; degrees of freedom = 3; $P = .004$.
*Comparison versus spontaneous labor with the Fisher exact test.
Abbreviation: NS, Not significant.
(Courtesy of Ravasia DJ, Wood SL, Pollard JK: Uterine rupture during induced trial of labor among women with previous cesarean delivery. Am J Obstet Gynecol 183:1176-1179 2000.)

▶ It is useful to recall the information demonstrated nicely in this case control study of VBAC attempted in 2119 women in Alberta, Canada. Twenty-seven percent had induction of labor for the usual reasons, that is, gestational age at or past 41 weeks, low amniotic fluid index, spontaneous rupture of membranes, and medical complications. The incidence of uterine rupture was 0.45% among women with spontaneous onset of labor, entirely comparable to the results of several other investigators. Among those undergoing induction of labor, the rate of rupture was 1.4%—almost all attributable to the 575 women whose inductions included 172 patients with PGE$_2$ vaginal gel application. Forty-five percent of those pregnancies also had oxytocin-based inductions. The effects of PGE$_2$ on the uterus and cervix are unpredictable with respect to the force of uterine contractions and, in some cases, PGE$_2$ pretreatment tends to increase the likelihood of oxytocin hyperstimulation of the uterus. Though low gestational age and low parity exist as confounding factors of induction of labor, PGE$_2$ is best avoided in VBAC, and other means of cervical ripening are better employed when induction with oxytocin is deemed necessary.

T. H. Kirschbaum, MD

Vaginal Birth After Cesarean: To Induce or Not to Induce

Sims EJ, Newman RB, Hulsey TC (Med Univ of South Carolina, Charleston)
Am J Obstet Gynecol 184:1122-1124, 2001   7–2

Background.—The induction of labor may be linked with a need for cesarean delivery versus vaginal delivery. The safety and success of labor induction in women who now were anticipating vaginal delivery after having had a previous cesarean delivery (vaginal birth after cesarean, VBAC) were evaluated.

Methods.—The 505 women observed prospectively presented for delivery consecutively. Of these, 236 women underwent a trial of labor. The 3 cohorts evaluated were 269 women who had repeat cesarean without trial of labor, 179 women with a spontaneous trial of labor, and 57 with an induced trial of labor.

Results.—Patients who had spontaneous labor achieved vaginal delivery at a significantly higher rate than women whose labor was induced (77.1% for the former, 57.9% for the latter). VBAC success was influenced by previous vaginal delivery, previous VBAC, and favorable cervical score, with both previous vaginal delivery and spontaneous onset of labor independent predictors of success in achieving VBAC. Patients who had not given birth vaginally in a previous pregnancy were at significantly higher risk of a repeat cesarean when labor was induced. The risk of cesarean delivery was not increased in women who had delivered vaginally in a previous pregnancy. Indications for repeat cesarean were similar, whether labor was induced or spontaneous. Uterine scar separation occurred significantly more often in women with induced labor than in those with elective repeat cesarean but did not differ in the other groups. Method of induction had no effect on success or safety of induction, but use of oxytocin in women who spontaneously entered labor was linked to a significant reduction in the likelihood that vaginal delivery would be accomplished.

Conclusions.—The induction of labor in women who are planning to deliver vaginally after having had a previous cesarean delivery carries a significantly reduced rate of success. In addition, the risk of separation of the uterine scar is increased in these women, leading to the recommendation that labor be induced only when the maternal or fetal indications are compelling.

▶ In studies of VBAC larger than this, with enough cases to explore results based on the indication from the first or prior cesarean section, a previous abdominal birth because of failure of cervical progression has long appeared as an unfavorable sign for success in later VBAC. Here that cannot be affirmed, but it exists as an uncontrolled independent variable that might account for the results of this retrospective case control study of 236 women undergoing VBAC. In 24% of the women, labor was induced for indications that are not stated. Successful trial of labor occurred in 77.1% of those entering labor spontaneously and in 57.9% of those whose labors were induced. Further, the induction subset exhibited a 7% incidence of uterine dehiscense compared with 1.5% in those with spontaneous onset of labor. Both rates seemed high for unclear reasons. Some of the dehiscence incidents may have been derived from the use of vaginal misprostol and dinoprostone with adjunctive oxytocin, a practice not to be recommended. Without providing data, the authors claim that they can find no differences in the safety or efficacy based on the mode of induction. This study does provide a reminder that, among VBAC candidates, there is a subset of uncertain size destined to constitute repeated failures of labor induction because of unknown structural or functional characteristics of their uteri.

T. H. Kirschbaum, MD

Is Vaginal Birth After Cesarean Safe? Experience at a Community Hospital

Blanchette H, Blanchette M, McCabe J, et al (Metro West Med Ctr, Framington, Mass)
Am J Obstet Gynecol 184:1478-1487, 2001   7–3

Introduction.—The growing rate of cesarean deliveries in the United States became a cause for concern in the 1980s, and trials of labor after a previous cesarean birth were increased in the 1990s in an attempt to reduce the cesarean rate. The results of a 4-year program in which a trial of labor after previous cesarean (TOLAC) was promoted were reported.

Methods.—The study was conducted at a 350-bed community hospital in Massachusetts. The hospital had a total cesarean rate of 20% in 1995 and a repeat cesarean rate of 7.3%. During the period of review, 1996 through 1999, 1481 women who delivered at the hospital had a history of cesarean birth. Physicians were encouraged to offer TOLAC to all patients except when medically contraindicated. Outcomes were compared for the 727 women who elected repeat cesarean section and the 754 who attempted TOLAC. The latter cohort was further divided into successful vaginal birth after cesarean (VBAC) and unsuccessful VBAC. All uterine ruptures were recorded and analyzed.

Results.—The incidence of maternal complications across the 3 cohorts (elective repeat cesarean, successful VBAC, and unsuccessful VBAC) was very small. Patients for whom a trial of labor failed, however, and who underwent an emergency cesarean, had significantly greater blood loss. The unsuccessful VBAC group included 12 patients with uterine rupture. Eleven of the ruptures involved induction or augmentation of labor (Table 5). Both neonatal deaths that occurred resulted from catastrophic uterine rupture, but neonatal outcomes were otherwise similar in the 3 cohorts. The VBAC attempt rate was 50.9% and declined significantly during the last 2 years of the study, whereas the elective repeat cesarean rate increased significantly during the last 2 years of the study.

Conclusion.—The VBAC attempt rate was not increased at a community hospital in which physicians were encouraged to reduce the rate of repeat cesarean births. After 2 fetal losses occurred, many practitioners counseled their patients to consider repeat cesarean delivery. Although

TABLE 5.—Method of Labor and Relationship to Uterine Rupture

	Spontaneous Labor Alone	Augmented Labor Alone	Induced Labor (2 With Augmentation)
No.	292	288	174
Uterine rupture	1	4	7
Percent with rupture	0.3	1.4	4.0*

*Significant by chi-square, $P = .004$.
(Courtesy of Blanchette H, Blanchette M, McCabe J, et al: Is vaginal birth after cesarean safe? Experience at a community hospital. *Am J Obstet Gynecol* 184:1478-1487, 2001.)

TABLE 1 (discussion).—Rates of Uterine Rupture During VBAC

Series	Type of Labor	Uterine Rupture No.	%	Comment
Flamm et al (Kaiser, Los Angeles)	Spontaneous labor	33/4569	0.7%	All 6 cases of rupture had prostaglandin gel plus oxytocin
	Induced labor	6/453	1.3%	
McNally and Turner (Dublin)	Spontaneous labor	0/560	0.0%	Oxytocin plus amniotomy; only 9 cases had prostaglandin E_2
	Induced labor	2/103	2.0%*	
Zelop et al (Harvard)	Spontaneous labor	16/2214	0.7%	Oxytocin plus prostaglandin E_2; 4.5% rupture rate
	Induced labor	13/560	2.3%*	
Fleischman et al (Yale)	Spontaneous labor	13/560	2.3%	Oxytocin with or without dinoprostone or misoprostol
	Induced labor	11/203	5.4%*	
Bebbington and Waterman (Vancouver)	Spontaneous labor	11/2590	0.4%	Oxytocin with or without prostaglandin E_2
	Induced labor	8/1097	0.7%	
Blanchette et al (current study) (Framingham, Mass)	Spontaneous labor	4/580	0.7%	Oxytocin with or without misoprostol
	Induced labor	8/174	4.6%*	

*Significant at $P < .01$.
Abbreviation: VBAC, Vaginal birth after cesarean.
(Courtesy of Blanchette H, Blanchette M, McCabe J, et al: Is vaginal birth after cesarean safe? Experience at a community hospital. *Am J Obstet Gynecol* 184:1478-1487, 2001.)

VBAC can be safe, a repeat elective cesarean may be safer, especially if labor is induced (Discussion Table 1).

▶ This report of the attempt to reduce a 20% cesarean section rate by use of VBAC from 1996 to 1999 is similar to the results reported by others but is informative in pointing out a hazard that, in retrospect, may have been overlooked. In the initial year of VBAC, 51% of 148 eligible women accepted a trial or labor with a 76% success rate. Assuming an annual delivery incidence of 2800 women per year, this yields a 13% incidence of gravidas with a prior cesarean section, some with more than 1 prior section. Comparisons between successful and unsuccessful trials of labor showed only an increased mean estimated blood loss and reduced Apgar scores among the latter, explicable by the presence of 12 uterine ruptures, all but 1 of which occurred in women undergoing labor induction or oxytocin augmentation and misoprostol. Clearly, this is a dangerous combination. There was no surplus neonatal morbidity or mortality as a result of trial of labor. The overall uterine rupture rate of 1.6% is high compared with the experience of others, but the author and his discussants from the Pacific Coast Obstetrical and Gynecological Society meeting, where the paper was presented, provide an abstract of 5 other reports with rupture rates with oxytocin and a prostoglandin uteronic ranging from 0.7% to 5.4%. The authors conclude that the induction/augmentation is not safe in VBAC. Almost certainly, the risk may be diminished by using oxytocin alone, but the safety of induction of labor in patients undergoing VBAC is something to concern all of us.

T. H. Kirschbaum, MD

Temporal Changes in Rates and Reasons for Medical Induction of Term Labor, 1980-1996
Yawn B, Wollan P, McKeon K, et al (Mayo Clinic, Rochester, Minn)
Am J Obstet Gynecol 184:611-619, 2001   7–4

Objective.—Although the rate of labor induction has more than doubled in the last decade, there have been few studies about the risks and benefits of elective induction of labor. Temporal shifts in the relative rates of induction, indications for induction, and apparent modifications to the definition applied to those indications were retrospectively investigated in a population-based cohort of women with term deliveries.

Methods.—All 1293 women with term pregnancies, who were induced between 1980 and 1995, were identified. Demographic and personal data, prenatal data, data from labor and delivery, and highest blood pressure were analyzed. Changes with time for induction were grouped for the years 1980 to 1982, 1986 to 1988, 1990 to 1992, and 1993 to 1995. The Mantel-Haenszel test was used to determine trends.

Results.—Maternal age and weight increased during the study period, while the percentage of primiparous women who had labor induced declined, even though the numbers of primiparous women who had labor

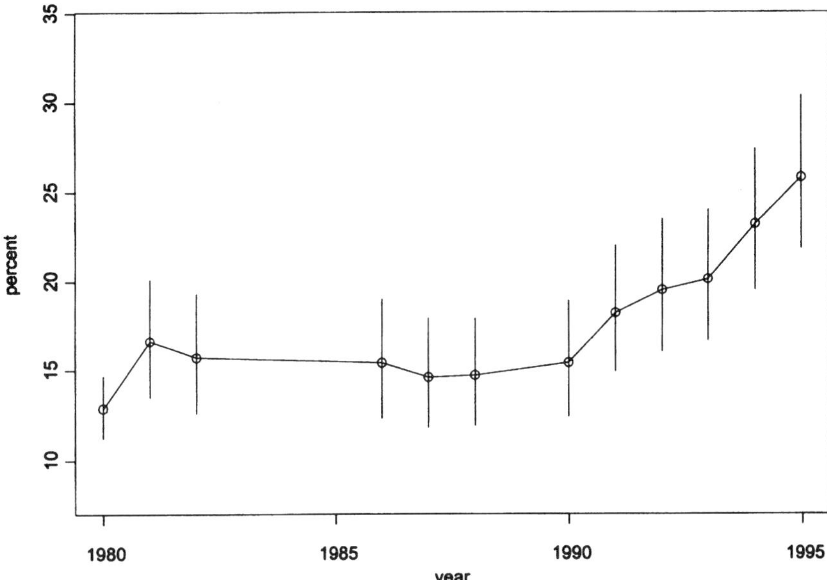

FIGURE 1.—Temporal trends in percentage of term pregnancies induced. (Courtesy of Yawn B, Wollan P, McKeon K, et al: Temporal changes in rates and reasons for medical induction of term labor, 1980-1996. *Am J Obstet Gynecol* 184:611-619, 2001.)

induced increased. The annual rate of term pregnancies that were induced increased significantly (Fig 1). Reasons for induction, including postdate gestation, large for gestational age (LGA) fetus, maternal or fetal problems, and choice increased significantly from 1980 to 1995. Induction for premature rupture of membranes decreased significantly during the same period. Gestational age at delivery declined significantly in postterm induction births (Table 3). Methods of induction with the use of intravenously administered oxytocin declined from 99% to 67%, while the use of prostaglandin vaginal inserts, and orally, vaginally, and rectally administered misoprostol increased. The percentage of cesarean deliveries after induction increased during the study period, while the percentage of cesarean deliveries among women with spontaneous labor at term declined.

TABLE 3.—Gestational Age at Delivery in Those Pregnancies With Labor Induced for the Stated Reason of Postterm Gestation

Postterm Inductions in Period (%)	<40 wk	40-40.9 wk	41-41.9 wk	≥42 wk
1980-1982 (n = 83)	3.6	7.2	30.1	59.0
1986-1988 (n = 73)	0.0	4.1	54.8	41.1
1990-1992 (n = 96)	4.2	13.5	68.8	13.5
1993-1995 (n = 123)	3.3	26.0	61.8	8.9

(Courtesy of Yawn B, Wollan P, McKeon K, et al: Temporal changes in rates and reasons for medical induction of term labor, 1980-1996. *Am J Obstet Gynecol* 184:611-619, 2001.)

Conclusion.—The incidence of induced labor for premature rupture of membranes has declined, and the number of inductions for elective reasons has increased significantly. The risks and benefits of the increasing use of induction need to be evaluated.

► If you feel, as I do, that inductions of labor at term are increasing in number and increasingly involve pregnancies with unsupportable indications, you will be pleased with this chart study of 1293 women induced at term in Olmsted County in southern Minnesota. The time interval studied was from 1980 to 1995; prior to 1980, Minnesota birth certificates did not yield information regarding induction or augmentation of labor, and after that they did not give an indication for the procedure. This omission necessitated extensive chart reviews which were managed with reviews of delivery logs and partial record reviews evaluated for completeness, alternating with complete reviews for some years (1980 for example) and full reviews of every third chart abstracted in later years. In this way, 41% of the available 4100 cases were abstracted and 1293 records or 31.5% composed the basis for this study. Ninety two percent of the women were Caucasian.

Over the 15 years reported, inductions doubled in incidence from 12.9% to 25.8% of all term births. These incidence figures virtually duplicate those reported by the Bureau of Health Statistics for 1955.[1] The incidence of premature rupture of membranes as an indication for term induction declined from about 4.3% to 0.2% at birth, a value that exceeds the 2.1% figure that would be expected from doubling the denominator composed of total term induction during the period of 1980 to 1995. The result is not clear and the observation suggests underreporting in record abstracting. The bulk of the increase in term inductions came from postdatism, which increased 2.3 times in number, composed largely of pregnancies averaging 41 weeks' gestational age (see Table 3). Only 2.3% of term deliveries reached 42 completed weeks of gestation during this time interval versus 19.2% in the same category for 1980. Elective inductions, that is, those for which no indication was discernible, doubled in relative frequency during this interval. Inductions for suspected macrosomia increased from virtually none in 1980 to 3.4% of term births in 1995, most of them infants with birth weights less than 4 kg.

We are left with a decrease in the relative frequency of term indications for premature rupture of membranes for which there is evidence of maternal and fetal benefit, and increases in induction for gestational age at or prior to 42 completed weeks of pregnancy, suspected macrosomia, and elective inductions without objective support. Because induction resulted in longer hospitalization and spontaneous labor onset in this and other studies, along with a greater likelihood of abdominal birth, these data raise questions about induction practices, at least in Olmsted County, and whether they might not indicate contemporary trends in obstetrical practice nationwide.

T. H. Kirschbaum, MD

Reference

1. Ventura SJ, Martin JA, Kurtin SC, et al: Report of final neonatal statistics, 1995. *Mon Vital Stat Rep* 45(1):1-80, 1997.

Prolonged Pregnancy: Induction of Labor and Cesarean Births
Alexander JM, McIntire DD, Leveno KJ (Univ of Texas, Dallas)
Obstet Gynecol 97:911-915, 2001   7–5

Background.—Labor is induced in about 20% of pregnant women, with most inductions occurring in women who have the longest gestations. Studies have been done that link an increased incidence of cesarean birth with labor induction because of prolonged gestation, but the women studied had numerous other complicating factors and varying periods of gestation. Women whose gestation was 41 to 41 6/7 weeks and whose only complication was prolonged pregnancy were studied in an attempt to determine the effects of labor induction on cesarean delivery in women with this specific condition.

Methods.—The women studied were scheduled for labor induction at 42 weeks, having reached 41 weeks already. The rates of cesarean delivery

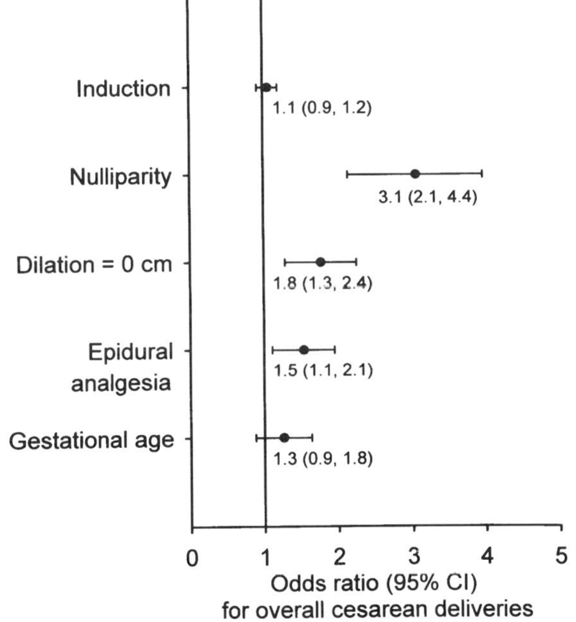

FIGURE 1.—Odds ratio for overall cesarean delivery related to induction of labor corrected for nulliparity, cervical dilatation, gestational age, and epidural analgesia. *Abbreviation: CI,* Confidence interval. (Reprinted with permission from The American College of Obstetricians and Gynecologists from Alexander JM, McIntire DD, Leveno KJ: Prolonged pregnancy: Induction of labor and cesarean births. *Obstet Gynecol* 97:911-915, 2001.)

TABLE 4. Summary of Retrospective Studies Published During the 1990s Dealing Specifically With the Effects of Labor Induction on Cesarean Delivery

Author(s)	Year	Women Studied (N)	Does Induction Increase Cesarean Rate?
Macer et al	1992	506	No
Xenakis et al	1997	597	Yes
Prysak and Castronova	1998	922	No
Seyb et al	1999	1561	Yes
Yeast et al	1999	7224	Yes
Maslow and Sweeney	2000	1135	Yes

(Reprinted with permission of The American College of Obstetricians and Gynecologists from Alexander JM, McIntire DD, Leveno KJ: Prolonged pregnancy: Induction of labor and cesarean births. *Obstet Gynecol* 97:911-915, 2001.)

were compared between those who had spontaneous labor and those whose labor was induced.

Results.—Six hundred eighty-seven of the 1325 women enrolled in the study underwent spontaneous labor before inductions were done. Labor was longer and epidural analgesia more frequent among women in whom labor was induced than in those with spontaneous labor. In addition, cesarean delivery was used more often for women who had induced labor. With adjustment for cervical dilation, gestation age, nulliparity, and epidural analgesia (Fig 1), the odds ratio for cesarean delivery associated with labor induction was 1.1. In 4 other studies excess cesarean births occurred with induction, and in 2 studies no link was found (Table 4). Nulliparity and undilated cervices accounted for the increased use of cesarean section in women who underwent labor induction.

Conclusions.—Risk factors that are associated with the patient and the condition of the pregnancy are linked to an increased incidence of cesarean delivery among women with prolonged pregnancies rather than labor induction.

▶ This study illustrates nicely the difference between univariate and multivariate analysis and says something important about induction of labor in women in danger of postdatism, that is, pregnancy persisting beyond 42 completed weeks of pregnancy. The primary objective here is to explore the relationship between induction for pregnancies at an average of 42 completed weeks and the risk of cesarean section. Other confounding variables related both to induction and to cesarean section, particularly cervical dilatation, nulliparity, and the use of epidural anesthesia, complicate the issue. Over 27 months, 1325 women were accepted into the study, having completed between 41 and 41 6/7 weeks of pregnancy and destined for induction of labor to begin at 42 weeks. Vaginal PGE2 gel was administered on an afternoon and oxytocin induction was begun the following morning if the patient did not go into labor. Fifty-two percent of such women did go into labor spontaneously before oxytocin use; they form the control group for the calculation of odds ratios for cesarean sections between women induced and those who entered into labor spontaneously but modified by the administration of PGE2. The induction group showed a 40% increase in incidence of cesarean section, largely because of failure of cervical progression, and had a greater likelihood of prolonged labor and epidural anesthesia. When multivariate analysis was employed to deal with confounding variables, it demonstrated that induction per se was not a cause of increased risk of cesarean section but that nulliparity, unripe cervix, and epidural anesthesia were independent risk factors for abdominal birth. The appropriate conclusion, which the authors failed to derive, seems clear. To minimize the risk of cesarean section in induction of labor for women close to postdatism, the decision to induce or not should be based on parity and cervical dilatation, which are important in the risk of failed induction, and the duration of pregnancy is irrelevant as judged by the subsequent cesarean section incidence.

T. H. Kirschbaum, MD

Postoperative Morbidity Associated With Cesarean Delivery Among Human Immunodeficiency Virus–Seropostive Women

Rodriguez EJ, Spann C, Jamieson D, et al (Emory Univ, Atlanta, Ga)
Am J Obstet Gynecol 184:1108-1111, 2001   7–6

Background.—Mothers infected with HIV have a heightened risk of transferring HIV to their infants during birth, and for that reason the use of elective cesarean delivery has been recommended. However, the risk-benefit ratio of cesarean delivery has not been clarified for these mothers. The complication rates associated with cesarean delivery among HIV-seropositive women were evaluated, and the potential effects of immuno-compromise and antiretroviral therapy on operative morbidity in this population were assessed.

Methods.—This study was conducted at a large, urban teaching institution where 86 HIV-seropositive women underwent cesarean delivery and were matched to a control group of 86 HIV-seronegative women who also underwent this procedure. Complications of the operation were classified as either major or minor and then further stratified among HIV-positive women to maternal disease status and use of retroviral therapy.

Results.—The areas that differed between the seropositive and seronegative women were that tobacco and recreational drugs were used more often among the HIV-positive women than among controls and preoperative antibiotic therapy was used for HIV-positive women significantly less often than for controls. Minor postoperative complications occurred more commonly among the HIV-seropositive women than among seronegative women (odds ratio, 2.73; 66.3% vs 41.8%). Febrile morbidity was the most common complication. There appeared to be no correlation between CD4+ count and overall complication rate. HIV-seropositive women who had viral loads between 1001 and 10,000 ran a higher risk of complications than those whose viral loads were undetectable. No differences related to antiretroviral therapy were noted.

Conclusions.—Overall, the postoperative morbidity among HIV-seropositive women who underwent cesarean delivery did not differ from that noted in HIV-seronegative women who had this procedure. Cesarean delivery appeared to be safe for these mothers, with only minor complications that were easily managed.

▶ Recommendations that HIV-1–positive gravidas be treated with elective cesarean section to reduce the risk of fetal HIV infection during vaginal transit assume no significant increase in maternal risks of postoperative complications in these sometimes immune-suppressed women (see 1999 YEAR BOOK OF OBSTETRICS, GYNECOLOGY, AND WOMEN'S HEALTH, pp 75-77, and 2000 YEAR BOOK, pp 93-99). This study offers some reassurance and sharpens the area of increased maternal risk. Of the 86 HIV-1–seropositive women, compared with controls matched for age, race, time of delivery, and indication for section, 17% had CD4 counts 200 or less per cubic millimeter of blood: of 44 women for whom HIV RNA copy numbers were determined, 59% had more than 1001 per millliter. Unfortunately, only 75% of HIV-1–positive women received prophylactic preoperative antibiotics, significantly fewer than the 97.7% of controls, a difference that may be reflected in the greater incidence of minor infectious complications among HIV-1–positive postoperative women. Temperature elevation, endometritis, and wound and genitourinary infections generally lasting less than 48 hours were more common among HIV-positive women, but the incidence of major complications was the same in both groups. Those women with RNA copy numbers from 1001 to 10,000 per cubic millimeter had an increased likelihood of minor complications not seen in women with greater than 10,000 copy numbers per milliliter, presumably because of inadequate subject numbers. It is reassuring that HIV-positive women may have only an increased risk of minor postsection infections, which are usually readily managed.

T. H. Kirschbaum, MD

Subsequent Birth Outcomes After an Unexplained Stillbirth: Preliminary Population-Based Retrospective Cohort Study

Robson S, Chan A, Keane RJ, et al (Univ of Adelaide, South Australia; Dept of Human Services, Adelaide, South Australia)
Aust N Z J Obstet Gynaecol 41:29-35, 2001   7–7

Background.—Generally, the cause of stillbirth can be determined in up to 70% of cases, and the risk of recurrence is related to cause. It has been hypothesized that for women who have a stillbirth, the risk of future stillbirth is about 10 times higher than for the general population. An attempt was made to determine whether women who have had an unexplained stillbirth or other adverse outcome are actually at greater risk of recurrence than those who have never had these problems.

Methods.—The population studied was drawn from the South Australian perinatal database. A total of 316 subsequent births to women who had an unexplained stillbirth were compared with 3160 births to women who had no previous stillbirth, with analysis relying on logistic regression techniques.

Results.—No increased rate of stillbirth was noted, nor was there a statistically significant increased rate of perinatal or neonatal death for subsequent pregnancies among the women who had a previous stillbirth. Certain abnormalities were noted to occur with increased frequency in these women, including abnormal glucose tolerance or gestational diabetes, need for labor induction and elective cesarean delivery, fetal distress and postpartum hemorrhage, need for forceps or emergency cesarean delivery, and preterm birth. All of these were independent of the added risk associated with labor induction. The fetus's gestational age at birth and birth weight were also reduced.

Conclusions.—Women who have had a stillbirth or other adverse fetal outcome should be closely monitored for the development of the complications noted. However, the risk of a subsequent pregnancy resulting in another stillbirth or adverse fetal outcome is not increased in this population.

▶ Clearly, management of a pregnant woman with a prior history of fetal death tends to differ as a consequence, and this retrospective cohort study examines the rationality of that systematic difference. Data from the South Australian Pregnancy Outcome Unit was searched for instances of fetal death followed by subsequent pregnancy. Two hundred twenty four such women were identified from records collected from 1986 to 1995; cases with evidence of fetal anomaly, maternal medical or obstetrical complications, birth trauma, and fetal and neonatal abnormality associated with fetal death were excluded. Also excluded were multiple pregnancies and pregnancies in indigenous women. Patients with the same exclusions whose pregnancies resulted in normal infants made up the control group. Univariant analysis in the form of odds ratio for a wide range of obstetric and neonatal abnormalities in the subsequent pregnancy in comparison with the control was followed by stepwise multiple regression analysis, with particular attention to confounding by age and parity.

Patients with prior fetal death showed no significant difference in the incidence of subsequent fetal death or neonatal or perinatal death when compared with controls. Multivariant analysis demonstrated an increased likelihood of abnormal glucose tolerance and diabetes mellitus in women with a prior stillbirth. On the other hand, the results of differences in management were seen fairly clearly. In those patients with a prior fetal death there was an increased risk of operative birth, labor and birth complications, preterm birth, postpartum hemorrhage, and decreased mean birth weight at gestational age, apparently a reflection of management decision based on physician concern. There is no objective evidence here of any basis for extraordinary management decisions that seem to be based on physician anxiety. This is important information for patient counseling and for physician reflection in the management of such women.

T. H. Kirschbaum, MD

Human Neutrophil Collagenase (Matrix Metalloproteinase 8) in Parturition, Premature Rupture of the Membranes, and Intrauterine Infection
Maymon E, Romero R, Pacora P, et al (Natl Inst of Child Health and Human Development, Bethesda, Md; Wayne State Univ, Detroit; Seoul Natl Univ, Korea)
Am J Obstet Gynecol 183:94-99, 2000

7–8

Introduction.—The leading causes of preterm birth are preterm labor and premature rupture of the fetal membranes. Microbial invasion of the amniotic cavity is implicated in 30% to 40% of cases of preterm membrane rupture. Recent investigations implicate endogenous host enzymes in the process of membrane rupture in the setting of intra-amniotic infection. This study sought to determine whether matrix metalloproteinase 8 (MMP-8), or human neutrophil collagenase, is present in amniotic fluid, and whether its concentrations vary in preterm and term labor and in membrane rupture with and without intra-amniotic infection. Also examined were the amniotic fluid concentrations of MMP-8 in lower and upper uterine compartments in term labor.

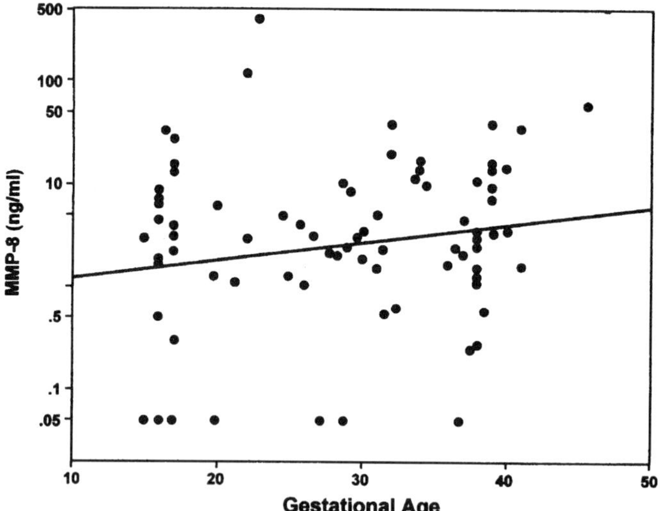

FIGURE 1.—No significant relationship was found between amniotic fluid concentrations of metalloproteinase 8 (*MMP-8*) and gestational age (Spearman $\rho = 0.2$; $P = .06$). (Courtesy of Maymon E, Romero R, Pacora P, et al: Human neutrophil collagenase (matrix metalloproteinase 8) in parturition, premature rupture of the membranes, and intrauterine infection. *Am J Obstet Gynecol* 183:94-99, 2000.)

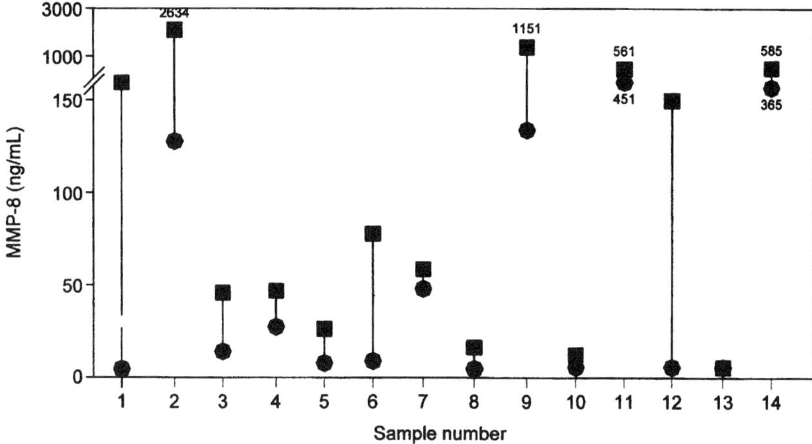

FIGURE 2.—Amniotic fluid concentrations of metalloproteinase 8 (*MMP-8*) in upper and lower compartments of the uterine cavity in women in labor with intact membranes at term. Median amniotic fluid concentrations of MMP-8 were significantly higher in fluids obtained from forebag (*squares*) than in fluid contained from upper uterine compartment (superior cavity, *circles*) (66.2 ng/mL; range, 7.4-170; vs 13.3 ng/mL; range 2-170; *P* <.01; paired *t* test). (Courtesy of Maymon E, Romero R, Pacora P, et al: Human neutrophil collagenase (matrix metalloproteinase 8) in parturition, premature rupture of the membranes, and intrauterine infection. *Am J Obstet Gynecol* 183:94-99, 2000.)

Methods.—Search of a clinical database and bank of biological specimens identified 5 categories of women who underwent transabdominal amniocentesis in the following categories: (1) midtrimester, (2) preterm labor in the presence or absence of microbial invasion of the amniotic cavity, (3) preterm premature rupture of the membranes in the presence or absence of microbial invasion of the amniotic cavity, (4) term patients in labor and not in labor, and (5) term premature rupture of membranes. In addition, samples of amniotic fluid were obtained from lower and upper uterine compartments of 14 women in spontaneous labor with intact membranes at term.

Results.—An enzyme-linked immunosorbent assay detected MMP-8 in 249 of 261 (95.4%) amniotic fluid samples. Concentrations of MMP-8 did not change with gestational age (Fig 1). In both term and preterm gestation, spontaneous parturition was associated with a significant increase in amniotic fluid concentrations of MMP-8; concentrations were significantly higher at term labor than at term without labor. Median MMP-8 concentrations were significantly higher in forebag compartment fluid than in upper compartment fluid (Fig 2). A major finding was that intra-amniotic infection is associated with a marked increase in amniotic fluid concentrations of MMP-8 in women with intact and ruptured membranes.

Conclusion.—This is the first study to demonstrate increased availability of MMP-8 in the amniotic fluid of women with spontaneous premature rupture of membranes, intra-amniotic infection, and spontaneous term and preterm labor. Higher concentrations of MMP-8 in the forebag compartment region may explain the predilection for membrane rupture near the lower pole of the uterus.

▶ MMP-8 is a glycoprotein product of neutrophil origin released by chemotoxic stimulation by a variety of cytokines and prostanoids. It is 1 of 3 MMP isotypes active in enzymatic degradation of collagen I, the predominant source of tensile strength in placental membranes. Because of its properties, MMP-8 provides a functional measure of neutrophil infiltration and activation in vivo. Here the enzyme was detected in 95.4% of the 232 samples collected by amniocentesis in a varied assortment of patient types, sampled to explore the relationship of MMP-8 to gestational age, preterm labor, rupture of membranes, and culture-proven amnionitis.

The concentration of amniotic fluid MMP-8 was independent of gestational age in the absence of labor or rupture of membranes. Its concentration was increased during labor at any gestational age, with spontaneous preterm rupture of membranes whenever culture-positive amniotic fluid was found, but not coincident with normal term labor. In the 25 women in spontaneous labor at term, MMP-8 was present in much higher concentrations in fluid collected from the forewaters between the presenting part and the intact membranes than in amniotic fluid obtained above the fetus, in the hind waters.

This latter observation was made by of Paul C. MacDonald who found the same differential distribution of prostaglandin F2-α and P prostaglandin E$_2$ in women laboring at term (see 1995 YEAR BOOK OF OBSTETRICS, GYNECOLOGY, AND WOMEN'S HEALTH, pp 31-32 and 1994 YEAR BOOK, pp 19-21). The findings demonstrate the active inflammatory process within placental forewaters associated with cervical dilatation, descent of the presenting part, and contact through intact membranes with the bacterial flora of the vagina. The authors' data confirm the role of inflammation associated with preterm premature rupture of membranes and absence of inflammatory reaction products where rupture of membranes occurs at term prior to the onset of normal labor. Undoubtably, amnionitis stimulates an abundance of cytokines and inflammatory cell products, which are discernible here. Although useful, nothing here enables us to separate the role of inflammation as a cause or an effect of the onset of preterm labor.

T. H. Kirschbaum, MD

Risk Factors for Third Degree Perineal Ruptures During Delivery
de Leeuw JW, Struijk PC, Vierhout ME, et al (Ikazia Hosp, Rotterdam, The Netherlands; Erasmus Univ Hosp, Rotterdam, The Netherlands)
Br J Obstet Gynaecol 108:383-387, 2001   7–9

Objective.—After third-degree perineal tears, as many as 85% of women have persistent anal sphincter problems. Episiotomy has been shown to have no prophylactic effect. Risk factors for the occurrence of

TABLE 1.—Analysis of Potential Risk Factors for the Occurrence of Third-Degree Perineal Ruptures (n = 284,783)

Risk Factor	Present	%	Relative Risk (%)	Logistic Regression Adj. OR (95% CI)	
Parity					
Multiparity	2173/159903	1.35	1		
Primiparity	3355/124880	2.69	1.99	2.39	(2.24-2.56)
Fetal presentation					
Occipito-anterior	5082/264426	1.92	1		
Occipitoposterior	250/7624	3.28	1.71	1.73	(1.52-1.98)
Breech presentation	103/9842	1.05	0.54	1.00	(0.78-1.26)
Other presentation	93/2891	3.21	1.67	1.59	(1.28-1.98)
Episiotomy					
No episiotomy	4185/183919	2.28	1		
Mediolateral episiotomy	1234/97250	1.27	0.56	0.21	(0.19-0.23)
Median episiotomy	109/3614	3.02	1.33	0.81	(0.66-0.98)
Induction of labour					
No induction	4556/238383	1.91	1		
Induced labor	972/46400	2.09	1.10	1.19	(1.11-1.28)
Assisted vaginal delivery					
No intervention	4052/238503	1.70	1		
Fundal expression*	191/9176	2.08	1.23	1.83	(1.57-2.14)
Fundal expr. + vacuum	74/2661	2.78	1.64	1.78	(1.40-2.28)
Fundal expr.+ forceps	27/522	5.17	3.04	4.62	(3.09-6.89)
Vacuum extraction*	646/21254	3.03	1.79	1.68	(1.52-1.86)
Vacuum. + forceps	51/656	7.77	4.58	4.74	(3.49-6.45)
Forceps delivery*	348/7478	4.65	2.73	3.53	(3.11-4.02)
Intevention: for shoulder dytocia*	46/1180	3.89	2.29	2.03	(1.49-2.74)
Breech extraction*	27/1284	2.10	1.24	2.91	(1.88-4.51)

Present is defined as number of women with third degree rupture/total number of women.

*Applied with exclusion of any other type of assisted vaginal delivery.

(Courtesy of de Leeuw JW, Struijk PC, Vierhout ME, et al: Risk factors for third degree perineal ruptures during delivery. *Br J Obstet Gynaecol* 108:383-387. Copyright 2001 Elsevier Science, publisher.)

third-degree perineal ruptures was investigated in a population-based observational study using the Dutch National Obstetric Database (LVR).

Methods.—There were 289,578 vaginal deliveries listed in the LVR for the years 1994 and 1995. The incidences of third-degree perineal ruptures were calculated for each potential risk factor (Table 1).

Results.—The risk for third-degree perineal rupture was 1.94% (5528 of 284,783). Primiparity was a significant risk factor for rupture, as was fetal occipitoposterior position and presentations other than breech presentation. The episiotomy rate was 35.4%, with mediolateral episiotomy conferring a strongly protective factor (odds ratio [OR], 0.21) and median episiotomy conferring a weak protective factor. All types of assisted vaginal delivery significantly increased the risk for third-degree rupture. Vacuum extraction significantly increased the risk for rupture, but to a lesser extent. Forceps delivery posed the greatest risk for rupture. Increasing birth weight increased the risk of rupture (Fig 1). Length of labor was significantly related to risk for rupture (OR, 1.12) (Fig 2).

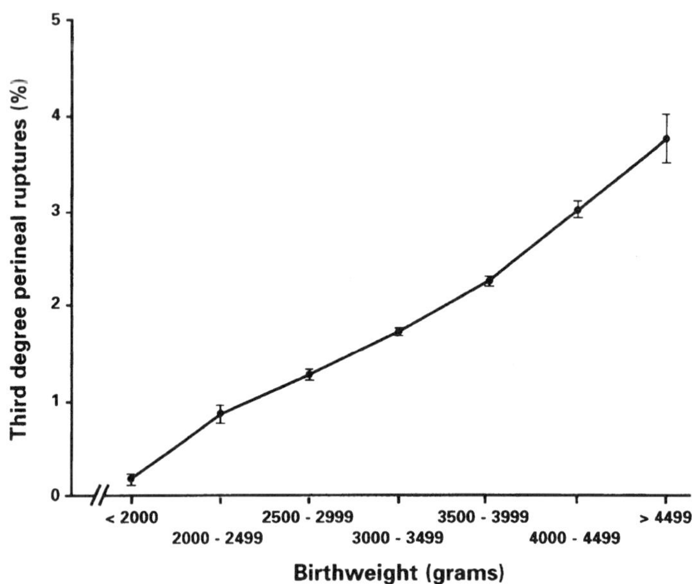

FIGURE 1.—Risk of third-degree perineal ruptures per 500 g birth weight. (Courtesy of de Leeuw JW, Struijk PC, Vierhout ME, et al: Risk factors for third degree perineal ruptures during delivery. *Br J Obstet Gynaecol* 108:383-387. Copyright 2001 Elsevier Science, publisher.)

Conclusion.—Primiparity, assisted vaginal delivery, vacuum extraction, forceps delivery, length of labor, and increasing birth weight increased the risk of third-degree perineal ruptures during delivery.

▶ This study, based on records held by the LVR for 1994 and 1995, yields interpretations using univariant statistics for 284,783 vaginal births, or 82.5% of all Dutch births during that time. Certainly the largest modern study of its sort, it is destined to be referenced for decades to come. About 39% of women were delivered in primary care facilities by midwives and general practitioners and the rest at secondary care facilities staffed by obstetrician specialists. The overall rate for third-degree lacerations was 1.94%; episiotomy was done in about one third, only about 1.3% of which were median in type. The incidents of primiparity was 44%. The incidence of third-degree tears for each variable known to be related to such complications was calculated and ORs struck against items occurring most often in normal labor and delivery (see Table 1).

Third-degree tears were found to be significantly increased in risk ratio in primigravidas, with fetal malpresentation other than breech presentation and in occiput/posterior positions at birth. Mediolateral episiotomy generated reduced risk ratios for third-degree tears and median episiotomy was also protective, but the reduction in risk was small. Similarly, labor induction was associated with a small increase in risk ratio and all assisted delivery techniques, including both fundal pressure and operative vaginal birth, were associated with increased risk of periueal ruptures. The third-degree lacera-

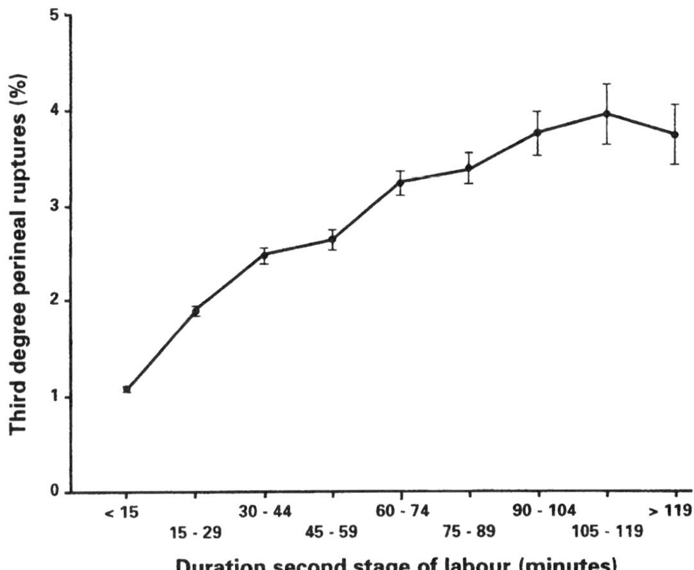

FIGURE 2.—Risk of third-degree perineal ruptures per 15-min duration of the second stage of labor. (Courtesy of de Leeuw JW, Struijk PC, Vierhout ME, et al: Risk factors for third degree perineal ruptures during delivery. *Br J Obstet Gynaecol* 108:383-387. Copyright 2001 Elsevier Science, publisher.)

tion incidence varied directly in relation to birth weight and the duration of the second stage. The failure to look for confounding relations with multi-variant analysis among supposedly independent variables here is a weakness in this study.

Aside from its authoritativeness, this report gains significantly from the growing realization that complaints and evidence of puerperal fecal incontinence are more often associated with inadequate sphincter repair than with neurologic dysfunction (see 2001 YEAR BOOK OF OBSTETRICS, GYNECOLOGY, AND WOMEN'S HEAITH, pp 207-208). Supervised instruction in the repair of first- and third-degree lacerations is a very important part of modern obstetrical pedagogy.

T. H. Kirschbaum, MD

8 Puerperium

Epidemiology of Transmission of Cytomegalovirus From Mother to Preterm Infant by Breastfeeding
Hamprecht K, Maschmann J, Vochem M, et al (Univ Hosp of Tübingen, Germany)
Lancet 357:513-518, 2001   8–1

Introduction.—Although cytomegalovirus (CMV) is known to be present in human breast milk, the role played by milk cells and cell-free virus in CMV transmission remains uncertain. Few studies have addressed the transmission of CMV from nursing mothers to their preterm infants. A large sample of breast-fed, preterm infants were studied to assess the epidemiology and clinical outcomes of postnatal CMV transmission.

Methods.—The prospective study included 176 preterm infants of 151 mothers. All infants were born before 32 weeks' gestational age or weighed less than 1500 g at birth. At baseline, the mothers underwent screening for CMV by serology, viral culture, and PCR. The infants were followed up for CMV transmission, and the contributions of cell-free and cell-associated CMV excretion during lactation were assessed.

Results.—Sixty-nine mothers (control group) were seronegative at baseline. None of these had CMV DNA detected in their breast milk, and none of their 80 infants excreted CMV in urine. Among the 76 seropositive mothers, CMV reactivation occurred in 96%. Viral DNA appeared in milk whey at a median of 3.5 days postpartum in transmitters compared with 8 days in nontransmitters. Median times to appearances of infectious virus in milk whey for transmitters and nontransmitters were 10 and 16 days, respectively. Viral transmission was more likely when both of these events occurred early on. The cumulative transmission rate was 37%, with a mean incubation time of 42 days to infection of the neonates. Although about half of the infants were asymptomatic, sepsis-like symptoms occurred in 4.

Conclusions.—Among mothers who are seropositive for CMV, the rate of CMV reactivation during lactation is nearly 100%. Early appearance of viral DNA and infectious virus in milk whey are the major risk factors for CMV transmission to preterm infants (Fig 2A). Compared with term infants, preterm infants appear more likely to develop symptomatic CMV infection. Techniques for inactivation of CMV in seropositive breast milk to prevent transmission to preterm infants are being investigated.

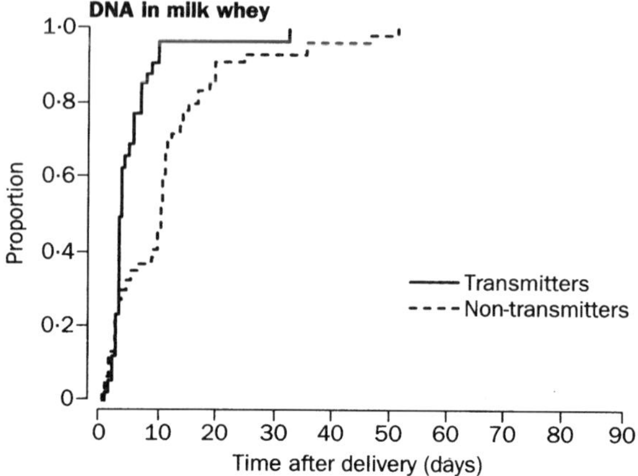

FIGURE 2A.—Onset of cytomegalovirus reactivation in different milk compartments of maternal transmitters (n = 27) and nontransmitters (n = 46). A, Maximum likelihood estimates of proportion with viral DNA in milk whey based on log-normal distribution. (Courtesy of Hamprecht K, Maschmann J, Vochem M, et al: Epidemiology of transmission of cytomegalovirus from mother to preterm infant by breastfeeding. *Lancet* 357:513-518, 2001. Copyright by The Lancet Ltd, 2001.)

▶ Though viral isolation from breast milk in CMV-infected women has been known for decades, it has attracted little attention because of the consistent lack of evidence of newborn transfer to nursing term infants. These authors, however, provide evidence of reason to be concerned about preterm infants breast fed by women who are CMV-antibody positive. All infants selected were born prior to the 32nd week of gestation, had birthweights less than 1.5 kg, and were delivered at a mean gestational age of 29 weeks. In a series of 76 CMV IgG-positive women, newborn infection was excluded by negative cord blood serology, ear and throat swabs negative for CMV virions, negative DNA PCR in cord blood, and absent newborn IgM in specimens obtained within 2 hours of birth. Repeat exams of breast milk, both spun cells and whey, were evaluated by CMV culture and DNA PCR through 3 months of newborn age. Vaginal contamination during delivery was minimized, because 87% of the gravidas studied were delivered abdominally. A control group of 80 gravidas seronegative for CMV IgG and uninfected women were examined during lactation. No evidence of infection in mother or newborn controls was seen.

The incidence of viral activation among seropositive puerpera exhibiting viral DNA and virions in breast milk occurred in 96% of the 76 women. Among those who failed to show CMV virions in breast milk, only 1 of 15 infants showed evidence of puerperal transmission marked by recovery of CMV virus and DNA from plasma and white cells, urine specimens, and appearance of IgM to CMV. Women who were both DNA positive and showed CMV virions in breast milk constituted 34% of the 76 cases and resulted in 32 infected infants. Half of those neonatally infected infants were symptomatic, and in 12.5%, a septic pattern devoid of evidence of bacterial infection with occasional thrombopenia was noted.

This group is exploring the possible development of a means of viral inactivation of breast milk from CMV IgG-positive nursing puerperas. Until such a method is established, they have given us reason to become concerned with puerperal CMV infection of newborns weighing 1.5 kg or below at birth.

T. H. Kirschbaum, MD

Ultrasonographic Evaluation of the Postpartum Uterus

Edwards A, Ellwood DA (Univ of Sydney, Canberra, Australia)
Ultrasound Obstet Gynecol 16:640-643, 2000   8–2

Objective.—The most common cause of postpartum complications, which occur in 10% of births, is hemorrhage. US, the preferred means of evaluating the uterus of women with a secondary postpartum hemorrhage, can reveal an echogenic mass within the endometrial cavity. How often an echogenic mass is present in healthy women experiencing an uncomplicated postpartum recovery was investigated.

Methods.—Transabdominal US was performed in 40 women, aged 17 to 40 years, on postpartum days 7, 14, and 21. Half of the women were primiparous. Uterine cavity and cavity volume were assessed (Fig 1). Women recorded the amount of vaginal bleeding they experienced for 6 weeks or until bleeding had stopped for 1 week.

Results.—A total of 105 scans was performed. Of the deliveries, 33 were vaginal deliveries, 4 were forceps deliveries, and 3 were vacuum extractions. An echogenic mass was found in 51% of women at 7 days, 21% at 14 days, and 6% at 21 days. Uterine volume and cavity volume decreased significantly from 7 to 14 days and from 14 to 21 days. The average duration of postpartum bleeding was 24.5 days. Women reported the amount of bleeding to be within their expectations. Duration of bleeding and uterine volume were not related. Amount of bleeding and cavity volume were not related. Neither uterine volume, cavity volume, nor duration of bleeding was related to parity at any time point. Bleeding duration or amount was not related to the presence or absence of a uterine cavity echogenic mass at any time point.

Conclusion.—There was no difference between women with a uterine cavity echogenic mass and those without in terms of the duration or amount of bleeding.

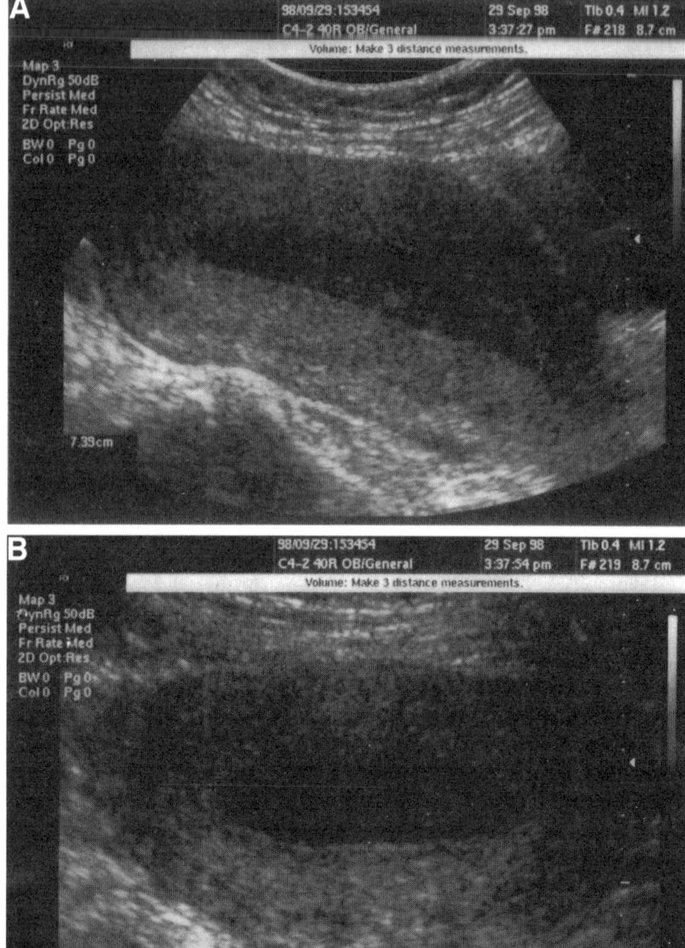

FIGURE 1.—Estimation of cavity volume. **A,** Longitudinal view, **B,** transverse view. The cavity is measured in 3 planes and volume is calculated by the US machine's internal software. In this case, at 7 days postpartum, the cavity content was generally hypoechoic with some scattered echoes, and had an estimated volume of 47 mL. This was a common appearance in our study population, for which the day 7 cavity volume range was 2.6 to 88 mL. (Courtesy of Edwards A, Ellwood DA: Ultrasonographic evaluation of the postpartum uterus. *Ultrasound Obstet Gynecol* 16:640-643, 2000. Reprinted by permission of Blackwell Science, Inc.)

▶ Shortly after delivery of the placenta, hormonal support for the decidualized endometrium begins to decline and vaginal bacterial florae quickly flow into the uterine cavity, where they participate in the protolytic necrosis or lipolysis and fragmentation of what quickly becomes the lochial discharge. A couple of weeks later, proliferation of endometrial surface epithelium, proceeding from glandular epithelium in the endometrial stratum basalis begins to undermine the usually thrombosed decidual vessels which formerly subserved the placental intervillous space. This tissue is shed by defoliation leaving little endometrial stroma scarring to interfere with subsequent endometrial function. The end of the process is marked by a cessation of lochial discharge and a return to normal vaginal discharge characteristics. In this group of 40 puerperas, half of them primipara, the duration of the process ranged from 14 to 45 days, with a mean of 24.5 days.

The results of uterine US in the first 21 days of the puerperium are useful in evaluating scans done during this time, scans largely motivated by refractory pelvic infection or bleeding. In normal nulliparas there is abundant (sometimes surprisingly abundant) echogenic material left adherent to the myometrial walls. Such findings are normal and not necessarily related to complaints of bleeding, and should not, in themselves, constitute indications for curettage.

T. H. Kirschbaum, MD

9 Genetics And Teratology

Second-Trimester Ultrasound to Detect Fetuses With Down Syndrome: A Meta-Analysis
Smith-Bindman R, Hosmer W, Feldstein VA, et al (Univ of California, San Francisco; Univ of Oxford, England; California Pacific Med Ctr, San Francisco)
JAMA 285:1044-1055, 2001   9–1

Objective.—Second-trimester US is widely performed as a screening study for fetal Down syndrome. However, the accuracy of the various proposed sonographic "markers" for Down syndrome is uncertain. A meta-analysis was performed to assess the accuracy of prenatal US in screening for Down syndrome.

Methods.—The analysis included 56 studies of second-trimester US markers for Down syndrome. All studies included information on chromosomal findings and clinical outcomes; a total of 1930 affected and 130,365 unaffected fetuses were included. Diagnostic performance was evaluated for a wide range of proposed markers, classified by whether they were noted in isolation or in combination with fetal structural abnormalities.

Results.—In the absence of structural malformations, all of the markers had a low sensitivity (1% to 16%), and most fetuses with these isolated markers did not have Down syndrome. The most accurate marker for differentiating between affected and unaffected fetuses was thickening of the nuchal fold. A thickened nuchal fold was associated with a 17-fold increase in the likelihood of Down syndrome. Still, the number of cases needed to screen to detect 1 infant with Down syndrome on the basis of this marker would be nearly 16,000 for average-risk women and 7000 for high-risk women. In isolation, the other markers analyzed—choroid plexus cyst, echogenic intracardiac focus or echogenic bowel, renal pyelectasis, and humeral and femoral shortening—were of little or no help in assessing the risk of Down syndrome. All of these markers were present in only a small number of Down syndrome fetuses. Thus, a normal finding did not significantly reduce the risk of Down syndrome.

Conclusions.—This meta-analysis questions the value of isolated second-trimester US "markers" of Down syndrome. Although a thickened nuchal fold significantly increases the likelihood that the fetus is affected, even this marker is too insensitive as a practical screening test. If these markers were used on their own in deciding to perform amniocentesis, the number of fetal losses would exceed the number of cases detected.

▶ These investigators employ meta-analysis to attempt to evaluate the role of ultrasonic observation of fetal nuchal fold thickness in improving the predictive capacity of maternal biochemical screening for Down syndrome. The screening makes use of second trimester measurements of maternal alpha fetoprotein, human chorionic gonadatropin, estriol, and inhibin A to support the use of amniocentesis for karyotypic diagnosis. The sensitivity of that approach varies around 60% to 65% with a 7% false-positive rate. False positives are important because of the risk of fetal mortality following amniocentesis of 0.5 to 1.0 percent. The relationship between Down syndrome and nuchal thickness greater than 6 mm in the second trimester is well-established (see 1994 YEAR BOOK OF OBSTETRICS, GYNECOLOGY, AND WOMEN'S HEALTH, pp 206-207, and 1996 YEAR BOOK, pp 111-112), but estimates of the clinical usefulness of the finding vary (see 1999 YEAR BOOK, pp 200-202, and 2001 YEAR BOOK, pp 227-229). The usefulness of first trimester US measurement is unconfirmed (see 1997 YEAR BOOK, pp 130-133).

The authors selected case reports from the literature from 1980 to 1999 based on second trimester ultrasound with data sufficient to calculate sensitivity and specificity figures on the basis of outcomes showing either Down syndrome, other karyotypic abnormalities, or unaffected infants. Of 132,295 case reports of screening, there were 1930 cases of Down syndrome, an incidence of 1.5% among women with a mean age of 34 years. In addition to nuchal thickening, the authors also studied chorionic cysts, echogenic endocardiac foci, shortened femur and humerus, renal pyelectasis, echogenic bowel, and fetal structural abnormalities but found only nuchal thickening to be helpful in predicting or excluding Down syndrome.

The sensitivity of nuchal thickening varied among published reports from 7% to 75%, depending largely on differences in experimental design and whether the finding was an isolated one or part of several indicators. The sensitivity of Down syndrome detection with isolated nuchal thickening was 4%, the prospective positive value, 2.4%, and the false-positive rate, 97%. The incidence of Down syndrome in fetuses with nuchal thickening was 2% among low-risk women and 5% among women at high risk. The likelihood ratio of 17 for the finding means that nuchal thickening increases the chances of Down syndrome 17 times, but the abnormality occurs so rarely that 16,000 women would have to be screened to diagnose a case in women at low risk and 6818 women at high risk. The number of probable fetal losses occurring from the amniocentesis in this population would be 0.6 and 0.2 per detected case for low and high risk, respectively. The authors conclude that "nuchal fold thickening has sensitivity too low for it to be a practical screening test for Down syndrome"; most, I think, would agree.

T. H. Kirschbaum, MD

Prenatal Detection of Fetal Down's Syndrome From Maternal Plasma

Poon LLM, Leung TN, Lau TK, et al (Chinese Univ of Hong Kong, Shatin)
Lancet 356:1819-1820, 2000   9–2

Background.—Fetal DNA has been found in maternal plasma at concentrations much higher than those present in the cellular fraction, suggesting new possibilities for noninvasive prenatal diagnosis. The feasibility of prenatal detection of fetal trisomy 21 by maternal plasma analysis was studied.

Methods and Findings.—Three women carrying fetuses with trisomy 21 and 10 women carrying euploid fetuses were studied. Cells with 3 chromosome-21 signals were clearly seen in all 3 women with trisomy 21 fetuses. The trisomic cells comprised 0.4% to 0.8% of the nuclei examined. Further analysis showed that trisomic fetal cells were present in maternal plasma before the invasive procedure was done.

Conclusions.—Fetal cells with 3 chromosome-21 signals were identified in plasma samples obtained from 3 women carrying affected fetuses. Noninvasive detection of fetal chromosomal aneuploidy by maternal plasma analysis appears to be feasible.

▶ This interesting preliminary development in the study of maternal plasma DNA for fetal diagnosis may constitute a real cost benefit saving for the non-invasive diagnosis of fetal Down syndrome and some other aneuploidies. This group is very experienced in the analysis of fetal soluble DNA in maternal blood (see 2000 YEAR BOOK OF OBSTETRICS, GYNECOLOGY, AND WOMEN'S HEALTH, pp 57-59, pp 103-104, and pp 207-208). With previous demonstration by van Wijk et al[1] that some fetal DNA in maternal plasma rests in apoptotic or normal fetal cells, they explored the possibility of applying fluorescent in situ hybridization (FISH) to fetal cells available by that route. Preliminary results are provided here based on 3 women bearing Down syndrome fetuses and 10 healthy control subjects. Fetal cells were harvested by centrifugation of diluted maternal blood samples collecting cells in the remaining plasma sample concentrated by differential density centrifugation. The authors collected and fixed these cells and used DNA probes for chromosomes 13, 18, 21, and Y in FISH (see 1995 YEAR BOOK, pp 209-211, and 2000 YEAR BOOK, pp 211-212). All 3 women with fetuses with trisomy 21 were correctly identified; gender was accurately predicted and no false-positive indication of Down syndrome or other trisomies was seen in the healthy control subjects. Noteworthy is the suggestion that genetic diagnosis from more or less intact fetal cells in the maternal circulation may be obtained by simple centrifugation, avoiding the costly equipment needed for cell separation and enhancement, as previously reported. If wider experience confirms these results, it means that noninvasive fetal genetic diagnosis will become much more widely available at less cost and effort than at present.

T. H. Kirschbaum, MD

Reference

1. van Wijk IJ, Dehoon AC, Jurajwan R, et al: Detection of apoptotic fetal cells in plasma of pregnant women. *Clin Chem* 46:729-731, 2000.

Dietary Folate and the Prevalence of Neural Tube Defects in the British Isles: The Past Two Decades

Murphy M, Whiteman D, Stone D, et al (Univ of Oxford, England; Univ of Glasgow, Scotland; Univ of Leeds, England)
Br J Obstet Gynaecol 107:885-889, 2000   9–3

Introduction.—Until the past 2 decades, the rates of neural tube defects in England, Scotland, Wales, and Ireland were among the highest in the world. Whether the rate of neural defects is affected by genetics or environmental factors is not known. The change in folate consumption that has taken place since fortification of breakfast cereals and breads with this supplement began in 1985 and 1991, respectively, was compared with the prevalence of neural tube defects in the British and Irish populations during the past 2 decades.

Methods.—The average daily dietary intake of folate for Britain for the period from 1980 to 1998 was estimated from the National Food Survey.

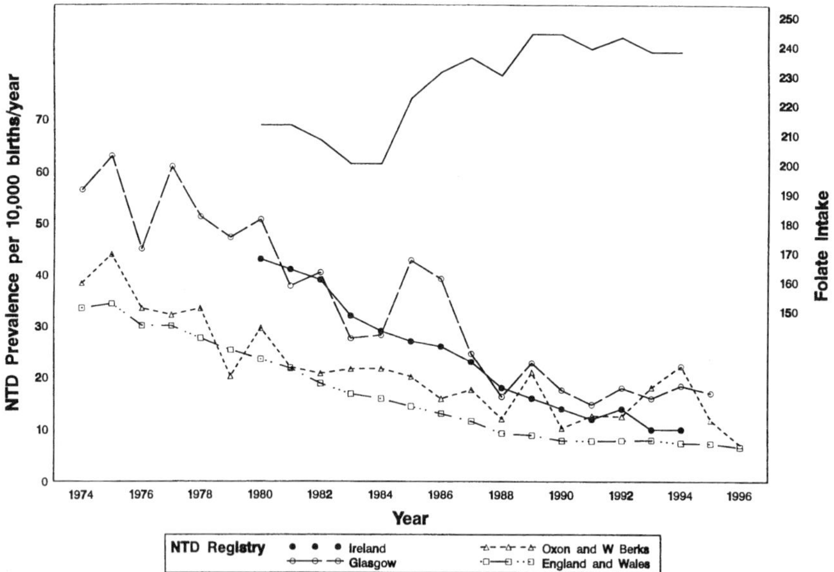

FIGURE 1.—Prevalence of neural tube defect in 4 registries in the British Isles (1974-1996), and estimated folate intake levels for the period 1980-1994. Oxfordshire and West Berkshire denominator populations for 1995 and 1996 are estimated. *Filled circle* indicates Ireland; *open circles* indicate Glasgow; triangles indicate Oxon and West Berkshire; and squares indicate England and Wales. (Courtesy of Murphy M, Whiteman D, Stone D, et al: Dietary folate and the prevalence of neural tube defects in the British Isles: The past two decades. *Br J Obstet Gynaecol* 107:885-889, 2000, Elsevier Science, publisher.)

The annual tube defect prevalences for the same time period were obtained from the Oxford Record Linkage Study neural tube defect registry, the Glasgow EUROCAT Register, and the 3 Irish EUROCAT registers in Belfast, Dublin, and Galway.

Results.—Dietary folate consumption rose on average by 1.6% per annum in Scotland and Wales, and 1.4% in England during the evaluation period. The annual rate of reduction in neural tube defect prevalence averaged 10.4% in the Irish population, 8.2% in Glasgow, and 5.2% in the Oxfordshire and West Berkshire registers (Fig 1).

Conclusion.—The reduction in neural tube defect prevalence seen in all British and Irish populations since the early 1970s has continued with the introduction of folate fortification of cereals, which provides measurable increases in average daily folate consumption. It is possible that further declines in neural tube defect prevalence may be observed by targeting folate supplementation during the periconceptual period. It must be remembered that this strategy of food fortification is not without risk to some individuals: those taking medication for epilepsy or at risk for subacute combined degeneration of the spinal cord.

▶ For decades, the prevalence of neural tube defects in the United Kingdom, especially Scotland and Ireland, has been among the highest reported by national natology-registers throughout the world. From 1976 to 1996, there was a striking monotonic reduction in incidence throughout the UK,[1] perhaps in part reflecting British folate supplementation of breakfast cereals introduced from 1985 to 1991 and of breads in 1991. Dietary folate ingestion per household was estimated by the National Food Survey of the Ministry of Agriculture, Fisheries, and Food based on food purchasing data through 1985, supplemented by folate measurements performed since then. Note that the decline in neural tube defects has been progressive since 1974 and was not strikingly altered by the introduction of the dietary supplementation beginning in 1985. It is unlikely that changes in gene frequencies responsible for neural tube defects could have changed in such a short time. Though there is no proof of a direct relationship between folate ingestion and neural tube defect prevalence, such a relationship is a plausible explanation for at least part of the improvement that has been seen.

T. H. Kirschbaum, MD

Reference

1. Lo YMD, Tein MSC, Lau TK, et al: Quantative analysis of fetal DNA in maternal plasma and serum: implications for noninvasive prenatal diagnosis. *Am J Hum Genet* 62:768-775, 1998. (1999 Year Book of Obstetrics, Gynecology, and Women's Health, p 193.)

Fetal DNA in Maternal Plasma Is Elevated in Pregnancies With Aneuploid Fotucoe

Zhong XY, Bürk MR, Troeger C, et al (Univ of Basel, Switzerland; Jefferson Med College, Philadelphia)
Prenat Diagn 20:795-798, 2000

9–4

Introduction.—Demand is increasing for prenatal diagnosis. However, couples are frequently reluctant to expose mother and child to the risk of invasive procedures, including amniocentesis or chorion villus sampling. The current noninvasive screening methods for prenatal diagnosis of fetal aneuploidies are limited by low sensitivities and high false-positive rates. A novel noninvasive approach for prenatal diagnosis of fetal genetic characteristics is the use of free extracellular DNA, which can be detected by polymerase chain reaction (PCR) in the serum or plasma of pregnant females. Real-time quantitative PCR has been used to demonstrate that circulatory male fetal DNA in maternal plasma is increased in pregnancies with trisomy 21 infants. These findings were evaluated to determine if they could be extended to other fetal aneuploidies.

Methods.—Twenty-eight plasma samples from a singleton male aneuploid fetus were compared with 29 samples taken from normal pregnancies with a male fetus. Average gestational age at sampling was 14 weeks. The samples were blinded to all personnel taking part in their preparation and analysis. The DNA was extracted from samples and underwent the TaqMan real time PCR analysis.

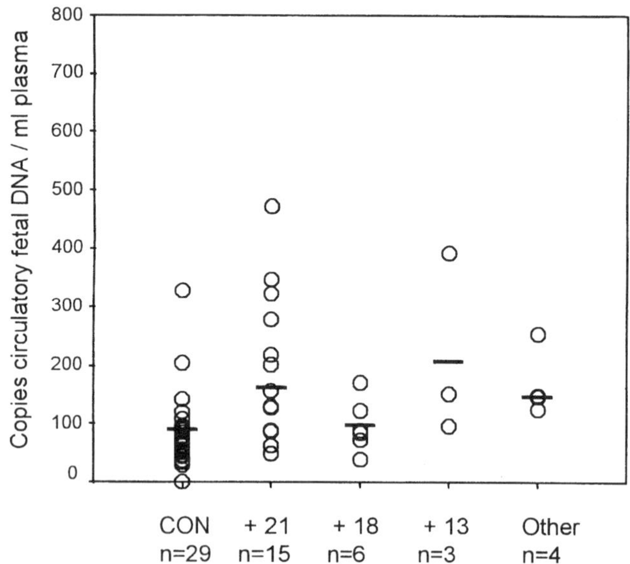

FIGURE 1.—Level of fetal DNA in maternal plasma in normal and aneuploid pregnancies. *Abbreviation:* CON, Controls. (Courtesy of Zhong XY, Bürk MR, Troeger et al: Fetal DNA in maternal plasma is elevated in pregnancies with aneuploid fetuses. *Prenat Diagn* 20:795-798, 2000. Copyright John Wiley & Sons Limited. Reproduced with permission.)

Results.—Fetal DNA samples were taken as follows: 29 from controls, 15 from trisomy 21, 6 from trisomy 18, 3 from trisomy 13, and 4 from other aneuploidies. The mean fetal DNA levels were significantly elevated in the 15 plasma samples analyzed from fetuses with trisomy 21 (mean = 83.1 copies/mL of maternal plasma) (Figure 1). The fetal plasma DNA levels were not significantly elevated from the normal level in fetuses with trisomy 18 (95.5 copies/mL compared with 83.1 copies/mL). For cases with trisomy 12 and the 4 other chromosomal aberrations evaluated, the levels of fetal DNA were also elevated at a mean of 213.2 and 168.7 copies/mL of maternal plasma. Although there were only 2 cases with 47 + XXY, the levels of fetal DNA (125.3 and 146.9 copies per/mL of maternal plasma, respectively), both were above the mean observed in control samples.

Conclusion.—The amount of fetal DNA in maternal plasma is significantly elevated in pregnancies with certain fetal aneuploidies, especially trisomy 21.

▶ This report constitutes independent confirmation of the finding of elevated DNA copy numbers in the blood of women bearing Down syndrome infants (see 2001 YEAR BOOK OF OBSTETRICS, GYNECOLOGY, AND WOMEN'S HEALTH, pp 217-219). Again, the method involves identification of fetal DNA by recognizing Y chromosome-based sequences in the PCR product of the blood of women bearing male fetuses and with TaqMan realtime PCR for quantitation of DNA as previously described (see 1999 YEAR BOOK, pp 193-196). Note the mean quantity of fetal DNA in 15 cases of Down syndrome pregnancy is larger than the mean value for 25 normal controls at an average 14.5 weeks gestational age. Note also the extensive overlap with control values makes DNA quantitation as currently available of little predictive value in case management. Note also no significant difference is claimed for mean DNA copy numbers per unit in maternal blood for 6 cases with trisomy 18 and that data from those with trisomy 13 is too few and too heterogeneous to warrant comment. As before, no explanation is available for the increase in fetal DNA in the blood of preeclamptics (see 2000 YEAR BOOK, pp 103 104). This is undoubtedly a real phenomenon not yet of clinical utility but with enormous potential value when its underlying mechanisms become clear.

T. H. Kirschbaum, MD

Detection of Fetal Rhesus D and Sex Using Fetal DNA From Maternal Plasma by Multiplex Polymerase Chain Reaction

Zhong XY, Holzgreve W, Hahn S (Univ of Basel, Switzerland)
Br J Obstet Gynaecol 107:766-769, 2000   9–5

Introduction.—The presence of male fetal DNA in the serum and plasma of pregnant women, detectable by polymerase chain reaction (PCR) with primers specific for the Y chromosome, has recently been discovered. Although this finding has limitations, it suggests a new approach to prenatal diagnostic procedures. The sensitivity, specificity, and reproducibility of using fetal DNA obtained from plasma of pregnant women by PCR was tested for the simultaneous detection of both fetal gender and rhesus (Rh) D genotype.

Methods.—Blood samples were collected from 22 rh D–negative women about to undergo an invasive procedure. The DNA was extracted from the plasma fraction and analyzed by means of multiplex nested PCR using Y chromosome– and Rh D–specific primers. These findings were compared with those obtained from the analysis performed on samples taken during the invasive procedure.

Results.—The sensitivity of the plasma PCR-based method showed a high degree of accuracy (almost 100%) in correctly determining fetal gender and Rh D status. A false-positive result for Rh D was observed on initial evaluation; subsequent testing revealed a negative result.

Conclusion.—The ease and rapidity with which the plasma PCR-based method can be conducted makes it a possible method for assessing multiple fetal loci, including Rh D and gender.

▶ Fetal genetic diagnosis based on the isolation of fetal red cells from maternal blood, employing cell-separation techniques and fluorescent in situ hybridization or PCR, consumes considerable time and effort and generates equivalent costs.[1,2] This is an exploration of the usefulness of the presence of fetal DNA in solution in maternal plasma during pregnancy for fetal diagnosis[3,4,5] (see 1999 YEAR BOOK OF OBSTETRICS, GYNECOLOGY, AND WOMEN'S HEALTH, pp 193-196, 2000 YEAR BOOK, pp 207-208, 210-211). The method is applicable only to instances in which the DNA of interest is present in the fetal but not the maternal genome. Here DNA is extracted from maternal plasma and exposed to PCR using primers appropriate to the Rh D gene and the SRY gene present on the Y chromosome. Primers for a beta globin gene segment were employed for quality control. Fetal male sex was successfully identified in 9 cases and female gender in 13 cases by exclusion. Rh D–positive status was correctly identified in 18 cases, with 1 false positive out of 19 in an Rh-negative fetus. Fetal Rh D negativity was correctly diagnosed in 4 cases. Proving feasibility is an important first step in evaluation of this promising approach and further experience should result in improvement in precision of this approach to noninvasive fetal genetic diagnosis.

T. H. Kirschbaum, MD

References

1. Bianchi DW, Williams JM, Sullivan LM, et al: PCR quantitation of fetal cells in maternal blood in normal and aneuploid pregnancies. *Am J Hum Genet* 61:822-829, 1997. (1999 YEAR BOOK OF OBSTETRICS, GYNECOLOGY, AND WOMEN'S HEALTH, p 191.)
2. Bischoff FZ, Lewis DE, Nguyen DD, et al: Prenatal diagnosis with use of fetal cells isolated from maternal blood: Five-color fluorescent in situ hybridization analysis on flow-sorted cells for chromosomes X, Y, 13, 18, and 21. *Am J Obstet Gynecol* 179:203-209, 1998. (2000 YEAR BOOK OF OBSTETRICS, GYNECOLOGY, AND WOMEN'S HEALTH, p 211.)

3. Lo YMD, Tein MSC, Lau TK, et al: Quantative analysis of fetal DNA in maternal plasma and serum: Implications for noninvasive prenatal diagnosis. *Am J Hum Genet* 62:768-775, 1998. (1999 YEAR BOOK OF OBSTETRICS, GYNECOLOGY, AND WOMEN'S HEALTH, p 193.)
4. Xu K, Shi ZM, Veeck LL, et al: First unaffected pregnancy using preimplantation genetic diagnosis for sickle cell anemia. *JAMA* 281:1701-1706, 1999. (2000 YEAR BOOK OF OBSTETRICS, GYNECOLOGY, AND WOMEN'S HEALTH, p 208.)
5. Fass BHW, Beuling EA, Christiaens GCML, et al: Detection of fetal RHD-specific sequences in maternal plasmas. *Lancet* 352:1196, 1998. (2000 YEAR BOOK OF OBSTETRICS, GYNECOLOGY, AND WOMEN'S HEALTH, p 210.)

Significant Fetal-Maternal Hemorrhage After Termination of Pregnancy: Implications for Development of Fetal Cell Microchimerism

Bianchi DW, Farina A, Weber W, et al (Tufts Univ, Boston; Genzyme Genetics, Framingham, Mass; Genzyme Genetics, Cambridge, Mass; et al)

Am J Obstet Gynecol 184:703-706, 2001   9–6

Background.—Recent research links fetal cell microchimerism to autoimmune disease. Many researchers are now investigating the persistence of fetal cells post partum. Most of these studies, however, have focused on term pregnancies. Pregnancies of a shorter duration have not received much attention. The efficacy of quantitative polymerase change reaction amplification to determine the presence of fetal-maternal hemorrhages after elective termination of pregnancy was investigated.

Methods.—Within 1 hour after elective abortion, peripheral venous blood samples were taken from 23 women suspected of carrying male fetuses. Twenty-one of the fetuses were male and two were female. At the time of venipuncture, gestational ages ranged from 6 to 23 weeks. Samples were analyzed by quantitative polymerase chain reaction amplification, using Y-chromosome primers. Weighted linear regression analysis was used to evaluate results, which were equilibrated to 16 mL. Using this method, the correlation between gestational weeks and male fetal nucleated cell equivalents was determined.

Results.—No male fetal nucleated cells were detected in samples from the mothers of female fetuses. The samples from mothers of male fetuses showed between 50 and 37,618 fetal nucleated cells equivalents (median = 1552). A significant positive correlation between fetal age and the amount of male fetal nucleated cells was found ($P < 0.001$).

Conclusions.—A large fetal-maternal transfusion after elective abortion was shown to occur even in women who were not pregnant to term. Thus, the population of women who might be affected by fetal cell microchimerism is much larger than was once suspected.

▶ Chimerism is defined by the presence of more than one genotype present in a single individual; in microchimerism, the number of atypical cells is small. Microchimerism has now been identified in humans in instances of scleroderma (see 1997 YEAR BOOK OF OBSTETRICS, GYNECOLOGY, AND WOMEN'S HEALTH, pp 202-203, 1999 YEAR BOOK, pp 189-191, and 2000 YEAR BOOK, pp

99-100), and chimerism may exhibit long persistence extending into adult life for up to 27 years in the form of Y chromosome-bearing cells in parous women (see 2001 YEAR BOOK, pp 219-220). The inordinate incidence of scleroderma and autoimmune disease in parous women compared with males suggests that the known fetal-to-maternal trafficking of cells during pregnancy may be responsible (see 1999 YEAR BOOK, pp 191-193). Since female fetal cells are difficult to identify among maternal phenotypes and since males don't achieve pregnancy, all that is known about cell trafficking during pregnancy is based on the identity of genes of the Y-chromosome, as expressed in female blood and tissue. Here the question is whether women undergoing therapeutic abortion between 6 and 23 weeks of gestational age provide sufficient numbers of copies of fetal DNA transferred to the mother in the course of the procedure to make them candidates for microchimerism.

The semiquantitative PCR amplification employing the TaqMan realtime procedure previously described here (see 1999 YEAR BOOK, pp 193-196) uses a fluor coupled to 2 sets of primers appropriate to gene quenching and activating segments of DNA on the long arm of the Y-chromosome. By plotting increasing fluorescence with time, the authors estimate the quantity of amplified Y-chromosome DNA. Comparison with standard curves of known amounts of DNA added in parallel allows conversion of fluorescent intensity to picograms of DNA, and these authors accept a conversion factor of 5 pg per DNA-containing cell to estimate cell numbers. In that case, fetal DNA corresponding to between 3.1 and 235 .1 cells/mL of maternal blood was seen. When modal DNA concentrations are employed, the result is 1552 cells/mL of maternal blood. In earlier work (see 1999 YEAR BOOK, pp 191-193), Dr. Bianchi found a mean of 2 cell units of DNA per mL of maternal blood in pregnancy would range from 0 to 5.7 cells/mL, assuming 6.6 pg of DNA is equivalent to 1 cell. Clearly there is an abundance of fetal to maternal DNA transfer during abortion sufficient to make microchimerism a possibility following the procedure. This study confirms her earlier work, demonstrating that transfer amounts increase with increasing gestational age.

T. H. Kirschbaum, MD

Early Diagnosis of Cystic Fibrosis Through Neonatal Screening Prevents Severe Malnutrition and Improves Long-Term Growth
Farrell PM, and the Wisconsin Cystic Fibrosis Neonatal Screening Study Group (Univ of Wisconsin, Madison; et al)
Pediatrics 107:1-13, 2001   9–7

Introduction.—Cystic fibrosis (CF) is difficult to diagnose in early childhood, despite the fact that it is a relatively common autosomal recessive disease and the sweat test is readily available. Delays in diagnosis can cause severe malnutrition, lung disease, and death. The benefits and risks of early diagnosis through screening were investigated in the Wisconsin CF Neonatal Screening Project. The incidence of CF was calculated, and the validity of the randomized method was assessed by comparing 16 demographic variables.

Methods.—Dried newborn blood specimens underwent immunoreactive trypsinogen analysis for determination of CF risk from 1985 to 1991, and from 1991 to 1994, the analysis was coupled to DNA-based detection of the ΔF508 mutation. The blood specimens of 650,341 newborns were randomized into 2 groups when the specimens arrived at the Wisconsin screening laboratory: (1) an early diagnosis, screened cohort and (2) a standard diagnosis or control group. To prevent selection bias, a unique unblinding method was created to precisely identify control subjects. Because sequential analysis of nutritional outcome measures showed significantly better growth in screened patients during 1996, the unblinding was accelerated and completely identified the control group by April 1998. Every member in this cohort was enrolled and evaluated for at least 1 year. A comprehensive surveillance program was completed, and another statistical analysis of the anthropometric indices was performed that included all patients with CP who did not have meconium ileus.

Results.—The incidence of CF diagnosed by means of a sweat chloride value of 60 mEq/L or greater was 1:4189. By incorporating other patients with CF born during the randomization period, including 2 diagnosed by autopsy and 8 probable patients, a maximum incidence of 1:3938 was calculated. Despite the fact that there were group differences in the proportion of patients with ΔF508 genotypes and with pancreatic insufficiency, validity of the randomization plan was confirmed when 16 demographic variables were analyzed, and no significant differences after adjusting for multiple comparisons were found. For patients without a meconium ileus, a marked difference in the mean deviation age of diagnosis for screened patients was 13 weeks, compared with the standard diagnosis group (100 weeks). Anthropometric indices of nutritional status were significantly higher at diagnosis for the screened group than for the standard diagnosis group, including length/height, body weight, and head circumference. During 13 years of evaluation, analysis of nutritional outcomes demonstrated significantly greater growth associated with early diagnosis, despite similar nutritional therapy and the inherently better pancreatic status in the control group. The screened group had a substantially lower proportion of patients with body weight and height data below the 10th percentile throughout childhood.

Conclusion.—The screened group had a higher proportion of patients with pancreatic insufficiency, yet their growth indices were significantly better, compared with the control group during 13 years of follow-up.

▶ The demonstration of a putative gene for CF responsible in homozygous mutated state on chromosome number 7 stimulated hopes for programs of genetic screening and early diagnosis for one of our most common somatic recessive illnesses (see 1991 YEAR BOOK OF OBSTETRICS, GYNECOLOGY, AND WOMEN'S HEALTH, pp 151-152, and 1994 YEAR BOOK, pp 209-210). Subsequent experience in preimplantation diagnosis (see 1995 YEAR BOOK, pp 218-220, and 1997 YEAR BOOK, pp 204-205) and gene therapy (see 1997 YEAR

Book, pp 175-176) followed. It was soon recognized that there were many different mutation sites in this large transmembrane conductance regulator gene among disease victims, and that the most common site of mutation, at locus ΔF508, accounted for no more than 75% of cases of CF. Cautions against general screening for CF on this basis stemmed from the low prevalence of the disease in 1:2000 births, the inefficiency of screening directed only at the ΔF508 site, and the uncertainty about the value of early detection. Only in the Australian continent and in Wisconsin were universal screening programs instituted, and this is the definitive report of the operation of 2 CF Neonatal Screening Centers operating in Wisconsin from 1985 to 1998.

The experimental design was complex and changed with time. Originally, universal screening was done with immunologic testing for trypsinogen, present in low concentrations in infants with CF by virtue of their pancreatic insufficiency. The diagnosis was then confirmed by demonstrating elevated concentrations of chloride in sweat samples. After 1991, DNA analysis for the ΔF508 locus was added. In all, 650,341 infants were enrolled, omitting newborns with meconium ileus, which serves as an early sign of CF, and divided into control and test groups of equal sizes. From 1994 to 1998, a standard diagnosis and treatment program was instituted for infants suspected of having CF, and randomization ceased as evidence of benefit of early diagnosis was evinced. Therapy took the form of administration of fat-soluble vitamins, fatty acids, pancreatic enzymes, employment of a high-caloric high-fat diet, chest physiotherapy, and antibiotics for recurrent bronchitis. Screening data from control subjects was then made available on patient request or with the presumptive clinical diagnosis of CF or attainment of 4 years of age. These constituted the late diagnosis group.

Comparisons are made between infants with an early diagnosis of CF (mean, 13 weeks of postnatal age) and late diagnosis (mean, 107 weeks of postnatal age). In this study, the ultimate incidence of CF was 1:4000 and the incidence of meconium ileus among 151 children with CF diagnosed by sweat analysis was in the range of 20% to 25%. What emerged was clear benefit in height and body weight of those 75 infants with early diagnosis compared with the later diagnosis group (see Figure 3 in the original article). Dietary analysis showed greater protein and caloric intake in children with CF with pancreatic insufficiency in both the screened and control groups.

This study demonstrates the presence of severe nutritional impairment in CF with little evidence of catch-up growth without specific therapy begun once the diagnosis was made. Clearly the earlier that therapy is instituted, the greater is the chance for normal long-term infant nutritional development. A difference in mean age of diagnosis of 94 weeks postnatal age accounts for measurable differences in growth parameters when evaluated at the age of 13 years. These results add to the strength of the argument in favor of routine screening in a process of evaluating the cost-benefit ratio of such an approach.

T. H. Kirschbaum, MD

Association of the C677T Methylenetetrahydrofolate Reductase Mutation and Elevated Homocysteine Levels With Congenital Cardiac Malformations

Wenstrom KD, Johanning GL, Johnston KE, et al (Univ of Alabama, Birmingham)

Am J Obstet Gynecol 184:806-817, 2001   9–8

Objective.—A mutation in the gene for the enzyme methylenetetrahydrofolate reductase (MTHFR) results in neural tube defects. Mothers with this mutation have abnormally high levels of homocysteine in amniotic fluid. High homocysteine levels have also been associated with premature cardiovascular disease and hereditary thrombophilia in adults. Whether the C677T *MTHFR* mutation and high amniotic fluid levels of homocysteine are causally linked to isolated congenital cardiac malformations was investigated in patients with pregnancies complicated by isolated fetal cardiac defects.

Methods.—Homocysteine levels and *MTHFR* genotype were determined in the amniotic fluid obtained from 26 patients with pregnancies complicated by isolated fetal cardiac defects and from 116 healthy controls.

Results.—Homocysteine levels and the number of C677T *MTHFR* mutations were significantly higher in complicated pregnancies than in normal pregnancies (Table 2). The developmental influence is most likely mediated through the effect of the homocysteine pathway and the C677T *MTHFR* gene on methionine. Only 1 methyl group distinguishes homocysteine from methionine, which is the precursor for S-adenosylmethionine, the major intracellular methyl donor for DNA, protein, and lipid reactions.

Conclusion.—The C677T *MTHFR* mutation and high homocysteine levels are responsible at least in part for congenital cardiac defects.

▶ Following the clue that women treated with supplementary folic acid to prevent recurrent neural tube defects have infants with less than the expected incident rates of ventricular septal defects, conotruncal, and other ventricular outflow tract anomalies (see 1993 YEAR BOOK OF OBSTETRICS, GYNECOLOGY, AND WOMEN'S HEALTH, pp 193-194), these authors have confirmed the partial responsibility of the C to T mutation in the gene for 5 MTHFR in isolated nonsyndromic congenital cardiac lesions. They have also provided us new hypotheses regarding a broad range of potential anomalies in genetic environmental interactions in general. Using archival amniotic fluid material and a computer-based patient data bank, the authors identified 26 women seen between 1988 and 1998 with infants demonstrating isolated cardiovascular anomalies identified by ultrasound and then subjected to amniocentesis. Infants with other anomalies were excluded. For controls, they randomly selected 116 women from the same patient population with infants normal by karyotype, ultrasound, and neonatal examination whose amniotic fluid samples were used as control material. Controls were

TABLE 2.—Amniotic Fluid Homocysteine Levels and *MTHFR* Mutation Status in Case Patients With Congenital Cardiac Defects and in Control Subjects

	Case Patients (n = 26)	Control Subjects (n = 116)	Statistical Significance	Odds Ratio	
				Value	95% Confidence Interval
Homocysteine level (µmol/L, mean ± SD)	1.7 ± 1.7	1.0 ± 0.7	$P = .07$	—	—
Samples with homocysteine level >90th percentile* (No.)	7/26 (27%)	11/116 (9%)	$P = .02$	3.5	1.2-10.2
Samples heterozygous or homozygous for C677T *MTHFR* (No.)	9/26 (35%)	12/93 (13%)	$P = .01$	3.6	1.3-9.8
Samples both heterozygous or homozygous for C677T *MTHFR* and homocysteine level >90th percentile (No.)	3/26 (12%)	0/116 (0%)	$P = .006$	34.7	1.7-694.3
Samples either heterozygous or homozygous for C677T *MTHFR* or homocysteine level >90th percentile (No.)	13/26 (50%)	23/116 (20%)	$P = .003$	4.0	1.6-9.9

*>1.85 µmol/L.

(Courtesy of Wenstrom KD, Johanning GL, Johnston KE, et al: Association of the C677T methylenetetrahydrofolate reductase mutation and elevated homocysteine levels with congenital cardiac malformations. *Am J Obstet Gynecol* 184:806-817, 2001.)

matched for race and duration of storage of amniotic fluid at less than 20°C (a mean of 4.9 years) and compared with respect to homocysteine concentration and the incidence of MTHFR replacement mutation based on PCR and restriction fragment polymorphisms of DNA isolated from amniotic fluid cell pellets. The incidence of either increased homocysteine concentration or mutation abnormality was 50% in the 26 index patients versus 20% in the control population, a statistically significant difference.

It is important that the C677T mutation is a precursor to more than cardiac defects. Folate therapy fails to prevent 28% of repeat neural tube defects in women treated after a first anomalous infant. Folate supplementation and diet are capable of superceding the impairment of the *MTHFR* gene defect that functions to methylate homocysteine to form methionine. Methionine is an important component for DNA methylation and acts in epigenetic control of gene expression. DNA methylation is active in regulating cell proliferation and differentiation, cell transport, extracellular matrix formation, and production of a wide range of biochemical products. This makes it important in the general control of fetal development. Inadequate methionine-based methylation has been associated with chromosomal instability and abnormal mutational control. It is not surprising that folic acid presumably acting to ensure adequate MTHFR and methionine activity has been reported to reduce the occurrence rates for cleft palate and lip, urinary tract and limb anomalies, Down syndrome, and a wide range of gastrointestinal anomalies, genital defects, schizophrenia, and depression. These are important concepts that will provide the basis for future research in the important area of human teratogenesis. Fairly clearly, the *MTHFR* mutation appears unrelated to pregnancy hypertension (see 2001 YEAR BOOK, pp 104-105).

T. H. Kirschbaum, MD

Genetic Susceptibility to Preeclampsia: Roles of Cytosine-to-Thymine Substitution at Nucleotide 677 of the Gene for Methylenetetrahydrofolate Reductase, 68-Base Pair Insertion at Nucleotide 844 of the Gene for Cystathionine β-Synthase, and Factor V Leiden Mutation

Kim YJ, Williamson RA, Murray JC, et al (Univ of Iowa, Iowa City; Wake Forest Univ, Winston-Salem, NC; Ewha Women's Univ, Seoul, Korea)
Am J Obstet Gynecol 184:1211-1217, 2001   9–9

Background.—A familial tendency toward development of preeclampsia has been noted, but the exact genes responsible have not been identified. The tendency of patients with preeclampsia to have vascular or thrombotic disorders has suggested several candidates. Gene mutations present in common vascular or thrombotic disorders were evaluated to see whether there was any connection with preeclampsia.

Methods.—Whole blood or cheek swab samples were taken from 360 women in the control group who had gone through at least 2 term pregnancies without preeclampsia and from 281 women with preeclampsia. Deoxyribonucleic acid was extracted from these samples. The 2 groups were compared with respect to mutation frequencies, with a *P* value less than .05 considered significant.

Results.—Homozygosity for cytosine-to-thymine substitution at nucleotide 677 in the gene for methyltetrahydrofolate reductase (MFTR) was noted in 11.7% of the women with preeclampsia, 11.4% of those with severe preeclampsia, and 11.4% of those in the control group. Heterozygosity for the insertion of 68 bases at position 844 in the gene for cystathionine β-synthase was found in 15.5% of those with preeclampsia, 12.6% of those with severe preeclampsia, and 17.5% of those in the control group. Heterozygosity for the Leiden mutation in the gene for factor V was present in 6.0% of those with preeclampsia, 6.5% of those with severe preeclampsia, and 4.7% of the women in the control group.

Conclusions.—None of the mutations studied showed a significant correlation with an increased risk for preeclampsia.

▶ A genetic basis for preeclampsia has long been recognized (see 1988 YEAR BOOK OF OBSTETRICS, GYNECOLOGY, AND WOMEN'S HEALTH, p 175, and 1990 YEAR BOOK, pp 50-51). This well-conducted study uses recombinant DNA techniques to explore the possibility that expression of a gene deficiency involving 1 of 2 mutations is responsible for hyperhomocysteinemia, an agent known to result in endothelial dysfunction, and the Leiden mutation, leading to production of clotting factor V resistant to activated protein C resulting in thromboembolic phenomena in pregnancy. Both have been suspected of a role in the pathophysiology of preeclampsia (see 1998 YEAR BOOK, pp 210-211, 2000 YEAR BOOK, pp 119-120, and 2001 YEAR BOOK, pp 104-105). Blood homocysteine concentration increases in folate deficiency (see Abstract 2–2) or in the presence of a mutation of the enzyme 5 MTHFR, both of which interfere with the reduction of homocysteine to methionine, as does the mutated gene for cystathione β-synthetase, a common cause of homocystinuria. The factor V mutation is suspect because of the thrombotic vaso-occlusive pathology of severe preeclamspsia.

The approach here was to use DNA from clinical blood samples from 281 preeclamptic women and 369 control normal gravidas obtained from 1996 to 1999. Samples were subjected to polymerase chain reaction with primers specific to the 3 defective gene sites and normal mutant alleles sequenced to look for subtle variants in women with preeclampsia. Comparisons with control samples were carried out, looking for heterozygous and homozygous genotypes and abnormal alleles among preeclamptic nulligravidas and multiparas, properly a misnomer, in women categorized as preeclamptic, severely preeclamptic, or exhibiting HELLP syndrome. No significant differences were noted from women with normotensive pregnancies. Mutated MTHFR gene was more prevalent in "multiparous preeclamptics" because the incidence of chorionic hypertension is far greater in multiparas than it is in primigravid preeclampsia.[1] In any event, it seems appropriate to give up hope of finding any real causal relationship between preeclampsia and any of these 3 mutations.

T. H. Kirschbaum, MD

Reference

1. Chesley CL: Recognition of the long term sequela of eclampsia. *Am J Obstet Gynecol* 189:249, 2000.

Paternal and Maternal Components of the Predisposition to Preeclampsia

Esplin MS, Fausett MB, Fraser A, et al (Univ of Utah, Salt Lake City)
N Engl J Med 344:867-872, 2001   9–10

Objective.—A familial predisposition to preeclampsia has been reported, and the paternal genes may play a role in the pathophysiology of preeclampsia and in placentation. Because preeclampsia occurs more often in first pregnancies or after a change in partners, an interaction between maternal antibodies and paternally derived fetal antigens is suggested. Whether the offspring of men and women who were born to mothers with preeclampsia were more likely also to be born to preeclamptic mothers was investigated in a prospective study.

Methods.—Using the Utah Population Database, the incidence of preeclampsia was investigated in offspring born to a cohort of women and a cohort of men, born between 1947 and 1957, to mothers with preeclampsia. A control group of 596 men and 474 women, born between 1947 and 1957, was used for comparison. Characteristics of index pregnancies among women or partners of men were compared using the Student's *t*-test. An adjusted odds ratio (OR) for the development of preeclampsia during each pregnancy was calculated using backward logistic regression analysis.

Results.—Of 210,313 live births during the study period, 1900 women had preeclampsia. There were 947 offspring born to 298 males and 830 offspring born to 237 females between 1970 and 1992. In the male study group, 26 (2.7%) offspring were born to mothers with preeclampsia

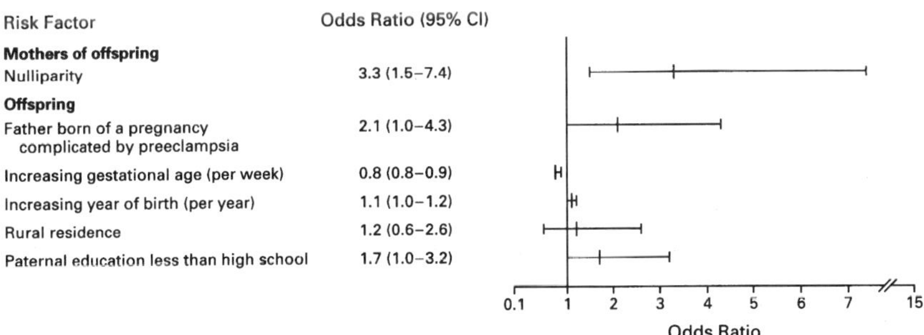

FIGURE 2.—Odds ratios among the partners of the male study group as compared with the partners of the male control group. The scale of the abscissa differs on either side of unity. *Abbreviation: CI,* Confidence interval. (Reprinted by permission of The New England Journal of Medicine from Esplin MS, Fausett MB, Fraser A, et al: Paternal and maternal components of the predisposition to preeclampsia. *N Eng J Med* 344:867-873, 2001. Copyright 2001, Massachusetts Medical Society. All rights reserved.)

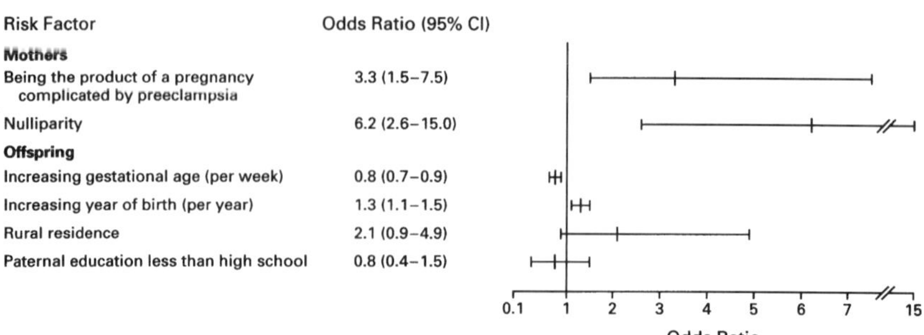

FIGURE 3.—Odds ratios for preeclampsia in the female study group as compared with the female control group. The scale of the abscissa differs on either side of unity. *Abbreviation: CI,* Confidence interval. (Reprinted by permission of The New England Journal of Medicine from Esplin MS, Fausett MB, Fraser A, et al: Paternal and maternal components of the predisposition to preeclampsia. *N Eng J Med* 344:867-873, 2001. Copyright 2001, Massachusetts Medical Society. All rights reserved.)

compared with 1.3% in the male control group (OR, 2.1) (Fig 2). In the female study group, 39 (4.7%) of 830 offspring were born to mothers with preeclampsia compared with 1.9% in the female control group (OR, 3.3) (Fig 3). First pregnancy increased the risk of preeclampsia significantly (OR, 6.2). Female partners (n = 52) of men born of mothers with preeclampsia who also had preeclamptic pregnancies were identified. Birth records available for 41 of these women showed that they had not been born of mothers with preeclampsia, ruling out a maternal history of preeclampsia.

Conclusion.—Men and women who had been born to mothers with preeclampsia were significantly more likely to have a child who was the product of a preeclamptic pregnancy, especially when it was a first birth. This study establishes that both the genotype of the fetus and a paternal component contribute to the development of preeclampsia.

▶ Given the frequently cited hypothesis that preeclampsia stems from deficiencies in the immunologic factors that render the fetal allograft free of rejection, both the maternal and paternal haplotypes of the fetal genotype might be expected to play some role. Assuming preeclampsia is an expression of a single gene (see 1988 YEAR BOOK OF OBSTETRICS, GYNECOLOGY, AND WOMEN'S HEALTH, p 175), an analysis suggests a simple recessive inheritance pattern to which both maternal and paternal alleles are required for expression.

The Salt Lake Valley has long offered an unparalleled resource for genealogic data aggregates, originally collected as information important to the Mormon faith. With wide recognition of the Utah Population Database's usefulness in the evaluation of familial patterns of disease and as a substratum for epidemiologic research, it has gained wide support from state and several federal grantees as well as the University of Utah's Huntsman Cancer Institute. Here, it is used to explore the possible role of a paternal component to add to the well-known evidence of maternal inheritance of the syndrome.

Birth certificate data was used to identify approximately 1000 male and 889 female infants born between 1947 to 1957, to women with preeclampsia. Of those approximately 1900 individuals, 298 males were listed as fathers in 947 deliveries from 1970 to 1992, all complicated by preeclampsia. In the same time span, 237 women born of preeclamptic mothers in the earlier time period delivered 830 infants as products of preeclamptic pregnancies. ORs for the likelihood of preeclampsia occurring to men and women delivered of preeclamptic mothers were struck using a control group delivered in 1947 to 1957 of normotensive women of roughly twice as many pregnancies matched for sex, county residence, maternal age, year of birth, and birth order. Siblings of test subject pregnancies were excluded. Multivariant analysis was used to correct for 15 confounding variables. The incidence of preeclampsia in women born of preeclamptic mothers was 4.7% versus 1.9% in controls. In men with the same heritage, 2.7% resulted in preeclamptic pregnancies with a control incidence of 1.3%. Pregnancies in women with preeclamptic mothers were 3.3 times more likely to have preeclampsia than were controls; for men, the incremental risk was 2.1 at times, but the significance of the latter figure was not robust. Nulliparity in preeclamptic women delivered from 1947 to 1957 strangely increased the incidence of preeclampsia in the next generation.

A mechanistic intermediate in the increased predisposition for preeclampsia among male offsprings of preeclamptic mothers can only be speculative, but this is one more test that any theory of the origin of preeclampsia must ultimately meet. This is, however, strong evidence that a modest paternal component in the familial incidence of preeclampsia does exist.

T. H. Kirschbaum, MD

10 Newborn

Adverse Effects of Early Dexamethasone Treatment in Extremely-Low-Birth-Weight Infants
Stark AR, for the National Institute of Child Health and Human Development Neonatal Research Network (Brigham and Women's Hosp, Boston; et al)
N Engl J Med 344:95-101, 2001   10–1

Introduction.—The early administration of high doses of dexamethasone may decrease the risk of chronic lung disease in premature infants. Infants in trials with high-dose dexamethasone experienced adverse effects, including hypertension or hyperglycemia. Treatment with a moderate dose of dexamethasone was evaluated to determine whether it could reduce the risk of chronic lung disease and have minimal adverse effects in infants with birth weights ranging from 501 to 1000 g who were treated with mechanical ventilation within 12 hours after birth.

Methods.—The study included 220 very low birth weight infants who were randomized to treatment with either dexamethasone or placebo with either routine ventilatory support or permissive hypercapnia. Dexamethasone was administered within 24 hours after birth at 0.15 mg/kg of body weight per day for 3 days, then tapered over 7 days. The main outcome measures were death or chronic lung disease at 36 weeks' postmenstrual age.

Results.—Compared with placebo, the relative risk of death or chronic lung disease was 0.9 in the dexamethasone group. The effect of dexamethasone did not differ with respect to ventilatory approach, so the dexamethasone and placebo groups were combined. In comparison with the placebo group, infants in the dexamethasone group were less likely to require oxygen supplementation at 28 days after birth ($P = .004$), receive open-label glucocorticoid treatment during hospitalization (34% vs 51%; $P = .01$), more likely to have hypertension ($P < .001$), and more likely to receive insulin treatment for hyperglycemia ($P = .02$). During the first 14 days, infants in the dexamethasone group were also more likely than those in the placebo group to have spontaneous gastrointestinal perforation (13% vs 4%; $P = .02$). Dexamethasone-treated infants had lower body weight ($P = .02$) and a smaller head circumference ($P = .04$) at 36 weeks' postmenstrual age, compared with placebo-treated infants.

Conclusion.—The early administration of dexamethasone in moderate doses had no effect on death or chronic lung disease in very low birthweight preterm infants; it was associated with gastrointestinal perforation and diminished growth.

▶ Though glucocorticoid administration to gravidas in preterm labor 24 hours prior to delivery confers genuine benefit on the newborn as it makes its respiratory transformation from fetal life, the problem of pulmonary dysplasia and the prolonged need for supplementary oxygen remains in very low birth weight infants after the immediate neonatal period. This is an effort by the Neonatal Research Network of NICHD to explore the effectiveness and safety of neonatal dexamethasone administration of 0.15 mg/kg daily for 3 days followed by decremental dosage for 7 days. This moderate dose was chosen since prior work using dexamethasone doses 0.5 mg/kg or more per day generated reports of serious cardiovascular and carbohydrate regulatory problems in the infants. A total of 220 newborns of 0.5 to 1.0 kg birthweight treated with ventilatory support for the first 12 hours of life but free of anomaly, congenital infection, or evidence of acidosis and hypoxia at birth were enrolled and randomly assigned to dexamethasone at the dose prescribed or to placebo. Two systems of respiratory therapy were employed, one allowing relative hypercarbia, but no differences in outcome measurements, that is, neonatal death or the need for supportive chronic lung disease past 36 weeks of age, were noted between them.

Compared with the control group, dexamethasone, as prescribed, made no difference in those 2 outcome measurements. Dexamethasone therapy appeared to decrease the need for supplemental neonatal oxygen, further corticoid therapy, and yielded decreased evidence of pulmonary interstitial emphysema. No impact on the incidence of patent ductus arteriosus, pulmonary hemorrhage, or pneumothorax was noted. When, however, at 14 days of life, the incidence of intestinal perforation proved to be 13% in dexamethasone recipients and 4% in the control group, the Independent Data Safety Monitoring committee closed the study. Perforations occurred primarily in infants also receiving indomethacin, probably to facilitate ductus arteriosis closure. Dexamethasone, however, becomes of its independent role in decreasing prostaglandin production and as a result of the decrease in cardiac output associated with ductus arteriosus closure, appeared to intensify the deleterious effects.

Because of evidence of neonatal injury in the absence of clear evidence of benefit in this weight range, the NICHD Network feels dexamethasone therapy for this indication and this dosage is not warranted and offers particular caution regarding the simultaneous use of indomethacin.

T. H. Kirschbaum, MD

Antenatal Steroids and Neonatal Periventricular Leukomalacia

Canterino JC, Verma U, Visintainer PF, et al (New York Med College, Valhalla)
Obstet Gynecol 97:135-139, 2001   10–2

Background.—The use of antenatal steroids is partly responsible for recent improvements in neonatal survival. This treatment reduces the risk of respiratory distress syndrome (RDS), intraventricular hemorrhage (IVH) necrotizing enterocolitis, and neonatal death. However, the effect of antenatal steroids on periventricular leukomalacia (PVL) has not been established.

Methods.—A cohort of 1161 neonates with gestational ages of 24 to 34 weeks and birth weights of 500 to 1750 g was studied retrospectively. The mothers of 400 neonates had received antenatal steroids, and the mothers of 761 had not. Neonatal neurosonograms were obtained at 3 and 7 days of life.

Findings.—Twenty-three percent of the infants exposed to antenatal steroid treatment had PVL or IVH, compared with 31% of those not receiving such treatment. This difference was significant. PVL with IVH occurred in 5% and 11% of those with and without antenatal steroid treatment, respectively, and isolated PVL occurred in 3% and 7%, respectively. These differences were also significant. In a logistic regression analysis adjusting for confounding maternal and neonatal characteristics, antenatal steroid therapy was associated with a 56% lower likelihood of PVL with IVH and a 58% lower likelihood of isolated PVL (Table 1).

TABLE 1.—Relationship Between the Use of Antenatal Steroids
and Selected Characteristics

Characteristic	Steroids ($n = 400$)	No Steroids ($n = 761$)	P
Maternal age (y)	29.2 ± 6.0	28.7 ± 6.0	.18
Preterm delivery	299 (74.8)	576 (75.7)	.72
Gestational age (wk)	29.0 ± 2.8	29.0 ± 2.8	.98
Birth weight (g)	1187.8 ± 328.0	1198.2 ± 344.0	.62
Clinical chorioamnionitis	32 (8.0)	95 (12.5)	.02
Histologic chorioamnionitis	165 (41.1)	314 (41.4)	.98
Apgar score at 5 min <7	62 (15.8)	198 (26.5)	.001
RDS	141 (35.4)	376 (49.5)	.001
Neonatal death	32 (8.0)	80 (10.5)	.17
Any lesion	92 (23.0)	234 (30.8)	.005
PVL with IVH	18 (4.6)	83 (11.0)	.001
PVL only	9 (2.8)	40 (7.1)	.009

Note: Data are given as mean ± SD or n (percent).
(Reprinted with permission from the American College of Obstetricians and Gynecologists, courtesy of Canterino JC, Verma U, Visintainer PF, et al: Antenatal steroids and neonatal periventricular leukomalacia. *Obstet Gynecol* 97:135-139, 2001.)

Conclusions.—Antenatal steroid treatment reduces the incidence of PVL in preterm neonates by more than 50%. The increased use of antenatal steroid treatment may also improve long-term neurologic outcomes.

▶ This appears to be an example of newborn RDS and its treatment serving as a confounding variable between maternal antenatal steroid administration and evidence of neonatal brain injury. The apparent relationship between 2 variables is confounded if both of the variables are mutually related to a third variable. This often results in the spurious suggestion of a direct relationship between the variables of original interest. In this cohort study of infants born prior to 34 weeks' gestational age, pregnancies not treated with antenatal corticoids showed a larger incidence of clinically suspected, but not laboratory confirmed, chorioamnionitis. There were increased rates of occurrence of RDS and decreased 5-minute Apgar scores in those infants whose mothers were not so treated. At a mean gestational age of 29 weeks, those infants with RDS were undoubtedly subjected to NICU admission and likely received respiratory supportive therapy. Neither the incidence of neonatal ICU admission or respiratory assist are provided in the article. The positive relationship of respiratory support of premature infants to IVH is well known[1,2] and has likely accounted for the increased incidence of brain injury in the group whose mothers were not treated with steroids. Before the authors consider direct glucocorticoid effects on the fetal cerebral vasculature, they need to exclude respiratory supportive therapy as the immediate causal agent.

T. H. Kirschbaum, MD

References

1. Perlmore VM, Goodwans, Kreufser KL: Reduction in intraventricular hemorrhage by eliminating cerebral blood flow velocity in preterm infants with RDS. *N Engl J Med* 312:1353, 1985.
2. Volpe JJ (ed): *Neurology of the Newborn*, ed 3. Philadelphia, WB Saunders, pp 437-438, 1995.

Growth Restriction in Dexamethasone-Treated Preterm Infants May Be Mediated by Reduced IGF-I and IGFBP-3 Plasma Concentrations
Bloomfield FH, Knight DB, Breier BH, et al (Univ of Auckland, New Zealand)
Clin Endocrinol (Oxf) 54:235-242, 2001   10–3

Background.—Restricted growth often occurs in preterm infants who are given dexamethasone for chronic lung disease (CLD) of prematurity. The mechanism that causes retarded growth, however, has not yet been determined. The association between dexamethasone dose and insulin-like growth factor binding protein 3 (IGFBP-3) and IGF-I levels, and the association between these levels and linear growth of bones were investigated.

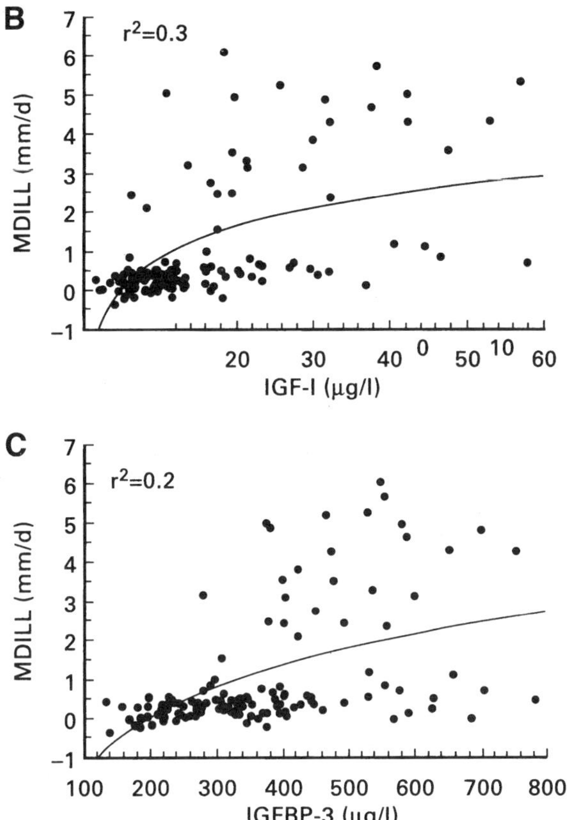

FIGURE 2.—Regression plots: B, IGF-I vs MDILL; C, IGFBP-3 vs MDILL. Data were log-transformed prior to linear regression analysis, then back-transformed for graphing. Each dot represents a paired measurement. Regression lines and correlation coefficients (r^2) shown. *Abbreviations*: MDILL, mean daily increase in lower leg length. (Courtesy Bloomfield FH, Knight DB, Breier BH, et al: Growth restriction in dexamethasone-treated preterm infants may be mediated by reduced IGF-I and IGFBP-3 plasma concentrations. *Clin Endrocrinol (Oxf)* 54: 235-242, 2001. Reproduced by permission of Blackwell Science, Inc.)

Methods.—The study included 40 preterm infants with a birthweight 1250 g or less, aged 7 days, who were ventilated and were randomly given either a long course (42 days) of tapering dexamethasone or a 3-day repeatable pulse course of treatment with dexamethasone. Nineteen infants were included in the pulse group, and 21 were included in the long-course group. Knemometry was used to measure linear growth of the lower leg 3 times per week. IGFBP-3 and IGF-1 levels were assessed on days 1 (prior to treatment), 14, 42, and at 36 weeks postmenstrual age (PMA). Variable interactions were analyzed using stepwise regression analysis and covariance analysis (ANCOVA). Correlation coefficients were used to assess associations between variables.

Results.—IGFBP-3 levels were significantly (using ANCOVA) influenced by the mean daily dose of dexamethasone per kilogram body weight

(MDDD) and by the treatment group to which the infants were assigned ($P - .0009$ and $P = .017$, respectively). IGF-1 levels were also influenced by these variables ($P = 0.098$ and $P = 0.07$). Mean daily increase in lower-leg length (MDILL) was also significantly influenced by MDDD. ($P < .01$). Levels of IGFBP-3 and IGF-1 also correlated to MDILL in a significant fashion (ANACOVA, $P < .01$). Figure 2, parts (B) and (C) show the regression plots for IGF-1, IGFBP-3, and MDILL (Fig 2). Correlation coefficients of 0.2 and 0.3 were shown for IGFBP-3, and IGF-1 correlated with MDILL (both, $P < .0001$). Increasing PMA was found to significantly increase both IGFBP-3 and IGF-1 levels ($P < .0001$). A high correlation was also noted between IGFBP-3 and IGF-1 levels ($r^2 = 0.52$, $P < .0001$). Females exhibited significantly higher IGF-1 levels ($P = 0.036$).

Conclusions.—Suppression of the IGF axis may, at least partially, mediate some of the growth-restricting effects of dexamethasone therapy. Both MDDD and dexamethasone treatments for both dose strategies influence the levels of circulating IGF-1 and IGFBP-3.

▶ In exploring the relationships between dexamethasone, growth hormone concentration, and those of the somatomedins IGF1 and IGF2 as well as their plasma binding proteins, these authors offer a tentative explanation of growth retardation associated with prophylactic steroid therapy for the prevention of respiratory distress syndrome in preterm infants. IGF-1 is a regular correlate and presumed regulator of fetal growth. IGF-1 concentration is regulated in part by the concentration of its major binding protein, IGFBP3, and by nutrient availability. In prenatal life, fetal growth hormone regulates the activity of IGF-1 and, in turn, fetal growth. In a study of 40 newborns weighing 1.25 kg or less at birth, the authors demonstrate that both the concentration of exogenous dexamethasone and the pattern of its administration, either in a pulse dose or in a decremental 3-day dosage schedule of a 42-day low-dose exposure, reduce the concentration of both IGF-1 and IGFBP3. These changes were paralleled by a serial decrease in mean daily increase in lower leg length determined ultrasonically. The pattern of IGF-1 change is to decrease with acute dexamethasone exposure and then increase in activity as dexamethasone decreases with time and catabolism, stimulating catch-up growth in the fetus. Whether the changes are due directly to altered neonatal growth hormone release itself is not determined here. This is, in any event, convincing evidence of a probable mechanism for growth impairment noted by other clinicians in infants exposed to betamethasone antenatally (see Abstract 3–3).

T. H. Kirschbaum, MD

Neurologic and Developmental Disability After Extremely Preterm Birth

Wood NS, for the EPICure Study Group (Univ of Nottingham, England; et al)
N Engl J Med 343:378-384, 2000
10–4

Background.—Being born an extremely preterm infant has been shown to lead to a greater incidence of neurologic and developmental disabilities. All children born at 25 weeks of gestation or earlier in the United Kingdom and Ireland during the period from March to December of 1995 were assessed. Evaluation was conducted when the median age of these children was 30 months (corrected for gestational age).

Methods.—Although 314 children were discharged home, a formal assessment conducted by an independent examiner was done for each of 283 surviving children. The Bayley Scales of Infant Development served as the measure of development; standardized examination was the basis for determining neurologic function. Predetermined criteria were used to evaluate disability and severe disability.

Results.—Referenced to a population mean of 100, on the Bayley Mental Index the mean score was 84, while that on the Psychomotor Developmental Index was 87. Severely delayed development indicated by scores over 3 SD below the mean was noted in 19% of these children; another 11% had scores 2 to 3 SD below the mean. Severe neuromotor disability was seen in 10%, 2% were blind or perceived light only, and 3% had hearing loss that required hearing aids or could not be corrected. Overall 49% had disability of some degree, 23% of whom were severely disabled (Table 1 and Fig 1). Based on evaluations from local pediatricians, 49% of the 314 infants discharged home were without disability. Boys were more likely to be disabled than girls.

TABLE 1.—Summary of Outcomes Among Infants Born Alive at 22 Through 25 Weeks of Gestation

Outcome	22 Wk (N = 138)	23 Wk (N = 241)	24 Wk (N – 382)	25 Wk (N = 424)
		number (percent)		
Died in delivery room	116 (84)	110 (46)	84 (22)	67 (16)
Admitted to NICU	22 (16)	131 (54)	298 (78)	357 (84)
Died in NICU	20 (14)	105 (44)	198 (52)	171 (40)
Survived to discharge	2 (1)	26 (11)	100 (26)	186 (44)
Died after discharge	0	1 (0.4)	2 (0.5)	3 (0.7)
Lost to follow-up	0	0	1 (0.3)	1 (0.2)
Had severe disability at 30 mo	1 (0.7)	8 (3)	24 (6)	40 (9)
Had other disabilities at 30 mo	0	6 (2)	28 (7)	44 (10)
Survived without overall disability at 30 mo				
As a percentage of live births	1 (0.7)	11 (5)	45 (12)	98 (23)
As a percentage of NICU admissions	1 (5)	11 (8)	45 (15)	98 (27)

Note: Three infants, all of whom died, were admitted at less than 22 weeks of gestational age. For infants who died in the delivery room, gestational age was based on the estimate used in the delivery room. For infants who were admitted to the neonatal ICU (*NICU*), gestational age was confirmed postnatally.

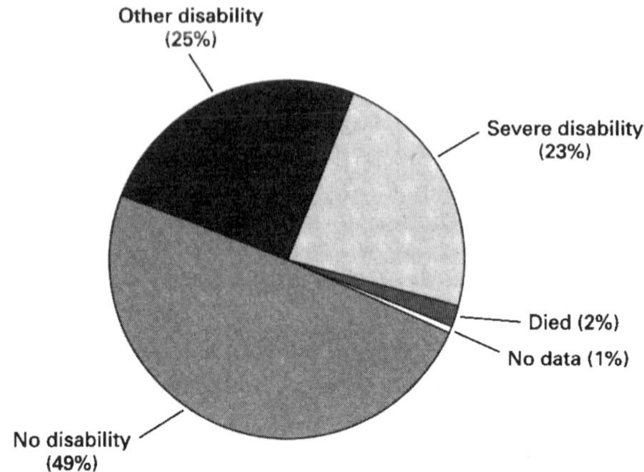

FIGURE 1.—Summary of outcome with respect to overall disability at 30 months for 314 children born at 22 through 25 weeks of gestation. (Reprinted by permission of *The New England Journal of Medicine* courtesy of Wood NS, for the EPICure Study Group: Neurologic and developmental disability after extremely preterm birth. *N Engl J Med* 343:378-384, 2000. Copyright 2000, Massachusetts Medical Society. All rights reserved.)

Conclusion.—Nearly half of the extremely preterm infants studied had deficits in the realms of mental and psychomotor development, neuromotor function, or sensory and communication function at approximately age 30 months (corrected). This may translate into later behavioral, fine-motor, and educational difficulties for these children. Thus, the results of this study should be useful in planning appropriate interventions.

▶ In terms of intact survival of the human newborn, the interval from 23 to 26 weeks' gestational age is critically important. There is no time in gestation where an added week of survival in utero is a more sensitive determinant of live birth and the absence of permanent disability. That conclusion is clear from this analysis of births registered in the United Kingdom and Ireland over a 10-month interval in 1995. Births occurring from 20 to 25 weeks' gestation were analyzed, a subset comprising 1% to 1½% of births constituting about 50% of neonatal deaths and encumbering vast resources, inpatient facilities, and personnel efforts as well as family anguish.

Results are categorized by gestational age, not birth weight, to avoid confusion with uncontrolled growth retardation. Rates are calculated based on live births to avoid inclusion of induced abortion specimens as part of the basis for comparison. Only 30% of total births in this gestational age range were live born. About 30% of live births expired prior to neonatal ICU admission, and 61% of the 811 infants admitted to the neonatal ICU expired prior to discharge. The remaining 308 infants' survival was sufficient for multiphase evaluation of function and disability at a median of 30 weeks of age.

Table 1 demonstrates that intact survival at 22 weeks with an expectant mean birth weight of 500 g is negligible and small at 23 weeks' gestation. One week later at 24 weeks, the chances of being live born and neurologically intact has increased 2½-fold. One week more of in utero life and the favorable odds double again. By 26 weeks' gestational age, the improved chances for intact survival accelerate even more.[1]

Intact survival rates here are not as great as in comparable data provided by others (see 1989 YEAR BOOK OF OBSTETRICS, GYNECOLOGY, AND WOMEN'S HEALTH, pp 185-187, 1991 YEAR BOOK, pp 179-180, and 1995 YEAR BOOK, pp 238-240). That likely stems from failure of a uniform policy regarding intent and content of resuscitation efforts among centers and unspecified employment of neonatal surfactant administration. Nonetheless, the message is clear. A week of continued intrauterine life at this gestational age range will shorten neonatal ICU residence by months if it can be attained.

T. H. Kirschbaum, MD

Reference

1. Copper RL, Goldenberg RL, Creasy RK, et al: A multicenter study of preterm birth weight and gestational specific neonatal mortality. *Am J Obstet Gynecol* 168:78, 1993.

Neurodevelopmental Outcome of Infants Treated With Head Cooling and Mild Hypothermia After Perinatal Asphyxia

Battin MR, Dezoete JA, Gunn TR, et al (Natl Women's Hosp, Auckland, New Zealand; Univ of Auckland, New Zealand)
Pediatrics 107:480-484, 2001

10–5

Objective.—Prolonged, moderate hypothermia can provide neuroprotection even in cases of severe asphyxia. There are few data on the long-term outcome of infants with perinatal asphyxia cooled in the neonatal period. The neurodevelopmental outcome was studied in a group of term infants treated with selective head cooling versus controls after hypoxic-ischemic encephalopathy.

Methods.—Infants of gestational age more than 37 weeks, a 5-minute Apgar score 7.09 or less, and encephalopathy were randomly allocated to no head cooling (n = 25) or head cooling (n = 13) to 34.5°C (n = 7), 35.5 to 35.9°C (n = 6), or 36 to 36.5°C (n = 6) from 6 hours after birth to 72 hours. Infants were slowly rewarmed at 0.5°C. Infants were followed up in a blinded fashion, with neurologic testing and developmental testing using the revised Bayley scales, until aged 18 months. Infants with major congenital abnormalities and metabolic diseases were excluded.

Results.—There were 6 deaths: 3 in the control group, 2 in the minimally cooled group, and 1 in the mildly cooled group. There was 1 late-infancy death in a control infant with severe spastic quadriparesis. There were 28 infants evaluated at 18 months. Six control, 1 minimally cooled, and 4 mildly cooled infants had stage 1 encephalopathy, and 1 had an adverse outcome. Four (44%) control, 4 (80%) minimally cooled, and 4 (26%) mildly cooled infants with stage 2 or 3 encephalopathy had an adverse outcome (odds ratio, 0.46 vs the control group).

Conclusion.—Infants with perinatal asphyxia, treated with head cooling, show no adverse effects at 18 months. Infants with more severe encephalopathy tended to show improvement after head cooling.

▶ After demonstration by this productive group of Auckland investigators of the biphasic response to acute cerebral ischemia in experimental animals and an interval of 24 hours or so before irreversible neuronal loss was seen, the search for preventive measures useful during that 24 hours or so began in earnest. An early treatment, effective in experimental animals, consisted of cooling the extradural space to 32°C (see 1998 YEAR BOOK OF OBSTETRICS, GYNECOLOGY, AND WOMEN'S HEALTH, pp 231-235), followed by a small pilot study to explore short-term safety of cooling in human beings.[1] This is a larger study using 4 levels of cooling that fails to demonstrate deleterious effects but yields some small indications of success. Originally, 33 infants with 5-minute Apgar scores of 6 or less with umbilical artery blood pH 7.09 or less and with some evidence of encephalopathy graded 1 to 3 after Sarnet and Sarnet were studied.[2] Excluding infants with anomalies or metabolic defects, infants were randomly divided into 15 uncooled controls and 3 groups of 6 each subjected to cooling after cerebral ischemia and treated within 6 hours of birth. The investigators used 10°C water flow to a helmet sufficient to lower rectal temperature into 3 ranges of temperature of approximately 36.5°, 35.5°, and 35°C; later a fourth group of 7 infants cooled to 34.5° was added, bringing the total treated to 25. All infants were examined by US, CT of the head, and EEG and were followed up by investigators to 18 months of age, when they were evaluated by a developmental psychologist blinded to treatment.

The clearest result is that head cooling produced no evidence of worsening of the status of the 25 treated infants. Short-term mortality rate before discharge consisted of 3 control infants, all Sarnet 3 infants, 2 Sarnet 1 infants and 1 Sarnet 2 infant. The majority of infants with mild asphyxia (alert, normal Moro and stretch receptors, normal sympathetic tone, and EEG) recovered fully. Of those with moderate to severe injury in the range of Sarnet 2 to 3, all were deemed no worse than expected and some somewhat better. The group at Sarnet 3 level showed stupor, flaccidity, depressed brain stem and autonomic function, and isopotential EEG with infrequent discharges. Adverse effects occurred in 28% of those treated with hypothermia versus 44% of untreated controls. Of the 11 Sarnet class 2 to 3 infants cooled to the lowest range at 34.5° to 35°C, 8 were normal at 18 months.

Despite these encouraging findings, long-term benefit is unproven. The severity of brain injury varies within Sarnet class and is fundamentally important in determining ultimate outcome. Infant inclusion criteria are probably not stringent enough because 11 of 15 control cases, 6 of them Sarnet 1, were normal on follow-up without treatment. The time of the CNS insult is critical to locating the window of opportunity for therapy, known for certain in experimental animals and usually uncertain in humans. Power analysis shows that to show a 30% reduction in death or disability with a 50% incidence in controls, 350 infants, half untreated, would be required.

Nonetheless, this work is important as a preliminary to mounting just such a prospective clinical trial.

T. H. Kirschbaum, MD

References

1. Gunn AJ, Gluckman PD, Gunn TR, et al: Selective head cooling in newborn infants after prenatal asphyxia: A safety study. *Pediatrics* 102:885, 1998.
2. Sarnet HB, Sarnet MS: Neonatal encephalopathy following fetal distress. *Arch Neurol* 33:696, 1976.

Cerebral Glucose Metabolism Measured by Positron Emission Tomography in Term Newborn Infants With Hypoxic Ischemic Encephalopathy
Thorngren-Jerneck K, Ohlsson T, Sandell A, et al (Univ Hosp, Lund, Sweden)
Pediatr Res 49:495-501, 2001   10–6

Background.—Birth asphyxia among term infants has remained a significant problem, with high rates of mortality and physical impairment. The clinical grading of hypoxic ischemic encephalopathy (HIE) after perinatal asphyxia has been shown to be a useful prognostic tool in assessing the term infant. Infants with mild HIE typically have a normal outcome, while severe HIE will result in death or cerebral palsy. However, infants with moderate HIE can experience either cerebral palsy or a normal outcome. Because early interventions for birth asphyxia soon may be possible, the early prediction of future handicap is important. Among the techniques that have been used to investigate the cerebral pathology in relation to perinatal asphyxia is positron emission tomography (PET) with measurement of total and regional cerebral glucose metabolism (CMRgl) with 2-(^{18}F) fluoro-2-deoxy-D-glucose (^{18}FDG). In this study, cerebral glucose metabolism in the subacute period after asphyxia was correlated with neurologic clinical scoring of HIE in the term newborn infant after perinatal asphyxia.

Methods.—Using PET, CMRgl was measured with ^{18}FDG in 20 term infants with HIE after perinatal asphyxia. Signs of perinatal distress were evident in all the infants, and 15 of them were severely acidotic at birth. Six of the infants had mild HIE, while 12 developed moderate HIE and 2 developed severe HIE in the first days of life. The PET scans were performed at a median age of 11 days. Quantification of CMRgl was based on a new method, which used the glucose metabolism of the erythrocytes and required only 1 blood sample.

Results.—The most metabolically active areas of the brain in all the infants were the deep subcortical parts, the thalamus, the basal ganglia, and the sensorimotor cortex. The frontal, occipital, and parietal cortex areas were less metabolically active. There was an inverse correlation of total CMRgl with the severity of HIE. Five of the six infants who developed cerebral palsy had a mean CMRgl of 18.1 μmol/min^{-1}/100 g^{-1}, compared with a mean of 41.5 μmol/min^{-1}/100 g^{-1} in infants who had no neurologic sequelae at 2 years.

Conclusions.—The measurement of CMRgl in the subacute period after perinatal asphyxia in term infants was found to be highly correlated with the severity of HIE and short-term outcome.

▶ Because hypoxic-ischemic insults as measured by blood composition and blood flow rates are transient and often quickly normalized, prediction of the extent of cerebral injury, which may take days to evolve, is difficult. Magnetic resonance spectroscopy using ^{31}P or ^{1}H may be used to evaluate brain injury in real time based on cell energetics. PET allows a second approach based on the capture of positrons, positively charged subatomic particles approximately of electron mass, a second approach to estimating localized changes in brain glucose metabolism. The method involves an indicator molecule, ^{18}FGD, which functions as a positron emitter in response to metabolism of its glucose terminus. Within an hour after injection of the tracer, 2 10-minute scans are used to sense brain positron emissions. In an effort to make quantitative estimates of glucose oxidation, blood glucose concentration, tracer dose, and time of scan are divided by a constant that corrects for the difference between tracer and actual glucose metabolism, and the integral with respect to time of concentration of tracer is calculated. These calculations require 2 additional computational devices subject to some possible introduction of error to avoid multiple infant blood sampling and to afford normalization among individual examinees. In 20 cases of presumed examples of HIE, examined at 4 to 24 days of life, severity of injury was graded clinically after the criteria of Sarnet and Sarnet.

The results showed that CMRgl was maximal in deep cerebral structures in the sensory-motor cortex surrounding the cerebral central sulcus. General metabolic activity was inversely related to clinically predicted severity after Sarnet and Sarnet, and CMRgl increased with gestational age. The degree of apparently decreased glucose metabolism activity measured in this way correlates fairly well with abnormal brain function at 2 years of life. This is a pilot study, and improvements in quantitation and sensitivity may be expected. Obstetricians should be aware of this approach and follow the evolving story, which may ultimately allow another avenue to the fine discrimination of cerebral injury after, and perhaps before, birth.

T. H. Kirschbaum, MD

Reference

1. Sarnet HB, Sarnet MS: Neonatal encephalopathy following fetal distress. *Arch Neurol* 33:696-705, 1976.

High Incidence of Respiratory Distress Syndrome (RDS) in Infants Born to Mothers With Placenta Previa

Bekku S, Mitsuda N, Ogita K, et al (Univ of Tokushima, Japan; Osaka Univ, Japan)
J Matern Fetal Med 9:110-113, 2000   10–7

Background.—Preterm infants of women with placenta previa are at high risk of respiratory distress syndrome (RDS), especially those who are born by cesarean section. A previous small study found a high rate of RDS among infants with low birth weight whose mothers had placenta previa. In this larger study, the incidence of RDS in infants born of women with or without placenta previa was retrospectively compared, and risk factors for RDS in this population were examined.

Methods.—The subjects were 99 women with placenta previa (mean age, 30.5 years) and 102 controls with preterm labor (but not placenta previa) who were matched for year of birth (mean age, 30.3 years). All women were delivered by cesarean section at 30 to 35 weeks' gestation, because of either placenta previa (in the cases) or to a previous cesarean section or a breech presentation (in the controls). Additionally, levels of cortisol, epinephrine, and norepinephrine in umbilical cord blood were measured in 11 cases and 17 controls, none of whom received antepartum corticosteroid therapy. Maternal outcomes (preeclampsia, premature rupture of membranes [PROM], histologic chorioamnionitis, and corticosteroid therapy) and neonatal outcomes (gestational age, sex, birth weight, Apgar score, neonatal asphyxia, and incidence of RDS) were compared between the 2 groups.

Results.—Compared with controls, the placenta previa group had a significantly lower incidence of preeclampsia (2% vs 14.7%), PROM (7.1% vs 17.6%), and histologic chorioamnionitis (14.1% vs 30.4%) (Table I). However, significantly more patients with placenta previa re-

TABLE 1.—Maternal Characteristics

	Placenta Previa (n = 99)	Control (n = 102)	P Value*
Maternal age (years)	30.5 ± 4.9	30.3 ± 5.2	NS
Gravidity	2.3 ± 2.0	1.7 ± 1.3	<0.05
Parity	1.2 ± 1.0	1.0 ± 0.8	<0.05
Preeclampsia (%)	2.0	14.7	<0.01
PROM (%)	7.1	17.6	<0.05
Histological chorioamnionitis (%)	14.1	30.4	<0.01
Corticosteroid therapy (%)	56.6	36.3	<0.01

Abbreviations: NS, Not significant.
Data are presented as mean ± SD or as n.
*Student *t* test, Fisher exact test, or χ^2 test.
(Courtesy of Bekku S, Mitsuda N, Ogita K, et al. High incidence of respiratory distress syndrome (RDS) in infants born to mothers with placenta previa. *J Matern Fetal Med* 9:110-113, 2000. Reprinted by permission of Wiley-Liss, Inc., a subsidiary of John Wiley & Sons, Inc.)

<table>
<tr><td colspan="4" align="center">TABLE II.—Neonatal Outcomes</td></tr>
<tr><td></td><td align="center">Placenta Previa
(n = 99)</td><td align="center">Control
(n = 102)</td><td align="center">P value*</td></tr>
<tr><td>Gestational age
(weeks)</td><td align="center">32.9 ± 1.7</td><td align="center">32.9 ± 1.7</td><td align="center">NS</td></tr>
<tr><td>Birth weight (g)</td><td align="center">2016 ± 402</td><td align="center">1892 ± 488</td><td align="center">NS</td></tr>
<tr><td>Apgar score (1 min)</td><td align="center">6.8 ± 1.8</td><td align="center">7.1 ± 1.6</td><td align="center">NS</td></tr>
<tr><td>Apgar score (5 min)</td><td align="center">8.4 ± 1.1</td><td align="center">8.7 ± 1.1</td><td align="center">NS</td></tr>
<tr><td>Gender (% male)</td><td align="center">46.5</td><td align="center">44.1</td><td align="center">NS</td></tr>
<tr><td>Low cord pH and/or
low Apgar score
(%)</td><td align="center">37.3</td><td align="center">25.4</td><td align="center">NS</td></tr>
<tr><td>RDS (%)</td><td align="center">29.3</td><td align="center">6.9</td><td align="center"><0.0001</td></tr>
</table>

Abbreviations: NS, Not significant.
Data are presented as mean ± SD or as n.
*Student *t* test.
(Courtesy of Bekku S, Mitsuda N, Ogita K, et al. High incidence of respiratory distress syndrome [RDS] in infants born to mothers with placenta previa. *J Matern Fetal Med* 9:110-113, 2000. Reprinted by permission of Wiley-Liss, Inc., a subsidiary of John Wiley & Sons, Inc.)

ceived corticosteroid therapy (56.5% vs 36.3%). The only significant between-group difference in neonatal outcomes was that infants in the placenta previa group had a significantly higher incidence of RDS (29.3% vs 6.9%) (Table II). Umbilical cord blood cortisol levels sampled from the placenta previa group were significantly lower than those sampled from the controls (median 7.3 vs 10.6 mg/dL). Epinephrine and norepinephrine levels did not differ significantly between groups.

Conclusions.—In these 2 groups of women delivered by cesarean section at 30 to 35 weeks' gestation, the incidence of RDS was 4 times higher in the infants born of mothers with placenta previa than in infants whose mothers did not have placenta previa. Furthermore, almost one third of the infants born of mothers with placenta previa had RDS, even though slightly more than half of the mothers in this group received antepartum corticosteroid therapy to accelerate fetal lung maturity. Previous studies have shown that pregnancy-induced hypertension tends to accelerate fetal lung maturation, and the women with placenta previa in this study had a significantly lower incidence of stressors (preeclampsia, PROM, and chorioamnionitis) than the controls. Furthermore, stress stimulates the secretion of cortisol by fetal adrenal glands, and umbilical cord blood cortisol levels were significantly lower in the infants in the placenta previa group. Taken together, these findings suggest that the development of RDS in infants born of women with placenta previa may be related to decreased fetal stress.

▶ This is an interesting retrospective cohort study with an unexpected conclusion that makes sense on reflection. Women undergoing abdominal birth for placenta previa at 30 to 35 weeks' gestational age after ultrasonic diagnosis were compared with a group of women delivering during the same gestational age range after the onset of preterm labor and in the presence of breech presentation and/or prior cesarean section. In that way, instances of abruption, fetal anomaly, and abnormal fetal heart rate patterns were excluded from the control group.This group was used solely to control for gestational age and the presence of placenta previa. Despite the appropriate use of acute antenatal corticoids in 56.6% of cases of previa, a larger fraction than in the control women, the incidence of RDS was 4 times higher in newborns in women with previa than in controls. The authors point to the lower incidence of pregnancy-induced hypertension and of premature rupture of membranes in patients with placenta previa, both of which are associated with evidence of an increased fetal cortisol production. The incidence of histologic chorioamnionitis was significantly less in pregnancies with previa, in which both premature rupture of membranes and prolonged labor were relatively infrequent. Because previa is an accident of implantation in which, in the absence of maternal hypotension, fetal physiology is preserved intact, it's understandable why fetal blood cortisol concentrations tend to be lower in these fetuses than in the control group. This relative lack of endogenous fetal cortisol, which might otherwise protect the fetuses against the risk of RDS, likely determines the results.

T. H. Kirschbaum, MD

Neonatal Pulmonary Hypertension: Urea-Cycle Intermediates, Nitric Oxide Production, and Carbamoyl-Phosphate Synthetase Function
Pearson DL, Dawling S, Walsh WF, et al (Vanderbilt Univ, Nashville, Tenn)
N Engl J Med 344:1832-1838, 2001   10–8

Background.—A vital component in the reduction in pulmonary vascular resistance after birth is the endogenous production of nitric oxide. A urea-cycle intermediate, arginine, is the precursor of nitric oxide. For this study, it was hypothesized that low concentrations of arginine would be found to be correlated with the presence of persistent pulmonary hypertension in newborns. It was further hypothesized that the supply of arginine would be affected by a functional polymorphism in carbamoyl-phosphate synthetase, which is known to control the rate-limiting step of the urea cycle.

Methods.—The study group comprised 65 near-term neonates in respiratory distress. Plasma concentrations of amino acids and genotypes of the carbamoyl-phosphate synthetase variants were determined in the neonates, and plasma nitric oxide metabolites were measured in a subgroup of 10 patients. The results of assessment by ECG in infants with pulmonary hypertension were compared with results in infants without pulmonary hypertension, and the frequencies of carbamoyl-phosphate synthetase genotypes in the study population were assessed for the Hardy-Weinberg equilibrium.

Results.—Infants with pulmonary hypertension had lower mean plasma concentrations of arginine and nitric oxide metabolites compared with infants without pulmonary hypertension (Fig 2). In a comparison with the general population, the infants in the study group were found to have a

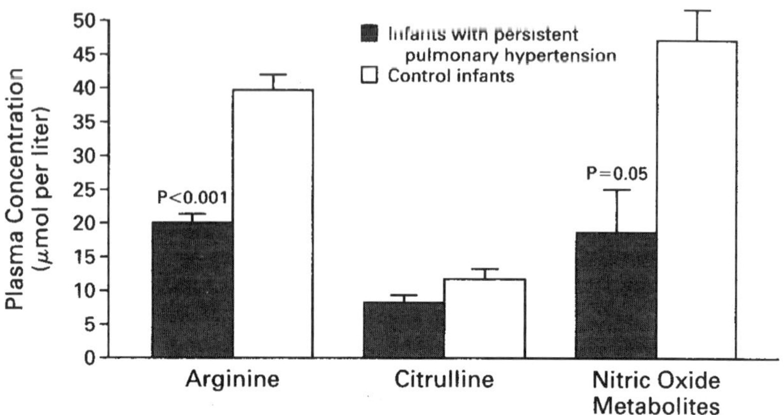

FIGURE 2.—Mean (+SE) concentrations of nitric oxide precursors and metabolites in the infants with persistent pulmonary hypertension and in the control infants. *P* values are for the comparison with the concentrations in the control group. (Courtesy of Pearson DL, Dawling S, Walsh WF, et al: Neonatal pulmonary hypertension: Urea-cycle intermediates, nitric oxide production, and carbamoyl-phosphate synthetase function. *N Engl J Med* 344:1832-1838. Copyright 2001, Massachusetts Medical Society. All rights reserved.)

significantly skewed distribution of the genotypes for the carbamoyl-phosphate synthetase variants at position 1405. None of the infants with pulmonary hypertension was found to be homozygous for the T1405N polymorphism.

Conclusions.—Low plasma concentrations of arginine and nitric oxide metabolites were present in infants with persistent pulmonary hypertension. The simultaneous presence of diminished concentrations of precursors and breakdown products suggests involvement of the inadequate production of nitric oxide in the pathogenesis of neonatal pulmonary hypertension. The preliminary observations in this study would suggest that the genetically predetermined capacity of the urea cycle may contribute to the availability of precursors for synthesis of nitric oxide.

▶ At the time of onset of neonatal air breathing, the infant normally replaces the complex fetal diffusional path for oxygen from mother's lung to placental intervillous space to placental trophoblasts with his or her own pulmonary diffusional surface and inspired air. The relatively low PO_2 of fetal life, vital to maintaining high pulmonary vascular resistance, is replaced by higher PO_2 in pulmonary artery blood, which results in pulmonary vasodilatation and ductus arteriosus closure. Endothelial nitric oxide production by pulmonary endothelium based on conversion of arginine to citrulline appears to be the final step in producing pulmonary vasodilatation. Clamping the umbilical cord raises fetal left ventricular and left atrial pressures, closing the foramen ovale; pulmonary artery PO_2 greater than 60 mm of mercury effectively closes the ductus arteriosus by inhibiting endothelial prostaglandin synthesis. However, in roughly 0.2% of cases, reduction in pulmonary vascular resistance does not occur normally. What then results is pulmonary hypertension with right-to-left shunts through the ductus arteriosus and foramen ovale, decrease in cardiac output, and hypoxemia resulting from the right-to-left shunting of the deoxygenated blood.

This group has identified a single base replacement mutation of the gene for carbamoyl-phosphate synthetase that plays a role in the production of arginine, an ultimate precursor for urea. In a series of 65 term neonates admitted on average at 36 hours of life, they found 31 with neonatal pulmonary hypertension based on low arterial PO_2 and US evidence of persistent right-to-left shunts on Doppler analysis of tricuspid valve regurgitation during systole. Infants with growth retardation, anomalous hearts, or sepsis were excluded from the study. Treatment of the infants with nitric oxide inhalation led to recovery in 30 out of 31; the remaining infant showed alveolar-capillary dysplasia, a structural and unrelated problem. Infants with neonatal pulmonary hypertension showed significantly lower concentrations of arginine and nitric oxide metabolites than did control subjects suggesting deficient arginine availability as a source for pulmonary endothelial nitric oxide production. Genetic analysis failed to show a higher incidence of the gene defect in cases than in control subjects, meaning there is likely to be more than 1 gene defect in the urea cycle that may be important in impairing neonatal nitric oxide production and regulating pulmonary artery pressure.

The importance to obstetricians is that these infants on admission bore diagnoses of perinatal asphyxia, meconium aspiration, hyaline membrane disease, and transient tachypnea of the newborn. Clearly, some of these cases result from genetically determined defects in the urea cycle necessary for optimal production of arginine and pulmonary endothelial nitric oxide. Others may be caused by the widespread use of nonsteroidal anti-inflammatory drugs which inhibit cyclooxygenases and may result in ductal obstruction in utero.[1] Certainly, it is a mistake to attribute all such problems in fetal neonatal pulmonary adjustments to obstetric management.

T. H. Kirschbaum, MD

Reference

1. Alano WA, Ngougcmc E, Ostrea EM: Analysis of nonsteroidal antiinflammatory drugs in meconium in its relationship to persistent pulmonary hypertension of the newborn. *Pediatrics* 107:519-523, 2001.

The Effectiveness of Risk-Based Intrapartum Chemoprophylaxis for the Prevention of Early-Onset Neonatal Group B Streptococcal Disease

Lin FYC, Brenner RA, Johnson YR, et al (Natl Inst of Child Health and Human Development, Bethesda, Md; Children's Hosp Med Ctr of Northern California, Oakland; Univ of Alabama, Birmingham; et al)
Am J Obstet Gynecol 184:1204-1210, 2001

10–9

Background.—Antibiotic prophylaxis has been the recommended strategy to prevent early-onset neonatal group B streptococcal infection. The retrospective case-control method was used to assess whether this approach has been successful.

TABLE 1.—Early-Onset Group B Streptococcal Disease in 6 US Academic Centers, 1992-1994: Attack Rates and Prevalence of Maternal Risk Factors Among Case Infants

Study Center	Early-Onset Disease (No.)	Total Births (No.)	Attack Rate Per 1000 Live Births	Presence of Risk Factor	
				No.	%*
Alabama	34†	15,791	2.2	21	64
California	42	27,403	1.5	29	69
Florida	27	10,513	2.6	17	63
New Jersey	17	18,557	0.9	7	41
New York	23	16,714	1.4	19	83
Texas	34‡	23,711	1.4	16	50
TOTAL	177	112,689	1.6	109	62

*Based on the number of available maternal records.
†One maternal chart was not available.
‡Two maternal charts were not available.
(Courtesy of Lin FYC, Brenner RA, Johnson YR, et al: The effectiveness of risk-based intrapartum chemoprophylaxis for the prevention of early-onset neonatal group B streptococcal disease. *Am J Obstet Gynecol* 184:1204-1210, 2001.)

Methods.—The women who received prophylaxis had 1 or more risk factors, including preterm labor, rupture of membranes, prolonged rupture of membranes (specifically over 18 hours), fever during labor, or birth of a previous child with group B streptococcal infection. Birth hospital and gestational age were used to choose case-matched controls. The effectiveness of the intrapartum prophylactic antibiotics was determined by review of medical records.

Results.—Early-onset group B streptococcal infection was found in 177 infants, for whom 174 maternal charts were available. Sixty-two percent of the affected infants were born to mothers with risk factors; only 22% of the mothers in the control group had risk factors. Attack rates ranged from 0.9 to 2.6 per 1000 live births (median 1.45:1000) (Table 1). Among the 109 affected infants, 37% were preterm, 63% had signs within 1 hour of birth, and 90% had symptoms within 12 hours. Twenty mothers of affected infants had received antibiotics; 70 of those in the control group had. Antibiotics were first given within 2 hours of delivery in 50% of the affected cases and 25% of the control cases (where this was recorded), meaning that 75% of the mothers in the control group received their first dose of antibiotics at least 2 hours before delivery, as did 50% of the mothers with affected infants (Table 3). When the effectiveness of the prophylaxis is broken down by risk factor, 72% effectiveness was found for mothers who had fever during labor, 80% for those with preterm labor or with membrane rupture at less than 37 weeks' gestation, and 90% for mothers whose membranes ruptured at least 18 hours before delivery. On the basis of a 70% prevalence of maternal risk factors when no antibiotic prophylaxis is given, the risk-based use of antibiotics could reduce the incidence of early-onset streptococcal disease by 60%.

Conclusions.—Basing the use of antibiotics prophylactically against neonatal streptococcal disease on maternal risk factors appears to be an effective strategy. The maximal preventive effect is achieved by giving the first dose of antibiotic at least 2 hours before delivery is anticipated.

TABLE 3.—Timing of First Dose of Intrapartum Antibiotics Administered to Case and Control Mothers

	Case (*n* = 109)		Control (*n* = 207)	
	No.	%	No.	%
Received any antibiotics	20	18	70	34
Received recommended regimen*	19	17	69	33
Length of time from first dose to delivery				
<2 h†	9	47	17	25
≥2 h†	9	47	50	72
Unknown	1	5	2	3
TOTAL	19	100	69	100

*Ampicillin, 2 g IV load and then 1 g IV every 4 hours until delivery, penicillin G 5 mU IV load and then 2.5 mU IV every 4 hours until delivery, erythromycin 500 mg IV every 6 hours until delivery, clindamycin 900 mg IV every 8 hours until delivery, or broad-spectrum antibiotics for amnionitis or chorioamnionitis.

†$P < 0.05$.

(Courtesy of Lin FYC, Brenner RA, Johnson YR, et al: The effectiveness of risk-based intrapartum chemoprophylaxis for the prevention of early-onset neonatal group B streptococcal disease. *Am J Obstet Gynecol* 184:1204-1210, 2001.)

▶ The history of the development of recommendations for antibiotic prophylaxis in gravidas to prevent early-onset group B streptococcal sepsis (EOGBSS) in newborn infants is complicated and colorful. In 1992, the American College of Obstetricians and Gynecologists (ACOG) recommended prophylactic antibiotics based on recognition of risk factors in parturients, specifically preterm labor, premature preterm rupture of membranes, membrane rupture more than 18 hours before delivery, maternal fever, GBS bacteruria, or a previous infant with group B streptococcal disease (see 1992 YEAR BOOK OF OBSTETRICS, GYNECOLOGY, AND WOMEN'S HEALTH, pp 32-33, and 2000 YEAR BOOK, pp 228-229). Subsequently, a conflicting set of recommendations was made by the American Academy of Pediatrics, and an attempt at conflict resolution was made in 1996 by the Centers for Communicable Disease Control (CDC). The latter recommended either the maternal risk–based approach of the ACOG or treatment given women with positive cervical vaginal cultures for GBS done at 35 to 37 weeks of gestational age. The results of implementing these recommendations have been reported (see 2001 YEAR BOOK, pp 233-236) and are excellent, documenting a nearly 90% reduction of cases of EOGBSS with implementation of the CDC guidelines.

This study is a massive retrospective case-control investigation based on 11 hospitals and 6 academic centers operating from 1992 to 1994, during which time only 1 center had an operative protocol for GBS antibiotic prophylaxis. Here the study design was to identify the 109 infants with complete records of EOGBSS and to compare the incidence of adequate antepartum antibiotic therapy among women who had risk factors in labor with 207 matched parturients with normal infants.

Of the aggregate of 112,689 deliveries, there were 111 cases of EOGBSS (an incidence of 0.16%). Among pregnancies resulting in sepsis, the incidence of preterm birth was 36%, and 62% of the parturients had 1 or more risk factors. Only 22% of the controls exhibited risk factors. Newborn signs and symptoms of EOGBSS were seen within 1 hour of birth in 63% of the cases and within 12 hours of birth in 90%. Antibiotic dosage of acceptable time and amount was seen in 17% of the women whose infants had sepsis and in 33% of the controls. The calculated effectiveness of prophylactic antibiotic therapy for women with risk factors was 86%, the same as the result of the CDC study referenced. If antibiotics were given 2 or more hours before birth, efficacy in prevention was 89%. This study makes clear the virtue of the ACOG recommendations, now nearly 10 years old, and the equivalent merits of the CDC recommendations made 5 years ago in the management of this dreaded newborn complication of pregnancy.

T. H. Kirschbaum, MD

Newborn Screening for Human Immunodeficiency Virus Infection in the Bronx, NY, and Evolving Public Health Policy

McNeeley DF, Laroche L, Bhutra S, et al (Lincoln Med and Mental Health Ctr, Bronx, NY; Cornell Univ, New York)
Am J Perinatol 16:503-507, 1999   10–10

Introduction.—Progress in the diagnosis and treatment of HIV infection is a driving force in the public understanding of HIV infection and the administration of public health law. During the past decade, New York State has moved from a policy of blind newborn screening for seroprevalence data to mandatory HIV testing as a component of the statewide Newborn Screening (NBS) Program. A new statewide program of expedited HIV testing (48-hour turn-around results) of pregnant women and newborns (whose HIV status is not known at the time of delivery) was initiated in the summer of 1999. The experience with the new NBS program from February 1, 1997, to January 31, 1999, was examined to ascertain what benefit the newly expedited testing program has for HIV-exposed/infected children.

Methods.—A retrospective review of the NBS registry for the first 24 months for which HIV testing was part of the statewide NBS program was conducted to collect data regarding total number of HIV-exposed/infected infants born, mother's HIV status at the time of delivery (if known), amount of time between blood sampling and return of test results, and medical follow-up of infants with positive test results.

Results.—There were 104 newborns with positive HIV antibody, and a polymerase chain reaction test of viral DNA verified that 13 (12.5%) were infected with HIV. Of these, 65 (62.5%) were born to mothers who were known to be infected with HIV before delivery; 39 (37.5%) were not expected. Four (30%) of the 13 HIV-infected infants were born to mothers known to be infected with HIV before delivery, and 9 (70%) were born to mothers whose HIV status was not known at the time of delivery (Table 1). Although 20% of the HIV-infected infants received follow-up care at another institution, they were not "lost" from the NBS program. The average time between collection of blood samples and receipt of results for all blood tests was 16 days (range, 10–141 days).

TABLE 1.—Newborn Screen Results: 104 HIV-Exposed/Infected (HIV Antibody-Positive) and Maternal History of HIV Infection at Delivery

	Maternal HIV Infection Known	Maternal HIV Infection Unknown
HIV Antibody-Positive N = 104	65 (62.5)*	39 (37.5)
HIV Infected (PCR-positive) N = 13	4 (30)	9 (70)

*Number in parentheses represents percentage.

(Reprinted with permission of American Journal of Perinatology from McNeeley DF, Laroche L, Bhutra S, et al: Newborn screening for human immunodeficiency virus infection in the Bronx, NY, and evolving public health policy. *Am J Perinatol* 16:503-507, 1999. Thieme Medical Publishers, Inc.)

Conclusion.—In about 40% of the newborns who acquired HIV infection from their mothers, the findings were not anticipated because of the unknown HIV status of the mothers at the time of delivery. These unanticipated HIV-infected newborns represent a missed opportunity for prevention of mother-to-child transmission of HIV infection and early therapeutic intervention for the HIV-infected infants.

▶ Because of the personal, economic, and social implications of HIV infection, the balance between the perceived need for personal concealment in contrast to the universal screening and disclosure customary in the management of most communicable diseases of this magnitude has been slow to shift toward universal screening. In the high-risk New York area, state public policy has changed over the past 20 years, and this retrospective cohort study brings us up to August 1999 to estimate the benefit from a new policy of mandatory maternal screening and universal 48-hour turn-around introduced then. The NBS program is aimed at the detection of previously unrecognized HIV-1 and hepatitis C virus (HCV) infection in infants and their mothers. The first change in the previously laissez-faire policy occurred in 1989, when blinded newborn screening was adopted primarily to protect nursing personnel from unrecognized exposure to infected infants. In 1990, reporting of HIV-positive test results to guardians, foster parents, and prospective adoptive parents was mandated for similar reasons. In 1997, mandated testing of all newborns for HIV-1 and HCV was introduced, and this report describes the results from 1997 to 1999. The diagnosis of newborn infection was based on 2 positive HIV-DNA-PCR results before the age of 15 months or a positive HIV-1 antibody by ELISA confirmed by Western blot after the age of 18 months, the time appropriate to rule out passive newborn antibody transfer.

One hundred four infants exposed to HIV-1–positive gravidas were reported with an incidence of vertical transmission of 12.5%. Of those, 70% (or 8.75% of all infants) were infected by the 3 of 8 women not known to be infected before delivery and newborn screening. It is at this population that the 24-hour turn-around diagnostic capability is aimed, allowing rapid newborn treatment. As the public health implications of the growing number of anticipated deaths from HIV-1 grow with time, mandatory infant and maternal testing can be anticipated to become increasingly widespread.

T. H. Kirschbaum, MD

Fetal and Childhood Growth and Hypertension in Adult Life

Eriksson J, Forsén T, Tuomilehto J, et al (Natl Public Health Inst, Helsinki; Univ of Southampton, England)
Hypertension 36:790-794, 2000

10–11

Objective.—Low birth weight, associated with increased blood pressure later in life, results from retarded fetal growth. There is some evidence that the effects of retarded fetal growth on later cardiovascular disease are moderated by postnatal growth. The highest rates of coronary heart disease in Finnish men occurred in those who were thin at birth but gained weight in an accelerated rate in early childhood. The relation between birth weight and later hypertension was investigated in a cohort of individuals born in Finland between 1924 and 1933.

Methods.—Among a cohort of 7086 individuals, 1958 (975 men) were treated for hypertension. Of the 471 individuals with type 2 diabetes, 250 also had hypertension. The association between hypertension and accelerated weight gain was analyzed by multivariate logistic regression.

Results.—The cumulative incidence of hypertension declined with increasing birth weight for both men and women. Children who were later diagnosed with hypertension were significantly taller and heavier than other children between the ages of 7 and 15 (Fig 1). The incidence of hypertension increased significantly with increasing maternal body mass index and with maternal age. The incidence of hypertension decreased significantly with the number of inhabitants in the home and increased significantly with social class (39.6% in the upper social class vs 29.7% in

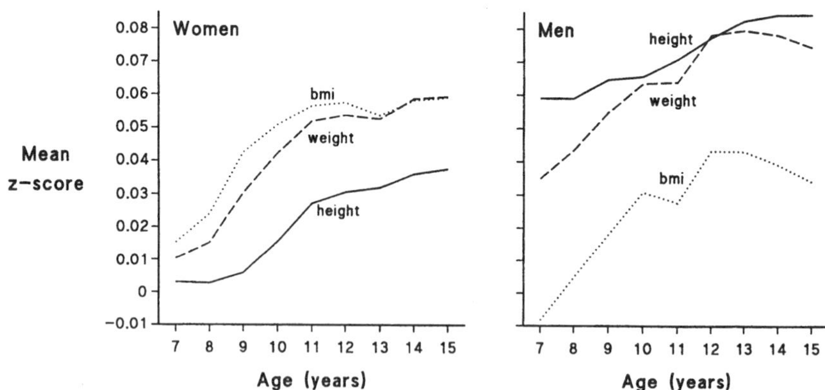

FIGURE 1.—Z scores for height, weight, and body mass index from 7 to 15 years in 975 boys and 983 girls who later had hypertension develop. Mean values for all 7086 subjects in cohort are zero. (Courtesy of Eriksson J, Forsén T, Tuomilehto J, et al: Fetal and childhood growth and hypertension in adult life. *Hypertension* 36:790-794, 2000.)

the lower social class). The incidence of hypertension with or without type 2 diabetes decreased significantly with increasing birth weight, length, and ponderal index for men and women. The incidence of hypertension and type 2 diabetes decreased with increasing placental weight. As the ratio of placental weight to birth weight rose, so did the cumulative incidence of hypertension alone. Retarded fetal growth may result in fewer cells in organs such as the kidney. Subsequent accelerated growth may place excessive metabolic demand on these limited cells.

Conclusion.—Individuals with hypertension in this cohort had reduced fetal growth and accelerated weight gain before age 7. The incidence was highest among those in the highest social strata in the least crowded homes. Those who also had type 2 diabetes had a smaller placental size and continued growth acceleration after age 7.

▶ This is one of more than 60 publications by this group published over the past 5 years in support of a hypothesis that growth retardation in term infants predisposes to hypertension and other problems in later life (see Abstracts 3–1 and 3–2). The data is epidemiologic and presented in a fairly uniform format. In this case birth records of 7086 infants born at the Helsinki Central Hospital between 1924 and 1933 were reviewed in 1971 in regard to the later life incidence of hypertension. Birth data includes weight, length, placental weight, and head circumference. It is not clear what fraction of the total number of births during this 10-year interval in Helsinki are reported or how the distribution of birth characteristics among all births corresponded with those reported here. For this reason, accession bias cannot be excluded. Socioeconomic status was estimated from birth records, not from data collected from individuals aged 38 to 47 in 1971 or subsequently. The incidence of hypertension was based not on examination in adult life but by evidence of registry in the Social Insurance Institutions' registry of partial state reimbursement for antihypertensive medication. This likely underestimates the incidence of hypertension because of uncertain ascertainment of the diagnosis in the entire population and the presence of hypertension not treated by antihypertensive medication in the 40 to 45 years of life of the study subjects. A total of 1958 individuals were found to have received support for hypertensive medications, an incidence of 27.6%. Although there was a significant inverse trend for cumulative, not discrete, hypertension by birth weight, no relation to newborn length, ponderal index, or placental weight was seen. By using school measurements of height and weight between ages of 6 to 16, Z scores were used to adjust to different means and variances in successive years, and deviations from all cases, given a reference Z score value of 0, were displayed as continuous functions of age from 7 to 15 years. No differences in growth estimated in this way were seen until ages 7 to 15 years, during which time subsequent hypertensives became taller and heavier than controls. Hypertension was unrelated to social class reflected in birth certificate data, but the incidence of hypertension was inversely related to the number of inhabitants per room at home, certainly a very crude measure of socioeconomic status.

The authors' hypothesis is that low birth weight at term followed by catch-up weight to normal beginning at 7 years with growth more rapid than average to age 15 is associated with an increased risk of hypertension. Data analysis for the incidence of diabetes in this population has been reviewed here earlier (see Abstract 1–4). It is important to recognize that the authors, because of the uncertain precision of recorded birth and infancy data, possible accession bias, and the uncertain diagnosis of hypertension make claim only to the associations among variables and not to proof of relation among them; their language reflects this. For instance, "the associations" between low birth weight and hypertension are described, short body length and thinness "may reflect the effects of fetal under nutrition." "One may speculate" that timing of malnutrition during gestation may be important and rapid increase in height and weight is associated with hypertension in later life. Remember this is a hypothesis frequently defended by its proponents but utterly lacking in objective controlled observations in its support.

T. H. Kirschbaum, MD

Birth Weight and 24-Hour Ambulatory Blood Pressure in Nonproteinuric Hypertensive Pregnancy

Waugh J, Perry IJ, Halligan AWF, et al (Univ of Leicester, England; Univ College Cork, Ireland)
Am J Obstet Gynecol 183:633-637, 2000   10–12

Background.—According to the Barker intrauterine programming hypothesis, a higher birth weight is linked to the development of hypertension and other cardiovascular conditions later in life. However, this relation may be influenced by the mother's blood pressure during pregnancy. Maternal blood pressure is inversely related to birth weight in normotensive nulliparous women. The relation between maternal blood pressure (as measured by 24-hour ambulatory monitoring) during pregnancy and birth weight among pregnant women with hypertension but not preeclampsia was prospectively studied.

Methods.—The subjects were 234 pregnant women (mean age 29.9 years) with a singleton pregnancy at more than 20 weeks' gestation. All patients had hypertension during their pregnancy ($\geq$140/90 mm Hg), but none had significant proteinuria (24-hour total urinary protein concentration >0.3 g or 2 consecutive urine dipstick readings $\geq$1+). Each patient participated in 1 ambulatory blood pressure monitoring session, during which blood pressure was measured every 30 minutes for 24 hours. Differences in predicted birth weights (as determined from published sources) were plotted as a function of ambulatory blood pressure measurements. Analyses of the relation between birth weight and maternal blood pressure were adjusted for gestational age and sex.

Results.—Mean blood pressures were 129.8/82.1 mm Hg during the daytime (10 AM-8 PM) and 116.5/68.3 mm Hg during the nighttime (12 AM-6 AM). Univariate analyses revealed significant inverse associations

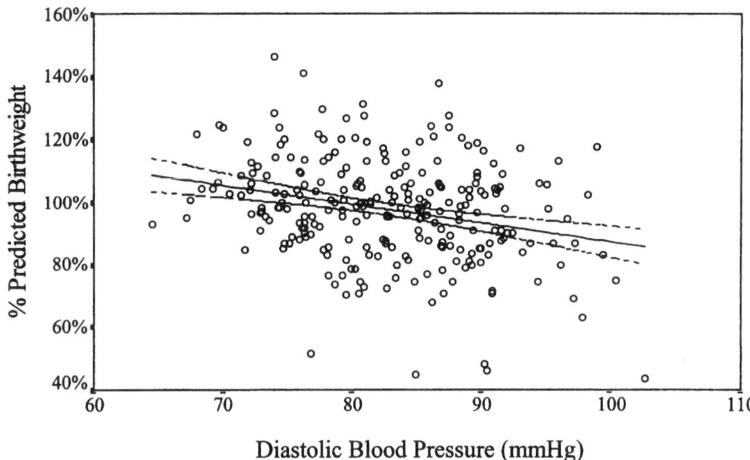

FIGURE 1.—Scatter plot and regression line (*solid line*) with 95% confidence interval (*dashed lines*) for relation between percentage of predicted birth weight and daytime ambulatory diastolic blood pressure monitor measurement (gradient ± SE, –0.6 ± 1.14; $P < .001$). (Courtesy of Waugh J, Perry IJ, Halligan AWF, et al: Birth weight and 24-hour ambulatory blood pressure in nonproteinuric hypertensive pregnancy. *Am J Obstet Gynecol* 183:633-637, 2000.)

between birth weight and ambulatory systolic and diastolic blood pressure measurements. The magnitude of the association was greater with diastolic pressures than with systolic pressures. Multivariate analysis indicated that the daytime diastolic ambulatory blood pressure measurement was the strongest predictor of birth weight (Fig 1). For each 5-mm Hg increase in daytime mean ambulatory diastolic blood pressure, there was a 67.5-g decrease in birth weight.

Conclusions.—Even after data adjustment for gestational age at delivery, sex, gestational age at referral, and the mother's weight, age, smoking status, and parity, there was a significant inverse association between daytime mean ambulatory diastolic blood pressure and birth weight in these hypertensive, nonproteinuric pregnancies. These data provide further support that maternal blood pressure confounds the relation between birth weight and the development of cardiovascular disease in adult life and should be accounted for in investigations of the Barker hypothesis.

▶ This study raises the possibility that familial hypertension may be a confounding variable in the relation between low birth weight and later life development of hypertension and related cardiovascular disease—the Barker hypothesis (see Yearbook 2002, Abstract 4–5). The authors studied 234 hypertensive nulliparous women excluding those known to have prepregnancy hypertension, multiple pregnancies, or receiving antihypertensive therapy. Women past 20 weeks' gestational age without albuminuria were also rejected from the study, sharply reducing but not entirely eliminating those with preeclampsia. Gravidas were examined periodically by auscultatory methods, and each wore an automated 24-hour recording blood pressure monitor for a single day. Blood pressure values were adjusted for gestational age and infant sex and deviations from anticipated normal blood pressures, similarly adjusted, were calculated with data published by Oxford University investigators.[1] When deviations from normal birth weight were plotted as a function of recorded diastolic blood pressure, what resulted was a statistically significant inverse linear correlation. What this means is that women with neither pregnancy induced hypertension nor diagnosable chronic renovascular hypertension tend to produce small infants to the extent that their diastolic blood pressures are higher than average on 24-hour surveillance. Their infants are likely recipients of whatever genetic predisposition their mothers possess. It is this genetic complement, not in utero adaptation to impaired nutrition as Barker posits, that tends to increase their later life development of hypertensive cardiovascular disease. The authors propose that both maternal nutrition and maternal blood pressure need to be considered simultaneously as data on in utero adaptation in relation to later life disease are developed and evaluated.

T. H. Kirschbaum, MD

Reference

1. Yudkin PL, Aboualfa M, Eyre JA, et al: Newborn birth weight and head circumference percentiles for gestational ages 24-42 weeks. *Early Hum Devel* 15:45, 1987.

Antenatal Magnesium Sulphate Exposure Is Associated With Prolonged Parathyroid Hormone Suppression in Preterm Neonates
Rantonen T, Kääpä P, Jalonen J, et al (Univ of Turku, Finland)
Acta Paediatr 90:278-281, 2001   10–13

Background.—To prevent seizures in women with preeclampsia and inhibit premature uterine contractions, women are given magnesium sulfate ($MgSO_4$). Infants born to these mothers have transient hypermagnesemia for the first few days of life. This can be potentiated in distressed premature infants, and it can cause neonatal respiratory depression, generalized lethargy, and muscle hypotonia from the ages of 1 to 3 days, with possible long-term consequences (increased infant mortality and bone mineral disturbances). This study evaluated neonatal mineral status for up to 2 weeks after birth among those infants exposed to $MgSO_4$ antenatally.

Methods.—Eight exposed and 27 control infants born prematurely (33 weeks' gestation or less) constituted the study population. Mothers had received an initial infusion of 5 g of $MgSO_4$, and then continued on doses of 1 to 2 g/hour, with a mean total infusion time of 44 hours and a mean interval between the end of the infusion and delivery of 1 hour. Samples of cord blood and capillary blood were obtained from the infants at the ages of 3, 7, and 14 days and were analyzed for total magnesium, calcium, phosphorus, and parathyroid hormone (PTH). Urine samples were similarly analyzed.

Results.—During the first week of life, serum and urinary magnesium concentrations increased in both control and exposed infants, with a significantly higher concentration noted in those exposed to magnesium antenatally. In both groups, the serum calcium concentration fell transiently at 3 days and serum phosphorus at 7 days. Urinary levels of both magnesium and calcium were increased over the first 3 days of life in exposed infants, and phosphorus level was decreased throughout the 14 days. PTH in exposed infants was significantly decreased, falling below detection levels by 2 weeks. PTH in controls at 3 days was significantly higher than in cord blood samples but fell and was maintained over the rest of the 2-week period. Cord/peripheral serum magnesium levels had a significant correlation with urinary magnesium levels throughout the 2-week period in both groups.

Conclusions.—The use of maternal MgSO$_4$ therapy produces neonatal hypermagnesemia early in the infant's life along with a high level of both magnesium and calcium in the urine and blunted production of PTH. Thus it is prudent to monitor the use of such therapy.

▶ The usual large doses of magnesium sulfate for tocolysis and seizure suppression in pregnancy-induced hypertension inevitably expose the fetus and often the neonate to periods of hypermagnesemia. The potential for newborn hypotonia, respiratory depression, and altered calcium and phosphorous metabolism exists, but they appear uncommonly except in preterm infants in whom immature renal function might delay excretion of the surplus magnesium load. This study of 35 infants born at or before 33 weeks' gestational age, with a mean birth weight of 1352 grams, shows the changes in newborn blood and urine throughout the first 2 weeks of life.

Cord blood and first urine samples showed the elevated serum magnesium and urine magnesium excretion that one might predict. Serum calcium concentration is normal, but the urinary calcium level is significantly increased, probably associated with and likely caused by significantly depressed serum para-hormome concentration. The depression in PTH becomes more apparent over the first week of life because the normal increase in parathyroid hormone in early neonatal life is not seen in specimens from magnesium-exposed infants. The low concentration of parathyroid hormone in magnesium-treated infants appears to play a role in inhibiting urinary calcium excretion to allow the relatively low early neonatal serum calcium concentrations to return to normal by 7 days of life. The lesson here is that PTH is suppressed for several days by exposure of pregnant women to magnesium, an important factor in increasing the risk of hypocalcemic tetany and seizures to which premature infants are predisposed.

T. H. Kirschbaum, MD

In Utero Remodeling of the Fetal Lamb Ductus Arteriosus: The Role of Antenatal Indomethacin and Avascular Zone Thickness on Vasa Vasorum Proliferation, Neointima Formation, and Cell Death

Clyman RI, Chen YQ, Chemtob S, et al (Univ of California, San Francisco; McGill Univ, Montreal)

Circulation 103:1806-1812, 2001

10–14

Background.—Preterm newborn infants whose mothers are given indomethacin just before birth have a higher rate of patent ductus arteriosus (PDA) after delivery that is resistant to indomethacin therapy given postnatally. Why this should be so is not yet clear. One hypothesis is that the constriction in utero resulting from exposure to indomethacin increases the thickness of the avascular zone of the ductus arteriosus. This enhanced thickness progressively increases vascular endothelial growth factor (VEGF) expression, increases nitric oxide (NO) production, and leads to the loss of medial smooth muscle cells. These changes then impair the ductus arteriosus' ability to contract. The validity of this hypothesis was evaluated.

Methods.—Fetal lambs were infused with indomethacin over 48 hours to constrict the ductus arteriosus and increase the thickness of the ductus' avascular zone. Tissue samples were tested by Western blot analysis for endothelial nitric oxide synthase (eNOS) and VEGF, and immunohistochemical and contraction studies were run.

Results.—The duct was patent 24 hours after the beginning of infusions. Of the 8 indomethacin-infused fetuses, marked constriction was seen in 5, moderate constriction in 2, and wide patency in 1. The control ducts were all patent. After 48 hours of infusion, the partial pressure of oxygen in arterial blood (PaO$_2$) was essentially equal in the 2 groups, but the pressure gradient was 14 mm Hg in infused animals and 2 mm Hg in control animals. Thickness of the avascular zone related directly to the degree of constriction of the ductus arteriosus. More VEGF was expressed by fetuses having the indomethacin infusion than by control animals. This increased expression correlated with the avascular zone's thickness, with a progressive increase in VEGF expression by the muscle media when the avascular zone exceeded 500 µm. Associated with the increased VEGF expression was an increased number of vasa vasorum and a resulting increase in eNOS. Indomethacin-infused animals formed neointima in 10 of 13 cases, whereas a neointima developed in only 1 control fetuses. By 24 hours after the infusions were stopped, the pressure gradient had returned to control values in fetuses with moderate constriction, but in those with marked constriction it did not fall below 6 mm Hg. Prostaglandin production by the indomethacin-exposed ductus arteriosus returned to control values by 24 hours after infusion. With moderate constriction the production of NO was increased, inhibiting contractility in the ductus. With marked constriction, tissue distensibility and contractile capacity were inhibited.

Conclusions.—Once the ductus arteriosus has been exposed to indomethacin in utero, it becomes resistant to postnatal therapy with this agent. Thus, the patency of the ductus arteriosus is no longer under the primary control of prostaglandins at this point.

▶ The fetal ductus arteriosus, together with shunting in the right atrium, allows the 2 ventricles to function in parallel, largely bypassing the high-resistance pulmonary circuit and allowing the fetus's cardiac output to reflect the sum of the outputs of both ventricles. With lung expansion and ductal closure, cardiac output decreases to equal the lesser of the 2 ventricular outputs, with the ventricles now arranged in series through the pulmonary circulation. At this point, the neonatal pulmonary circuit has become a low-resistance structure by virtue of the increase in pulmonary artery partial pressure of oxygen (PO_2), which functions to inhibit ductus endothelial prostaglandin production. Ductal patency depends on low blood PO_2 and extensive ductal endothelial prostaglandin production. Indomethacin given to gravidas as a tocolytic infuses the ductus and, by inhibiting prostaglandin synthetase, causes the ductus arteriosus to constrict. Since pulmonary blood PO_2 is not increased, cardiac output decreases in the face of increasing resistance, reflected in decreased fetal glomerular filtration rate, amniotic fluid volume, and decreased mesenteric and cerebral blood flow. The authors site a meta-analysis of 6 publications demonstrating that newborns exposed to indomethacin as fetuses have an increased incidence of neonatal patent ductus arteriosus requiring surgical ligation because of refractoriness to indomethacin given to neonates.[1] In a well-documented study in fetal lambs at 0.9 term, the authors demonstrate that changes in the ductus arteriosus in such newborns exposed in utero to indomethacin reflect the same changes seen with spontaneous ductus arteriosus closure in newborns.

In 8 fetal lambs, infusion of 0.2 mg/K/hour of indomethacin produced ductal closure to less than 50% of normal volume in all but 1 case. This resulted in increased pressure gradient across the ductus from 2 to 14 mm of mercury after 48 hours of infusion. Constriction increased ductal wall thickness from a mean of 1.05 mm to 1.23 mm and increased the avascular region, which relies on diffusion from endothelial surfaces and deep vasa vasora, from 0.50 to 0.68 mm. Within that expanded zone, ischemia stimulates VEGF production, cell apoptosis and fibroplasia, and the development of neointima in the narrowed ductus. Because of increased shear stress due to vasoconstriction and increased ductus arteriosus blood velocity, eNOS is produced in increasing amounts (see Abstract 4–10). In 10 of 13 cases, ductus arteriosus segments retained in vitro rigidity and lack of compliance for at least 24 hours after exposure to indomethacin, as a result of the restructuring of the vessel's media layer and increased NO synthetase. The results nicely explain the complications in neonatal patent ductus arteriosus dynamics that follow indomethacin tocolysis, an additional reason to avoid its use in that role.

T. H. Kirschbaum, MD

Reference

1. Karunasiri M, Nasbaum H, Pinhero J: Tocolysis with indomethacin is associated with patent ductus arteriosus refractory to therapy. *Pediatr Res* 39:221A, 1996.

A Prospective Study of Smoking During Pregnancy and SIDS

Wisborg K, Kesmodel U, Henriksen TB, et al (Aarhus Univ, Denmark)
Arch Dis Child Fetal Neonatal Ed 83:203-206, 2000   10–15

Background.—Numerous case-control and registry-based studies indicate a strong association between maternal smoking and sudden infant death syndrome (SIDS). Nonetheless, the former type of study can be plagued by recall bias, and the latter type may not control for all possible confounders. A large, prospective 7-year study that controlled for obstetric, sociodemographic, and lifestyle factors to examine the independent association between smoking and SIDS in Denmark was performed.

Methods.—Data were collected from 24,986 Danish mothers who delivered a single, live-born child between September 1989 and August 1996. Subjects completed 3 questionnaires while pregnant, the first 2 before the first antenatal visit at 16 weeks' gestation, and the last 1 before the visit at 30 weeks' gestation. The first questionnaire (100% completion rate) gathered information on medical and obstetric history, maternal age, smoking habits before and during pregnancy, and alcohol intake during pregnancy. The second questionnaire (74% completion rate) gathered information on marital status, education, employment status during pregnancy, and caffeine intake during pregnancy. Women who reported smoking 1 or more cigarettes/day on either of the first 2 surveys were classified as smokers; the remainder were considered nonsmokers. The third questionnaire (66% completion rate) focused on smoking habits during pregnancy. Information regarding an infant's death during the first year of life was gathered from national registries, and case records were reviewed to confirm the cause of death.

Results.—The 17,536 nonsmokers (70%) included 2642 women (15%) who had stopped smoking during the first trimester. Of the 7450 women who smoked during pregnancy (70%), 44% smoked 1 to 9 cigarettes/day and 56% smoked 10 or more cigarettes/day. Of the 24,986 live births, 20 infants died of SIDS during their first year of life, for an overall rate of 0.80 per 1000 live births. Of these 20 infants, 12 had mothers who smoked during pregnancy. In crude analyses, compared with infants of nonsmokers, infants of smokers had more than 3 times the risk of SIDS. Risk was not affected by data adjustment for parity, alcohol, or caffeine intake during pregnancy, maternal height or weight before pregnancy, education, employment status during pregnancy, marital status, or the number of antenatal visits. However, data adjustment for mother's age had a slight effect in reducing the strength of the association between smoking and SIDS (adjusted odds ratio [OR], 3.5). Furthermore, the risk of SIDS increased significantly as the number of cigarettes smoked per day increased (adjusted OR 3.4 for 1 to 9 cigarettes/day, 3.7 for 10 or more cigarettes/day). Further data adjustment for birth weight (which was an average of 323 g less in children who died of SIDS than in survivors) and gestational age at birth also slightly reduced the strength of the association between smoking and SIDS (adjusted OR 2.9).

Conclusions.—The results of this large, prospective study, which accounted for possible confounders, are clear: Infants whose mothers smoke during pregnancy have 3 times the risk of SIDS compared with infants whose mothers do not smoke while pregnant. Furthermore, the risk of SIDS increases as the number of cigarettes per day increases. Note that these data may underrepresent the true association between smoking and SIDS because 15% of the mothers classified as nonsmokers smoked before pregnancy but quit during the first trimester. The authors estimate that 30% to 40% of deaths from SIDS could be avoided if mothers stopped smoking during pregnancy.

▶ The presumption that maternal smoking increases the risk of SIDS is based on case-controlled studies, which are prone to accession bias because the presence of SIDS tends to increase recall of smoking data. This large prospective study conducted from 1989 to 1996 provided detailed questionnaire data on maternal health and habits including smoking, alcohol and coffee intake, as well as demographic status of parturients. The prospective data collection was designed to allow evaluation of confounding relations between smoking and SIDS, an important deficiency in earlier case-controlled studies. In an experience based on roughly 25,000 live births, 30% of them of women who smoked, the incidence of SIDS was more than 3 times higher among smoking mothers than among nonsmokers, and the risk ratios among smokers were proportional to the number of cigarettes smoked per unit of time. Logistic regression analysis was used to correct for differences in maternal height and weight, education, marital status, number of prenatal visits, and alcohol and caffeine use between smokers and nonsmokers. This is an important step in proving the role of maternal smoking in increasing the incidence of SIDS independent of other related maternal variables and not influenced by fetal positioning.

T. H. Kirschbaum, MD

Neonatal Withdrawal Syndrome After In Utero Exposure to Selective Serotonin Reuptake Inhibitors

Nordeng H, Lindemann R, Perminov KV, et al (Univ of Oslo, Norway; Ullevål Univ, Oslo, Norway; Central Hosp of Akershus, Nordbyhagen, Norway)
Acta Paediatr 90:288-291, 2001   10–16

Background.—Cases of mild to moderate depression are generally treated with selective serotonin reuptake inhibitors (SSRIs). Women who are pregnant may experience such depression and may be taking these agents, but no major anomalies have been associated. However, use of SSRIs during the third trimester may be a factor in a pattern of symptoms detected in infants exposed in utero. These symptoms appear to constitute a neonatal withdrawal syndrome, occurring when the infants are abruptly removed from exposure at birth. Five case reports of infants with this withdrawal syndrome were reviewed.

> *Case Reports.*—All 5 infants were initially breast-fed, although 1 had to be tube-fed after the age of 5 days. Daily scoring by using the National Abstinence Score (NAS), with a score over 4 indicating withdrawal symptoms and a score over 8 indicating withdrawal symptoms requiring medical attention, was performed. The SSRIs being used by the mothers were paroxetine (10 to 40 mg, cases 1 to 3), citalopram (30 mg, case 4), and fluoxetine (20 mg, case 5). Four of the infants (cases 1, 2, 3 and 5) were born at term with weights of 3300 to 4230 g and good Apgar scores. The preterm infant (case 4) weighed 860 g and was born at 27 weeks' gestation. Apgar scores were 9/9 at 1 and 5 minutes for this boy. NAS values were above 8 in cases 1 to 4, and symptoms were marked. NAS values were 4 to 6 in case 5, in which the symptoms were light, consisting of increased tonus of the extremities and neck and jitteriness.

Results.—Infants exhibited symptoms of irritability, constant crying, shivering, increased tonus, eating and sleeping difficulties, and convulsions during the first few days of life. These lingered for up to a month postnatally. Chlorpromazine was required for treatment in 4 of the 5 infants; the infant in case 4 was given phenobarbital for 1 week while the diagnosis was uncertain.

Conclusions.—Physicians should be advised that neonatal withdrawal syndrome can occur with third-trimester use of SSRIs by the mother. The symptoms resolved over time, but it is important to follow up infants exposed in utero to SSRIs and to watch for the development of this withdrawal syndrome.

▶ These authors provide a series of 5 case reports of newborns exhibiting what appear to be withdrawal symptoms after delivery from women using SSRIs, presumably for symptoms of anxiety and depression. The newborns exhibited irritability, agitation, tremors, frequent crying, tachypnea, hypertonus, and disturbances in feeding and sleeping. The diagnosis was structured around the Neonatal Abstinence Score and confirmed by response to time and the use of such agents as chlorpromazine and phenobarbital. In this era when psychotropic agents are used so freely, neonatal withdrawal syndrome is something to look for as you follow up your patients' newborns.

T. H. Kirschbaum, MD

GYNECOLOGY

11 Gynecologic Urology

Tension-Free Vaginal Tape for Primary Genuine Stress Incontinence: A Two-Centre Follow-Up Study
Moran PA, Ward KL, Johnson D, et al (Northampton Gen Hosp, England; Royal Victoria Infirmary, Newcastle Upon Tyne, England)
BJU Internatl 86:39-42, 2000   11–1

Background.—The tension-free vaginal tape (TVT) procedure is a new treatment for genuine stress incontinence (GSI). This procedure involves implantation, under local anesthesia, of polypropylene (Prolene) tape around the mid-urethra. Initial experience has been very promising. The use of the TVT procedure, outcome, and potential complications are discussed.

Methods.—The study group consisted of 40 women, aged 33 to 86 years, with primary GSI refractory to conservative therapy. None had previous continence surgery. All patients had dual-channel subtracted cystometry with uroflowmetry. All patients were treated with the TVT procedure. Catheters were not routinely inserted. The women were followed up for 6 to 24 months after the TVT procedure with subjective symptom analysis, repeat cystometry and uroflowmetry, a 1-hour pad test, and complication assessment.

Findings.—The average operative duration was 42 minutes, and 93% of patients resumed spontaneous voiding immediately afterwards without any catheterization. The mean inpatient stay was overnight. Subjectively, more than 97% of women considered themselves cured or significantly improved. GSI was objectively cured in 95% of women who received the TVT procedure. Symptomatic detrusor instability was detected in 15% of women in the study group and voiding dysfunction in 5%. No healing problems or tape rejections were noted.

Conclusions.—After approximately 1-year of follow-up, the tension-free vaginal tape procedure appears to be safe and effective for the treatment of genuine stress incontinence in women. Longer-term follow-up studies and those that compare TVT with the Burch procedure are awaited to further validate this method.

A Comparison of Bladder Neck Movement and Elevation After Tension-Free Vaginal Tape and Colposuspension

Atherton MJ, Stanton SL (St George's Hosp, London)
Br J Obstet Gynaecol 107:1366-1370, 2000

11–2

Background.—The tension-free vaginal tape (TVT) procedure is a new treatment for genuine stress incontinence (GSI) that supports the mid-urethra. Treatment with TVT was compared colposuspension by using transperineal US to determine the effect on bladder neck position and mobility.

Methods.—The study group consisted of 30 consecutive British women who had either TVT (n = 17) or colposuspension (n = 13) for primary GSI between March 1998 and June 1999. Treatment assignment was not randomized overall during the study. Before treatment, patients had clinical and urodynamic assessment by cystometry, uroflowmetry, urethral pressure profilometry, and transperineal US of the bladder neck. These tests were repeated 3 to 4 weeks after surgery. Bladder neck elevation, angle, and movement were the main outcomes.

Findings.—After both TVT and Burch procedures, the bladder neck angles at rest and valsalva were more acute than before the procedures. Postoperative linear movement on valsalva was less than pre-operative movement. After the Burch procedure only, postoperative rotational movement on valsalva was significantly less. Angles and movement were significantly less postoperatively, and the resting bladder neck position was significantly higher after the Burch procedure compared with TVT.

Conclusions.—Both TVT and the Burch colposuspension decrease bladder neck angles at rest and valsalva, reduce linear movement on valsalva, and elevate the bladder neck, but TVT causes significantly less profound changes than the Burch procedure. This suggests that the continence mechanism of the TVT procedure is more likely dependent on mid-urethral support and is less dependent on bladder neck change than the colposuspension procedure.

▶ TVT has taken Europe by storm over the past 5 years since its first description by Ulmsten et al in 1996.[1] Performed primarily by gynecologic surgeons, TVT is becoming increasingly popular in North American centers also. The report from Northampton and Newcastle Upon Tyne in the United Kingdom by Moran et al is fairly typical of outcomes reported thus far. The obvious attractions of the procedure include (1) its performance under local anesthesia, so that its effects can be assessed intraoperatively; (2) rapid recovery; (3) early return of voiding function; and (4) cure rates comparable to the more complicated Burch colposuspension. The report by Atherton and Stanton documents that there is significantly less bladder neck elevation and more bladder neck movement postoperatively after a TVT than after a Burch, supporting TVT's unique mode of action at the mid urethra. Despite occasional poorly documented allusions to catastrophic vascular injuries and an appreciable intraoperative bladder perforation rate with few sequelae when detected before the plastic sheaths are removed, and despite infrequent nerve injuries, the acute safety of the procedure seems acceptable and is comparable with other continence procedures. Those of us who have not yet taken the plunge still await documented long-term efficacy from well-designed surgical outcomes studies and long-term follow-up, proving that this prolene tape can avoid the chronic erosion problems that have plagued every other synthetic material inserted vaginally for prolapse or incontinence.

R. C. Bump, MD

Reference

1. Ulmsten U. Henriksson L, Johnson P, et al: An ambulatory surgical procedure under local anaesthesia for treatment of female urinary incontinence. *Int Urogynecol J Pelvic Floor Dysfunct* 7:81-86, 1996.

Cadaveric Versus Autologous Fascia Lata for the Pubovaginal Sling: Surgical Outcome and Patient Satisfaction
Brown SL, Govier FE (Virginia Mason Med Ctr, Seattle)
J Urol 164:1633-1637, 2000   11–3

Objective.—Each of the various materials used to perform the pubovaginal sling procedure has advantages and disadvantages. Cadaver fascia lata should offer many of the same benefits as autologous fascia, without the drawbacks associated with intraoperative harvesting. An initial study with cadaver fascia lata for the pubovaginal sling procedure was discussed, including a comparison of cadaver fascia with autologous fascia.

Methods.—The study included 121 consecutive patients from 1997 to 1999 (group 1) who underwent a pubovaginal sling procedure and were operated on using cadaver fascia lata. The results were compared with those of 46 consecutive women from 1994 to 1997 (group 2) undergoing a pubovaginal sling procedure using autologous fascia lata. Mean follow-ups were 12 and 44 months, respectively. A detailed survey was mailed to all patients at follow-up.

Results.—The questionnaire response rate was 86% in the cadaver fascia group and 65% in the autologous fascia group. In the cadaver fascia group, 85% of patients said they were cured of stress incontinence. Eighty-three percent reported improvement in urinary control, and 74% said they had minimal or no leakage. The women remained catheterized for a median of 9 days. Eighty-nine percent said they were satisfied with the results of the cadaver fascia sling procedure, and 83% said they would recommend it to other patients.

In the autologous fascia group, 90% of patients said they were cured of stress incontinence. Ninety percent reported improved urinary control, and 73% reported minimal or no leakage. The median catheterization was 14 days. Patient satisfaction and recommendation rates were similar to those in the cadaver fascia groups.

Conclusions.—The use of cadaver fascia lata for the pubovaginal sling procedure was effective and met with a high degree of patient satisfaction.

▶ This article has many of the shortcomings typical of the continence surgical literature. It is a retrospective cohort study that tries to compare 2 surgical procedures that were not performed contemporaneously or randomly. The follow-up interval was, by definition, not equal, and follow-up was via a nonvalidated questionnaire with no objective testing or examination. Fourteen percent of subjects in group 1 and 35% in group 2 did not respond to the survey. Finally, the groups are not comparable, because there were different indications for a sling in the 2 groups, leading to a 1.2 per month procedure rate for the early group and a 4.2 per month procedure rate for group 1. The authors claim that the results for the 2 procedures were comparable, but no attempt is made to account for the many confounders.

As sling procedures have become more widely advocated, a large number of variations of technique have been developed for a variety of medical, economic, and commercial reasons. Some of these (eg, certain synthetic sling materials and bone-anchoring techniques) have resulted in significant complication rates and have been abandoned or withdrawn from the market after brief and often geographically localized popularity.[1-3] In an effort to avoid the added operative time and discomfort associated with harvest of autologous rectus fascia or fascia lata and the complications associated with synthetic materials, the use of donor fascia lata has become increasingly popular with both gynecologic and urologic surgeons. While the ability to obtain biologic sling materials from tissue banks has expanded the ease of performing sling procedures, there is some evidence that success rates with donor fascia (50%-75%)[4] may fall substantially below those generally attributed to procedures using autologous harvested slings (89%-95%).[5,6] Failures with donor materials have been attributed both to graft autolysis[4] and suture pull through when less than full-length slings are employed.[7] A recent report on donor slings concluded that a prospective randomized comparison of autologous and donor slings is needed.[8]

R. C. Bump, MD

References

1. Bent AE, Ostergard DR, Swick-Zaffuto M: Tissue reaction to expanded polytetrafluoroethylene suburethral sling for urinary incontinence: Clinical and histologic study. *Am J Obstet Gynecol* 169:1198-1204, 1993.
2. Leach GE, Kobashi CK, Mee SL, et al: Erosion of woven polyester synthetic ("Protegen") pubovaginal sling. *J Urol* 161:106A, 1999.
3. Bologan RA, Gordon DA, Trager SL, et al: Osseous complications with pubic bone anchors post urethral sling surgery. *J Urol* 161:202A, 1999.
4. Fitzgerald MP, Mollenhauer J, Bitterman P, et al: Functional failure of fascia lata allografts. *Am J Obstet Gynecol* 181:1339-1346, 1999.
5. Urinary Incontinence Guideline Panel. *Urinary Incontinence in Adults: Clinical Practice Guideline*, AHCPR Pub. No. 92-0038. Rockville, MD: Agency for Health Care Policy and Research, Public Health and Human Services. 1992, pp 1-11.

6. Urinary Incontinence Guideline Panel. *Urinary Incontinence in Adults: Acute and Chronic Management*, AHCPR Pub. No. 96-0682. Rockville, MD: Agency for Health Care Policy and Research, Public Health and Human Services. 16:51-52, 1996.
7. Chaikin DC. Blaivas JG: Weakened cadaveric fascial sling: An unexpected cause of failure. *J Urol* 160:2151-2152, 1998.
8. Amundsen CL, Visco AG, Ruiz H, et al: Outcome in 104 pubovaginal slings using freeze dried allograft fascia lata from a single tissue bank. *Urology* 56:2S-8S, 2000.

Comparison of Biomechanical Properties of Periosteal Suture Fixation and Bone Anchor Fixation to the Pubic Bone

Winters JC, Fontenot C, Glowacki C, et al (Louisiana State Univ, New Orleans)

Urology 55:866-870, 2000

11–4

Background.—Surgery for stress urinary incontinence aims to establish urethral support and prevent urethral descent during Valsalva maneuvers. The strength of fixation using bone anchors (BAs) was compared with that of direct suture placement in the periosteum.

Methods.—The anterior bony pelves from 21 female cadavers were used. Bone anchor suture fixation was done with Conch anchors on 1 side of each pubic bone, and direct periosteal suture fixation (PSF) was done on the contralateral side. No. 1 polyproprolene sutures were used in all specimens.

Findings.—Among the BA-fixed pelves, the failure modes were 11 pull-out, 1 midsuture failure, and 9 sutures cut by BA. Among the PSF pelves, failure modes were 6 suture pull-outs through the bone, 14 midsuture failures, and 1 suture cut at the bone. Compared with BA pelves, PSF pelves required significantly greater loads to induce failure. In many specimens, both PSF and BA were adequate fixation points. The major mechanism of failure was suture rupture. Among pelves with suture failure, the load required to induce failure was significantly greater in the PSF than in the BA group. When the suture failed, PSF was the better procedure, because BA fixation broke some sutures.

Conclusions.—In this study, biomechanical testing showed that BA suture fixation was not superior to PSF fixation. Because BAs induced suture failure in many cases, PSF appears to be the better procedure.

▶ Bone anchors seem to be gadgets looking vainly for an application in continence and pelvic reconstructive surgery. Surgeons have recommended the use of anchors to secure the pubic bone point of fixation for slings and urethropexies and the sacral point of fixation for sacral colpopexies. The basic premise for anchor use is that anchors provide stronger points of fixation, a premise challenged by the findings of this article. The specific anchors used were not stronger and predisposed to easier suture failure than the direct placement of sutures. Any surgeon familiar with the security of a well-placed suture through Cooper's ligament or the anterior longitudinal sacral ligament has a hard time appreciating any added advantage of an anchor. Most suspensory failures are related more to the tensile strength of the tissues being suspended than to a deficiency in the integrity of the site of fixation. Finally, the devastating complication of osteomyelitis observed on occasion with bone anchors is yet another reason to temper enthusiasm for their use in a clean but contaminated operative field.

R. C. Bump, MD

Burch Procedure Compared With Sling for Stress Urinary Incontinence: A Decision Analysis

Weber AM, Walters MD (Cleveland Clinic Found, Ohio)
Obstet Gynecol 96:867-873, 2000   11–5

Background.—There is no consensus on the best surgical treatment for women with genuine stress incontinence (GSI) and urethral hypermobility, although it is generally accepted that anterior repairs and needle suspension procedures are less effective than Burch retropubic colposuspensions and sling procedures. The relative risks and benefits of Burch and sling procedures for primary genuine stress incontinence with urethral hypermobility in women were explored with the use of a decision analytic model.

Methods.—The decision analytic model was developed by defining a population of women with GSI and urethral hypermobility for whom surgery was planned. Burch colposuspension or sling procedure outcomes were estimated. This model included a second set of treatments and outcomes for women who were not initially cured. The main outcome was treatment effectiveness, that is, cure of incontinence, persistent stress incontinence, incontinence caused by de novo detrusor instability, and permanent urinary retention. Secondary treatments included repeat surgery, collagen injection, medical treatment, and urethrolysis. Risks and benefits were estimated from published literature. One-way sensitivity analyses were conducted to estimate the effect of varying each characteristic through its range.

Findings.—The overall cost and effectiveness of Burch and sling procedures were similar. One-way sensitivity analysis indicated that the Burch procedure was more effective when the risk of retention after sling was higher than 9.0% or when the risk of de novo detrusor instability after sling was greater than 10.3% (Fig 2). Conversely, if the risk of de novo detrusor instability after Burch was greater than 6.8%, the sling procedure was more effective. Therefore, efficacy was influenced by the relative risks of complications.

Conclusions.—Decision analysis indicates that the retropubic Burch colposuspension and sling procedures are equally effective for primary surgical treatment of women with genuine stress incontinence, although relative effectiveness is strongly influenced by the risk of complications. Until data from randomized, controlled clinical trials are available, this

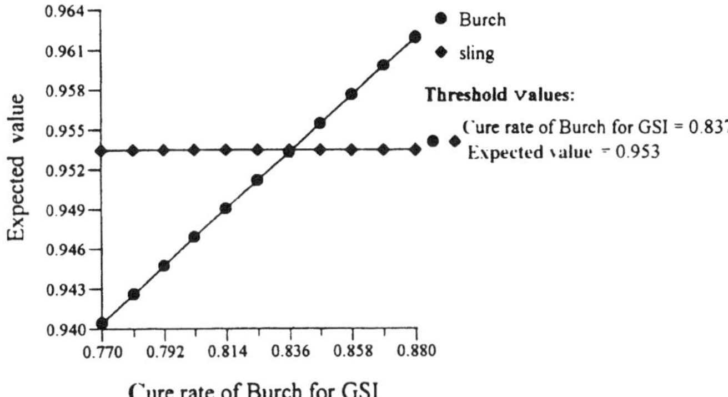

FIGURE 2.—One-way sensitivity analysis demonstrating the threshold value of 83.7% (*dashed line*) for the estimated probability of cure after Burch colposuspension for genuine stress incontinence (GSI). If the cure rate after Burch was lower than 83.7%, the overall effectiveness (cure rate of incontinence after initial and secondary treatments [expected value]) of the sling procedure arm of the model was higher than that of the Burch arm of the model. Conversely, if the cure rate after Burch was higher than 83.7%, the effectiveness of Burch was higher. The overall effectiveness of the Burch and sling arms of the model was equivalent when the cure rate after Burch equaled 83.7%. (Courtesy of Weber Am, Walters MD: Burch procedure compared with sling for stress urinary incontinence: A decision analysis. Reprinted with permission from The American College of Obstetricians and Gynecologists *Obstetrics and Gynecology*, 2000, 96, 867-873.)

decision analysis may prove useful in assisting individual physicians and their patients in the decision process for treatment for GSI.

▶ Besides being a very thoughtful analysis of a contemporary topic of hot debate, this article can serve as a well-crafted primer on decision analytic methods for the practicing clinician. A large number of procedures have been developed to correct GSI, most of which have not been evaluated using contemporary standards for outcomes analysis. The 1996 update of the Agency for Health Care Policy and Research (AHCPR) Urinary Incontinence Clinical Practice Guidelines concluded that the surgical literature is deficient in standards "for describing the patient population, the type of incontinence, the methods for accurate diagnosis, the techniques of the surgical procedure, or the outcome in different domains."[1] These conclusions are substantiated by a comprehensive systematic review by Black and Downs[2] in which the authors document the poor methodologic quality of the stress incontinence surgical literature. They note that methodologic flaws make determinations speculative, both about the effectiveness of any surgery and about the relative effectiveness of different procedures for stress incontinence. They conclude that "recommendations as to the best clinical practice cannot be based on scientific evidence." The major methodologic flaws identified by Black and Downs included (1) variability in or a complete lack of case definition for stress incontinence; (2) failure to control for confounding by random assignment or to account for known confounders by reporting their distribution; (3) a lack of standardization of surgical technique; (4) variability in duration of follow-up; (5) low or indeterminate external validity (generalizability); (6) inadequate power to detect clinically important differences; (7)

a lack of comprehensive assessment of postoperative complications; and (8) marked variability in outcome assessment.

In spite of the limitations of the surgical literature reviewed, Black and Downs[2] did make the following speculative conclusions based on their review: (1) Colposuspension appears to be more effective than anterior colporrhaphy in curing and improving stress incontinence with about 85% of women being continent 1 year after colposuspension compared with 50% to 70% after anterior colporrhaphy. (2) Colposuspension appears to be more effective than needle suspension in curing and improving stress incontinence with about 85% of women continent 1 year after the former compared with 50% to 70% for the latter. The benefit of colposuspension seems to be maintained for at least 5 years, whereas the benefits of needle suspensions seem to diminish quite rapidly. (3) There is no convincing evidence that there is any difference in the effectiveness of colposuspension and sling procedures. All 4 underpowered prospective and 11 of 12 retrospective reports showed no difference in the effectiveness of slings and colposuspension. Only the study by Iosif[3] showed a difference, with the proportion cured following 135 colposuspensions (95%; 95% CI, 91%-98%) being significantly higher than the proportion cured following 164 slings (79%; 95% CI, 72%-85%).

The lack of scientifically valid studies has not prevented several generations of gynecologic and urologic surgeons from forming strong opinions, largely unencumbered by data, about the best surgical procedure for GSI associated with bladder neck hypermobility. Currently gynecologists, disappointed with unacceptably high failure and recurrence rates for anterior colporrhaphy, have gravitated toward retropubic suspension procedures applying the "gold standard" label to the Burch colposuspension. In contrast, urologists, disenchanted with high recurrence rates with various needle suspensions, recently have declared their allegiance in growing numbers to the sling as their gold standard.

The analysis by Weber and Walters concludes with two important recommendations: (1) Individual surgeons can best counsel their patients on the preferred surgical procedure based on a knowledge of their individual cure and complication rates. Implicit in this recommendation is that individual surgeons actually track these rates in a comprehensive manner. (2) Randomized controlled trials comparing Burch and sling procedures should be performed. The latter is the basis of a long-overdue protocol being sponsored in the NIH Urinary Incontinence Treatment Network.

R. C. Bump, MD

References

1. Urinary Incontinence Guideline Panel. *Urinary Incontinence in Adults: Acute and Chronic Management*, AHCPR Pub. No. 96-0682, Rockville, MD, Agency for Health Care Policy and Research, Public Health and Human Services. 1996 pp 51-52.
2. Black NA, Downs SH: The effectiveness of surgery for stress incontinence in women: A systematic review. *Br J Urol* 78:497-510, 1996.

3. Iosif CS: Results of various operations for urinary stress incontinence. *Arch Gynecol* 233:93-100, 1983.

Resolution of Urge Symptoms Following Sling Cystourethropexy
Schrepferman CG, Griebling TL, Nygaard IE, et al (Univ of Iowa, Iowa City; Univ of Kansas, Kansas City)
J Urol 164:1628-1631, 2000   11–6

Background.—The urge component of mixed incontinence is often bothersome for patients and frequently reduces quality of life. Although most women who undergo continence procedures such as sling cystourethropexy find that their urge symptoms resolve, some do not experience change or may even have worsened urge symptoms. The predictive power of preoperative video urodynamics was analyzed retrospectively to determine the likelihood that sling cystourethropexy will resolve urgency symptoms.

Methods.—From 1992 to 1997, a total of 84 women underwent pubovaginal sling cystourethropexy. Surgery was performed on candidates because of stress-related leakage of urine, urethral hypermobility, low abdominal leak point pressure measurements (less than 100 cm H_2O pressure), bladder necks that remained open at rest, and patient preference. Fourteen patients were eliminated from the study because they did not exhibit urge symptoms. The 70 remaining cases were divided into 2 categories: (1) sensory urge (subjective urge without detrusor instability), and (2) motor urge (subjective urge with detrusor instability). The motor urge group was subdivided into 2 further categories: (1) high-pressure (detrusor contractions > 15-cm H_2O pressure) and (2) low-pressure (detrusor contractions < 15-cm H_2O pressure). One patient died of myocardial infarction 5 days after surgery and was thus excluded from data analysis. Surgeons used either fascia lata and rectus fascia chosen by preference. Cadaver fascia or vaginal wall were not used. Urge symptom data was gathered postoperatively and was given one of the following 4 classifications: resolved, improved, unchanged, or worsened. Other follow-up data included use of medication, continence status, catheterization duration, and rates of complications.

Results.—Of 69 patients, 41 (59%) were found to have motor urge. Sensory urge was diagnosed in 28 (41%). Complete resolution of urge after surgery was found in 24 (58.5%) of the motor urge group and 11 (39.3%) of the sensory urge group. Improved urge was found in 7 (17.1%) motor urge patients and 9 (32.1%) sensory urge patients. A statistically significant difference in rate of resolution was observed between the two groups ($P < .05$). Within the motor urge group, complete resolution was observed in 21 (91.3%) of the 23 low-pressure patients but in only 5 (27.8%) of the 18 high-pressure patients. Improved urge was found in 2 (8.7%) of the low-pressure group and 5 (27.8%) of the high-pressure group. The difference between the 2 groups was significant ($P < .05$).

Conclusions.—A large number of women experienced complete resolution of urge after surgical treatment of incontinence. Reliable ways to predict those women who will experience complete resolution have not yet been established, but the findings suggest that urodynamic parameters can be used to predict postoperative urge resolution. Those with motor urges are more likely to have postoperative resolution. Also, within the motor group, those with low-pressure (<15-cm H_2O pressure) showed greater than 90% resolution while more than two thirds of the higher-pressure group exhibited residual urgency. Resolution rates for the 3 groups were high-pressure motor urge, 28%; low-pressure motor urge, 91%; and sensory urge, 39%.

▶ The condition of mixed incontinence, genuine stress incontinence (GSI), and detrusor instability (DI) in the same patient, has long been the subject of therapeutic controversy. Some experts advocate first treating the instability component pharmacologically and/or behaviorally, reserving operative management for those patients who have persistent bothersome stress incontinence after the urge component is controlled.[1] Others argue that many women with mixed incontinence have genuine stress incontinence (GSI) as their primary problem and that the DI results secondarily. They advocate primary operative correction of bladder neck support, reserving pharmacologic and/or behavioral therapy for those who have persistent urge incontinence after surgery.[2,3] The article by Schrepferman et al addresses this challenging clinical situation and includes women with both GSI and overactive bladder symptoms due either to DI or sensory urgency. The authors note that women with sensory urgency or high pressure DI are significantly less likely to have resolution of their urge symptoms than are women with low pressure DI. This observation may be useful clinically, but the authors' theory that urine forced into the urethra due to a stress incompetent bladder neck stimulates the detrusor contraction is probably not true. In a study from the laboratory at Duke University,[4] urethral perfusion stimulated DI only in women with DI but did not identify any patient with DI who was not diagnosed with standard urodynamics. No woman with GSI had DI induced by urethral perfusion. Based on the results of that study, it appears that some conscious women, just as some anesthetized animals, will exhibit detrusor activity in response to perfusion of fluid through the urethra. This response seems to be primarily the result of failure of voluntary cortical suppression of the micturition reflex, a failure that is felt to be the primary pathophysiologic basis for idiopathic DI in women. Conversely, most women with normal functioning of cerebral-brain stem loop, with or without an incompetent bladder neck, will not experience a detrusor contraction in response to urethral perfusion. While some women will experience resolution of urge symptoms following continence surgery, it is also true that some will develop de novo DI following such surgery. This latter effect seems often to be related to overcorrection of bladder neck support.[5] To date, there are no foolproof preoperative explanations for either of these outcomes.

R. C. Bump, MD

References

1. Karram MM, Bhatia N: Management of coexistent stress and urge urinary incontinence. *Obstet Gynecol* 26:250-256, 1989.
2. McGuire E J, Lytton B, Kohorn El, et al: The value of urodynamic testing in stress urinary incontinence. *J Urol* 124:256-258, 1980.
3. McGuire E J, Savastano JA: Stress incontinence and detrusor instability/urge incontinence. *Neurourol Urodyn* 4:313-316, 1985.
4. Bump, RC: The urethrodetrusor facilitative reflex in women: Results of urethral perfusion studies. *Am J Obstet Gynecol* 182:794-804, 2000.
5. Bump RC, and the Continence Program for Women Research Group. Understanding urinary tract function in women soon after bladder neck surgery. *Neurourol Urodyn* 18:629-637, 1999.

Intraoperative Cystoscopy in Conjunction With Anti-incontinence Surgery

Tulikangas PK, Weber AM, Larive AB, et al (Cleveland Clinic Found, Ohio)
Obstet Gynecol 95:794-796, 2000   11–7

Background.—Many surgeons perform cystoscopies after high-risk procedures to evaluate ureteral patency and to search for bladder injury. At the Cleveland Clinic, it is routinely done after anti-incontinence surgery. The frequency of bladder and ureteral injuries, as detected by cystoscopy, sustained during continence surgery was analyzed.

Methods.—The charts of 351 women undergoing continence surgery and routine intraoperative cystoscopy between 1995 and 1998 were re-

TABLE 2.—Procedures Performed

Incontinence procedures ($n = 347$)	
Laparoscopic Burch colposuspension	48 (14)
Open Burch colposuspension	138 (40)
Pubovaginal sling	161 (46)
Hysterectomy ($n = 110$)	
Abdominal	14 (13)
Vaginal	95 (86)
Laparoscopic	1 (1)
Culdeplasty ($n = 208$)	
Abdominal	24 (12)
Vaginal	173 (83)
Laparoscopic	11 (5)
Anterior colporrhaphy	168 (48)
Posterior colporrhaphy	233 (67)
Vaginal apex suspension ($n = 147$)	
Abdominal sacral colpopexy	12 (8)
Ileococcygeus fascia suspension	129 (88)
Laparoscopic sacral colpopexy	6 (4)
Paravaginal defect repair ($n = 48$)	
Abdominal	42 (88)
Laparoscopic	6 (13)

viewed (Table 2). Four records were incomplete, and these patients were excluded from further analysis.

Findings.—Nine injuries occurred in 347 patients, for an incidence of 2.6%. Four cystotomies occurring during laparoscopic Burch procedures were detected before cystoscopy was performed. The remaining 5 injuries were found at cystoscopy. Four injuries occurred during 161 pubovaginal sling procedures, for a 2.5% incidence. In 1 woman, cystoscopy enabled detection of sutures in the bladder from a previous procedure. No previously unrecognized injuries were detected by cystoscopy in a total of 186 Burch procedures.

Conclusions.—In the current series, the rate of injury to the lower urinary tract during continence surgery was 2.6%. All injuries occurring during Burch procedures were caught before cystoscopy.

▶ The worst lower urinary tract operative injury is the one that is unrecognized before the patient leaves the operating room. Increasingly, pelvic surgeons include a surveillance cystoscopy using intravenous indigo carmine dye at the conclusion of complex pelvic surgery, including many continence and prolapse procedures. The authors of this article confirmed a low unsuspected injury rate (1.5%) detected only by cystoscopy, all after pubovaginal sling procedures. No unsuspected injuries were found after Burch colposuspension. Despite this low yield, the authors defend routine cystoscopy because of the low morbidity of the procedure and because injuries detected and repaired at the time of the primary surgery result in less morbidity than those with delayed detection and repair. The majority of ureteral injuries occur with "simple" hysterectomy.[1] Using a decision analysis model from the hospital perspective, Taber et al[2] demonstrated that the cost-effectiveness of routine cystoscopy with hysterectomy is most dependent on the rate of ureteral injury. An injury rate of 2% rendered universal cystoscopy more cost-effective than no cystoscopy in a model that included no patient indirect costs or costs related to litigation.[2] Intravenous indigo carmine is the contrast agent of choice for visualization of ureteral spill, which should be observed bilaterally and equally within 10 minutes of injection. Observation of ureteral spill is facilitated by the instillation of 150 mL of 10% glucose into the bladder before cystoscopy.[3] The increased density of this solution compared with the urine allows the blue urine to rise from the ureteral orifices through the 10% glucose. Thus, pooling of the dyed urine over the trigone is avoided and independent assessment of each ureter is quite easy. A 70-degree cystoscope is optimal to visualize the trigone if there is any degree of bladder neck elevation; otherwise, a 30-degree cystoscope suffices.

R. C. Bump

References

1. Symmonds RE: Ureteral injuries associated with gynecologic surgery: Prevention and management. *Clin Obstet Gynecol* 19:623-643, 1976.

2. Taber K, Visco A, Weidner A, et al: Cost-effectiveness analysis of universal cystoscopy at the time of hysterectomy. *Int Urogynecol J & Pelvic Floor Dysfunct* 10(S2):S22, 1999.
3. Lin BL, Iwata Y: A modified cystoscopy to evaluate unilateral traumatic injury of the ureter during pelvic surgery. *Am J Obstet Gynecol* 162:1343-1344, 1990.

Suprapubic Bladder Drainage After Extraperitoneal Cystotomy
Karram M, Partoll L, Miklos J, et al (Univ of Cincinnati, Ohio)
Obstet Gynecol 96:234-236, 2000   11–8

Background.—Urinary tract injuries are not uncommon in obstetric and gynecologic surgery. Mismanagement of urinary tract injuries can cause significant morbidity for the patient. During abdominal operations, intentional cystotomy can be used for intravesical evaluation. Bladder drainage was retrospectively analyzed after 84 extraperitoneal cystotomy repairs to make recommendations on this use of this procedure and the length of continuous bladder drainage required afterwards.

Methods.—The study group consisted of 78 women with retropubic urethropexies and 6 women with retropubic paravaginal repairs. Intentional cystotomies were performed intraoperatively to ensure ureteral patency and bladder integrity and to detect any suture penetrations. All cystotomies were closed in 2 layers. Suprapubic catheters were placed intraoperatively. As soon as urine was clear, voiding trials were initiated. Catheters were removed when there was spontaneous voiding of at least 80% of total bladder volume. Women were followed up for 3 months after surgery.

Findings.—Voiding trials were begun on the first postoperative day for the majority of the women. Suprapubic catheters were discontinued an average of 4 days after surgery. Neither short- nor long-term complications were observed during the 3-month follow-up period.

Conclusions.—The bladders of women who had intentional extraperitoneal cystotomy during abdominal surgery to assess the status of their urinary tract healed rapidly and well, without adverse effects. Continuous bladder drainage was not required for more than 24 hours in the majority of these women, and catheters were removed an average of 4 days after surgery. These findings should allow surgeons to be more liberal in their use of intraoperative cystotomies when urinary tract status needs to be evaluated.

▶ Surgical injury to the lower urinary tract is described with virtually every continence procedure. Such injuries have been described with 3% to 6% of Burch colposuspensions.[1,2] The risk of injury can be minimized but not eliminated with experience and attention to the details of the technique. More importantly, the risk of unrecognized injury can be virtually eliminated with careful assessment of the integrity of the lower urinary tract during and after the performance of the procedure. As the authors of this article emphasize, it is the injury that is not recognized and managed before leaving the operating room that is the most dangerous for the patient. It is also the injury that is most likely to lead to litigation.

The performance of a controlled, high extraperitoneal cystotomy during abdominal retropubic procedures is an excellent technique to avoid more serious bladder, ureteral, or urethral injuries. Certainly, such a cystotomy is invaluable as the initial step in repeat retropubic procedures, in which significant scarring is often encountered. Karram and his coathors point out what most experienced pelvic surgeons already know; that is, such an extraperitoneal cystotomy will heal without complication and without prolonged catheter drainage. What is discouraging is that many young graduates of our residency programs have never performed and repaired such an intentional cystotomy, and when quizzed about the safest site for an intentional cystotomy, they will select the intraperitoneal dome of the bladder. Clearly, this is a technique that needs to be emphasized more to our gynecologic surgeons in training.

R. C. Bump, MD

References

1. Pow-Sang JM, Lockhart JL, Suarez A, et al: Female urinary incontinence: preoperative selection, surgical complications and results. *J Urol* 136:831-833, 1986.
2. van Geelen JM, Theeuwes GM, Eskes TKAB, et al: The clinical and urodynamic effects of anterior vaginal repair and Burch colposuspension. *Am J Obstet Gynecol* 159:137-144, 1988.

Obstetric Risk Factors for Stress Urinary Incontinence: A Population-Based Study
Persson J, Wølner-Hanssen P, Rydhstroem H (Univ Hosp, Lund, Sweden)
Obstet Gynecol 96:440-445, 2000   11–9

Objective.—The causative factors of stress urinary incontinence remain unclear, although trauma to the pelvic floor during childbirth may be an important contributor. Swedish national registry data were used to assess obstetric and maternal risk factors of stress urinary incontinence.

Methods.—Through the Hospital Discharge Registry, the investigators identified 10,074 women born between 1932 and 1977 who underwent surgery for stress urinary incontinence between 1987 and 1996. Cross-linkage to the Medical Birth Registry provided information on obstetric history for 4634 women with a history of operation for stress urinary incontinence who gave birth in 1973 or after. Information on total number of children was obtained from the Fertility Registry (Table 1). Statistical analyses were performed to identify obstetric and maternal risk factors for stress urinary incontinence and their associated odds ratios.

Results.—Risk factors for incontinence surgery included parity, (Table 2), birth weight, diabetes mellitus, body mass index, age at first delivery, and epidural anesthesia. Factors showing a negative association with incontinence surgery included cesarean section, forceps or vacuum extrac-

TABLE 1.—Maternal Characteristics

	Study Population	Total population
	n	*n*
Maternal age (y)		
≤19	146	74,459
20-24	598	334,156
25-29	755	357,123
30-34	329	117,206
35-39	107	29,430
40-44	7	4273
≥45	0	121
Number of births		
1	336	251,027
2	949	412,984
3	499	164,102
4	113	37,639
≥5	46	11,016
Any multiple birth		
No	1892	861,460
Yes	50	15,308

Note: Data from Swedish-born women who delivered their first child between 1973 and 1995, and women undergoing surgery for stress incontinence between 1987 and 1996 using the same criteria. Year of birth and maternal age refer to first birth.

(Reprinted with permission from The American College of Obstetrics and Gynecologists courtesy of Persson J, Wølner-Hanssen P, Rydhstroem H: Obstetric risk factors for stress urinary incontinence: A population-based study. *Obstet Gynecol* 96:440-445, 2000.)

tion, and episiotomy. Education, multiple births, age at last delivery, maternal smoking, large perineal tears, and breech presentations had no effect on incontinence risk. Elective cesarean section reduced the risk of incontinence surgery to a similar extent for nulliparous and uniparous women—the odds ratio associated with vaginal delivery was 4.76. The risk associated with vaginal delivery increased with the birth weight of the woman's largest infant.

Conclusions.—Vaginal delivery appears to be a significant risk factor for subsequent operation for stress urinary incontinence. This relationship is

TABLE 2.—Odds Ratios for Later Incontinence Surgery According to Parity

No. of Children	OR	95% CI
0	1.0	—
1	3.57	3.13, 4.00
2	5.26	4.76, 5.88
3	6.67	5.88, 7.14
≥4	7.14	6.67, 8.33
All parous women	5.56	5.00, 6.25

Note: Stratification for women's year of birth. Nulliparous women are used as reference. Calculations irrespective of mode of delivery.

Abbreviation: OR, Odds ratio.

(Reprinted with permission from The American College of Obstetrics and Gynecologists courtesy of Persson J, Wølner-Hanssen P, Rydhstroem H: Obstetric risk factors for stress urinary incontinence: A population-based study. *Obstet Gynecol* 96:440-445, 2000.)

strongest for initial births, and is significantly modified by various maternal factors and intrapartum interventions. Pregnancy itself is not a risk factor.

A Community-Based Epidemiological Survey of Female Urinary Incontinence: The Norwegian EPINCONT Study
Hannestad YS, Rortveit G, Sandvik H, et al (Univ of Bergen, Norway)
J Clin Epidemiol 53:1150-1157, 2000
11–10

Purpose.—Reported estimates of the prevalence of urinary incontinence vary significantly, depending on the definition, sample selection criteria, and survey methods used. The Epidemiology of Incontinence in the County of Nord-Trøndelag (EPINCONT) study was designed to estimate the prevalence of incontinence in an unselected population of Norwegian women.

Methods.—The study was based on a larger survey of more than 94,000 adult residents of a Norwegian county, performed in 1995-1997. Of 34,755 community-dwelling women, nearly 28,000 (a response rate of 80%) provided information on the prevalence and severity of urinary incontinence. Specifically, the women were asked whether they experienced involuntary urine loss. If they answered yes, they were asked additional questions about the frequency, volume, and duration of the leakage; associated events and urge to void; and how much of a problem it was.

Results.—Involuntary urine loss was reported by 25% of women, with a peak prevalence of 30% for women aged 50 to 54 years (Fig 1). About half of affected women had stress incontinence only, one third had mixed incontinence, and one tenth had urge incontinence only. Incontinence was rated severe in 17% of the stress group, 38% of the mixed group, and 28% of the urge group. Two thirds of women rated their incontinence as no problem to a minor nuisance, and one tenth as a major problem. Overall, incontinence was considered significant in 7% of the study population (Fig 3). The problem was reported bothersome by 24% of women with stress incontinence, 47% with mixed incontinence, and 36% with urge incontinence. Overall, 26% of the women had sought medical advice for incontinence, including 54% of those with severe incontinence, and 64% of those bothered by incontinence.

Conclusions.—These findings underscore the high prevalence of urinary incontinence. One fourth of Norwegian women report some involuntary urine loss, while 7% appear to have "significant" incontinence. This group should be regarded as potential patients, and those for whom incontinence is less problematic should receive education and self-care advice.

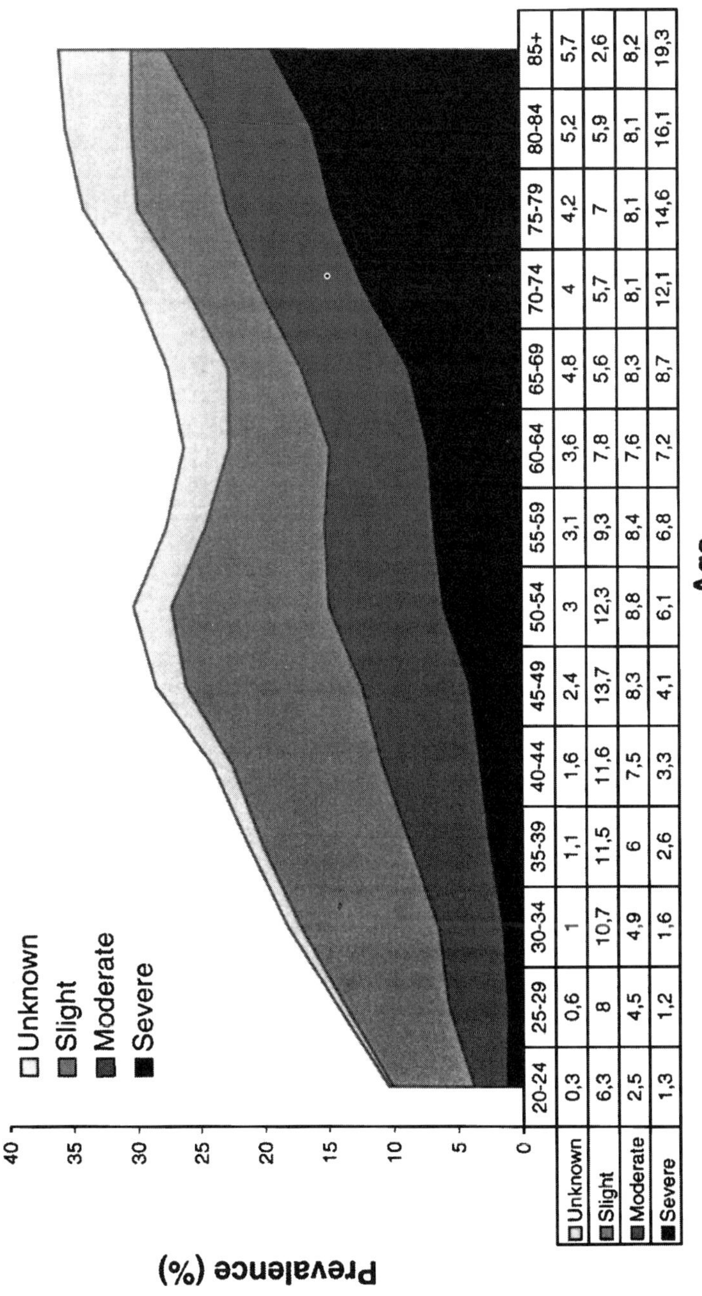

	20-24	25-29	30-34	35-39	40-44	45-49	50-54	55-59	60-64	65-69	70-74	75-79	80-84	85+
Unknown	0,3	0,6	1	1,1	1,6	2,4	3	3,1	3,6	4,8	4	4,2	5,2	5,7
Slight	6,3	8	10,7	11,5	11,6	13,7	12,3	9,3	7,8	5,6	5,7	7	5,9	2,6
Moderate	2,5	4,5	4,9	6	7,5	8,3	8,8	8,4	7,6	8,3	8,1	8,1	8,1	8,2
Severe	1,3	1,2	1,6	2,6	3,3	4,1	6,1	6,8	7,2	8,7	12,1	14,6	16,1	19,3

FIGURE 1.—Prevalence of urinary incontinence by age group and severity. (Courtesy of Hannestad YS, Rortveit G, Sandvik H, et al: A community-based epidemiological survey of female urinary incontinence: The Norwegian EPINCONT Study. *J Clin Epidemiol 53*:1150-1157. Copyright 2000, with permission from Elsevier Science.)

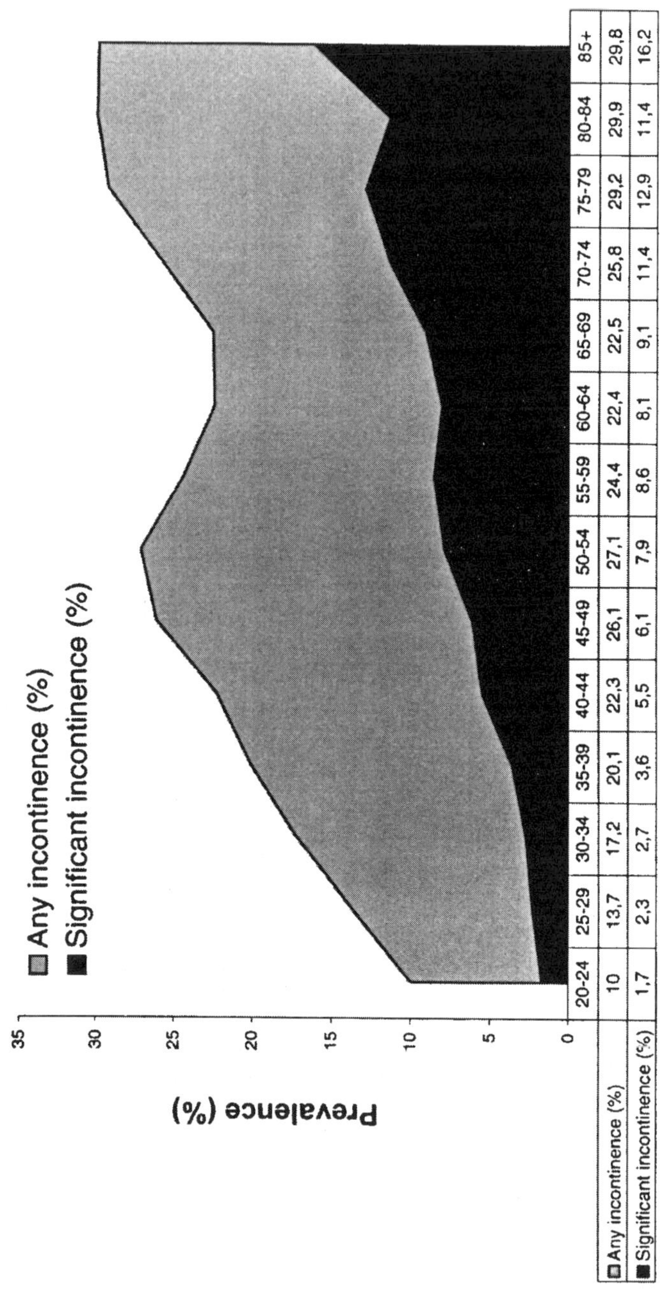

	20-24	25-29	30-34	35-39	40-44	45-49	50-54	55-59	60-64	65-69	70-74	75-79	80-84	85+
Any incontinence (%)	10	13,7	17,2	20,1	22,3	26,1	27,1	24,4	22,4	22,5	25,8	29,2	29,9	29,8
Significant incontinence (%)	1,7	2,3	2,7	3,6	5,5	6,1	7,9	8,6	8,1	9,1	11,4	12,9	11,4	16,2

FIGURE 3.—Prevalence of any (n = 6170) and significant (n = 1832) incontinence by age group (women with incomplete data on significance were excluded). (Courtesy of Hannestad YS, Rortveit G, Sandvik H, et al: A community-based epidemiological survey of female urinary incontinence: The Norwegian EPINCONT Study. *J Clin Epidemiol* 53:1150-1157. Copyright 2000, with permission from Elsevier Science.)

Risk Factors for Lower Urinary Tract Symptoms in Women 40 to 60 Years of Age

Møller LA, Lose G, Jørgensen T (Univ of Copenhagen)
Obstet Gynecol 96:446-451, 2000   11–11

Background.—Menopause is among the many interrelated variables proposed as risk factors for urinary incontinence and other lower urinary tract symptoms. Potential risk factors for lower urinary tract symptoms in women aged 40 to 60 years were evaluated.

Methods.—The population-based study included 502 Danish women aged 40 to 60 years who reported lower urinary tract symptoms more than once weekly in response to a questionnaire. Along with 742 asymptomatic control subjects, the women completed an additional questionnaire regarding possible associated factors including a wide range of obstetric and other medical variables.

Results.—Response rates were 97% for the symptomatic women and 76% for the control group (Table 1). Factors associated with stress incontinence included parity, odds ratio (OR) 2.2 for primiparas, 3.9 for para 2, and 4.5 for para 3; diuretic use, OR 2.2; and hysterectomy, OR 2.4.

TABLE 1.—Demographic Data

Characteristic	Cases	Controls	$P*$
History of high physical activity	275 (66.7)	381 (73.1)	0.034
BMI >25 kg/m^2	238 (48.9)	170 (30.1)	<.001
Abortion (one or more)	219 (46.0)	211 (37.7)	0.007
Parity (one or more)	454 (94.4)	494 (88.1)	0.001
Fetal weight >4000 g	92 (21.0)	99 (20.6)	0.875
History of episiotomy	275 (64.0)	321 (67.7)	0.332
Lesion of the anal sphincter	13 (3.4)	14 (3.0)	0.732
Repair of uterine prolapse	20 (4.2)	8 (1.5)	0.008
Cystocele repair	27 (5.6)	2 (0.4)	<.001
Hysterectomy	101 (21.4)	56 (10.1)	<.001
Constipation	144 (29.6)	110 (19.6)	0.002
Straining at stool	272 (56.8)	217 (40.1)	<.001
Hormonal inactivity	141 (29.6)	169 (30.3)	0.799
Use of diuretics	55 (11.3)	24 (4.3)	<.001
Cystitis treated with antibiotics	7 (1.4)	1 (0.2)	<.001†
Medication for noninfectious urinary symptoms	4 (0.8)	0 (0.0)	<.001†
County			
Copenhagen	239 (49.1)	263 (46.6)	0.280
Storstrøm	248 (50.9)	301 (53.4)	
Age (y):			
40	77 (15.8)	151 (26.8)	0.001
45	100 (20.5)	107 (19.0)	
50	99 (20.3)	117 (20.8)	
55	108 (22.2)	103 (18.3)	
60	103 (21.2)	86 (15.3)	

Note: Data are given as n (percentage).
*χ^2 test with 1 degree of freedom.
†Fisher exact test.
Abbreviation: BMI, Body mass index.
(Reprinted with permission from The American College of Obstetricians and Gynecologists courtesy of Møller LA, Lose G, Jørgensen T: Risk factors for lower urinary tract symptoms in women 40 to 60 years of age. *Obstet Gynecol* 96:446-451, 2000.)

Factors associated with urge incontinence were diuretic use, OR 4.0, and body mass index (BMI). Urgency was also associated with parity, OR 1.9 for primiparas, 3.0 for para 2, and 3.1 for para 3; diuretic use, OR 2.7; and body mass index. In general, women who reported straining at stool and constipation had more lower urinary tract symptoms. Anal sphincter lesions, episiotomy, fetal weight, physical activity, and hormone status were not significantly related to symptoms.

Conclusions.—For women aged 40 to 60 years, risk factors for incontinence include parity, body mass index, hysterectomy, and diuretic use. All types of lower urinary tract symptoms are related to straining at stool and constipation. The authors emphasize that most of the identified risk factors are preventable, reversible, or predictable.

▶ These 3 epidemiological studies (Abstracts 11–9 through 11–11) provide useful information and are recommended reading among the several hundred epidemiological studies that address urinary incontinence published over the past 2 decades. At the same time, these meticulously performed and analyzed data sets serve as examples of the limitations of such studies. These 3 studies, all from Scandinavian countries, add to an extensive number of reports from these homogeneous and overwhelmingly Caucasian populations. No comparable studies have been done in other racial and ethnic groups, and particularly no comprehensive surveys of African American or Hispanic groups in the United States have been done. What little data exist on racial and ethnic differences in incontinence suggest important differences that could have significant etiologic, preventative, diagnostic, and therapeutic implications. One clinical series showed that Caucasian subjects had a prevalence of pure Genuine Stress Incontinence on urodynamic testing 2.3 (95% CI, 1.4-4.0) times that of African American subjects.[1] In another study, Peacock et al demonstrated that correlations between symptoms, physical examination, and urodynamic findings were poor in an inner-city black population in Atlanta.[2] Greater inaccuracy in clinical diagnosis and differences in prevalence may place African American women at greater risk for inappropriate therapy, particularly unindicted surgery. Data also suggest that there may be important racial differences in factors that promote urinary incontinence, suggesting that continence prevention strategies may differ among racial and ethnic groups.[1] The only published study examining the prevalence of incontinence among Hispanic Americans demonstrated that Hispanic women with unstable bladders may be less likely to be seen with a symptom of urge incontinence than African Americans or whites.[3] The need to define epidemiologic parameters for incontinence in noncaucasian populations is finally being recognized and has been identified as a significant research objective by the National Institutes of Health.

The study by Persson et al (Abstract 11–9) linked a Swedish hospital discharge registry, fertility registry, and birth registry data to identify women who had undergone surgery for stress incontinence and look for an association with parity and specifics of the delivery process. The authors' findings are generally in line with those of prior studies regarding parity and obstetrical risk for stress incontinence, although the findings with respect to instrumented vaginal delivery and episiotomy are somewhat at odds with conventional popular opinion. The obvious limitation of such a study is that birth registries, even at their best, do not contain sufficient detail regarding the delivery process to allow meaningful specific recommendations to decrease the risk of birth injury to the continence mechanism. Such recommendations can only come from the meticulous prospective study of individual deliveries using innovative electrophysiologic and imaging techniques to determine which events cause specific lesions that contribute to the development of stress incontinence. Such studies are currently in progress. Until data from such studies are available, recommendations for cesarean delivery, episiotomy, or forceps delivery in specific clinical situations to prevent pelvic floor damage are premature.

Within epidemiological definitions, estimates of the prevalence of urinary incontinence in women vary widely depending upon the epidemiologic methods used and the population studied. In a recent review of the world's epidemiologic literature regarding urinary incontinence in women, Hampel et al[4] observed that the average prevalence estimate with Diokno's[5] "any incontinence in the prior year" definition was 40.5%; with Thomas'[6] "more than 2 incontinent episodes per month" definition it was 14.0%; and with the International Continence Society's[7] "social or hygienic problem and objectively demonstrable" definition it was 23.5%. The EPINCONT study (Abstract 11–10) sampled 80% of the 74% of the women who participated in the HUNT2 Survey. Thus, approximately 59% of women older than 20 years in Nord-Trøndelag County in Norway answered questions about urinary incontinence. The survey helps put into context the marked variability noted in incontinence prevalence estimates in various reports, accounting for both the severity and the bothersomeness of incontinence in this population sample. Although 25% of the participating women had incontinence, only 7% had incontinence that would likely warrant therapy. The ability of epidemiological studies to differentiate the type of incontinence is debatable. It is important to distinguish "type of symptoms" from "type of incontinence," because the latter term implies a pathophysiologic cause that cannot be discerned reliably from symptoms alone. This is particularly true of women who claim mixed symptoms, 75% of whom will have only genuine stress incontinence diagnosed on multichannel urodynamic testing.[8]

The Danish study reported by Møller et al (Abstract 11–11) is the only 1 of the 3 studies designed from its inception to examine lower urinary tract symptoms. It confirms that parity and obesity are significantly associated with lower urinary tract symptoms and provides some of the strongest evidence to date that constipation and straining at stool are significantly associated. Unfortunately, the cross-sectional nature of the study does not allow us to conclude that these associations (or the association observed for hysterectomy) are causal. Thus, we cannot determine if the injury that caused urinary incontinence also contributed to the development of constipation or if straining at stool caused nerve damage that contributed to the development of urinary incontinence. It is unfortunate that this well-designed study did not include questions about other putative risk factors for urinary incontinence, such as cigarette smoking, chronic lung disease, and diabetes mellitus. Finally, although the authors did ask about antibiotic use for cystitis, the positive response rate of only 0.7% leads me to believe that the question identified only a small fraction of women who would have had a urinary tract infection.

R. C. Bump, MD

References

1. Bump RC: Racial comparisons and contrasts in urinary incontinence and pelvic organ prolapse. *Obstet Gynecol* 81:421-425, 1993.
2. Peacock LM, Wiskind AK, Wall LL: Clinical features of urinary incontinence and urogenital prolapse in a black inner-city population. *Am J Obstet Gynecol* 171:1464-1471, 1994.
3. Mattox TF, Bhatia NN: The prevalence of urinary incontinence or prolapse among white and Hispanic women. *Am J Obstet Gynecol* 174:646-648, 1996.
4. Hampel C, Wienhold D, Benken N, et al: Definition of overactive bladder and epidemiology of urinary incontinence. *Urology* 50(suppl)6A:4-14, 1997.
5. Diokno AC, Brock BM, Brown MB, et al: Prevalence of urinary incontinence and other urological symptoms in the noninstitutionalized elderly. *J Urol* 136:1022-1025, 1986.
6. Thomas TM, Plymat KR, Blannin J, et al: Prevalence of urinary incontinence. *Br Med J* 281:1243-1245, 1980.
7. Abrams P, Blaivas JG, Stanton SL, et al: The International Continence Society Committee on Standardisation of Terminology. The standardisation of terminology of lower urinary tract function. *Scand J Urol Nephrol* 114S:5-19, 1988.
8. Weidner AC, Myers ER, Visco AG, et al: Which women with stress incontinence require urodynamics? *Am J Obstet Gynecol* 184:20-27, 2001.

A Longitudinal Cohort Study of Elderly Women With Urinary Tract Infections

Molander U, Arvidsson L, Milsom I, et al (Sahlgrenska Univ, Göteborg, Sweden)
Maturitas 34:127-131, 2000

11–12

Introduction.—Urinary tract infections and other urogenital complaints are common among elderly women. In the mid 1980s, the prevalence of urogenital complaints in a large, randomized sample of elderly Swedish women was reported. The long-term outcomes of women treated for urinary tract infections (UTIs) at that time, including the prevalence of recurrent UTIs, urinary incontinence, and overall mortality are described.

Methods.—The original study included a random sample of 6000 women born in Göteborg between 1900 and 1920 who were invited to complete a questionnaire about UTIs, urinary incontinence, (UI) and estrogen use. The response rate in that study was 70%. Ten years later, the investigators attempted to contact 688 women who reported treatment for a UTI. A similar questionnaire regarding UTI, UI, and estrogen use was sent to 434 women who were still alive. Of these women, 361 responded, a rate of 83%. Death certificate data were obtained to determine the causes of death for the 254 women who died. Mortality and causes of death for this group were compared with those of women from the original study who did not have UTIs.

Results.—Mortality among women with a history of UTI was 37%, compared with 28% for those who did not report a UTI during the original study. Causes of death did not differ significantly between groups. Sixty-one percent of surviving women with UTIs reported treatment for at least 1 additional UTI since the original study. In the original study, 30% of women with UTIs reported UI, compared with 17% of the total population sample (p < 0.001). At follow-up, the prevalence of UI among women with a history of UTIs had increased to 33%. Fifty-three percent of these women reported mixed incontinence, 30% urge incontinence, and 17% stress incontinence.

Conclusions.—These follow-up data suggest that elderly women with a history of UTI have a higher mortality than women of the same age without UTI. In addition, women with UTI are at elevated risk of repeat episodes of UTI. It is unclear whether UTI, per se, predicts a higher risk of mortality, or if women with UTI are more likely to have other diseases as well. The study includes no data on the prevalence of asymptomatic bacteriuria.

▶ The relationship between UTIs or asymptomatic bacteriuria and mortality in the elderly has been the subject of controversy for many years. Early studies suggested a relationship between bacteriuria and mortality[1,2] but a subsequent repeat study by 1 group did not support their original conclusions. In that 11-year nursing home study, persistent bacteriuria was not shown to significantly impact mortality.[3] In a 10-year observational study, Abrutyn et al[4] did not show UTI to be a significant independent cause of mortality after adjusting for age and other comorbidities. In a controlled trial attached to their longitudinal study, the authors also demonstrated that treatment of bacteriuria did not influence mortality. Now, in an elegant 10-year epidemiological study in a representative random population, Molander et al demonstrate increased mortality after 10 years in elderly women who were treated for UTIs in 1985-1986. The important limitations to this study are (1) there was no ability to control for any concomitant diseases or disabilities that might predispose both to UTI and to mortality; (2) there was no microbiological confirmation of UTI, noting that treatment for UTI does not always mean that a UTI was actually the cause of symptoms; and (3) there was no evaluation for asymptomatic bacteriuria. Thus, we are not really left with a message on which to act. We would all treat a woman with a symptomatic infection, the population of interest in this study. Such treatment is based on the discomfort of the patient not on the risk of subsequent mortality, which does not appear to be altered by treatment. Further, the issue of treating or not treating the pervasive problem of asymptomatic bacteriuria in elderly women is not addressed at all by the study. The study does not change the established clinical routine of treating symptomatic UTI and not treating uncomplicated asymptomatic bacteriuria in the elderly.

R. C. Bump, MD

References

1. Dontas AS, Kasviki-Charvati P, Papanayiotou DC, et al: Bacteriuria and survival in old age. *N Eng J Med* 304:939-943, 1981.
2. Sourander LB, Kasanen A: A 5-year follow-up of bacteriuria in the aged. *Geront Clin* 14:274-281, 1972.
3. Dontas AS, Tzonou A, Kasviki-Charvati P, et al: Survival in a residential home: and eleven-year longitudinal study. *J Am Geriatr Soc* 39:641-649, 1991.
4. Abrutyn E, Mossey J, Berlin JA, Boscia J, et al: Does asymptomatic bacteriuria predict mortality and does antimicrobial treatment reduce mortality in elderly ambulatory women? *Ann Intern Med* 120:827-833, 1994.

Effect of Postpartum Pelvic Floor Muscle Training in Prevention and Treatment of Urinary Incontinence: A One-Year Follow Up

Mørkved S, Bø K (Regional Hosp, Trondheim, Norway; Norwegian Univ, Oslo, Norway)
Br J Obstet Gynaecol 107:1022-1028, 2000   11–13

Background.—Pelvic floor muscle exercise has been recommended for the prevention and treatment of stress urinary incontinence (SUI). The objectives are to provide a structural support for the bladder and urethra and to develop the ability to prevent urethral descent and close the urethra during abrupt increases in intra-abdominal pressure. The 1-year follow-up results of a randomized controlled trial of pelvic floor muscle exercise for postpartum prevention and treatment of urinary incontinence are presented.

Methods.—The analysis included 81 matched pairs of women who had participated in a study of an 8-week pelvic floor muscle training program, starting in the eighth week after delivery. Women assigned to the exercise group attended once-weekly classes with a physiotherapist. They were also assigned home exercises, with instructions to perform 2 series of 8 to 12 maximum contractions, each held for 6 to 8 seconds, with 3 to 4 fast contractions at the end of each long contraction. Women in the control group received the usual postpartum instructions. The women's mean age was 28 years and mean number of deliveries 1.8. By the sixteenth week postpartum, the rate of SUI was 13/81 in the exercise group versus 24/81 in the control group (p<0.05).

For the current analysis, all women were contacted 1 year after delivery and interviewed about their continence status. Other assessments included a standardized pad test and clinical evaluation of pelvic floor muscle function and strength.

Findings.—Fifty-three percent of women in the exercise group continued to perform regular pelvic floor exercises during the follow-up period compared to 30% of those in the control group (p=.002). The mean increase in vaginal squeeze pressure during follow-up was 4.4 cm H_2O in the exercise group versus 1.7 cm H_2O in the control group (p=.001). This change was significantly related to the higher frequency of continued pelvic floor muscle training in the exercise group. The pad test showed

TABLE 5.—Number of Women With Stress Urinary Incontinence (SUI) Registered in the Structured Interview in the Training Group (TG) and the Control Group (CG) at the Tests 16 Weeks and 1 Year Postpartum

SUI Frequencies	TG (*n* = 81)	CG (*n* = 81)	*P**
16th week postpartum	13 (16)	24 (30)	0·039
<Once per week	12 (15)	17 (21)	
<Daily once per week	0 (0)	7 (9)	
Daily	1 (1)	0 (0)	
One year postpartum	13 (16)	25 (31)	0·026
<Once per week	9 (11)	18 (22)	
<Daily once per week	3 (4)	7 (9)	
Daily	1 (1)	0 (0)	

Note: Values are given as n (percentage), unless otherwise indicated.
*χ^2 test.
(Courtesy of Mørkved S, Bø K: Effect of postpartum pelvic floor muscle training in prevention and treatment of urinary incontinence. A one-year follow-up. *Br J Obstet Gynecol* 107:1022-1028. Copyright 2000 Elsevier Science, publisher.)

urinary leakage in 5/81 women in the exercise group versus 14/81 in the control group (p<.03). The percentage of women reporting urinary leakage remained significantly lower in the exercise group (Table 5).

Conclusions.—A postpartum pelvic floor muscle exercise intervention is effective in reducing the rate of urinary incontinence, and this benefit persists at 1 year after delivery. This report suggests that to be effective, the exercise must be intensive, and the mothers must have strong motivation and close follow-up.

▶ This article does provide evidence that the benefits of an intense post-partum pelvic floor muscle training program are maintained for 1 year. Of note, however, is the fact that the majority of incontinent women in both the treatment and control groups (70%) had less than 1 incontinent episode per week, only 1 (in the treatment group) had daily incontinence, and there were no group differences demonstrated in validated leakage or impact scales. Of incontinent control subjects, 20% said they were continent but had positive pad tests. Simply stated, the level of SUI was quite mild and may not have been enough motivation for either patients or control subjects to perform regular exercises. It is not known how many, if any, of the study group would have been seen with incontinence had they not been part of the study. A similar 10-month follow-up report this year from Switzerland[1] showed resolution of SUI in 10 of 16 exercise subjects compared with 1 of 9 control subjects. The 10-month postpartum SUI rates, however, were nearly identical, at 14% for the control group and 12% for the treatment group. In addition, there was no difference in resolution rates for anal incontinence and no difference between groups in 10-month pelvic muscle contraction strength, bladder neck mobility, or any urodynamic parameter. These negative results were observed despite an intense regimen that included 12 sessions that involved training instruction, 20 minutes of biofeedback, and 15 minutes of electrostimulation each. It is widely accepted that pelvic floor muscle training is a good thing to recommend postpartum; however, it is not clear how intense the training or how clinically significant the benefit may be.

R. C. Bump, MD

Reference

1. Meyer S, Hohlfeld P, Achtari C, et al: Pelvic floor education after vaginal delivery. *Obstet Gynecol* 97:673-677, 2001.

Is Intrinsic Sphincter Deficiency a Complication of Simple Hysterectomy?

Morgan JL, O'Connell HE, McGuire EJ (Univ of Melbourne, Australia; Univ of Texas, Austin)
J Urol 164:767-769, 2000

11–14

Introduction.—Type III stress urinary incontinence is also known as intrinsic sphincter deficiency. Various pelvic operations may lead to intrinsic sphincter deficiency, but a simple hysterectomy performed for benign conditions is not known to be one of them. The potential association between a simple hysterectomy and intrinsic sphincter deficiency was evaluated.

Methods.—The case–control study used data from a series of 387 consecutive women treated for incontinence over a 2-year period. The investigators matched 67 patients who had undergone hysterectomy for benign disease to 67 women with no such history (Table 1). The median ages were 59 and 50 years respectively. A significant number of women in both groups had histories of previous pelvic surgeries. In the hysterectomy group, 31% of patients had undergone anterior colporrhaphy, and 18% had undergone colposuspension or urethrocystopexy; in comparison, women in the control group had undergone minimal surgery for stress incontinence. All patients underwent fluoroscopic urodynamic studies, including measurement of abdominal leak point pressure. A separate com-

TABLE 1.—Demographic Data and Obstetric History

	Pts	Controls
Median age (range)	59 (31-92)	50 (16-92)
Median parity (range)	3 (0-7)	2 (0-5)
No. forceps delivery (%)	13 (19.4)	15 (22.4)
No. breech delivery (%)	0	4 (6.0)
No. twins (%)	4 (6.0)	2 (3.0)
No. perineal tear (%)	7 (10.4)	5 (7.5)
No. newborn greater than 9 lbs. (%)	5 (7.5)	7 (10.4)
No. multiparity 3 or more (%)	29 (65.9)	19 (32.2)
No. nulliparous (%)	23 (34)	8 (12)

(Courtesy of Morgan JL, O'Connell HE, McGuire EJ: Is intrinsic sphincter deficiency a complication of simple hysterectomy? *J Urol* 164:767-769, 2000.)

TABLE 2.—Abdominal Leak Point Pressure and Intrinsic
Sphincter Deficiency

	No. Pts. (%)	No. Controls (%)
Abdominal leak point pressure (cm. H_2O):		
Less than 60	14 (20.9)	4 (6.0)
60-75	18 (26.9)	12 (17.9)
Greater than 75 or no leakage	35 (52.2)	51 (76.1)
Intrinsic sphincter deficiency	32 (47.8)	18 (23.9)

(Courtesy of Morgan JL, O'Connell HE, McGuire EJ: Is intrinsic sphincter deficiency a complication of simple hysterectomy? *J Urol* 164:767-769, 2000.)

parison was performed for 29 cases and 53 control women with no risk factors for intrinsic sphincter deficiency.

Results.—Overall, 48% of women with hysterectomy versus 24% of control women had intrinsic sphincter deficiency (Table 2). The cases also had a higher incidence of grade 2 or 3 cystocele (52% vs 40%). Within the low-risk subgroup, the prevalence of intrinsic sphincter deficiency was 52% for patients versus 21% for controls. Despite the high prevalence of previous colporrhaphy (Table 4), cystocele and rectocele were common.

Conclusion.—Women with a history of hysterectomy for benign disease have an increased prevalence of intrinsic sphincter deficiency. This is so even among patients with no recognized risk factors for intrinsic sphincter deficiency. The authors plan a prospective study to confirm this association. Pending the results, the potential risk of intrinsic sphincter deficiency should be considered in clinical decision-making in situations in which the indications for a hysterectomy are equivocal.

▶ The effect of simple hysterectomy on lower urinary tract function is a matter of considerable contention. The conviction that hysterectomy causes de novo bladder and urethral dysfunction in previously normal women is pervasive in the urologic literature. However, most of the studies that are cited to support this conviction are anecdotal, retrospective, lack appropriate control groups, or are based solely on subjective parameters. In the largest report on the relationship between lower urinary tract dysfunction and hysterectomy, a retrospective questionnaire study that included 554 women, Vervest showed that women with gynecologic pathology necessitating

TABLE 4.—Incidence of Pelvic Surgery

Surgery	No. Pts. (%)	No. Controls (%)
Colporrhaphy	21 (31.3)	3 (4.5)
Suspension + urethrocystopexy	12 (17.9)	7 (10.4)
Colorectal surgery	3 (4.5)	0
Other	1 (1.5)	2 (3.0)
Total/Total No.	35/67 (52.2)	11/67 (16.4)

(Courtesy of Morgan JL, O'Connell HE, McGuire EJ: Is intrinsic sphincter deficiency a complication of simple hysterectomy? *J Urol* 164:767-769, 2000.)

hysterectomy have a higher prevalence of urologic symptoms than is seen in the general population.[1] In this study, 57% of women were symptomatic and 20% were incontinent prior to hysterectomy. The author warned against basing any conclusions on retrospective studies. Studies that have included preoperative and postoperative urodynamic testing have demonstrated contradictory, variable, often transient, and clinically inconsequential changes or no changes at all.[2-8]

The current article by Morgan et al is to be commended for including a control group and objective testing. However, the authors give us no hint as to how their controls were matched and give no information about other factors related to urodynamic measures of intrinsic sphincter deficiency (ISD) such as menopausal status, the use of hormones, or the number of women with concurrent detrusor instability. Moreover, it is remarkable to see an article published in 2000 that includes no statistical analysis of any sort, let alone the sophisticated analysis required to control for the many confounders that *are* revealed. It appears that there were significant differences in age (significance could not be calculated from data in the article), advanced parity ($P = .001$), and prior pelvic surgery ($P = .00002$) (P values derived from data in the article), lending doubt as to the adequacy of matching criteria.

Finally, the authors manipulation of both patients and data to define ISD in the majority of subjects with undefined stages of prolapse, make the validity of conclusions open to further question. The authors note in their discussion that their findings should help patients choose between hysterectomy and "a nonoperative solution." I suspect that this article will be widely cited by hysterectomy opponents, but adding ISD to the lists of reasons to oppose hysterectomy should await the publication of the authors' promised prospective case-control study.

R. C. Bump, MD

References

1. Vervest HAM, de Jonge MK, Vervest TMJS, et al: Micturition symptoms and urinary incontinence after non-radical hysterectomy. *Acta Obstet Gynecol Scand* 67:141-146, 1988.
2. Parys BT, Haylen BT, Hutton JL, et al: The effects of simple hysterectomy on vesicourethral function. *Br J Urol* 64:594-599, 1989.
3. Vervest HAM, van Venrooij GEPM, Barents JW, et al: Non-radical hysterectomy and the function of the lower urinary tract. *Acta Obstet Gynecol Scand* 68:221-229, 1989.
4. Wake CR: The immediate effect of abdominal hysterectomy on intravesical pressure and detrusor activity. *Br J Obstet Gynaecol* 87:901-902, 1980.
5. Lalos O, Bjerle P: Early and late effects of subtotal and total hysterectomy on bladder function. *Arch Gynecol* 237:140, 1985.
6. Lalos O, Bjerle P: Bladder wall mechanics and micturition before and after subtotal and total hysterectomy. *Eur J Obstet Gynecol Reprod Biol* 21:143-150, 1986.
7. Hansen BM, Bonnesen T, Hvidberg JE, et al: Changes in symptoms and colpocystourethrography in 35 patients before and after total abdominal hysterectomy: A prospective study. *Urol Int* 40:224-226, 1985.

8. Bump RC, Fantl JA: Acute (48-72 hour) and long-term (1 year) effects of vaginal hysterectomy on passive and dynamic urethral function. *J Pelvic Surg* 1:84-87, 1995.

Pelvic Floor Muscle Contraction During a Cough and Decreased Vesical Neck Mobility

Miller JM, Perucchini D, Carchidi LT, et al (Univ of Michigan, Ann Arbor; Universitaetsspital Zurich, Switzerland)
Obstet Gynecol 97:255-260, 2001

11–15

Background.—Having excessive vesical neck movement while coughing has been linked to stress urinary incontinence. Performing a contraction of the pelvic floor muscles immediately before and during a cough allowed less stress-related leakage of urine. This maneuver was termed the Knack, and it produced significant results. This study evaluated the amount of vesical neck displacement during a cough with and without the Knack maneuver, theorizing that the degree of displacement would be less when the Knack was used.

Methods.—Eleven young, continent, nulliparous women were trained to perform the Knack maneuver immediately before the data were collected. Eleven older, incontinent, parous women had completed an intervention extending for 6 months that was designed to assess the usefulness of the Knack in the management of incontinence. Subjects coughed with and without contracting their pelvic floor muscles. Perineal US was used to quantify vesical neck displacement at rest and during coughing.

Results.—The resting vesical neck positions differed significantly between the older, incontinent women and the younger, continent women. Vesical neck displacement during a cough without the Knack ranged from 1 to 21 mm, with a median of 5.4 mm. The median displacement with the Knack was 2.9 mm ($P < .001$). Displacement without the Knack was consistently in the dorsocaudal direction. By using the Knack, women could lift and maintain the vesical neck's cranioventral position relative to its resting state. At peak cough pressure with the Knack, the maximal cranioventral displacement was 7.3 mm and the maximal dorsocaudal displacement was 11.0 mm. Both age groups were able to reduce vesical neck displacement during coughing by using the Knack. For the older women, the median value without the Knack was 6.2 mm, but with it the value was 3.5 mm ($P = .003$). For younger women, the values were 4.6 mm without the Knack and 0.0 with it ($P = .007$). Thus, these older women reduced vesical neck displacement, and the younger women were able to control it completely.

Conclusion.—Use of the Knack allowed young, continent, nulliparous women to stabilize the vesical neck during the stress of coughing. Extension of the findings reveals that in most normal women, full activation of the muscle does not rely on reflex during coughing. The Knack improved stabilization among some women with stress urinary incontinence. Parous women's improved, but not total, control was believed to reflect the fact that volitional muscle action can influence vesical neck position only to the degree that it is unaffected by damage to fascial attachments, levator ani muscles, or innervating mechanisms.

Bladder Neck Mobility in Continent Nulliparous Women

Peschers UM, Fanger G, Schaer GN, et al (Ludwig-Maximilians Univ, Munich; Cantonal Hosp, Lucerne, Switzerland; Cantonal Hosp, Aarau, Switzerland et al)

Br J Obstet Gynaecol 108:320-324, 2001   11–16

Background.—Stress urinary incontinence is more likely to occur in patients who have bladder neck hypermobility. Maneuveurs to promote bladder neck hypermobility include the Valsalva maneuver and coughing. The ability of these 2 maneuvers to cause bladder neck mobility in healthy nulliparous women was compared using US.

Methods.—The study population consisted of 39 nulliparous women, aged 18 years or older, who had no history of recurrent urinary tract infection, disease of the upper or lower urinary tract, urinary incontinence, chronic constipation, or chronic coughing. Women were placed in the lithotomy position, and the bladder was filled with 200 mL of sterile water via catheter. The outer urethral meatus was observed for leakage during vigorous coughing in the supine position and in the standing position. Volunteers also performed Valsalva maneuvers according to a set protocol. During Valsalva and coughing, intrarectal pressure was determined. Using a 3.5 MHz curved linear array transducer, perineal US studies were done, and the bladder neck's position was evaluated by a standardized and reproducible method.

Results.—None of the women had leakage on coughing in either the supine or the standing position. During coughing, the vesical neck descent was significantly less (8 mm; SD 4) than during a Valsalva maneuver (15 mm; SD 10) in 25 women ($P < 0.005$). Test-retest reliability was evaluated in 20 women for bladder neck mobility during the Valsalva maneuver, and the results showed that the difference in descent was 5 mm or less (intraclass coefficient, $\alpha = 0.99$). Test-retest reliability during coughing yielded a maximum difference of 4 mm (intraclass coefficient, $\alpha = 0.956$).

Conclusion.—Mobility of the bladder neck is significantly greater during a Valsalva maneuver than during coughing, which could be attributed to pelvic muscle contractions during coughing stabilizing the pelvic floor and supporting the neck of the bladder. This helps to explain differences between cough and valsalva leak point pressures noted in other studies. Thus, normal, continent women have bladder neck mobility that is less during coughing than during Valsalva maneuvers.

▶ These articles used the same US techniques[1,2] to evaluate bladder neck mobility under 2 sets of experimental conditions. The latter article (Abstract

11–16) demonstrates that bladder neck mobility in a nulliparous population is less with an abrupt cough than it is with a more gradual Valsalva maneuver. It provides evidence for reflex contraction of the pelvic floor and increased stabilization of the urethra with a cough, compared with a strain. It helps explain why Valsalva leak point pressures tend to be lower than cough leak point pressures in women with stress incontinence. The former article (Abstract 11–15) shows that this reflex activation does not result in maximum contraction of the pelvic floor and that the reflex can be effectively augmented by training in the skill of "the Knack." Further, the articles together underscore the limitations of equating bladder neck hypermobility (for example, a maximum straining Q-tip axis of 40°) with stress incontinence in that the majority of healthy, continent women will have significant mobility in this circumstance. The critical issue is the woman's ability to use her pelvic floor muscles to stabilize this mobility in specific circumstances to avoid leakage.

One theory for using pelvic floor muscle training for the treatment of stress incontinence is that strengthening of the pelvic floor and urethral muscles will improve both sphincteric closure and bladder neck support. Continued training should result in hypertrophy of muscle over time, increasing mechanical pressure on the urethra and improving bladder neck support during stressful activity.[3] The second (Knack) theory is that patients can be taught and encouraged to contract the pelvic floor in anticipation of the physically stressful activities that usually cause urine leakage. This skill training has been shown to significantly reduce urine loss with medium (98.2% mean decrease in amount lost) and deep (73.3% mean decrease in amount lost) coughs within 1 week.[4] Both strength and skill training should be emphasized in a pelvic floor muscle-training program.

R. C. Bump, MD

References

1. Schaer GN, Koechli OR, Schuessler B, et al: Perineal ultrasound for evaluating the bladder in urinary stress incontinence. *Obstet Gynecol* 85:224-229, 1995.
2. Schaer GN, Koechli OR, Schuessler B, et al: Perineal ultrasound: Determination of reliable examination procedures. *Ultrasound Obstet Gynecol* 7:347-352, 1996.
3. Bö K: Pelvic floor muscle exercise for the treatment of stress urinary incontinence: An exercise physiology perspective. *Int Urogynecol J* 6:282-291, 1995.
4. Miller JM, Ashton-Miller JA, DeLancey JOL: A pelvic muscle precontraction can reduce cough-related urine loss in selected women with mild SUI. *J Am Geriatr Soc* 46:870-874, 1998.

Quantification of Intramuscular Nerves Within the Female Striated Urogenital Sphincter Muscle

Pandit M, Delancey JOL, Ashton-Miller JA, et al (Univ of Michigan, Ann Arbor)
Obstet Gynecol 95:797-800, 2000   11–17

Background.—Urethral sphincteric strength plays an important role in stress continence. Sphincter weakness, evidenced by reduced maximum urethral closure pressure, is associated with severity of stress incontinence. Thus, understanding the cause of sphincter weakness would improve understanding of the pathophysiology of stress urinary incontinence.

Methods.—Thirteen cadaveric urethras obtained from persons aged 15 to 78 years at the time of death were examined. Intramuscular nerves were identified by staining a sagittal histologic section with S100. The number of times a nerve was seen in the striated urogenital sphincter, as well as the number of axons in each nerve fascicle, were recorded.

Findings.—The number of intramuscular nerves in the striated urogenital sphincters varied markedly, ranging from 72 to 543. The number of axons ranged from 431 to 3523. Large nerve fascicles were primarily noted in the distal part of the striated urogenital sphincter. Decreased nerve density throughout the striated urogenital sphincter was associated with fewer muscle cells. Nerve density declined with increasing age.

Conclusion.—The quantity of intramuscular nerves varied greatly in the specimens studied. Those with sparse intramuscular nerves had fewer striated muscle cells. In addition, the density of intramuscular nerves decreased with advancing age.

▶ This histologic study of the striated urogenital sphincter provides morphological support for the accumulating electrophysiologic evidence for a neurogenic basis for stress urinary incontinence and other forms of pelvic floor dysfunction.[1-4] The authors demonstrated a significant correlation between the loss of nerves and a decrease in muscle cells as well as a significant decrease in nerve density with increasing age. Unfortunately, a lack of precise historical data from the study population did not allow the authors to assess for potentially important confounders to the age association. Nonetheless, there are 2 important clinical messages from this basic science paper. First, there is likely a progressive deterioration in the urethral sphincteric mechanism with aging that would explain the increased risk of incontinence (and recurrent incontinence after successful treatment) in older women. Second, the sphincteric mechanism does not remain "like new" through a woman's life, and none of our surgical interventions for stress incontinence regenerate nerve or muscle. Thus, surgery is compensatory rather than restorative.

Compensatory mechanisms generally work quite well, but as the sphincteric mechanism progressively deteriorates (often with concurrent deterioration in detrusor function), more drastic treatment impact is needed if cure is to be effected. This more drastic treatment impact in an effort to eliminate stress incontinence can often result in undesirable complications such as obstructed voiding and/or irritative symptoms, including urge incontinence. Most surgeons take extra time to counsel the elderly patient about her increased risk for persistent incontinence or new obstruction/urge symptoms following continence surgery. Experience and basic science both support this conscientious approach.

R. C. Bump, MD

References

1. Snookes SJ, Badenoch DF, Tiptaft RC, et al: Perineal nerve damage in genuine stress urinary incontinence: An electrophysiological study. *Br J Urol* 57:422-426, 1985.
2. Allen RE, Hosker GL, Smith AR, et al: Pelvic floor damage and childbirth: A neurophysiological study. *Br J Obstet Gynaecol* 97:770-779, 1990.
3. Aanestad O, Flink R: Urinary stress incontinence: A urodynamic and quantitative electromyographic study of the perineal muscles. *Acta Obstet Gynecol Scand* 78:245-253, 1999.
4. Weidner AC, Barber MD, Visco AG, et al: Pelvic muscle electromyography of levator ani and external anal sphincter in nulliparous women and women with pelvic floor dysfunction. *Am J Obstet Gynecol* 183:1390-1401, 2000.

Long-term Results of Sacral Nerve Stimulation (S3) for the Treatment of Neurogenic Refractory Urge Incontinence Related to Detrusor Hyperreflexia
Chartier-Kastler EJ, Bosch JLHR, Perrigot M, et al (Univ Pierre et Marie Curie [Paris VI]; Université Paris-ouest, Garches, France; Erasmus Med Ctr, Rotterdam, The Netherlands; et al)
J Urol 164:1476-1480, 2000   11–18

Background.—Chronic sacral nerve stimulation for the treatment of neurogenic urge urinary incontinence has not gained much popularity since the first publication of 2 case reports by Schmidt in 1991. Incontinence in patients with spinal cord diseases with upper motor neuron lesions is usually caused by detrusor hyperreflexia. It has been demonstrated in chronic experimental models that a new sacral segmental reflex arc may become functional because of neuroplasticity. The most common spinal causes of hyperreflexic neurogenic bladder are spinal cord injuries, multiple sclerosis, spinal cord lesions, spinal tumors, and viral myelitis. There are several therapeutic options for detrusor hyperreflexia, including pelvic floor training, pharmacotherapy with oral anticholinergic drugs, and vesical instillation of vanilloid agents with or without clean intermittent self-catheterization. Electrical stimulation has been used for treatment of detrusor instability since the 1960s, and sacral nerve stimulation has been extensively developed and evaluated over the past 5 years. A test stimulation trial is performed before implantation of the sacral nerve stimulation device to test its effectiveness. The clinical and urodynamic results of sacral nerve stimulation were evaluated for patients with neurogenic urge incontinence and detrusor hyperreflexia resistant to parasympatholytic agents.

Methods.—Nine women (mean age, 42.6 years) were treated since 1992 for refractory neurogenic urge incontinence with sacral nerve stimulation. The mean time since diagnosis was 12 years. All the patients were incontinent with chronic pad use related to detrusor hyperreflexia. In 5 patients, intermittent self-catheterization for external sphincter detrusor dyssynergia was used. The social life of these patients was impaired, making them candidates for bladder augmentation. After a positive test stimulation trial, a sacral (S3) lead was surgically implanted and connected to a subcutaneous neurostimulator.

Results.—During a mean follow-up of 43.6 months, all 9 patients had clinically significant improvement in their incontinence, and 5 patients were completely dry. Five continued to use clean intermittent catheterization as their voiding mechanism. The average number of voids per day decreased from 16.1 to 8.2. Significant improvements from baseline in urodynamic parameters were seen at 6 months after implant-1 maximum bladder capacity increased from 244 to 377 mL, and volume at first uninhibited contraction increased from 214 to 340 mL. Maximum detrusor pressure at first uninhibited contraction was increased in 3 patients, stabilized in 2 patients, and decreased in 4 patients. When stimulation was inactivated, urodynamic parameters returned to baseline. All of the patients reported subjective improvement of at least 75% on visual analogue scale results at last follow-up.

Conclusions.—In selected patients with refractory urge incontinence related to detrusor hyperreflexia resulting from spinal lesions, sacral nerve stimulation can provide an effective, reversible treatment option.

▶ Over the past decade, the efficacy of chronic sacral nerve stimulation for the clinical management of refractory idiopathic urge urinary incontinence has been demonstrated in multiple cohort studies. The current article is one of the first to suggest the utility of the technique in women with detrusor hyperreflexia (bladder overactivity because of a central nervous system lesion). Nine women with detrusor hyperreflexia caused by multiple sclerosis, spinal cord injury, or myelitis were successfully treated, avoiding the much more complicated and morbid procedure of augmentation cystoplasty for up to 6 years. Recently, the first randomized, though nonblinded, comparison of sacral nerve stimulation was reported in patients with refractory urge incontinence not due to known neurological disease.[1] The control group continued their previously unsuccessful conservative management regimens. The treatment group had significantly better responses than the control group as measured by leakage episode frequency, pad usage, cystometric bladder capacity, and quality of life instruments. Still, fewer than half of the initial candidates (45.5%) responded to their percutaneous test stimulation trial and were candidates for permanent implants. Thus, although the utility of the technique is limited to a subset of a select population, some patients seem to realize significant and nearly miraculous clinical benefit. Finally, the technique has prompted basic scientific interest and multiple research efforts directed at afferent neuromodulation, a promising new treatment category for irritative lower urinary tract and pelvic floor disorders.

R. C. Bump, MD

Reference

1. Weil EHJ, Ruiz-Cerdá JL, Eerdmans PHA, et al: Sacral root neuromodulation in the treatment of refractory urinary urge incontinence: A prospective randomized clinical trial. *Eur Urol* 37:161-171, 2000.

Pressure Flow Analysis May Aid in Identifying Women With Outflow Obstruction
Lemack GE, Zimmern PE (Univ of Texas, Dallas)
J Urol 163:1823-1838, 2000   11–19

Background.—The role of complete urodynamic assessment for evaluating lower urinary tract symptoms in women has continued to evolve. However, several questions are still unanswered. The current authors report the development of pressure flow cutoff values for female bladder outlet obstruction and their subsequent application in a group of women undergoing urodynamic testing for various lower urinary tract symptoms.

Methods.—Eighty-seven women with clinical obstruction were studied. The suspected cause of obstruction was prolapse in 33 women, previous incontinence surgery in 25, and no apparent source in 29. Another 124 patients seen for assessment of stress urinary incontinence made up a control group.

Findings.—The mean maximum flow rate in the control group was 23 mL per second. The mean detrusor pressure was 21.9 cm water. The corresponding values in persons with clinical obstruction were 10.7 mL per second and 40.8 cm water (Fig 2). No differences were observed among the groups with different causes of obstruction. Receiver operating characteristics analysis demonstrated cutoff values of 11 mL per second or less and 21 cm water or more as optimal for selecting patients with bladder outlet obstruction. With these values, the prevalence of bladder outlet obstruction was 20% in a consecutive cohort of women undergoing urodynamic tests.

Conclusions.—Cutoff pressure flow values were determined to help identify women with bladder outlet obstruction. Such cutoffs should be used only in conjunction with the overall clinical picture. Neither pressure flow data alone nor clinical symptoms alone appear sufficient for diagnosing obstruction.

▶ It is hard to argue with the carefully worded conclusions and recommendations of this article. The authors raise our consciousness about the often ignored and underreported issue of bladder outlet obstruction in women and provide some useful guidelines for suspecting obstruction in women. This is especially important in instances in which a woman with obstruction pre-

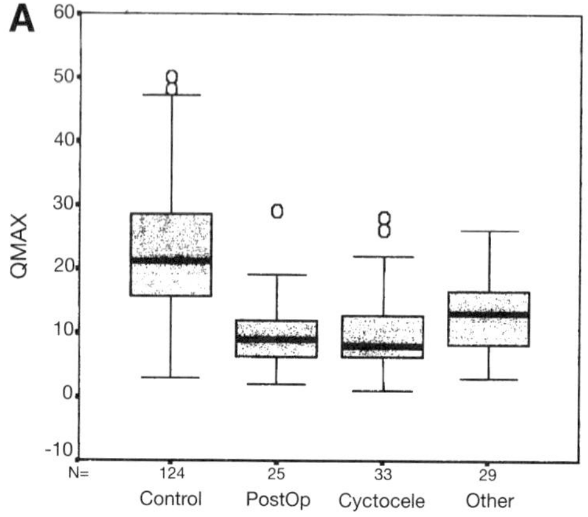

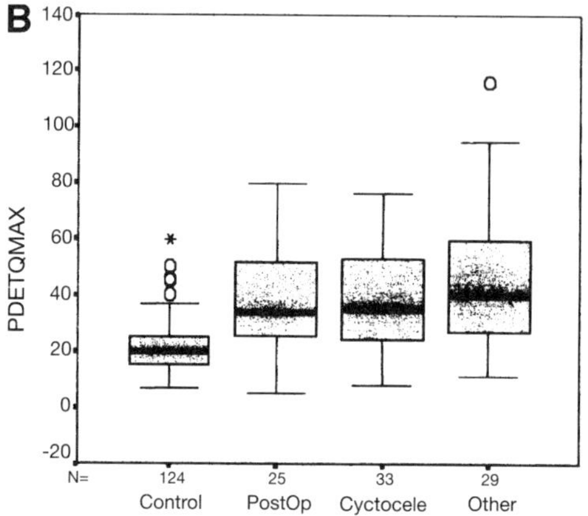

FIGURE 2.—Box and whiskers plot of 25th to 75th percentiles by disease category. *Thick lines* represent means. *Circles* and *asterisk* represent outliers. **A,** Maximum flow (QMAX). **B,** Detrusor pressure at maximum flow (PDETQMAX). (Courtesy of Lemack GE, Zimmern PE: Pressure flow analysis may aid in identifying women with outflow obstruction. *J Urol* 163:1823-1838, 2000.)

sents with symptoms of reactive bladder overactivity. It is such women and those who have detrusor hyperactivity with impaired contractility[1] who are at greatest risk of severe iatrogenic urinary retention when they are empirically given anticholinergic therapy. There are several shortcomings to this study as a comprehensive study of female emptying-phase dysfunction. First, the authors excluded an important subtype of obstructed voiding, vesicosphincter dyssynergia (a nonrelaxing rhabdosphincter in the face of a detrusor contraction), Second, much obstruction in women is dynamic, that is, accentuated when urethral resistance is augmented by straining, as is the case with advanced stages of anterior-superior segment pelvic organ prolapse and in some women after continence surgery.[2,3] These effects are largely eliminated because the authors excluded patients who strained over 10 cm water during their void. Next, the authors do not provide information about postvoid residual volumes in these patients. It is possible that a maximum flow rate from a noninstrumented uroflow combined with a postvoid residual volume could be as useful, and less invasive and prone to artifact, in raising the suspicion of obsruction. Finally, the authors' control group of women with stress incontinence is likely to have higher flow rates with lower detrusor pressures than the general population because of abnormally low outlet resistance, leading to artificially high flow and low pressure cutoff values for obstruction. Despite these methodologic shortcomings, the article presents useful guidelines for suspecting bladder outlet obstruction in women.

R. C. Bump, MD

References

1. Resnick NM, Yalla SV: Detrusor hyperactivity with impaired contractile function. *JAMA* 257:3076-3081, 1987.
2. Bump RC, Fantl JA, Hurt WG: Dynamic urethral pressure profilometry pressure transmission ratio determinations following surgery for stress incontinence: Understanding the mechanism of success, failure, and complications. *Obstet Gynecol* 72:870-874, 1988.
3. Bump RC, Hurt WG, Addison WA, et al: Understanding urinary tract function in women soon after bladder neck surgery. *Neurourol Urodynamics* 18:629-637, 1999.

A Survey of Pessary Use by Members of the American Urogynecologic Society
Cundiff GW, Weidner AC, Visco AG, et al (Duke Univ, Durham, NC)
Obstet Gynecol 95:931-935, 2000   11–20

Background.—Much of the research on pessaries consists of case reports of complications associated with pessary use, prompting some authorities to believe that pessaries are obsolete and even dangerous. The National Institutes of Health recently called for research to compare pessaries with surgical intervention for the treatment of pelvic organ prolapse. However, the lack of consensus on the appropriate use of pessaries has hindered the design of meaningful investigations. A survey was conducted to determine trends in pessary use for pelvic organ prolapse.

Methods.—The members of the American Urogynecologic Society received an anonymous survey. Forty-eight percent (359) of the 748 members returned their surveys.

Findings.—Seventy-seven percent of the respondents reported using pessaries as first-line treatment of prolapse. Twelve percent reserved pessary use for patients who were not surgical candidates. Eighty-nine percent used a pessary for anterior defects, 60% for posterior defects, 74% for apical defects, and 76% for complete procidentia. Twenty-two percent of the respondents reported using the same pessary, usually a ring, for all support defects. Among those who tailored pessary use to the defect, the use of support pessaries for anterior and apical defects was more common,

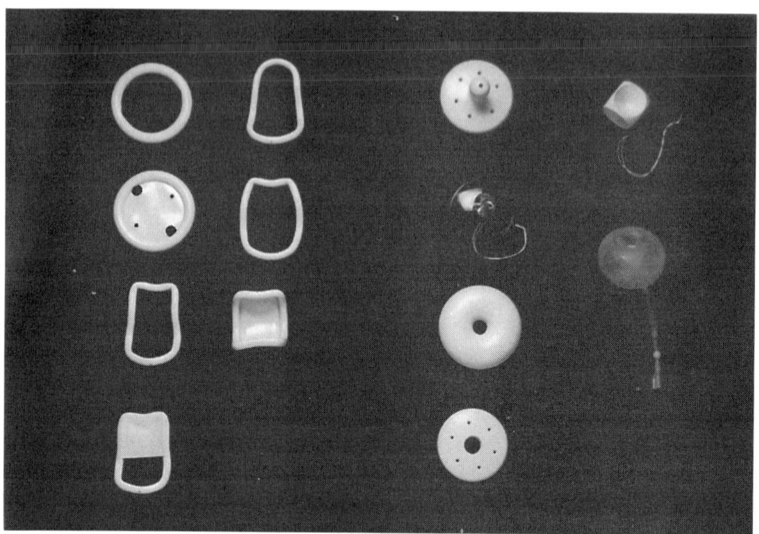

FIGURE 1.—Pessary types: support pessaries (columns 1 and 2 from left) and space-filling pessaries (columns 3 and 4 from left). (Reprinted with permission from The American College of Obstetricians and Gynecologists [Cundiff GW, Weidner AC, Visco AG, et al: A survey of pessary use by members of the American Urogynecologic Society. *Obstet Gynecol* 95(6):931-935, 2000.])

whereas the use of space-filling pessaries was more common for posterior defects (Fig 1 and Table 2). Fewer than half of the respondents considered previous hysterectomy or sexual activity to contraindicate pessary use. Sixty-four percent considered hypoestrogenism to be a contraindication. Ninety-two percent of the respondents believed that pessaries alleviate symptoms associated with pelvic organ prolapse. Forty-eight percent believed that pessaries also had therapeutic benefits in addition to alleviating symptoms.

Conclusions.—Trends in pessary use were identified in the current survey study. However, no clear consensus was observed on indications for support versus space-filling pessaries or on the use of a single pessary for all support defects versus tailoring the pessary to the specific defect. Randomized clinical studies are needed to determine optimal pessary use.

TABLE 2.—Top 3 Choices of Pessary by Support Defects Among Physicians Who Tailor the Pessary to the Support Defects

Choice	Anterior Defect (n = 247)	Apical Defect (n = 207)	Posterior Defect (n = 174)	Procidentia (n = 216)
First	Ring 124 (50%)	Donut 52 (25%)	Ring 82 (47%)	Gellhorn 84 (39%)
Second	Hodge 57 (23%)	Ring 41 (20%)	Hodge 33 (19%)	Donut 41 (19%)
Third	Gehrung 37 (15%)	Gellhorn 27 (13%)	Gellhorn 31 (18%)	InflatoBall 26 (12%)

(Reprinted with permission from the American College of Obstetricians and Gynecologists [Cundiff GW, Weidner AC, Visco AG, et al: A survey of pessary use by members of the American Urogynecologic Society. *Obstet Gynecol* 95(1):931-935, 2000.])

▶ This article introduces some of the controversies surrounding the use of pessaries and comprehensively surveys the limited literature on this oldest of methods for managing pelvic organ prolapse. The authors then proceed to report the results of the first reported pessary survey of experts on pelvic floor disorders. The results of the survey reveal that pessaries seem no longer relegated for use only by patients medically unfit for surgery, those waiting for surgery, or those refusing surgery.[1] The majority of responders used pessaries as first line therapy for prolapse of all vaginal segments. However, although the authors did not analyze for significant differences, my analysis confirms that responders were significantly less likely to use pessaries for posterior defects (rectoceles) than for anterior (cystoceles) or apical (vault or uterine) support defects. This may be testimony to the fact that it is easier for a pessary to hold something up (eg, a bladder or a uterus) than to hold something back (ie, the rectum). It is noteworthy that the cube pessary did not make the "top 3" list for any of the defects. Although the cube is very likely to stay in position, it is also significantly more likely to cause severe erosions,[2] often after only a few days. I suspect that many of the experienced clinicians in this survey had discovered this the hard way.

The authors did not ask in their survey how the responders themselves were instructed on using pessaries. I suspect that many learned by trial and error or by observing an older partner after they joined a practice. Many residents leave training without much experience with pessaries; as with many other aspects of medicine, as the prescriber gains experience, the treatment seems to become more effective. This article concludes with the observation that the death knell of pessaries may well be the economic hardship they impose on medical practices. With current Medicare reimbursement schemes often covering less than one- third to one- half of the practice's cost for pessaries, providing pessaries to older patients has become an act of charity that some practices and clinics may not be able to afford.

R. C. Bump, MD

References

1. Sulak PJ, Kuehl TJ, Shull BL: Vaginal pessaries and their use in pelvic relaxation. *J Reprod Med* 38:919-923, 1993.
2. Wu V, Farrell SA, Baskett TF, et al: A simplified protocol for pessary management. *Obstet Gynecol* 90:990-994, 1997.

Urodynamic Outcome After Surgery for Severe Prolapse and Potential Stress Incontinence
Klutke JJ, Ramos S (Univ of Southern California, Los Angeles)
Am J Obstet Gynecol 182:1378-1381, 2000
11–21

Background.—Paradoxically, women with severe prolapse may be continent, because of urethral kinking. Currently, urethropexy is commonly performed in women with prolapse when stress incontinence is observed on preoperative reduction of the prolapse. Urodynamic outcomes after reconstructive surgery that included suspending urethropexy were compared with outcomes after reconstruction alone.

Methods.—Between 1991 and 1997, 55 patients underwent urethropexy in addition to repair of the prolapse and 70 had reconstruction only. Charts were reviewed. Twenty-three patients in the first group and 20 in the second group were available at a mean 3.5 years for urodynamic follow-up assessment.

Findings.—Thirty percent of the patients in the urethropexy group had de novo detrusor instability, and 4% had stress incontinence. Five percent of the patients in the reconstruction-alone group had detrusor instability, and none had stress incontinence.

Conclusions.—Preoperative barrier assessment is helpful for identifying patients who do not need an anti-incontinence procedure. Prophylactic Burch retropubic urethropexy appears to increase the incidence of bladder instability.

▶ Using a pessary reduction test, the authors predicted genuine stress incontinence (GSI) in 44% of 125 women with advanced-stage pelvic organ prolapse (POP) and performed urethropexy on all of them. The remaining patients had vaginal prolapse surgery without urethropexy. Forty-two percent of the former group and 29% of the latter were evaluated 1 to 7 years after surgery in this retrospective study. Both groups had minimal risk of GSI, whereas the urethropexy group had significantly more detrusor instability.

It has long been recognized that surgical correction of severe POP may create symptomatic GSI in some women.[1] Severe POP, when accentuated by stress, will descend and obstruct the urethra, preventing stress incontinence.[2-4] Successful surgical correction of POP can eliminate this mechanical stress continence mechanism in some women. Preoperative physical reduction of the prolapse prevents this stress-activated urethral obstruction and reveals so-called occult or potential stress incontinence in from 36% to 80% of women with advanced prolapse.[2-5] The incidence of de novo postoperative GSI in this situation differs dramatically in various clinical series, however. Beck et al[1] reported that stress incontinence developed in only 10% of continent women undergoing vaginal prolapse surgery without suspending urethropexy. In contrast, Gordon et al[6] observed an 87% incidence of de novo GSI after vaginal surgery with Kelly plication of the bladder neck in 30 women who underwent vaginal surgery for advanced POP.

In the only randomized controlled trial addressing this issue, barrier testing predicted potential stress incontinence in 10 of 15 (67%) subjects who underwent vaginal prolapse surgery with endopelvic fascia plication of the bladder neck without a suspending urethropexy. However, GSI was observed in only 1 (7%) at 6 months. Formal suspending needle colposuspension increased the short-term complications, including prolonged retention and urgency incontinence due to detrusor instability, without providing additional protection for the development of de novo GSI.[7] In the same study, intrinsic urethral deficiency (ISD) was predicted by the barrier test in 7 of 29 women (24%), but only 1 of 7 (14%) actually demonstrated ISD 6 months after vaginal prolapse surgery that did not include a sling.

The fact that severe prolapse may mask potential GSI should be appreciated by every reconstructive pelvic surgeon. It should also be appreciated that a major aim of reconstructive surgery is for the patient to leave the operating room with durable and preferential support to the bladder neck. However, testing that will identify persons who *must* have that support provided by a formal urethropexy or sling has yet to be developed, standardized, or validated. As Klutke and Ramos aptly emphasize, older women with advanced POP often have deceptively precarious lower urinary tract function and may be more likely to experience complications of urethropexy (eg, urge incontinence or emptying-phase dysfunction) than they are to develop GSI for lack of a urethropexy.

R. C. Bump, MD

References

1. Beck RP, McCormick S, Nordstrom L: A 25-year experience with 519 anterior colporrhaphy procedures. *Obstet Gynecol* 78:1011-1018, 1991.
2. Richardson DA, Bent AE, Ostergard DR: The effect of uterovaginal prolapse on urethrovesical pressure dynamics. *Am J Obstet Gynecol* 146:901-905, 1983.
3. Bump RC, Fantl JA, Hurt WG: The mechanism of urinary continence in women with severe uterovaginal prolapse: Results of barrier studies. *Obstet Gynecol* 72:291-295, 1988.
4. Bergman A, Koonings PP, Ballard CA: Predicting postoperative urinary incontinence development in women undergoing operation for genitourinary prolapse. *Am J Obstet Gynecol* 158:1171-1175, 1988.
5. Rosenzweig BA, Pushkin S, Blumenfeld D, et al: Prevalence of abnormal urodynamic test results in continent women with severe genitourinary prolapse. *Obstet Gynecol* 79:539-542, 1992.
6. Gordon D, Groutz A, Wolman I, et al: Development of postoperative urinary stress incontinence in clinically continent patients undergoing prophylactic Kelly plication during genitourinary prolapse repair. *Neurourol Urodyn* 18:193-198, 1999.
7. Bump RC, Hurt WG, Theofrastous JP, et al: Randomized prospective comparison of needle colposuspension versus endopelvic fascia plication for potential stress incontinence prophylaxis in women undergoing vaginal reconstruction for stage III or IV pelvic organ prolapse. *Am J Obstet Gynecol* 175:326-335, 1996.

Urethral Diverticulum in Women: Diverse Presentations Resulting in Diagnostic Delay and Mismanagement

Romanzi LJ, Groutz A, Blaivas JG (Cornell Univ, New York)
J Urol 164:428-433, 2000   11–22

Background.—Urethral diverticulum in women is rare and is often seen with nonspecific, refractory, lower urinary tract symptoms that make diagnosis difficult. The authors' experience with 46 symptomatic women with urethral diverticulum was described.

Study Design.—The study consisted of a retrospective review of 46 consecutive symptomatic women with urethral diverticulum seen over a 6-year period. Most of the patients were referrals for refractory lower urinary tract symptoms. Clinical evaluation included history, physical examination, urinalysis and culture, 24-hour voiding diary, 24-hour pad test, video urodynamics, and urethrocystoscopy. Management was tailored to clinical findings. The women in the study group were aged 17 to 67 years.

Findings.—The most common symptoms were chronic, intermittent pain in 48%, urinary incontinence in 35% of patients, dyspareunia in 24%, and frequency/urgency in 22%. The interval between symptom onset and diagnosis ranged from 3 months to 27 years. Diverticula were palpable in 52%, and the content of the diverticulum could be "milked" through the urethral meatus in only 6 patients. There was malignancy in the diverticulum in 2 patients. Voiding cystourethrography was diagnostic in 65%, double balloon positive pressure urethrography in 11%, and transvaginal US in 15%. Diagnosis was incidental to vaginal operations in 9%. Transvaginal excision of the diverticulum with anti-incontinence and reconstructive procedures was performed for 75% of these patients.

Follow-up in this group ranged from 6 months to 6 years. All but 2 of the 22 women with pain symptoms became symptom-free. Pubovaginal sling was performed for 14 women, all of whom were postoperatively continent. Urethral reconstruction was required for 7 patients. One of them, who had a Tanagho reconstruction, had urge incontinence postoperatively. Five patients declined surgical treatment.

Conclusion.—Urethral diverticulum in women may have nonspecific, refractory lower urinary tract symptoms that make diagnosis difficult. A high index of suspicion is needed to diagnose this condition, especially when it is not palpable. A variety of imaging techniques may be necessary for diagnosis, but voiding cystourethrography is a good place to start. Treatment is usually by surgical excision, but reconstructive and continence measures need to be considered. Surgical treatment usually eliminates symptoms for women with urethral diverticulum.

▶ This article makes a number of useful observations regarding the presentation and evaluation of neglected or atypical urethral diverticula; however, it is unlikely that this report is generalizable to the majority of urethral diverticula. Clearly, 46 women referred to a busy tertiary urology service over a period of 6 years represents only a small fraction of all diverticula, given that the prevalence is estimated to be as high as 5% in women. It is possible that the authors did not see many women with the classic "3D" symptom complex of dysuria, dyspareunia, and dribbling because such women received their diagnoses without referral. Nonetheless, an important lesson from this series is to suspect a diverticulum as a cause of enigmatic chronic and episodic urethral, vaginal, and urinary symptoms.

In my clinical experience, many diverticula go undiagnosed because the diagnosis was never considered. The authors cite and confirm the statement of Davis and Telinde[1] that "the most important single diagnostic instrument for the discovery of a suburethral diverticula is a high index of suspicion." Imaging plays an important role in establishing or confirming the diagnosis and in establishing the complexity or multiplicity of the diverticulum so that complete operative removal can be ensured.

Voiding cystourethrography with a postvoid film will confirm most wide-mouthed diverticula, especially those associated with postvoid dribbling, but may not reveal the complexity of the diverticulum. Positive pressure urethrography and, increasingly, MRI seem the best techniques for this purpose. The latter is expensive but not prohibitively so, especially if one considers the cost of the single-use, double-balloon urethrography catheters; of the urologist or urogynecologist time required by the procedure; and of a lower positive and negative predictive value related to urethrography. Since a diverticulum will not cause classic stress urinary incontinence, any incontinence should be evaluated concurrently with the diverticulum evaluation so that definitive surgery can be directed at both problems if indicated. Finally, it should be emphasized that some diverticula are entirely incidental findings and may remain asymptomatic.

R. C. Bump, MD

Reference

1. Davis HJ, Telinde RW: Urethral diverticula: An assay of 121 cases. *J Urol* 80:34, 1958.

12 Infection

Effect of Condoms on Reducing the Transmission of Herpes Simplex Virus Type 2 From Men to Women

Wald A, Langenberg AGM, Link K, et al (Univ of Washington, Seattle; Chiron Corp, Emeryville, Calif; Westover Heights Clinic, Portland, Ore; et al)
JAMA 285:3100-3106, 2001

12–1

Background.—To date, no prospective study has shown that condom use reduces the transmission of herpes simplex virus type 2 (HSV-2). The risk factors for the acquisition of HSV-2 and the efficacy of condoms in preventing its transmission were reported.

Methods.—Data were obtained on 528 couples enrolled in a randomized, double-blind, placebo-controlled, 18-month follow-up trial of ineffective candidate HSV-2 vaccine conducted from 1993 to 1996. The couples were discordant for HSV-2 infection. Two hundred sixty-one men and 267 women were susceptible to HSV-2.

Findings.—Twenty-six women (9.7%) and 5 men (1.9%) acquired HSV-2 during follow-up. The rate per 10,000 sex acts for women and men were 8.9 and 1.5, respectively. A multivariate analysis showed that increased risk of HSV-2 acquisition was associated with younger age; seropositivity for HSV-1 and HSV-2, as opposed to HSV-2 alone in the source partner; and more frequent sexual activity. Condom use during more than 25% of sex acts protected women, but not men, from HSV-2 transmission. In the first 150 days, the risk of HSV-2 transmission was 8.5 per 100 person-years, declining to 0.9 in the final 150 days, concurrent with a decline in sexual activity and the proportion of sex acts taking place while the source partner had genital lesions.

Conclusion.—Condom use significantly protects susceptible women from HSV-2 transmission. Changes in sexual behavior after counseling to avoid sex in the presence of lesions were associated with a decrease in HSV-2 acquisition over time.

▶ It has been estimated that 22% of persons older than age 12 in the United States are infected with HSV-2. It is also estimated that about 500,000 uninfected people in the United States acquire HSV-2 each year, and 350,000 of them are women. The results of this study demonstrate that the use of a condom by a HSV-2–infected male partner during more than 25% of acts of sexual intercourse will significantly reduce the rate of HSV-2 transmission to the female partner by 75%. Therefore, uninfected women having sexual activity with a HSV-2–infected male partner should have the partner use a condom.

D. R. Mishell, Jr, MD

Vaginal Clindamycin and Oral Metronidazole for Bacterial Vaginosis: A Randomized Trial
Paavonen J, Mangioni C, Martin MA, et al (Univ of Helsinki; Ospedale S Gerardo di Monza, Italy; Pharmacia & Upjohn, Kalamazoo, Mich)
Obstet Gynecol 96:256-260, 2000   12–2

Introduction.—The standard treatment for bacterial vaginosis (BV) is metronidazole, 500 mg orally twice daily for 7 days. Clindamycin cream, 2% administered topically for 7 days, is as effective as standard metronidazole treatment for BV. The safety and efficacy of clindamycin vaginal ovules and oral metronidazole in the treatment of BV were compared.

Methods.—In this controlled, double-masked trial conducted at 23 European sites, women were randomly assigned to treatment with either 100-mg ovules of clindamycin (intravaginally for 3 consecutive days) plus placebo capsules (orally twice daily for 7 days) or metronidazole 500 mg (2 250-mg capsules orally twice daily for 7 days) plus placebo ovules (intravaginally for 3 consecutive days). The planned sample gave a probability of .84 of correctly concluding that the success rate of clindamycin ovules is not more than 15% less than the expected 75% success rate for metronidazole. Patients were evaluated at baseline and at 12 to 16 days and 28 to 42 days after initiation of treatment. A vulvovaginal examination was performed, and vaginal discharge was described. Additional examinations included pH, odor, and clue cells.

Results.—Of 399 women enrolled, 233 were available for determination of efficacy. Seventy-seven of 113 patients (68.1%) were cured with clindamycin treatment and 80 of 120 (66.7%) were cured with metronidazole (P = .810). Treatment-related adverse events were more common in the metronidazole group than in the clindamycin group (16.3% vs 10.3%; P = .104). Most of the difference between groups was due to systemic symptoms, including nausea and altered taste.

Conclusion.—A 3-day regimen of clindamycin, administered as intravaginal ovules, was as effective as and better tolerated than a 7-day regimen of oral metronidazole, 500 mg administered twice daily, for treatment of BV.

▶ Both oral metronidazole and vaginal clindamycin are effective therapies for BV. There appear to be fewer gastrointestinal side effects with vaginally administered clindamycin than with oral metronidazole. Clindamycin can be administered vaginally as 2% vaginal cream or as the vaginal ovules described in this report. One applicator (5-g) of vaginal cream and 1 ovule each contains 100 mg of clindamycin phosphate. Either formulation may be inserted at bedtime for at least 3 consecutive days to treat BV.

D. R. Mishell, Jr, MD

Metronidazole for Bacterial Vaginosis: A Comparison of Vaginal Gel vs Oral Therapy

Hanson JM, McGregor JA, Hillier SL, et al (Univ of Colorado, Denver; Univ of Pittsburgh, Pa; Univ of Washington, Seattle; et al)
J Reprod Med 45:889-896, 2000

12–3

Background.—Metronidazole vaginal gel is the treatment currently recommended by the Centers for Disease Control for bacterial vaginosis (BV). The efficacy rates of this treatment range from 78% to 87% 1 to 2 weeks after treatment and from 63% to 73% 4 to 5 weeks after treatment. The efficacy, patient tolerance, and patient use characteristics associated with 0.75% metronidazole vaginal gel and oral metrondazole tablets in the treatment of clinical BV in nonpregnant women were compared.

Methods.—One hundred twelve women were enrolled in the study. By random assignment, the women received 0.75% metronidazole vaginal gel, 5 g twice daily for 5 days, or oral metronidazole, 500 mg twice daily for 7 days. The patients were assessed approximately 2 and 5 weeks after initial treatment.

Findings.—At the first follow-up evaluation, BV was clinically eliminated in 83.7% of those receiving intravaginal treatment and in 85.1% of those receiving oral treatment. At the last follow-up visit, BV was eliminated in 70.7% and 71.1%, respectively. Gastrointestinal problems occurred in 51.8% of the oral treatment group and in 32.7% of the intravaginal treatment group, a significant difference.

Conclusion.—The efficacy of 0.75% metronidazole vaginal gel for women with BV is comparable to that of standard oral metronidazole. The intravaginal treatment was associated with significantly fewer gastrointestinal problems.

▶ When a single dose of 5 gm of 0.75% gel of metronidazole is administered vaginally, the maximum serum concentration is about 2% of that following ingestion of a 500 mg tablet. Thus, one would expect that gastrointestinal side effects would be less with the vaginal than with the oral administration of metronidazole. This randomized trial found that the vaginal administration of the gel twice daily for 5 days was as effective as ingestion of 500-mg metronidazole tablets twice daily for 7 days with less side effects. A recent study reported that once-daily dosing with the vaginal gel was as effective as twice-daily dosing. Thus, clinicians can use a single dose of 5-gm topical 0.75% vaginal gel of metronidazole daily for 5 days to treat BV with similar effectiveness to 7 days of twice daily oral therapy and have fewer gastrointestinal side effects.

D. R. Mishell, Jr, MD

Efficacy of Maintenance Therapy With Topical Boric Acid in Comparison With Oral Itraconazole in the Treatment of Recurrent Vulvovaginal Candidiasis

Guaschino S, De Seta F, Sartore A, et al (Univ of Trieste, Italy)
Am J Obstet Gynecol 184:598-602, 2001

12–4

Background.—The best treatment for recurrent vulvovaginal candidiasis is still debated. The efficacy of topical long-term treatment with boric acid was compared with that of oral long-term treatment with itraconazole in curing and preventing recurrent vulvovaginal candidiasis.

Methods.—Twenty-two patients were recruited for the prospective, nonrandomized study. Group 1 was treated with itraconazole, and group 2 was treated with boric acid. Follow-up extended for 1 year.

Findings.—During treatment, the 2 groups were comparable in positive culture results and in signs and symptoms. Six months after treatment cessation, relapses were common in both groups, at a mean 54.5%.

Conclusion.—Boric acid appears to be promising for treating vaginal infection and preventing recurrent vulvovaginal candidiasis. However, its efficacy ends with treatment cessation.

▶ About 5% of women who have a single episode of vulvovaginal candidiasis will have multiple episodes of infection during the following year. Recurrent vulvovaginal candidiasis is difficult to treat. The results of this small comparative study indicate that use of vaginal administration of 300 mg of boric acid daily for 5 days after the beginning of menses in each cycle is an effective and inexpensive method for the prevention of episodes of recurrent vulvovaginal candidiasis. The first episode of vulvovaginal infection with candidiasis was effectively treated with daily vaginal administration of 300 mg of boric acid for 14 doses.

D. R. Mishell, Jr, MD

Relationship of Bacterial Vaginosis and Mycoplasmas to the Risk of Spontaneous Abortion

Donders GGG, Van Bulck B, Caudron J, et al (Katholieke Universiteit Leuven, Belgium; Erasmus Hosp; Algemen Ziekenhuis St Blasius)
Am J Obstet Gynecol 183:431-437, 2000

12–5

Introduction.—There is increasing evidence of an association between anaerobic vaginal flora and bacterial vaginosis (BV) with intrauterine infection, intrauterine growth restriction, premature rupture of membranes, and preterm delivery. The vaginal flora of women was examined during early pregnancy to ascertain its relationship to subsequent spontaneous early loss of pregnancy.

Methods.—Between March 1989 and March 1994, 228 unselected women seen for routine pregnancy checkup at less than 14 completed gestational weeks who had living singleton fetuses underwent standardized vaginal speculum examination for microbiologic flora of the vagina. BV was evaluated either clinically (Amsel et al criteria), microscopically (clue cells), or by culture of BV-associated bacteria. Univariate (relative risk) and multivariate analyses were conducted.

Results.—The presence of BV at the first prenatal visit was strongly correlated with subsequent early pregnancy loss (relative risk, 5.4). Multivariate analyses revealed that *Gardnerella vaginalis, Mycoplasma hominis,* and *Ureaplasma urealyticum* but not other microorganisms were associated with increased risk of miscarriage.

Conclusion.—BV, particularly when *G vaginalis* or Mycoplasma was cultured, was correlated with a 5-fold increased risk of spontaneous abortion. The most likely mechanism is an ascending spread of infection followed by an inflammatory reaction.

▶ The results of this study indicate that the presence of BV diagnosed clinically or by cultures of *Gardnerella vaginalis, Ureaplasma urealyticum,* or *Mycoplasma hominis* in the vaginal secretions significantly increased the risk of early pregnancy loss after a viable fetus was visualized sonographically. The presence of other pathogenic organisms, including *Chlamydia trachomatis,* did not increase the rate of miscarriage. It remains to be determined whether appropriate therapy to treat BV or these other organisms in early pregnancy will effectively lower the rate of spontaneous miscarriage. Until such studies are performed, clinicians may wish to determine whether BV or any of these other organisms are present in the vaginal secretions of women with a history of unexplained recurrent abortion. If any are present, appropriate therapy can be given before conception is attempted.

D. R. Mishell, Jr, MD

13 Endocrinology

Outcome in Patients With Eating Disorders: A 5-Year Study
Ben-Tovim DI, Walker K, Gilchrist P, et al (Flinders Med Centre, Adelaide, Australia)
Lancet 357:1254-1257, 2001   13–1

Introduction.—Trials examining the outcomes of patients with eating disorders, including anorexia nervosa and bulimia, have been limited by technical and sampling problems. Predictors of outcome and effectiveness of available treatments were prospectively examined in a 5-year investigation of a representative sample of patients with eating disorders.

Methods.—Females 15 years of age or older who were making first contact with secondary or tertiary services for treatment of an eating disorder were evaluated within 48 hours of index contact and at 6 months and 5 years. There were 95 patients with anorexia nervosa, 88 with bulimia nervosa, and 37 with eating disorders not otherwise specified (EDNOS). Patients were grouped according to those who had and those who had not received treatment in specialist units and reached a safe body weight. They were further classified according to the intensity of any treatment they received. Clinical symptoms, body-related attitudes, and psychosocial function were evaluated.

Results.—There were 216 patients (98%) who were available for follow-up after 5 years. There were 5 deaths, 3 in patients with anorexia nervosa and 2 in patients with EDNOS. At 5-year follow-up, 65 (74%) patients with bulimia, 29 (78%) with EDNOS, and 53 (56%) with anorexia had no diagnosable eating disorder. A few patients in each group had poor Morgan-Russell Hayward scores. The final outcome was predicted by the extent and intensity, not the duration, of baseline symptoms among patients with anorexia nervosa and by initial body-related attitudes and impaired psychosocial functioning among patients with bulimia. The outcome of patients with EDNOS could not be predicted. Outcome was not affected by treatment in any group.

Conclusion.—Clear differences were observed in overall outcomes and the characteristics that predicted those outcomes in patients with bulimia and anorexia nervosa. These findings offer support for separate identities for anorexia and bulimia.

▶ Eating disorders are not uncommon among young women. These disorders are disabling, unpredictable, and difficult to treat. The main findings of this 5-year prospective study are that anorexia nervosa is a much more serious disorder than bulimia, and treatment of anorexia nervosa has little effect upon its prognosis or outcome. However three fourths of the women with bulimia had no evidence of eating disorders 5 years after enrollment in the study and, in contrast to anorexia nervosa, no woman with bulimia died during the follow-up period.

D. R. Mishell, Jr, MD

Long-Term Follow-Up of 246 Hyperprolactinemic Patients

Touraine P, Plu-Bureau G, Beji C, et al (Hôpital Necker, Paris)
Acta Obstet Gynecol Scand 80:162-168, 2001

13–2

Background.—A major cause of infertility in women is hyperprolactinemia, and many of these cases are caused by pituitary adenoma. Numerous treatments for prolactin-secreting pituitary tumors have been advocated, including transsphenoidal surgery to remove the adenoma, long-term treatment with an antitumoral dopaminergic agonist, or observation (as many of these tumors regress spontaneously). The outcomes of all 3 of these methods were compared in a long-term retrospective study of women with hyperprolactinemia.

Methods.—The 246 women with hyperprolactinemia were examined between 1978 and 1994, primarily for menstrual disturbances (92%) and/or galactorrhea (69%). None of the patients had hypothyroidism, chronic renal failure, or a drug-related disturbance in prolactin level. Most patients underwent a thyrotropin-releasing hormone stimulation test for confirmation and imaging (CT or MRI) to identify the presence and size of any adenoma. Treatment consisted of bromocriptine in 191 patients, surgery in 32, and observation in 23 (most of the last had low prolactin levels and no adenomas). Patients were followed up for a mean of 99.9 months to assess changes in prolactin levels and adenoma size.

Results.—At the initial evaluation, the mean plasma prolactin level was 135.0 ng/mL. An adenoma was detected in 122 of 204 patients (60%) who underwent imaging (64% microadenoma, 36% macroadenoma). Larger tumors were significantly associated with higher prolactin levels and with amenorrhea (compared with oligomenorrhea). During follow-up, prolactin levels decreased significantly in the patients taking bromocriptine, from 99.6 to 20.0 ng/mL. Of the 96 patients with initial and follow-up imaging studies, the adenoma resolved during treatment in 43 patients (45%), did not change in size in 38 patients (40%), and was visualized at the last follow-up visit in 15 patients (15%). In all 96 patients, however, prolactin levels decreased significantly. Among the 32 patients treated surgically, 8 had a microadenoma and 24 had a macroadenoma. At follow-up, prolactin levels were less than 10 ng/mL in only 8 patients (28%), even though no tumor was detectable in 24 of the 25 patients (96%) who underwent imaging. Thus, bromocriptine was given to the remaining 24 patients, and in most cases, prolactin levels subsequently normalized. Among the 23 untreated patients, prolactin levels decreased significantly over follow-up, from 71.2 to 42.5 ng/mL. Existing adenomas did not change in size, nor did any new adenomas develop in this group.

Conclusion.—After a mean follow-up of more than 8 years, women with mild hyperprolactinemia who took bromocriptine had lower levels of prolactin than patients treated surgically or those who were not treated. Among the patients taking bromocriptine, prolactin levels decreased during follow-up in all patients, even though 15 adenomas developed during this period; this "increase" in adenomas was likely caused by the increased sensitivity of pituitary imaging in recent years. Most patients treated surgically did not respond to resection alone and required bromocriptine for normalization of prolactin levels.

▶ This long-term follow-up study adds to our body of knowledge which indicates that prolactin-secreting pituitary microadenomas do not enlarge and may resolve completely when bromocriptine treatment is utilized. Among the small number of women who did not receive therapy, the adenomas also did not enlarge and prolactin levels decreased. Clinicians treating women who have prolactin-secreting microadenomas with bromocriptine should discontinue therapy every 1 to 2 years to determine whether prolactin levels remain normal. If so, bromocriptine therapy can be discontinued.

D. R. Mishell, Jr, MD

Women With Polycystic Ovary Syndrome Gain Regular Menstrual Cycles When Ageing
Elting MW, Korsen TJM, Rekers-Mombarg LTM, et al (Research Inst of Endocrinology, Reproduction and Metabolism, Amsterdam; Free Univ, Amsterdam)
Hum Reprod 15:24-28, 2000   13–3

Background.—Treating enlarged polycystic ovaries by wedge resection can result in regular menstrual cycles in patients with polycystic ovary syndrome (PCOS). Whether reduction of the antral follicle cohort from aging also leads to regular menstrual cycles in such patients was investigated.

Methods and Findings.—Two hundred five patients with PCOS participated in a telephone survey. All were aged 30 years and older. A highly significant linear trend for a shorter menstrual cycle length with increasing age was noted (Fig 1). The influence of age on menstrual cycle regularity persisted after statistical adjustment for body mass index, weight loss, hirsutism, previous clomiphene citrate or gonadotrophin treatment, previous pregnancy, ethnic origin, and smoking status.

Conclusions.—Regular menstrual cycles develop with aging in women with PCOS. The development of a new balance between inhibin B and follicle-stimulating hormone in the polycystic ovary, resulting solely from

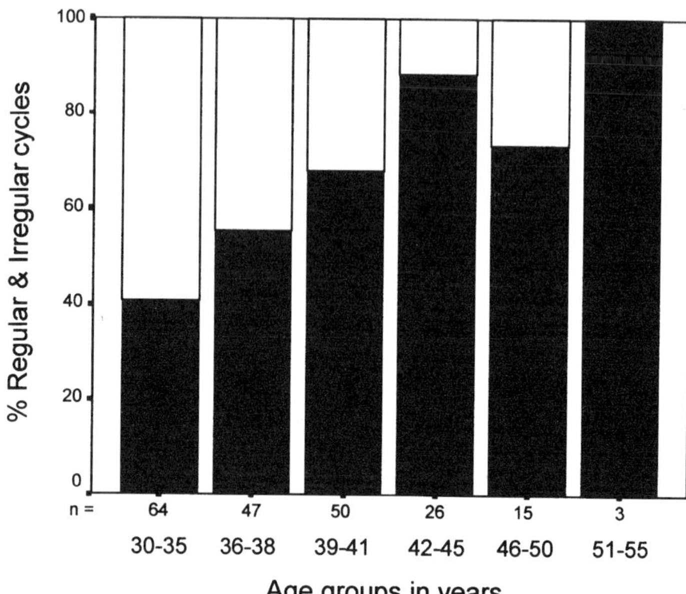

FIGURE 1.—Percentages of regular and irregular cycles in the various age groups, *n* is the number of patients in each age group. *black bars* indicate regular; *white bars* indicate irregular. (Courtesy of Elting MW, Korsen TJM, Rekers-Mombarg LTM, et al: Women with polycystic ovary syndrome gain regular menstrual cycles when ageing. *Hum Reprod* 15:24-28, 2000. Copyright, European Society for Human Reproduction and Embryology, by permission of Oxford University Press.)

follicle loss through ovarian aging, appears to explain the occurrence of these regular cycles.

▶ It appears that women with PCOS tend to develop regular ovulatory menstrual cycles as they age. However, if women with PCOS do not wish to conceive, it is beneficial to treat them with oral contraceptive to decrease circulating free testosterone levels as well as to prevent endometrial hyperplasia and endometrial adenocarcinoma.

D. R. Mishell, Jr, MD

Cardiovascular Disease in Women With Polycystic Ovary Syndrome at Long-Term Follow-Up: A Retrospective Cohort Study

Wild S, Pierpoint T, McKeigue P, et al (Univ College London)
Clin Endocrinol (Oxf) 52:595-600, 2000

13–4

Introduction.—Polycystic ovary syndrome (PCOS) is thought to be associated with increased risk of diabetes and coronary heart disease (CHD). Yet this has not been demonstrated in women with PCOS. The cardiovascular (CV) mortality and morbidity rates in middle-aged women in whom PCOS was diagnosed before 1979 were compared with age-matched controls in a retrospective cohort trial of women in the United Kingdom.

Methods.—Of 319 women in the cohort, 70 died before March 31, 1999. There were 1060 age-matched controls. National mortality rates were used to determine the expected number of deaths from the number of female-years at risk in each 5-year age group and 5-year calendar period. The general practitioners of all traced survivors of the cohort below the age of 75 years were contacted. Data were gathered from death certificates, general practitioners' records, and questionnaires with a measurement of CV risk factors in a subsample of questionnaire respondents.

Results.—Mean participant age was 56.7 years. The average follow-up since PCOS diagnosis was 31 years (range, 15 to 47 years) for patients with PCOS. All-cause and CV mortality in women with PCOS was similar to that of women in the general population (standardized mortality ratios, 93 and 78, respectively). Women with PCOS had higher levels of several CV risk factors: diabetes ($P = .002$), hypertension ($P = .04$), hypercholesterolemia ($P < .001$), hypertriglyceridemia ($P = .02$), and increased waist-hip ratio ($P = .004$). After adjustment for body mass index, odds ratios (OR) were 2.2, 1.4, and 3.2, respectively, for diabetes, hypertension, and hypercholesterolemia. A history of CHD was not significantly more frequent in women with PCOS (crude OR, 1.5). The crude OR for CV disease was 2.8. There were no between-group differences in prevalence of smoking, blood pressure, use of lipid-lowering or hormone replacement therapy, or proportion of women with undiagnosed diabetes ($P < .1$ for all variables).

Conclusion.—Women with PCOS have a higher rate of several CV risk factors, but no significant excess of CHD deaths or morbidity was identified among middle-aged women with PCOS. These findings indicate that control of weight and blood pressure in women with PCOS is important to decrease their excess risk of diabetes and CV disease.

▶ Women with PCOS have a higher incidence of risk factors for CV disease than age-matched controls without PCOS. However, despite the fact that women with PCOS are more likely to have diabetes, hypertension, hypercholesterolemia, hypertriglyceridemia, and an increased waist-to-hip ratio, the results of this study indicated that they were no more likely to die of CV disease than a control population. Women with PCOS should be encouraged to lose weight and exercise regularly as well as to control their blood pressure and glucose metabolism.

D. R. Mishell, Jr, MD

Troglitazone Improves Ovulation and Hirsutism in the Polycystic Ovary Syndrome: A Multicenter, Double Blind, Placebo-controlled Trial

Azziz R, for the PCOS/Troglitazone Study Group (Parke-Davis Pharmaceutical Res, Ann Arbor, Mich; et al)
J Clin Endocrinol Metab 86:1626-1632, 2001   13–5

Introduction.—Current therapies for polycystic ovary syndrome (PCOS) focus on suppressing androgen production or effect or on inducing ovulation. Several recent trials have demonstrated a beneficial effect of insulin-lowering agents for patients with PCOS. Troglitazone is an insulin-sensitizing agent of the thiazolidinedione class that has a postinsulin receptor mechanism of action. The effect of treatment with troglitazone on ovulatory dysfunction, hirsutism, hyperandrogenemia, and hyperinsulinemia was examined in 410 premenopausal women with PCOS in a multicenter, double-blind, placebo-controlled, randomized trial.

Methods.—Patients were randomly assigned to 44 weeks of treatment with either placebo (PBO) or troglitazone (150 mg/d [TGZ-150], 300 mg/d [TGZ-300], or 600 mg/d [TGZ-600]). Changes in ovulatory function were compared by monitoring the urinary levels of pregnanediol-3-glucuronide daily. Hirsutism was measured by a modified Ferriman-Gallwey scoring method. Assessment of hormone levels included measures of total and free testosterone, androstenedione, sex hormone–binding globulin, luteinizing hormone, lutein-stimulating hormone, and the luteinizing hormone/lutein-stimulating hormone ratio. Determination of glycemic parameters included fasting level of glucose, insulin, hemaglobin A_{1c}), and the glucose and insulin areas under the curve during an oral glucose challenge.

Results.—Of 410 patients recruited, 305 (74.4%) were included in the analyses. Baseline patient characteristics were similar across all 4 treatment arms. Ovulatory rates were significantly higher for patients who received TGZ-300 and TGZ-600, compared with PBO (0.42 and 0.58 vs 0.32; $P < .05$ and 0.0001, respectively). Of patients who were treated with TGZ-600, 57% ovulated over 50% of the time, compared with 12% of placebo-treated patients. There was a significant reduction in the Ferriman-Gallwey score in the TGZ-600–versus the PBO-treated patients (0.22 and -2.21; $P < .05$, respectively). Free testosterone decreased and sex hormone–binding globulin rose in a dose-related fashion with TGZ treatment. All 3 TGZ treatment groups differed significantly from placebo. Almost all glycemic parameters demonstrated dose-related reductions with TGZ treatment. Treatment groups were similar in the total number and severity of adverse events (including liver enzyme elevations) and the proportion of patients withdrawn from the trial because of adverse effects.

Conclusion.—Ovulatory dysfunction, hirsutism, hyperandrogenemia, and insulin resistance are improved in a dose-related fashion and with minimum adverse effects in patients with PCOS.

▶ Treatment of anovulation in women with PCOS who wish to conceive is difficult. Most women with PCOS do not ovulate following use of clomiphene citrate. Use of human menopausal gonadotropin or follicle-stimulating hormone with or without gonadotropin-releasing hormone analogues is expensive and requires very careful monitoring to avoid ovarian hyperstimulation. The use of 600 mg of TGZ daily, as reported in this large 44-week study, was a very effective method for inducing ovulatory cycles as well as reducing the amount of hirsutism in women with PCOS. This agent was also found to be safe. Thus, clinicians can treat anovulatory women with PCOS with 600 mg TGZ daily and expect a 60% rate of ovulation. This rate can probably be further increased with the use of periodic clomiphene citrate in addition to daily TGZ.

D. R. Mishell, Jr, MD

Metformin Increases the Ovulatory Rate and Pregnancy Rate From Clomiphene Citrate in Patients With Polycystic Ovary Syndrome Who Are Resistant to Clomiphene Citrate Alone

Vandermolen DT, Ratts VS, Evans WS, et al (Virginia Commonwealth Univ, Richmond; Washington Univ, St Louis; Univ of Virginia, Charlottesville)
Fertil Steril 75:310-315, 2001   13–6

Introduction.—Many women with polycystic ovary syndrome (PCOS) are resistant to insulin and have compensatory hyperinsulinemia. Hyperinsulinemia has a pathologic role in PCOS and seems to contribute to both chronic anovulation and hyperandrogenism. Obese women with PCOS are especially resistant to ovulation. Several trials of women with PCOS have revealed that when insulin-secretion is diminished with insulin sensitizing drugs, there is an increase in the rates of spontaneous ovulation and ovulation in response to clomiphene citrate (CC). Metformin, an insulin-sensitizing drug, was assessed for its ability to increase the ovulation and pregnancy rates in response to CC in women resistant to CC alone.

Methods.—All women in this randomized, double-blind, placebo-controlled trial were 18 to 35 years of age, wanted to become pregnant, and were anovulatory in response to a 5-day course of CC, 150 mg/day. To qualify for the study, patients also needed to have oligo-ovulation (fewer than 6 menstrual periods annually), hyperandrogenism, normal levels of thyroid-stimulating hormone, prolactin, 17-hydroxyprogesterone (less than 200 ng/dL), normal renal functioning, and normal liver function. Patients received either metformin, 500 mg 3 times daily for 7 weeks, or placebo. Data regarding reproductive steroids, gonadotropins, and oral glucose tolerance testing were collected at baseline and after treatment. Patients continued to receive either metformin or placebo, and CC treatment was initiated at 50 mg daily for 5 days. Ovulation was determined by a serum P level of 4 ng/mL or above. During ovulation, the daily CC dose was unchanged. With anovulation, the daily CC dose was increased by 50 mg for the next cycle. Patients completed their participation in the trial when they had 6 ovulatory cycles, became pregnant, or experienced an-

TABLE 2.—Ovulatory and Pregnancy Outcomes in Response to
Clomiphene Citrate

Outcome	Metformin Group	Placebo Group	P Value
No. of women who ovulated/total no. of women	9/12	4/15	.02
No. of women who ovulated (%)	(75)	(27)	
No. of women who conceived/total no. of women	6/11	1/14	.02
No. of women who conceived (%)	(55)	(7)	

Note: One patient each in the metformin and placebo groups who ovulated failed to complete the study protocol and was not included in the pregnancy rate analysis.

(Courtesy of Vandermolen DT, Ratts VS, Evans WS: Metformin increases the ovulatory rate and pregnancy rate from clomiphene citrate in patients with polycystic ovary syndrome who are resistant to clomiphene citrate alone. *Fertil Steril* 75:310-315, 2001. Reprinted by permission from the American Society for Reproductive Medicine.)

ovulation while receiving 150 mg of CC. The primary outcome measures were ovulation and pregnancy rates.

Results.—Nine of the 12 (75%) women in the metformin plus CC group and 4 of 15 (27%) in the placebo plus CC group ovulated ($P = .02$). Six of 11 participants (55%) in the metformin plus CC group and 1 of 14 (7%) in the placebo plus CC group became pregnant ($P = .02$) (Table 2). No significant changes in fasting insulin level, area under the curve for insulin, or fasting glucose-insulin ratio were observed in the metformin versus placebo group.

Conclusion.—The use of metformin significantly increased the ovulation rate and the pregnancy rate from CC treatment in anovulatory women with PCOS who were resistant to CC.

▶ It has been estimated that about one fourth of anovulatory women with PCOS do not ovulate when treated with CC. Various therapies, including the use of gonadotropin, partial ovarian destruction, and addition of dexamethasone, have been used to induce ovulation in these women. The results of this randomized trial provide evidence in addition to that suggested by earlier observational studies that use of the insulin-sensitizing agent metformin increases the ovulatory response to CC in a group of obese women with PCOS. Because of the result of these studies, clinicians may wish to administer metformin to anovulatory women with PCOS who do not ovulate with CC alone. Metformin should continue to be ingested until pregnancy occurs and perhaps throughout the duration of pregnancy, as suggested in the abstract that follows.

D. R. Mishell, Jr, MD

Continuing Metformin Throughout Pregnancy in Women With Polycystic Ovary Syndrome Appears to Safely Reduce First-Trimester Spontaneous Abortion: A Pilot Study
Glueck CJ, Phillips H, Cameron D, et al (Jewish Hosp, Cincinnati, Ohio)
Fertil Steril 75:46-52, 2001   13–7

Introduction.—Metformin is not considered a teratogenic drug by the Food and Drug Administration, but anecdotal experience shows that metformin therapy is usually discontinued during pregnancy in women with polycystic ovary syndrome (PCOS) who conceived while receiving the drug. Metformin was evaluated for its ability to safely decrease the rate of first-trimester spontaneous abortion without producing teratogenicity.

Methods.—Twenty-two previously oligoamenorrheic, nondiabetic women with PCOS who conceived while receiving metformin and continued therapy throughout pregnancy were evaluated in a prospective pilot trial. They were retrospectively compared with 125 women with PCOS who were not currently pregnant and who had 1 or more previous pregnancies while they were not receiving metformin. Patients in the prospective group took metformin, 1.5 to 2.55 g/day, throughout pregnancy. The primary outcome measures were rates of first-trimester spontaneous abortion and teratogenicity.

Results.—Before metformin, 10 women had 22 previous pregnancies with 16 first-trimester spontaneous abortions (73%). While taking metformin, these 10 women had 6 normal live births (60%), 1 spontaneous abortion (10%), and 3 normal ongoing pregnancies, all 13 weeks or more (30%; median gestation, 23 weeks). The first-trimester spontaneous abortion rate was 10% (1/10) while the women was receiving metformin, compared with a rate of 73% in 22 previous pregnancies when women were not taking metformin ($P < .002$). At final follow-up, among the 19 women who continued metformin therapy throughout pregnancy, there were 11 normal live births without defects (58%), 2 first-trimester spontaneous abortions (10.5%), and 6 ongoing normal pregnancies, all 13 or more weeks (32%; median gestation, 23 weeks). Sonography revealed normal fetal development without congenital defects in the 6 ongoing pregnancies. There were no maternal adverse effects. In women who received metformin before conception, decreases in insulin and plasminogen activator inhibitory activity were correlated ($r = .65; P - .04$). There were 265 pregnancies in the 125 women with PCOS who had 1 or more earlier pregnancies without metformin therapy. Of these, 39% of the pregnancies ended in first-trimester spontaneous abortions and 60% resulted in live births.

Conclusion.—Metformin therapy throughout pregnancy in women with PCOS decreases the otherwise high rate of first-trimester spontaneous abortion observed among women not receiving metformin. Metformin does not seem to have teratogenic effects.

▶ The results of this observational study suggest that administration of metformin in doses of 1.5 to 2.55 mg per day throughout pregnancy to women with PCOS may reduce the rate of spontaneous abortion. The authors postulate that this reduction may be due to metformin's ability to reduce plasminogen activator inhibitor activity. A randomized placebo-controlled trial with metformin needs to be undertaken to confirm whether this agent is able to reduce the high spontaneous abortion rate that occurs among women with PCOS who become pregnant.

D. R. Mishell, Jr, MD

▶ There is a growing awareness of the relationship between PCOS in women and what is variously called syndrome X or the dysmetabolic syndrome in men. The latter was originally described in men with accelerated atherosclerosis and early coronary heart disease who had insulin resistance, dyslipidemia (elevated LDL and decreased HDL), hyperlipidemia, and vascular hypertension in common. One hypothesis is that when syndrome X occurs in women, the associated biochemical hyperandrogenism results in anovulation, menstrual abnormalities, and infertility. Because the cyclic ovarian function of women during the reproductive period is lacking in men, this co-occurrence results in the definition of a second syndrome, PCOS. Whether syndrome X in men is associated with increased testosterone, androstenedione, and DHEA, as it is in PCOS, is both unclear and infrequently studied.

The use of metformin to reduce insulin resistance in type II gravid diabetics and to treat PCOS bears on this hypothesis and is the focus of this prospective pilot study. Women with PCOS treated with metformin have decreased insulin resistance and decreased serum insulin concentrations and resume normal menses in 90% of cases. Furthermore, they are spared the 40% to 50% incidence of spontaneous abortion in the event they become pregnant (rates seen in untreated women with PCOS). They also regain fertility.

Because metformin crosses the placenta, concerns regarding the deleterious effect of decreased insulin sensitivity in the fetus have arisen, and alternative means of treating insulin resistance in pregnant diabetics are being explored (see the 1998 YEAR BOOK OF OBSTETRICS, GYNECOLOGY, AND WOMEN'S HEALTH, pp 99-100 and the 2002 YEAR BOOK 4–3). However, these authors report 22 women who have conceived while receiving metformin for PCOS, 19 of whom continued the drug throughout pregnancy. In 3 other cases metformin was discontinued at 4 to 6 weeks of pregnancy. In an unblinded, nonrandomized cohort comparison with 118 nonpregnant women with PCOS not treated with metformin, we learned something about both PCOS and metformin effects on pregnancy.

In a previous study of 41 women with PCOS, these authors found elevated concentrations of platelet activator inhibitor (PAI), an inhibitor of fibrinolysis and therefore a thrombogenic agent possibly important in women who subsequently conceived and aborted.[1] They found PAI activity to be a significant independent factor for spontaneous abortion and found it reduced in maternal blood by treatment with metformin from a mean of 21 u/mL to 7 u/mL. Perhaps this accounts for the improved pregnancy survival in women conceiving after treatment of PCOS with metformin. Similarly, fasting serum insulin concentrations were reduced significantly in women with PCOS receiving metformin, and a reduction in thcir PAI concentration was directly correlated with that change. For all 19 women taking metformin throughout pregnancy, 89% had either normal newborns or were undelivered of fetuses without ultrasonic abnormality at publication date. Their incidence of spontaneous abortion was 10.5%, and there were no newborn abnormalities except for patent foramen ovale noted in 1 case.

This is suggestive evidence limited by small case numbers that metformin is effective in reducing insulin sensitivity in type II pregnant diabetics and reducing elevated PAI and then simultaneously reducing the risk of abortion from thrombotic events in early pregnancy. This may well be sufficient rationale for a major prospective study to explore possible fetal developmental abnormality associated with metformin use during pregnancy in view of the related apparent benefit in pregnancy survival that it affords.

T. H. Kirschbaum, MD

Reference

1. Gleuck CJ, Wang P, Fontaine RN, et al: Plasminogen activator inhibitor activity. *Metabolism* 48:1589-1595, 1999.

Spironolactone as a Single Agent for Long-Term Therapy of Hirsute Patients

Spritzer PM, Lisboa KO, Mattiello S, et al (Universidade Federal do Rio Grande do Sul, Brazil)
Clin Endocrinol (Oxf) 52:587-594, 2000   13–8

Introduction.—The 2 antiandrogens most frequently prescribed for hirsutism are spironolactone and cyproterone acetate (CPA). The general therapeutic effectiveness of these 2 drugs has been verified. Yet extended clinical trials conducted with either drug have yielded variable results. The androgen-suppressing effect of spironolactone and the use of this drug as a single agent in the long-term treatment of hirsute patients with either polycystic ovary syndrome (PCOS) or idiopathic hirsutism (IH) were examined in a prospective, randomized trial. Standard CPA treatment was used to monitor findings observed with spironolactone.

Methods.—Forty-four hirsute female patients aged 14 to 42 years werc evaluated. Nineteen had PCOS and 25 had IH. Patients were randomly assigned to 2 treatment groups and stratified for the presence of PCOS. Group 1 (21 patients, 10 with PCOS) received spironolactone, 200 mg/day 20 days per month for 12 months. Group 2 (23 patients, 9 with PCOS) received CPA, 50 mg/day 20 days per month for 12 months, in addition to ethinyl estradiol (35 µg/day) over the last 10 days of CPA treatment. Hirsutism was graded independently by 2 observers using the Ferriman Gallwey clinical score for hirsutism. Serum testosterone, androstenedione, and luteinizing hormone (LH) levels were obtained.

Results.—In patients with IH, hirsutism regressed equally with spironolactone and CPA (21 vs 23). In patients with PCOS, the mean score for hirsutism after 12 months of treatment was significantly lower with CPA than with spironolactone (12 vs 16). Testosterone levels remained the same with spironolactone. With CPA, these levels were reduced from baseline in PCOS (47% and 51% at 6 and 12 months); in patients with IH, these rates were 31% and 30%, respectively. Androstenedione levels were significantly reduced from baseline for CPA-PCOS–treated patients at 6 and 12 months (38% and 39%, respectively). These differences were not observed in spironolactone-treated patients with PCOS. The LH levels were reduced by 72% with CPA and not with spironolactone.

Conclusion.—Spironolactone used as a single agent was as effective as CPA combined with estradiol in the long-term treatment of patients with IH. In patients with PCOS, spironolactone was as effective as CPA in decreasing hirsutism. For the treatment of the hormonal or metabolic manifestations associated with PCOS, it may be important to combine spironolactone with either an antigonadotrophic agent or a drug that enhances peripheral insulin sensitivity.

▶ Spironolactone is a useful agent for treating IH as well as hirsutism associated with PCOS. Because spironolactone, when given alone, is associated with menstrual disturbances, it is usually given with a low androgenic estrogen containing oral contraceptive (OC). The estrogen in the OC raises sex hormone–binding globulin levels that bind endogenous testosterone and reduce the amount of bioactive testosterone. When given with an OC, the initial dose of spironolactone is usually 100 mg per day. If there is no decrease in the extent of hirsutism, then the dose can be increased to 200 mg/day.

D. R. Mishell, Jr, MD

14 Menopause

Soy Isoflavone Supplementation in Postmenopausal Women: Effects on Plasma Lipids, Antioxidant Enzyme Activities, and Bone Density
Hsu C-S, Shen WW, Hsueh Y-M, et al (Taipei Med Univ, Taiwan)
J Reprod Med 46:221-226, 2001   14–1

Background.—Soy protein appears to reduce lipid concentrations. Recent research has suggested that the components of soy protein underlying this effect are isoflavones. The effects of isoflavone supplementation on plasma lipids, erythrocyte antioxidant enzyme activity, and bone mineral density in postmenopausal women were studied.

Methods.—Thirty-seven postmenopausal women were included in the 6-month trial. Treatment consisted of 150 mg/d of isoflavone supplements given twice a day. No changes were made to the women's regular diet. Blood was obtained for analysis before and at 3 and 6 months after supplementation.

Findings.—The 3- and 6-month measures of plasma total cholesterol, high-density lipoprotein cholesterol, low-density lipoprotein cholesterol, triglyceride levels, and erythrocyte antioxidant enzyme activities did not differ significantly from baseline. In addition, isoflavone supplementation for 6 months did not affect calcaneus bone mineral density.

Conclusion.—In this study of postmenopausal women, isoflavone supplementation did not appear to have antioxidant effects. Supplementation with isoflavone alone may not have any hypocholesterolemic effects. Longer term studies are needed to clarify the bone-sparing effects of isoflavone supplementation.

▶ Many postmenopausal women wish to ingest soy or the isoflavones present in soy instead of estrogen because they believe soy or its components are a more natural source of estrogen than the estrogen compounds synthesized from plants or extracted from urine of pregnant mares. Published data, such as this report, indicate that unlike estrogen, soy protein or isoflavones do not have a similar beneficial effect upon risk factors for cardiovascular disease as estrogen and are not as beneficial as estrogen for the relief of vasomotor symptoms.

D. R. Mishell, Jr, MD

"

Cognitive Decline in Women in Relation to Non-Protein-Bound Oestradiol Concentrations

Yaffe K, Lui L-Y, Grady D, et al (Univ of California, San Francisco; Univ of Pittsburgh, Pa)
Lancet 356:708-712, 2000

14–2

Background.—Previous research has found no correlation between total serum estradiol concentrations and cognitive function. However, these measures may not indicate hormone concentrations available to the brain. Whether concentrations of non–protein-bound (free) and loosely bound (bioavailable) sex hormones correlate with cognitive function in older women was determined.

Methods.—Four hundred twenty-five women, aged 65 years and older, participated in the study. Free and bioavailable estradiol concentrations, as well as total and free testosterone, were assessed by radioimmunoassay in blood obtained at baseline. Cognitive performance was assessed by means of a modified mini mental status examination (mMMSE) at baseline and 6 years later.

Findings.—Initially, mMMSE scores did not differ by tertile of free estradiol, bioavailable estradiol, or testosterone. A cognitive decline of 3 or more points on the mMMSE occurred in 5% of the women in the high tertile for free estradiol and in 16% of those in the low tertile (Figure). The odds ratio remained at 0.3 after adjustment for age, years of education, body mass index, current estrogen use, history of surgical menopause, and baseline mMMSE score. The results for bioavailable estradiol were comparable. Cognitive impairment was not associated with serum testosterone levels.

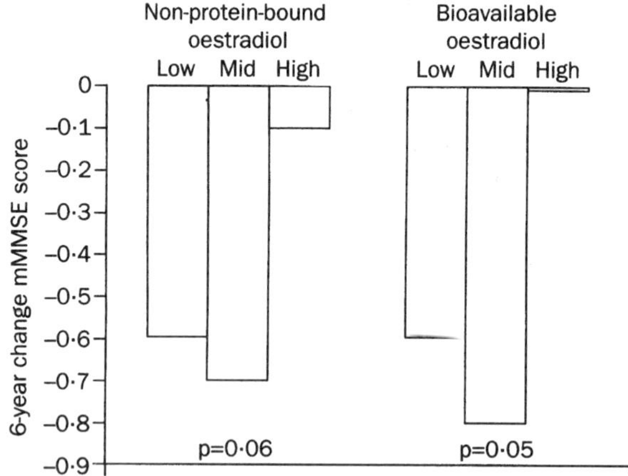

FIGURE.—Six-year decreases in the modified mini mental status examination (*mMMSE*) score according to tertile of estradiol concentration. (Courtesy of Yaffe K, Lui L-Y, Grady D, et al: Cognitive decline in women in relation to non–protein-bound oestradiol concentrations. *Lancet* 356:708-712, 2000. Copyright by The Lancet Ltd.)

Conclusion.—Women with high levels of free and bioavailable estradiol in serum appear to be less likely to have cognitive impairments than women with low concentrations. The current data are consistent with the hypothesis that greater levels of endogenous estrogens prevent cognitive decline.

▶ The results of this interesting study suggest that postmenopausal women with high levels of bioavailable endogenous estradiol are less likely to have impairment of mental function as they age than women with lower levels of bioavailable estradiol. Measurement of bioavailable estradiol levels in postmenopausal women may be of benefit in aiding their decision as to whether or not to take estrogen replacement. Women with low levels of bioavailable estradiol may have a greater benefit regarding their subsequent mental status from receiving exogenous estrogen than women with high levels of bioavailable estradiol.

D. R. Mishell, Jr, MD

Estrogen Replacement in Perimenopause-Related Depression: A Preliminary Report

Schmidt PJ, Nieman L, Danaceau MA, et al (NIH, Bethesda, Md)
Am J Obstet Gynecol 183:414-420, 2000   14–3

Introduction.—The potential role of estrogen in the treatment of depression was suggested more than 100 years ago. Yet, trials examining the use of synthetic forms of estrogen in the treatment of depression have had conflicting results. The effects of the short-term administration of estradiol replacement in 34 perimenopausal women meeting criteria for major or minor depression, especially in the absence of hot flushes, were examined.

Methods.—The age range of participants was 44 to 55 years. Women with perimenopausal-related depression were randomly assigned in double-blind parallel fashion to receive either 17β-estradiol or placebo for 3 weeks. Women receiving estradiol during the first 3 weeks continued to receive it for an additional 3 weeks. Those who received placebo crossed over to estradiol for 3 weeks. The outcome was evaluated by standardized mood rating scales and a visual analogue scale self-report instrument.

Results.—Initially, 16 patients received estradiol and 18 received placebo. After 3 weeks of estradiol, standardized mood rating scale and visual analogue symptoms scores (including sadness, anhedonia, and social isolation) were significantly reduced, compared with baseline scores ($P < .01$) and were significantly lower than scores in women receiving placebo ($P < .01$); the latter demonstrated no significant improvement (Fig 1). Neither the presence of hot flushes nor the duration of treatment (3 weeks vs 6 weeks) influenced outcome. A full or partial therapeutic response was observed in 80% of women receiving estradiol and 22% of those receiving placebo.

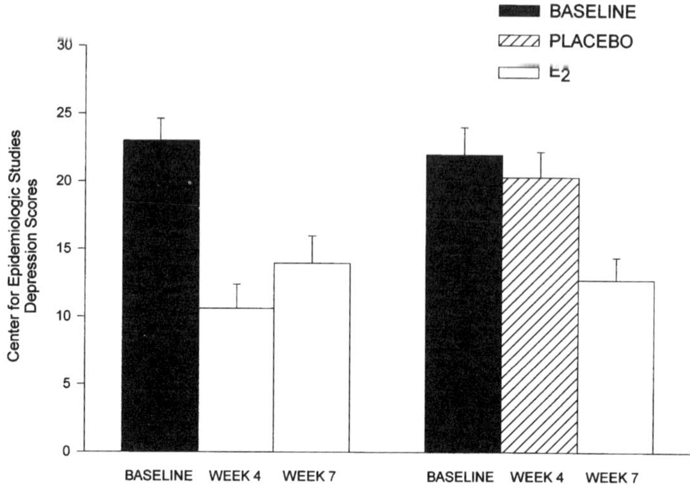

FIGURE 1.—Compared with baseline values, the scores of 16 women with perimenopausal depression experienced a significant decrease (the Center for Epidemiologic Studies–Depression Scale) after 3 weeks of estradiol administration (0.05 mg/d; $P < .01$). The decrease was maintained after 3 additional weeks of estradiol administration ($P < .01$). In contrast, 16 women with perimenopausal depression who received placebo during the first 3 weeks had no significant change in symptom scores until after estradiol treatment during the second 3 weeks of the study, when they experienced a significant decrease in symptoms scores compared with placebo ($P < .01$). *Filled columns* indicate Baseline; *hatched columns*, placebo; *open columns*, 17β-estradiol. (Courtesy of Schmidt PJ, Nieman L, Danaceau MA, et al: Estrogen replacement of perimenopausal-related depression: A preliminary report. *Am J Obstet Gynecol* 183:414-420, 2000.)

Conclusion.—Estradiol replacement effectively treated perimenopausal depression independent of its salutary effects on vasomotor symptoms. This response to estradiol occurred after 3 weeks of treatment; no further improvement was observed in mood after 6 weeks of estradiol replacement.

▶ Controversy exists as to whether administration of estrogen to postmenopausal women results in improvement of depression because previous studies have yielded conflicting results. The results of this well-done clinical trial provide a good level of evidence that estrogen is an effective agent for the treatment of major or minor depression in postmenopausal women.

D. R. Mishell, Jr, MD

Exploration of Cyclical Changes in Memory and Mood in Postmenopausal Women Taking Sequential Combined Oestrogen and Progestogen Preparations

Natale V, Albertazzi P, Zini M, et al (Univ of Bologna, Italy; Maternity Hosp, Bologna, Italy; Hull Royal Infirmary, England)
Br J Obstet Gynaecol 108:286-290, 2001   14–4

Objective.—Although estrogen has beneficial effects on mood and cognition, it must be used in conjunction with progesterone in postmenopausal women who have not had hysterectomies. Little is known about the effect of progesterone on cognition. The effects of progestogens added to estrogens in sequential combined hormone replacement therapy on memory, mood, sleep, and libido were evaluated.

Methods.—Between June and November 1999, 23 postmenopausal women, aged 46 to 70 years, taking sequential combined hormone replacement therapy for an average of 15 months, were each interviewed 3 times during the estrogen–progesterone part of the cycle and 3 times during the estrogen-only part of the cycle. Memory, mood (as evaluated by the Profile of Mood States [POMS]), sleep quality, and libido (as evaluated by the Sexuality Evaluation Schedule Assessment Monitoring) were assessed in both parts of the cycle.

Results.—Memory was significantly better during the estrogen–progesterone part of the cycle than in the estrogen-only part of the cycle. Women remembered more words during the former than during the latter (9.40 vs 8.65). Memory improved during the second cycle and worsened during the third. The combination phase lowered POMS mood scores significantly more than the estrogen-only phase (214.30 vs 194.58). Sleep was unaffected. The quality and frequency of sexual intercourse was significantly better during the estrogen-only phase than during the combination phase. All other measures of libido were unchanged.

Conclusion.—The combination of estrogen and progesterone significantly improved memory, significantly worsened mood compared with estrogen alone, but did not affect sleep or libido.

▶ Other studies have shown that progestins have a negative effect on mood and sense of well-being. For this reason, a lower dose of progestins given continuously is now being used with greater frequency than the intermittent cyclic use of high doses of progestin. The fact that progestins may enhance memory is of interest and needs to be confirmed in other studies.

D. R. Mishell, Jr, MD

Negative Mood Changes During Hormone Replacement Therapy: A Comparison Between Two Progestogens

Björn I, Bixo M, Strandberg Nöjd K, et al (Univ Hosp of Umeå, Sweden)
Am J Obstet Gynecol 183:1419-1426, 2000   14–5

Introduction.—Little is known about the psychological effects of progestogens. The addition of progestogens may cause negative mood swings during hormone replacement therapy. Women taking 0.625 mg of conjugated estrogens and 5 mg of medroxyprogesterone acetate have more negative psychological side effects than women taking 1.25 mg conjugated estrogens and placebo. The difference in effect on mood and physical symptoms between medroxyprogesterone acetate and norethindrone ac-

FIGURE 1

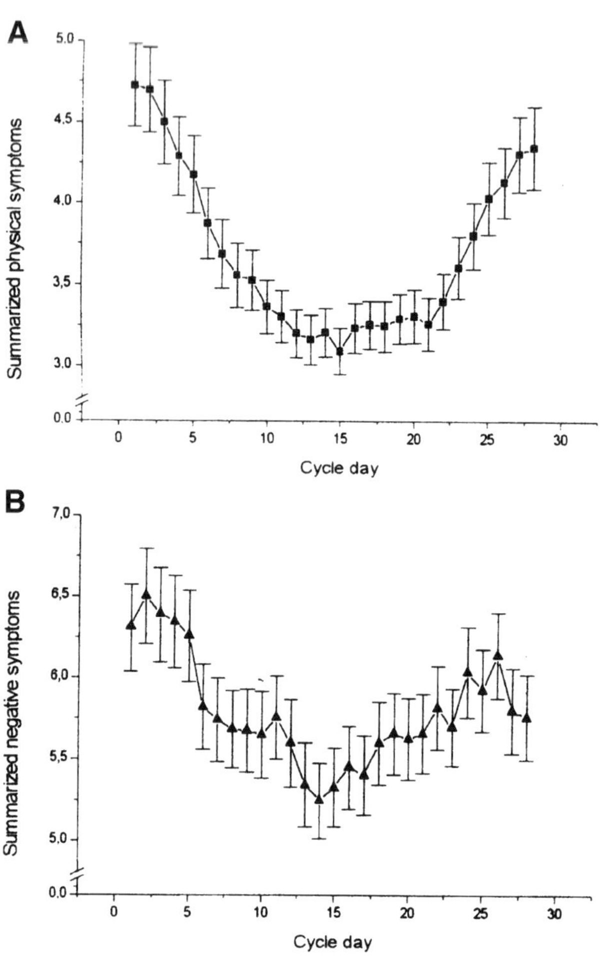

(Continued)

etate was examined in women with and without premenstrual syndrome (PMS).

Methods.—Fifty-one postmenopausal women were randomly assigned in a double-blind crossover trial to receive either 2 mg estradiol continuously during five 28-day cycles and 10 mg medroxyprogesterone or 1 mg norethindrone sequentially for 12 days of each cycle. The main outcome measure was daily symptom ratings.

Results.—Twenty-four of 46 participants who completed the trial reported a history of premenstrual symptoms (80% had moderate and 20% had severe PMS) during fertile life, with negative psychological symptoms affecting daily life. All symptoms of the Cyclicity Diagnoser demonstrated a significant difference between the worst and the best phase of a 28-day

FIGURE 1 (cont.)

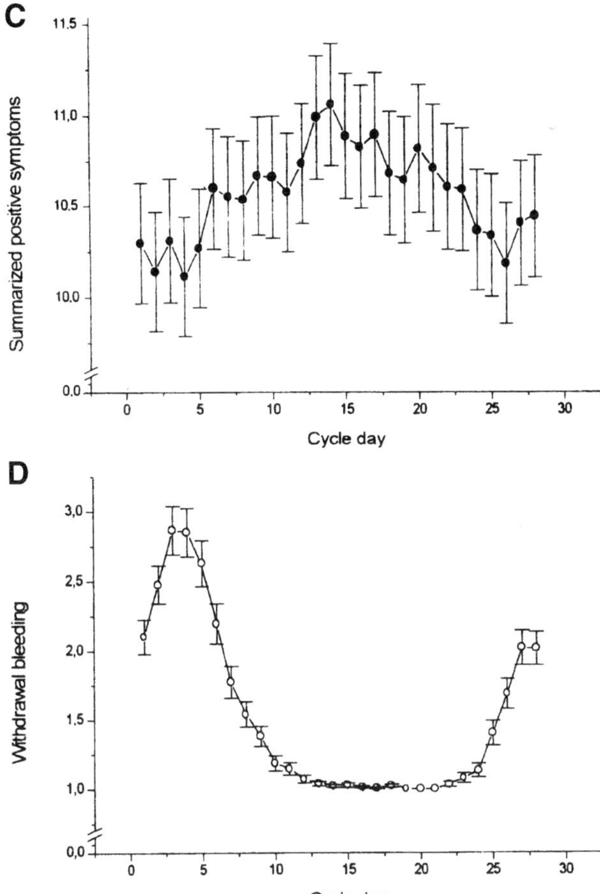

FIGURE 1.—Daily symptom ratings on 9-point Cyclicity Diagnoser of summarized physical (A) symptoms and of negative (B) and positive (C) mood symptoms and of withdrawal bleeding (D) during sequential estrogen-progestogen treatment. Each *point* represents the mean ± SEM of treatment cycles 2 through 5 among all women. All related symptom groups displayed significant cyclicity between best and worst phases of treatment cycle. (Courtesy of Björn I, Bixo M, Strandberg K, et al: Negative mood changes during hormone replacement therapy: A comparison between two progestogens. *Am J Obstet Gynecol* 183:1419-1426, 2000.)

cycle (Fig 1). Mood was at its highest and physical symptoms were at their lowest during midcycle (days 10-16). The worse period peaked during the late progestogen phase (days 25-28) and continued until the next cycle (days 1-3), after which it tapered off.

Negative mood symptoms began to rise at cycle day 18, the day after addition of a progestogen; physical symptoms began to rise at day 20. Positive mood symptoms diminished after day 20. Scores for breast tenderness, bloating, hot flushes, cheerfulness, friendliness, tension, fatigue, irritability, depression, effect on daily life, and libido were significantly cyclic.

During the progestogen phase, patients with PMS had significantly lower scores of positive symptoms, compared with those with no history of PMS. More physical symptoms were induced with norethindrone than with medroxyprogesterone ($P < .01$). Patients with no PMS history had more negative symptoms and fewer positive symptoms while taking norethindrone as compared with medroxyprogesterone ($P < .001$). Those with a PMS history had significantly more negative symptoms during medroxyprogesterone versus norethindrone treatment ($P < .001$).

Conclusion.—The addition of medroxyprogesterone to estrogen is preferable to that of norethindrone in terms of mood swings in women without a history of PMS.

▶ This study provides additional documentation that giving estrogen to postmenopausal women improves mood while administration of high-dose progestins sequentially has a deleterious effect upon mood. Women without a uterus should not be given progestin in addition to estrogen as there is no risk of adenocarcinoma of the endometrium. In women with a uterus there may be different effects upon mood with medroxyprogesterone acetate and norethindrone. Fortunately, combination formulations with estrogen plus either of these progestins, as well as norgestimate, are available to treat postmenopausal women with a uterus. For women with a uterus who do not tolerate any progestin, estrogen without a progestin can be administered for 5 days of each 7 days per week. The endometrial effect should then be monitored periodically by pelvic sonography or endometrial biopsy to determine whether endometrial hyperplasia has developed.

D. R. Mishell, Jr, MD

Transdermal Testosterone Treatment in Women With Impaired Sexual Function After Oophorectomy

Shifren JL, Braunstein GD, Simon JA, et al (Massachusetts Gen Hosp, Boston; Cedars-Sinai Med Ctr, Los Angeles; Women's Health Research Ctr, Laurel, Md; et al)
N Engl J Med 343:682-688, 2000   14–6

Background.—For premenopausal women, almost half of the circulating testosterone is provided by the ovaries. Bilateral oophorectomy in premenopausal women thus reduces serum levels of both estradiol and testosterone. Even with estrogen replacement therapy, many of these women report side effects associated with reduced testosterone levels, such as decreased libido, activity, and pleasure. Women who reported impaired sexual function after surgically induced menopause were studied to determine whether transdermal testosterone could improve their sexual function.

Methods.—The study included 75 women, aged 31 to 36 years, who had undergone bilateral salpingo-oophorectomy and hysterectomy before natural menopause between 1 and 10 years previously. All subjects had reduced testosterone levels (serum testosterone level < 32 ng/dL or serum free testosterone level < 1.8 pg/mL [normal range, 1.3-6.8 pg/mL]), and all were receiving conjugated equine estrogens (0.625 mg or more per day). In addition, all had been in a stable, monogamous heterosexual relationship for 1 year or more but reported less sexual activity or satisfaction since their surgery. During 3 consecutive 12-week treatments subjects were randomly assigned to receive either 2 placebo patches, 1 placebo patch and 1 transdermal testosterone patch (150 µg/day), or 2 testosterone patches (300 µg/day). For 28 days at baseline and for the last 28 days of each treatment period, subjects kept a daily diary of the frequency of sexual thoughts, desires, and activities. At baseline and at the end of each treatment period, subjects completed the Brief Index of Sexual Functioning for Women (BISFW) and the Psychological General Well-Being Index (PGWBI). Serum testosterone levels were measured at baseline and every 4 weeks, and serum estrogen levels were measured at baseline and at the end of each treatment period.

Results.—During the study, 18 women withdrew or were withdrawn because of adverse effects or poor compliance with the telephone diary. Intention-to-treat analysis included 65 women with at least 1 evaluation of efficacy during treatment. The mean serum free testosterone levels increased from 1.2 pg/mL during the placebo period, to 3.9 pg/mL during treatment with testosterone at 150 µg/day to 5.9 pg/mL during treatment with testosterone at 300 µg/day. The baseline mean composite score on the BISFW was 52% that of normal women. The mean composite BISFW scores increased with placebo and with the lower and higher doses of testosterone (72%, 74%, and 81%, respectively), with a significant difference also between values with higher-dose testosterone compared with those with placebo. In comparison with placebo, higher-dose testosterone was associated with significantly greater BISFW scores for the frequency of sexual activity and orgasm. The baseline mean composite score on the PGWBI was 78. The mean composite PGWBI scores increased by 1 point with placebo, 2 points with lower-dose testosterone, and 5 points with higher-dose testosterone ($P = .04$, higher dose vs placebo). Higher-dose testosterone was also associated with significantly better scores for depressed mood and positive well-being compared with those with placebo. Scores on the telephone-based diary did not change significantly during the study, nor did serum estrogen levels. The patches were well tolerated, with only 1 subject withdrawing because of an adverse effect (skin reaction with the placebo patch).

Conclusions.—Transdermally delivered testosterone at 300 µg/day, in combination with oral conjugated equine estrogens, increased testosterone levels and improved sexual functioning and well-being after surgically induced menopause in these women

▶ Bilateral oophorectomy in both premenopausal and postmenopausal women results in significantly decreased circulating testosterone levels. Decreased libido is a frequent symptom following bilateral oophorectomy. Parenteral administration of testosterone has been shown to increase libido, although there is no evidence that orally administered testosterone has a similar effect. The administration of testosterone by the transdermal patches used in this study increased total, free, and bioavailable testosterone levels and improved libido and sense of well-being without adversely affecting lipoprotein levels. When these patches become commercially available, they can be used to improve libido and sense of well being in women who have had bilateral oophorectomy and have problems with decreased libido and sexual enjoyment.

D. R. Mishell, Jr, MD

Hormone Replacement Therapy and Prevention of Nonvertebral Fractures: A Meta-Analysis of Randomized Trials
Torgerson DJ, Bell-Syer SEM (Univ of York, Heslington, England)
JAMA 285:2891-2897, 2001   14–7

Background.—The common belief that hormone replacement therapy (HRT) reduces fractures is based primarily on observational data. Evidence from randomized trials is sparse. A systematic review of all randomized studies of HRT that have reported or collected data on nonvertebral fractures without necessarily focusing on fracture prevention was presented.

Methods and Findings.—Several databases were searched for publications appearing between 1997 and 2000. Data from 22 studies were pooled. Overall, nonvertebral fractures were reduced by 27%. This effect was greater among women randomly assigned to HRT with a mean age younger than 60 years. Among those aged 60 years or older, this effect was diminished. The efficacy of HRT appeared to be more marked for hip and wrist fractures, especially among women aged younger than 60 years.

Conclusion.—This meta-analysis identified a significant reduction in nonvertebral fractures. This effect appears to be attenuated in women aged 60 years or older.

▶ This meta-analysis combined published and unpublished data from a wide variety of epidemiologic studies. The mean age of the women in the individual studies varied from 50 to 75 years. Some studies included only healthy women while others studied women with various diseases or only those who had had a hysterectomy. Some studies evaluated estrogen replacement in women with osteoporosis while others studied women with normal bone mineral density. Finally, despite the different types and different doses of estrogen used in the trials reviewed, the majority of the studies—15 of the 22 trials—reported a reduction in risk of nonvertebral fractures with estrogen use. When given to healthy women at the time of menopause, estrogen will prevent loss of bone and decrease the risk of vertebral and nonvertebral fracture.

D. R. Mishell, Jr, MD

Hormonal Replacement Therapy Reduces Forearm Fracture Incidence in Recent Postmenopausal Women—Results of the Danish Osteoporosis Prevention Study
Mosekilde L, Beck-Nielsen H, Sørensen OH, et al (Aarhus Univ, Denmark; Odense Univ, Denmark; Copenhagen Municipal Hosp; et al)
Maturitas 36:181-193, 2000   14–8

Background.—The more frequent occurrence of osteoporosis among women versus men is due primarily to the loss of endogenous estrogen production after menopause. In several studies, a protective effect of hormonal replacement therapy (HRT) against postmenopausal bone loss and fracture occurrence has been noted. However, with one exception, most previous fracture studies have been observational. In 2 recent prospective studies on the use of estrogen for the prevention of fractures, 1 demonstrated a reduction, whereas the other demonstrated no reduction in the occurrence of fractures. The Danish Osteoporosis Prevention Study (DOPS) was designed to study the primary prevention of fractures through the use of HRT in women in whom menopause had recently occurred. Total follow-up for the DOPS was 20 years. The DOPS was conducted as a partially randomized study, with a classic randomized controlled trial as 1 study arm and an observational study as the other study arm. Results concerning the risk of fractures in the first 5 years of the study are presented.

Methods.—In a prospective, controlled comprehensive cohort trial, 2016 healthy women aged 45 to 58 years were enrolled from a random sample of the background population. All participants were from 3 to 24 months past the last menstrual bleeding incident. The mean age of the participants was 50.8 ± 2.8 years, and the number of person-years followed was 9335.3. In the randomized study arm, 502 women were randomly assigned to HRT, and 504 were not; in the nonrandomized study arm, 221 women chose HRT and 789 did not. First-line HRT was oral sequential estradiol/norethisterone in women with intact uteri and oral continuous estradiol in women who had undergone hysterectomies.

Results.—The results after 5 years showed a total of 156 fractures in 140 women, and 51 forearm fractures occurred in 51 women. Intention-to treat analysis of 2016 women demonstrated a reduced overall fracture risk that was borderline statistically significantly, and a significant reduction in the risk of forearm fracture occurred with the use of HRT (Fig 3). When the analysis was restricted to women who had adhered to the initial

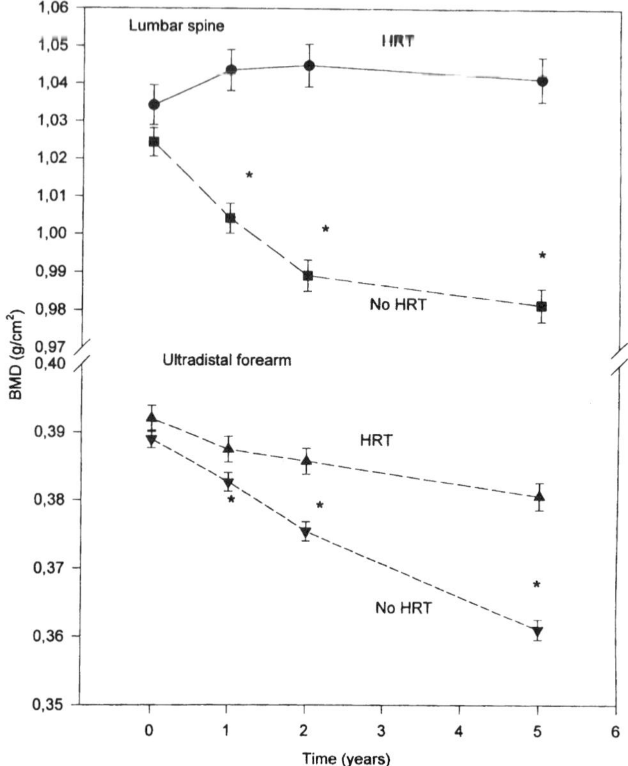

FIGURE 3.—Changes in lumbar spine bone mineral density (BMD) (L2-L4, g/cm²) in hormone replacement therapy (HRT) allocated (*n* = 723) and non-HRT allocated (*n* = 1293)—intention-to-treat. Figures are mean and one SEM. * denotes a significant difference between treated and untreated (*2P* < .05 by independent samples *t* test). (Reprinted from Mosekilde L, Beck-Nielsen H, Sørensen OH, et al: Hormonal replacement therapy reduces forearm fracture incidence in recent postmenopausal women—results of the Danish Osteoporosis Prevention Study. *Maturitas* 36(3):181-193, copyright 2000, by permission from Elsevier Science.)

allocation of either HRT or no HRT, a significant reduction was found in both the overall risk of fractures and the risk of forearm fractures (Table 3). The compliance with HRT after 5 years was 65%.

Conclusions.—The use of HRT in women in whom menopause had recently occurred may be an effective preventive measure to reduce the number of forearm fractures and possibly the total number of fractures in this population.

▶ This large, well-done prospective semirandomized clinical trial provides important information about the effects of estrogen on bone when estrogen is given soon after menopause to a group of healthy women. When estrogen therapy with a progestin (HRT) or unopposed therapy estrogen replacement therapy is given soon after menopause and is continued for 5 years, there is a significant reduction in forearm fractures and in all fractures compared with women who did not take estrogen. It was interesting that the risk of spinal

TABLE 3.—Factors of Significance to Fracture Occurrence: Risk Estimates and 95% CI

Parameter	Forearms*	Spine†	All Fractures‡
Intention-to-treat (all participants)			
Age at inclusion (years)	0.97 (0.88-1.07)	1.16 (1.01-1.33)**	0.95 (0.90-1.01)
BMD (g/cm²)§	2.24 (1.69-2.97)**	1.85 (1.21-2.82)**	1.47 (1.23-1.76)**
Treatment (HRT vs no HRT)‖	0.45 (0.22-0.90)**	1.80 (0.81-3.96)	0.73 (0.50-1.05)
Causal¶			
Age at inclusion (years)	0.91 (0.82-1.02)	1.11 (0.93-1.33)	0.91 (0.85-0.98)
BMD (g/cm²)§	2.24 (1.63-3.08)**	1.61 (0.94-2.77)	1.41 (1.15-1.72)**
Treatment (HRT vs no HRT)¶	0.24 (0.09-0.69)**	0.74 (0.20-2.70)	0.61 (0.39-0.97)**

*Cox regression, all independent variables entered, BMD of ultradistal forearm. Adjusted RR and 95% confidence limits.

†Logistic regression of all incident vertebral fractures (including symptomless ones), all independent variables entered, BMD of lumbar spine (L2-L4). Adjusted OR and 95% confidence limits. The dependent variable was occurrence of at least 1 incident vertebral fracture versus no vertebral fractures from baseline to the 5-year follow-up visit.

‡Cox regression with all independent variables entered. All fractures excluding symptomless vertebral fractures, BMD of lumbar spine (L2-L4). Adjusted RR and 95% confidence limits.

§Increase in fracture risk per 1 standard deviation *decrease* in BMD in actual region.

‖Intention to treat (all 2016 participants).

¶Comparison of the 395 who continued unchanged with the same HRT type versus the 977 who never received HRT during the 5-year follow-up.

**$P < .05$.

Abbreviations: BMD, bone mineral density; *HRT*, hormone replacement therapy; *RR*, relative risk.

(Reprinted from Mosekilde L, Beck-Nielsen H, Sørensen OH, et al: Hormonal replacement therapy reduces forearm fracture incidence in recent postmenopausal women—results of the Danish Osteoporosis Prevention Study. *Maturitas* 36(3):181-193. Copyright 2000 by Elsevier Science.)

fractures was increased among all participants who took estrogen compared with those who did not (relative risk [RR], 1.80; 95% CI, 0.81-3.96) but was decreased among the 395 women who continued with their hormones for 5 years compared with the 977 who never took hormones (RR, 0.74; 95% CI, 0.20-2.70). This finding indicates that women who stopped taking hormones before 5 years had an increased risk of spinal fractures. It is also reassuring that in this semirandomized study the risk of having breast cancer was insignificantly reduced among women taking hormones (RR, 0.68; 95% CI, 0.24-1.90) compared with those who did not. Studies of the effect of other agents, such as raloxifene, alendronate, and risedronate, on bone loss have been restricted to women who already have osteoporosis; the studies did not include healthy women, as was done in this study. These results support the findings observed in several other observational studies, that is, estrogen use in postmenopausal women without osteoporosis prevents bone loss and fractures.

D. R. Mishell, Jr, MD

Fracture Risk Reduction With Alendronate in Women With Osteoporosis: The Fracture Intervention Trial

Black DM, for the FIT Research Group (Univ of California, San Francisco; et al)
J Clin Endocrinol Metab 85:4118-4124, 2000   14–9

Introduction.—Recent treatment guidelines from the National Osteoporosis Foundation recommend that older women with osteoporosis should be treated with drugs to decrease fracture risk. The effect of alendronate treatment on fracture risk reduction in women with existing vertebral fracture was compared with that of women without extisting vertebral fracture, yet with a bone mineral density (BMD) T score of below -2.5. The World Health Organization defines osteoporosis as a BMD value over 2.5 standard deviations below the young adult peak. The effect of alendronate was examined with both groups of women combined.

Methods.—The effect of alendronate treatments on the risk of new fracture was examined in 3658 women with osteoporosis from 11 clinical centers in the United States who were enrolled in the Fracture Intervention Trial. The age range of participants was 55 to 80 years. All women had been postmenopausal for at least 2 years and had femoral neck BMD of 0.69 g/cm² or less. Women with existing vertebral fractures received alendronate for 3 years, and those without vertebral fractures received alendronate for 4 years. A true intention-to-treat analysis was performed.

Results.—Both groups had similar magnitudes of decreased fracture incidence with alendronate treatment, so the 2 groups were pooled for a more precise estimate of the effect of alendronate on relative risk of fracture (relative risk and 95% confidence interval, respectively): hip (0.47; 0.26-0.79), radiographic vertebral (0.52; 0.42-0.66), clinical vertebral (0.55; 0.36-0.82), and all clinical fractures (0.70; 0.59-0.82). The decreases in risk of clinical fracture were significant by 12 months into the trial.

Conclusion.—Decreases in fracture risk during treatment with alendronate are consistent in both women with existing vertebral fractures and those without such fractures yet with BMD in the osteoporotic range. Reductions in risk are evident early in the course of treatment.

▶ The results of this large, randomized trial provide a high level of evidence that administration of 10 mg of alendronate daily to women with osteoporosis without a prior fracture results in a rapid and significant decrease in subsequent incidences of fractures at many sites. Therefore, treatment of postmenopausal women with established osteoporosis with alendronate is advisable.

D. R. Mishell, Jr, MD

Skeletal Benefits of Alendronate: 7-Year Treatment of Postmenopausal Osteoporotic Women

Tonino RP, for the Phase III Osteoporosis Treatment Study Group (Univ of Vermont, Burlington)

J Clin Endocrinol Metab 85:3109-3115, 2000   14–10

Background.—Fractures related to osteoporosis are a significant health problem among elderly persons, particularly elderly women. Bone turnover increases and remains elevated about the time of menopause. This increase in bone turnover, combined with an imbalance favoring bone resorption over formation, leads to reductions in the amount (mass) and connectivity (microarchitecture) of bone tissue—a result that reduces bone strength. Bone mineral density (BMD) is an important indicator of skeletal health and reflects both the amount of bone tissue and the degree of mineralization. A progressive reduction in BMD and an increase in fracture risk occurs over time, particularly during menopause. This bone loss can be treated by inhibitors of bone resorption, which reduce fracture risk. Alendronate, a potent inhibitor of bone resorption, has been found to increase BMD, reduce bone turnover to premenopausal levels, and substantially reduce the incidence of vertebral and nonvertebral fractures among postmenopausal women. In previous studies, the incidence of new hip fractures among postmenopausal women was reduced by 63% within 18 months of the start of alendronate therapy. The results of a second 2-year extension of a clinical trial of alendronate among postmenopausal women are discussed.

Methods.—The extended study included 235 women who were blinded to treatment with alendronate (5 or 10 mg daily) and 115 women formerly treated with alendronate who were now switched to a blinded placebo.

Results.—Among women who were treated continuously with alendronate (10 mg daily) for 7 years, BMD in the lumbar spine was increased by 11.4% compared to baseline. After the initial 18 months of treatment, each additional year of treatment through 7 years indicated an increase in spine BMD of 0.8% for the 10-mg dose and 0.6% for the 5-mg dose, with significant increases from year 6 to year 7. During this same year, previously reported increases in BMD at other skeletal sites and decreases in biochemical markers of bone turnover remained stable. Among the women who had been taking alendronate for 5 years and were switched to placebo, no significant reduction in BMD at the spine or hip was observed; however, small but significant decreases in BMD at the forearm and total body, and small increases in biochemical markers, were noted. The safety and tolerability profiles of alendronate were similar to those of placebo.

Conclusions.—Long-term therapy with alendronate appeared to be well tolerated and effective at 7 years. Increases in BMD in the spine continued for at least 7 years, and other skeletal benefits were maintained. Discontinuation of alendronate therapy did not lead to accelerated bone loss, but better skeletal benefits were achieved with continuous treatment compared with shorter treatment.

▶ The results of this study indicate it is safe and effective to administer alendronate for 7 years to postmenopausal women to prevent bone loss. BMD of the lumbar spine continues to increase in the sixth and seventh year of alendronate therapy for postmenopausal women with established osteoporosis. Unlike estrogen, once alendronate is incorporated into bone it has an extremely long half-life. It was found in this study that after 5 years of treatment with alendronate, BMD did not decrease in the subsequent 2 years when placebo was given. When estrogen therapy is discontinued, there is a rapid decrease in BMD. Thus, alendronate has a longer duration of action than estrogen.

D. R. Mishell, Jr, MD

Effects of Alendronate and Hormone Replacement Therapy, Alone or in Combination, on Bone Mass in Postmenopausal Women With Osteoporosis: A Prospective, Randomized Study

Tiraş MB, Noyan V, Yildiz A, et al (Gazi Univ, Ankara, Turkey; McMaster Univ, Hamilton, Ont, Canada)
Hum Reprod 15:2087-2092, 2000

14–11

Introduction.—Vitamin D analogues, sodium fluoride, calcitonin, selective estrogen receptor modulators, and bisphosphonates may be used when patients do not wish to use hormone replacement therapy (HRT) or when its use is contraindicated. These alternative treatments lack the beneficial effect of HRT on the cardiovascular system, genitourinary tract, and mental status. Changes in bone mineral density (BMD) and bone

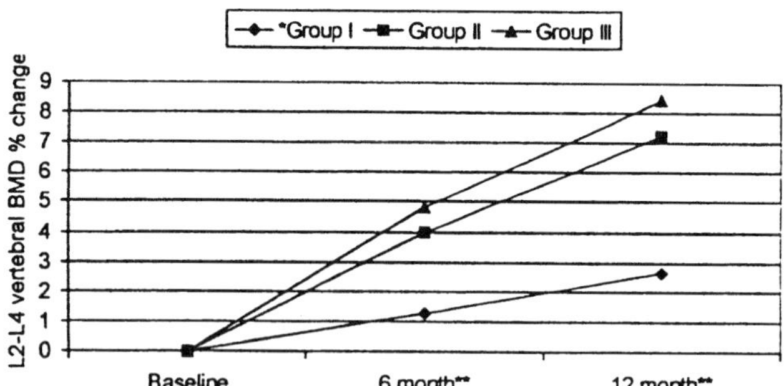

FIGURE 2.—Percentage changes of L2-L4 vertebral bone mineral density *(BMD)* from baseline. *Double asterisk* indicates $P = .001$ with analysis of variance. L2-L4 vertebral bone BMD (mean ± SEM) for 6th and 12th months, respectively, were group I (hormone replacement therapy [HRT], 1.324 ± 0.608 and 2.634 ± 0.636; group II (alendronate), 3.978 ± 0.472 and 7.233 ± 0.676; group III (HRT + alendronate), 4.816 ± 0.597 and 8.419 ± 0.944. (Courtesy of Tiraş MB, Noyan V, Yildiz A, et al: Effects of alendronate and hormone replacement therapy, alone or in combination, on bone mass in postmenopausal women with osteoporosis: A prospective, randomized study. *Hum Reprod* 15:2087-2092, 2000. Copyright, European Society for Human Reproduction and Embryology, by permission of Oxford University Press.)

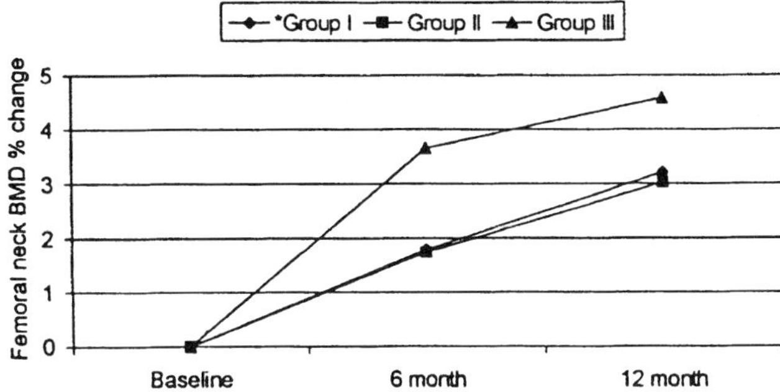

FIGURE 3.—Percentage changes of femoral neck bone mineral density (*BMD*) from baseline. Group I. hormone replacement therapy (HRT); group II, alendronate; group III, HRT + alendronate. Femoral neck BMD measurements (mean ± SEM) at 6th and 12 months, respectively, were as follows: group I, 1.780 ± 0.515 and 3.021 ± 0.440; group III, 3.651 ± 0.907 and 4.575 ± 0.979. (Courtesy of Tiraş MB, Noyan V, Yildiz A, et al: Effects of alendronate and hormone replacement therapy, alone or in combination, on bone mass in postmenopausal women with osteoporosis: A prospective, randomized study. *Hum Reprod* 15:2087-2092, 2000. Copyright, European Society for Human Reproduction and Embryology, by permission of Oxford University Press.)

turnover were followed up in patients with postmenopausal osteoporosis who were treated with HRT, alendronate, or a combination of HRT and alendronate.

Methods.—All 120 women had BMD of at least 2 standard deviations below the mean value for young premenopausal women. They were randomly allocated to treatment with 1 of the following: micronized 17β-estradiol 2 mg, and norethisterone acetate, 1 mg/d by mouth; alendronate 10 mg/d by mouth; or micronized 17β-estradiol (2 mg), norethisterone acetate (1 mg/d by mouth), and alendronate (10 mg/day, by mouth) for 1 year. All patients were given elementary calcium, 1500 mg/day. Ninety-five patients underwent measurement of spinal and femoral neck BMD and markers of bone mineral metabolism at baseline and 6 and 12 months after treatment.

Results.—At 12 months, significant increases in spinal and femoral neck BMD were observed in all 3 groups (Fig 2). Increases in spinal BMD were significantly higher among patients who were treated with alendronate or alendronate with HRT, compared with those who received HRT only (Fig 3). No significant between-group differences were seen in femoral neck BMD changes. Significant reductions in bone resorption and markers of bone formation were seen in all 3 groups.

Conclusion.—Alendronate was more effective than HRT alone and could be beneficial when added to the HRT regimen for patients with postmenopausal osteoporosis. Alendronate may also be used for postmenopausal women with osteoporosis when HRT use is contraindicated or when the patient is reluctant to use hormonal treatment.

▶ In this study, alendronate with or without HRT resulted in a significantly greater BMD increase in the spine in women with osteoporosis than did HRT alone. There was no difference in the increase in BMD in the hip between alendronate with or without HRT and HRT alone. There are no data showing that the combination of alendronate and HRT results in more of a decrease in subsequent fracture incidence in women with osteoporosis than occurs with the use of HRT alone. However, clinicians may decide to treat women with established osteoporosis with both antiresorptive agents rather than either alone because of the better effect upon spinal BMD with combination therapy.

D. R. Mishell, Jr, MD

Effect of Combined Risedronate and Hormone Replacement Therapies on Bone Mineral Density in Postmenopausal Women

Harris ST, Eriksen EF, Davidson M, et al (Univ of California, San Francisco; Univ of Aarhus, Denmark; Chicago Ctr for Clinical Research; et al)
J Clin Endocrinol Metab 86:1890-1897, 2001   14–12

Introduction.—Both hormone replacement therapy (HRT) and bisphosphonates are efficacious in preventing and treating postmenopausal osteoporosis. The safety and efficacy of a combined regimen of risedronate and HRT were examined in 524 postmenopausal women in a 1-year, double-blind, placebo-controlled trial.

Methods.—Participants received daily treatment with conjugated equine estrogens, 0.625 mg alone or in combination with risedronate, 5 mg. Women who had not undergone hysterectomy received medroxyprogesterone acetate up to 5 mg daily or cyclically at the discretion of their clinician. The primary efficacy end point was the percentage change from start of trial in mean lumbar spine bone mineral density (BMD) at 1 year. Changes in BMD at the proximal femur and forearm, bone turnover markers, and histology and histomorphometry were also evaluated.

Results.—At 12 months, significant ($P < .05$) increases from baseline in lumbar spine BMD were seen in both treatment groups (HRT only, 4.6%; combined risedronate-HRT, 5.2%). Between-group differences were not significant. Both therapies produced significant increases in BMD at 12 months at the femoral neck, trochanter, midshaft radius, and distal radius. The differences in BMD in the HRT-only and combined risedronate-HRT groups were significant at 6 months at the femoral neck and at the midshaft radius at 12 months. New vertebral fractures were observed at 12 months in 2.6% of patients in the HRT-only group and 1.8% of the combined group ($P = $ NS).

Both groups had significant reductions in biochemical markers of bone turnover, with somewhat greater reductions in the combined treatment group. Bone biopsies revealed normal bone structure and mineralization with both treatment groups. Expected reductions in bone turnover were observed and were greater in the combined treatment group (68%-79% decrease relative to baseline values; $P < .005$). Both groups had similar bone and gastrointestinal safety profiles.

Conclusion.—Combined risedronate-HRT administered for 1 year was well tolerated and produced increases in BMD at all skeletal sites. Both groups has similar increases in BMD at the lumbar spine, trochanter, and distal radius. The combined treatment group had slightly significantly greater increases in BMD at the femoral neck and midshaft radius.

▶ This study compared the effect of administering estrogen without a progestin and without risedronate to the effect of estrogen with and without a progestin combined with risedronate upon BMD in a group of postmenopausal women with and without evidence of bone loss. The results show that the combination of hormone therapy with risendronate resulted in a significantly greater increase in BMD in the radius and hip but not in the vertebral spine, as compared with hormone therapy without risedronate. Similar results have been reported when comparing the effect of estrogen and another bisphosphonate, alendronate, with estrogen alone when given to osteoporotic women. It remains to be determined whether addition of a bisphosphonate to estrogen replacement reduces the incidence of fractures in women with and without osteoporosis. Studies to date have not shown a significant difference in subsequent fracture incidence when a bisphosphonate is given in addition to estrogen, compared with estrogen alone.

D. R. Mishell, Jr, MD

Primary Prevention of Coronary Heart Disease in Women Through Diet and Lifestyle

Stampfer MJ, Hu FB, Manson JE, et al (Harvard Med School, Boston; Harvard School of Public Health, Boston)
N Engl J Med 343:16-22, 2000   14–13

Objective.—Diet and lifestyle can have a dramatic effect on coronary heart disease, the leading cause of death among men and women in the United States. The effect of a combination of lifestyle practices on risk of coronary heart disease and stroke was assessed for women participating in the Nurses' Health Study.

Methods.—When the Nurses' Health Study was established in 1976, a questionnaire, soliciting demographic information and specifically inquiring about height, body weight, and myocardial infarction (MI) in a parent aged less than 60 years, was mailed to 121,700 female US registered nurses.

In 1980 and beyond, inquiries about physical activity and diet were added to follow-up questionnaires. The low-risk group was defined as current nonsmokers with a body mass index less than 25, an average daily alcohol consumption of at least half a drink per day, and moderate-to-vigorous physical activity for at least 30 minutes a day. In addition, they scored in the highest 40th percentile of the cohort for consumption of fiber, marine n-3 fatty acid, and folate, with a high ratio of polyunsaturated to saturated fat, and consumed a diet low in transfat and sugar. Women were stratified by coronary heart disease risk group according to diet and lifestyle. Outcome measures were major coronary events occurring between 1980 and June 1, 1994.

Results.—During the 14-year follow-up, 1128 coronary events (832 nonfatal myocardial infarctions and 296 deaths from coronary heart disease) and 705 strokes occurred among the 84,129 women who entered into this substudy. Each component of the 5-factor low-risk profile was independently and significantly associated with risk, even after adjustment for confounding factors, such as pharmacologic agents, hypertension, age, family history, cholesterol level, and menopausal status. Within the 5-factor risk category, there was a gradient of risk, depending on the number of factors that were in the low-risk category for each woman. Women who were in the low risk category for all 5 factors had a relative risk of 0.17 compared with the rest of the women. The population-attributable risk was 82%, meaning that 82% of coronary events might have been prevented if all women were in the low-risk group.

Conclusion.—Women in the low-risk category for diet, exercise, nonsmoking, body mass index, and alcohol consumption had a very low risk of coronary heart disease.

▶ These data from a very large cohort of women followed up for a long duration provide a good level of evidence that moderate exercise, a low fat diet, and moderate alcohol intake together with lack of obesity and cigarette smoking substantially reduces the risk of major coronary artery events. When providing primary health care for women, clinicians should counsel their patients about adopting a lifestyle that will reduce the risk of the major cause of death of women.

D. R. Mishell, Jr, MD

Trends in the Incidence of Coronary Heart Disease and Changes in Diet and Lifestyle in Women

Hu FB, Stampfer MJ, Manson JE, et al (Harvard School of Public Health, Boston; Harvard Med School, Boston)
N Engl J Med 343:530-537, 2000   14–14

Objective.—Reductions in blood pressure and cholesterol levels have contributed to declines in the incidence and mortality rate of coronary heart disease (CHD). Data from the Nurses' Health Study were analyzed to assess the impact of diet and lifestyle factors on the incidence of CHD.

Methods.—The analysis included 85,941 female registered nurses, aged 34 to 59 years, with no history of diagnosed cardiovascular disease or cancer from 1980 to 1994. At baseline and at regular follow-up intervals, the women provided detailed information on their diet and other lifestyle factors. Diet and lifestyle variables were analyzed in relation to trends in the incidence of CHD.

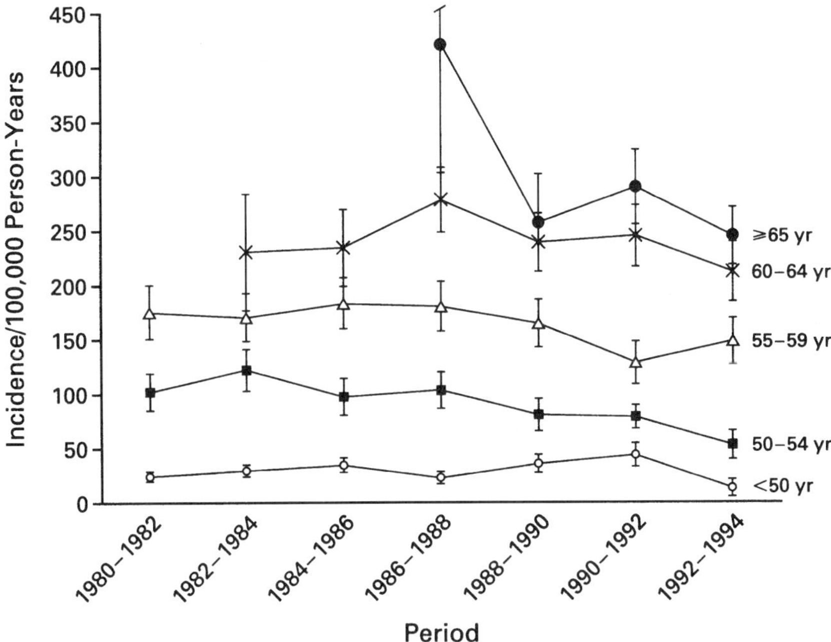

FIGURE 1.—Trends in the incidence of coronary disease according to age group in the Nurses' Health Study, 1980 to 1984. *I bars* indicate standard error. (Courtesy of Hu FB, Stampfer MJ, Manson JE, et al: Trends in the incidence of coronary heart disease and changes in diet and lifestyle in women. *N Engl J Med* 343:530-537, 2000. Copyright 2000 Massachusetts Medical Society. All rights reserved.)

Results.—With adjustment for age, the incidence of CHD declined by 31% between 1980 and 1982 and 1992 and 1994 (Fig 1). The number of subjects who currently smoked decreased by 41%. Other trends included a 175% increase in the proportion of postmenopausal women receiving hormone replacement therapy (HRT) and a 38% increase in the prevalence of being overweight (body mass index, 25 kg/m) (Fig 2).

Trends in diet improved significantly during the study period, including a decline in daily trans fat intake, an increase in the ratio of polyunsaturated to saturated fat, and an increase in cereal intake. The dietary trends accounted for 21% of the reduction in incidence of CHD, or 68% of the overall decline from 1980 to 1982 to 1992 to 1994. Reduced smoking accounted for 13% of the decrease in incidence of CHD, improved diet accounted for 16%, and increased use of HRT accounted for 9%. The rise in being overweight accounted for an 8% increase in the incidence of CHD.

Conclusion.—Recent declines in the incidence of CHD in women appear to result from lifestyle changes such as reduced smoking, better diet, and increased postmenopausal hormone replacement. Further declines have been prevented by the increasing prevalence of being overweight. Dietary and lifestyle practices have a major role to play in the primary prevention of CHD.

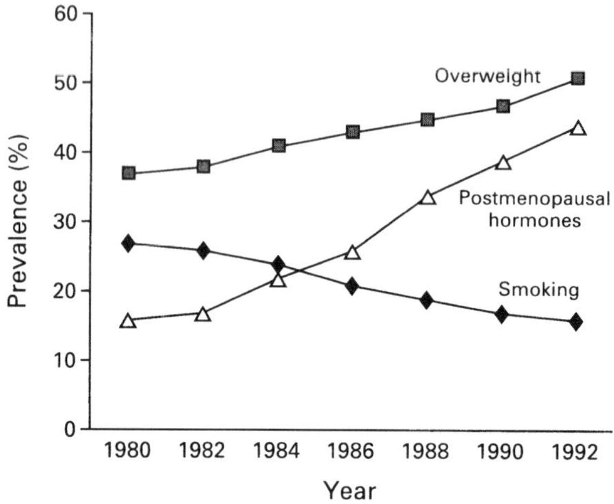

FIGURE 2.—Age-adjusted trends in the prevalence of smoking, being overweight (body mass index ≥25), and postmenopausal hormone use. Prevalences are standardized according to age distribution for the entire number of person-years of follow-up. The prevalence of postmenopausal hormone use was calculated for postmenopausal women only. All standard errors were less than 0.25% and thus would not be visible on the graph. (Courtesy of Hu FB, Stampfer MJ, Manson JE, et al: Trends in the incidence of coronary heart disease and changes in diet and lifestyle in women. *N Engl J Med* 343:530-537, 2000. Copyright 2000 Massachusetts Medical Society. All rights reserved.)

▶ The results of this large prospective observational study provide good evidence that smoking and obesity are risks for CHD, whereas a healthy diet and use of postmenopausal HRT lower the risk of CHD. Although HRT may not provide secondary prevention of coronary artery disease in older women with a prior history of CHD, as found in one randomized trial, there is much data from observational studies and one randomized trial that found that when HRT is given to healthy women it retards the development of coronary atherosclerosis.

D. R. Mishell, Jr, MD

Effects of Postmenopausal Hormone Replacement Therapy on Lipid, Lipoprotein, and Apolipoprotein (a) Concentrations: Analysis of Studies Published From 1974-2000

Godsland IF (Imperial College, London)
Fertil Steril 75:898-915, 2001

14–15

Background.—Measures of serum lipid and lipoprotein levels are important for assessing the safety of estrogen and progestogen use in postmenopausal hormone replacement therapy (HRT). Reference estimates of the effects of different HRT regimens on lipid and lipoprotein levels were determined.

Methods and Findings.—Publications identified by MEDLINE were included in the pooled analysis. Data from 248 studies on the effects of 42 different HRT regimens were obtained. All treatments with estrogen alone

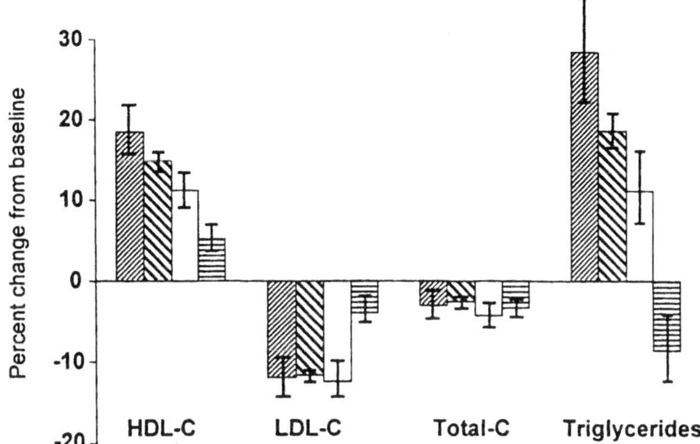

FIGURE 1.—Effects on lipid and lipoprotein levels of estrogen regimens commonly used in postmenopausal estrogen replacement therapy. Pooled mean percentage changes from baseline and 95% confidence intervals are shown. *Bars with left-slanted lines* indicate conjugated equine estrogens, 1.25 mg/d (268 patients); *bars with right-slanted lines* indicate conjugated equine estrogens, 0.625 mg/d (1513 patients); *white bars* indicate estradiol 17-beta 2.0 mg/d (283 patients); *bars with parallel lines* indicate transdermal estradiol 17-β, 0.05 mg/d (267 patients). (Reprinted by permission from the American Society for Reproductive Medicine courtesy of Godsland IF: Effects of postmenopausal hormone replacement therapy on lipid, lipoprotein, and apolipoprotein (a) concentrations: Analysis of studies published from 1974-2000. *Fertil Steril* 75:898-915, 2001.)

increased high-density lipoprotein (HDL) cholesterol and reduced low-density lipoprotein (LDL) and total cholesterol. Oral estrogen regimens increased triglyceride concentrations, and transdermal estradiol 17-β decreased triglyceride concentrations. Progestogens minimally affected estrogen-induced decreases in LDL and total cholesterol. Estrogen-induced increases in HDL and triglycerides were opposed depending on type of progestogen. In order from least to largest effect, these were dydrogesterone and medrogestone, progesterone, cyproterone acetate, medroxyprogesterone acctate, transdermal norethindrone acetate, norgestrel, and oral norethindrone acetate. Tibolone reduced HDL cholesterol and triglyceride concentrations. Raloxifene decreased LDL cholesterol concentrations. Data from 41 studies of 20 different formulation showed that HRT generally decreased lipoprotein(a) (Fig 1).

Conclusion.—Route of estrogen administration and type of progestogen determine the differential effects of HRT on lipid and lipoprotein concentrations in postmenopausal women. Further research is needed to interpret the clinical significance of these changes.

▶ This is an excellent summary of the published data regarding the effect of different types of estrogen, with and without different types of progestin, upon the lipid profile in healthy women. Pharmacologic agents, such as statins, which lower LDL cholesterol are associated with a decrease in myocardial infarction and major coronary artery events. One would expect that the beneficial changes caused by postmenopausal estrogen use upon the lipid factors is a major reason why estrogen replacement therapy given to healthy women has been associated with a reduced incidence of coronary heart disease. Clinicians should consider the extent of the attenuation of the beneficial effect of estrogen upon the lipid factors caused by different types, doses, and regimens of progestins when deciding which type and dose of progestin should be added to the estrogen component in postmenopausal women with a uterus.

D. R. Mishell, Jr, MD

A Prospective, Observational Study of Postmenopausal Hormone Therapy and Primary Prevention of Cardiovascular Disease

Grodstein F, Manson JE, Colditz GA, et al (Harvard Med School, Boston)
Ann Intern Med 133:933-941, 2000   14–16

Introduction.—Most primary prevention trials have reported that long-term users of postmenopausal hormone therapy are at lower risk of coronary events than their nonuser cohorts. Several questions remain. An adverse influence of hormone therapy on cardiovascular risk has been identified during the initial year of therapy. Few data are available regarding short-term hormone therapy. The cardiovascular effects of daily doses of oral conjugated estrogen lower than 0.625 mg are not known. Few trials have addressed estrogen plus progestin and its effect on cardiovascular disease. The duration, dose, and type of postmenopausal hormone therapy and primary prevention of cardiovascular disease were examined in the Nurses' Health Study (1976-1996) in a prospective, observational cohort trial.

Methods.—Of 70,533 postmenopausal women in the cohort, 1258 had major coronary events (nonfatal myocardial infarction or fatal coronary disease) and 767 had strokes. The details of postmenopausal hormone use were determined via a biennial questionnaire. Cardiovascular disease was reported by questionnaire and verified by review of medical records.

Results.—When all cardiovascular risk factors were considered, the risk of major coronary events was lower among current users (including short-term users) of hormone therapy than among never-users. Among women taking oral conjugated estrogen, the risk of coronary events was similarly decreased among those currently taking 0.625 mg daily (relative risk [RR], 0.54) and those taking 0.3 mg daily (RR, 0.58), compared with never-users. The risk of stroke was significantly higher among women taking 0.625 mg or more of oral conjugated estrogen daily and those taking estrogen plus progestin (RR, 1.35 mg/d vs 1.45 mg/d).

Conclusion.—In this large, observational, prospective trial, the risk of major coronary events seemed to be markedly reduced among current users of hormone therapy. For women taking oral conjugated estrogen, daily doses of 0.625 mg and 0.3 mg were related to decreased risk of heart disease, as was estrogen alone or in combination with a progestin. There was a modest increase in risk of stroke among women taking 0.625 mg or more of conjugated estrogen daily and those taking estrogen plus progestin.

▶ The Nurses Health Study is a large prospective observational cohort study involving more than 70,000 postmenopausal women who have been followed up since 1976. The results of this and many other observational studies of healthy women indicate that the use of estrogen, with or without a progestin, decreases the risk of coronary artery disease. To support the causal relationship of estrogen and reduction in cardiovascular disease, data show that oral estrogen has a beneficial effect on serum lipids as well as on coronary artery blood flow. Nevertheless, there is controversy about the beneficial effect of estrogen on coronary artery disease because a randomized controlled trial of women with existing cardiac disease did not show that estrogen reduced subsequent cardiac events compared with placebo. The results of this large observational study should enable clinicians to inform healthy postmenopausal women that both estrogen and estrogen plus progestin appear to reduce their likelihood of experiencing coronary artery disease but do not affect the possibility that they will have cerebrovascular disease.

D. R. Mishell, Jr, MD

Effects of Estrogen Replacement on the Progression of Coronary-Artery Atherosclerosis

Herrington DM, Reboussin DM, Brosnihan KB, et al (Wake Forest Univ, Winston-Salem, NC; Carolinas Med Ctr, Charlotte, NC; LeBauer Cardiovascular Associates, Greensboro, NC; et al)
N Engl J Med 343:522-529, 2000   14–17

Introduction.—Estrogen replacement therapy is commonly recommended for secondary prevention of heart disease in postmenopausal women. However, 1 recent study showed no significant reduction in the risk of cardiac events and death among women taking estrogen. This finding underscores the need for further information about how estrogen affects coronary atherosclerosis, including the possible modifying effects of concomitant progestin. The Estrogen Replacement and Atherosclerosis trial evaluated the effects of hormone replacement therapy on the progression of coronary atherosclerosis in postmenopausal women.

Methods.—The randomized double-blind trial included 309 postmenopausal women with coronary disease confirmed by angiography. The patients were assigned to receive conjugated estrogen, 0.625 mg/day, with or without medroxyprogesterone acetate (MPA), 2.5 mg/day, or placebo. Follow-up continued for a mean of 3.2 years, including quantitative coronary angiography to assess the progression of coronary atherosclerosis.

Results.—In both estrogen-treated groups, the low-density lipoprotein cholesterol level decreased significantly compared with the placebo group (by 9.4% in the estrogen-only group and 16.5% in the estrogen plus MPA group). Both treatments significantly increased high density lipoprotein cholesterol (by 18.8% and 14.2%, respectively). However, the progression of coronary atherosclerosis was similar among groups. With adjustment for baseline measurements, the mean minimal coronary artery diameter at follow-up was 1.87 mm in the estrogen-only group, 1.84 mm in the estrogen plus MPA group, and 1.87 mm in the placebo group. Other angiographic outcomes were also similar between groups, as were the clinical cardiovascular event rates.

Conclusion.—For postmenopausal women with coronary atherosclerosis, estrogen replacement therapy—with or without MPA—does not appear to influence the rate of atherosclerotic progression. Such patients should not expect cardiovascular benefit from the use of estrogen therapy. Estrogen replacement may still be effective in primary prevention of coronary disease, but this remains to be confirmed.

▶ The results of this randomized clinical trial suggest that estrogen has no effect on the progression of coronary artery disease in older (mean age, 68 years) women with established coronary artery disease despite having a beneficial effect on the lipid profile. For women with established coronary artery disease, statins or other treatments should be used to retard the progress of the disease. However, there is good evidence in animals and human beings that estrogens will retard the development of coronary artery atherosclerosis when given to young healthy postmenopausal women without evidence of coronary artery disease.

D. R. Mishell, Jr, MD

Increased Risk of Recurrent Venous Thromboembolism During Hormone Replacement Therapy: Results of the Randomized, Double-Blind, Placebo-Controlled Estrogen in Venous Thromboembolism Trial (EVTET)
Høibraaten E, Qvigstad E, Arnesen H, et al (Ullevål Univ, Oslo, Norway; Parexel Medstat, Lillestrøm, Norway; Novo Nordisk Pharma AS, Oslo, Norway)
Thromb Haemost 84:961-967, 2000   14–18

Introduction.—Evidence regarding the effect of hormone replacement therapy (HRT) on the risk of venous thromboembolism (VTE) is contradictory. Early epidemiologic trials failed to reveal an increased risk of VTE among HRT users; recent trials indicate a 2-to 4-fold increased risk for current users. A randomized, double-blind, placebo-controlled clinical trial using a triangular sequential design was initiated to determine whether estradiol treatment influences the risk of VTE.

Methods.—All participants were postmenopausal women younger than 70 years of age who had previous confirmed deep vein thrombosis (DVT) or pulmonary embolism (PE). Women were randomly assigned to treat-

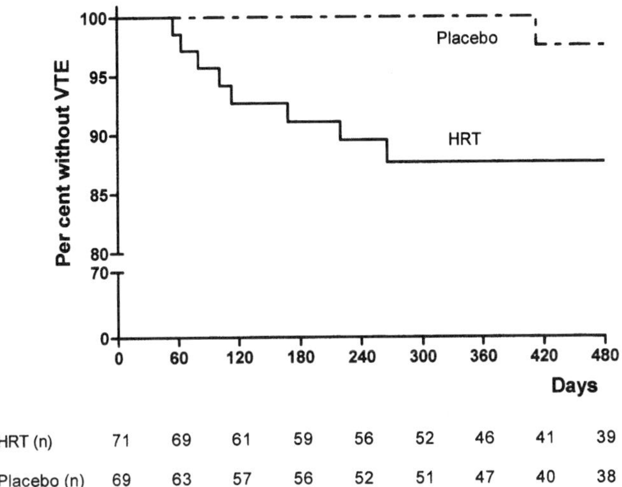

FIGURE 3.—Kaplan-Meier plot indicating the proportion of patients without recurrent VTE as a function of time from randomization by treatment group, ie, HRT (*continuous line*) and placebo. (Courtesy of Høibraaten E, Qvigstad E, Arnesen H: Increased risk of recurrent venous thromboembolism during hormone replacement therapy: Results of the randomized, double-blind, placebo-controlled estrogen in venous thromboembolism trial (EVTET). *Thromb Haemost* 84:961-967, 2000.)

ment with either 2 mg estradiol plus 1 mg norethisterone acetate, 1 tablet daily, or placebo. The main outcome measure was recurrent DVT or PE.

Results.—Of 140 women enrolled, 71 were allocated to receive HRT and 69 to receive placebo. Mean patient age was 55.8 years at baseline (range, 42 to 69 years). A positive screening test for thrombophilia was observed in 28% (20/71) of the women in the HRT group and 22% (15/69) of the women in the placebo group. There were 137 and 71 adverse events in the HRT and placebo groups. Mean follow-up was 485 days in the HRT group and 483 days in the placebo group. In the HRT group, 8 and 3 women, respectively, experienced recurrent VTE and PE. The incidence of VTE was 10.7% in the HRT group and 2.3% in the placebo group. An early excess risk of VTE related to HRT was evident according to a Kaplan-Meier plot (Fig 3). In the group treated with HRT, all 8 primary end points occurred within 261 days of treatment. The only primary end point in the placebo group was observed after 413 days of placebo. Thrombophilia was a significant risk factor for recurrence during HRT use (RR, 1.4).

Conclusion.—Postmenopausal women younger than 70 years with prior VTE who were receiving continuous HRT had an estimated 2- to 4-fold relative increased risk of VTE. It is recommended that this treatment be avoided in this patient group.

▶ Several recent observational studies have found that women taking postmenopausal HRT have a 2- to 4-fold greater risk of developing VTE. Women with a prior history of VTE are at increased risk of developing recurrent VTE. The results of this randomized trial show that the risk of a subsequent VTE is increased about 5-fold if women with a prior episode of VTE are given a high (2 mg) oral dose of estradiol daily as compared with a placebo control group. Thus, a prior history of VTE is at least a relative contraindication for oral HRT if the woman is not receiving anticoagulant therapy. It remains to be determined whether transdermal estrogen, which does not increase hepatic globulin production of factors that enhance thrombosis as much as oral estrogen, is also associated with an increased risk of VTE in women with a prior history of this problem. The effect of lower doses of oral estrogen on the risk of VTE in women with a history of VTE also remains to be determined. Clinicians need to counsel women with a history of VTE about the increased risks of a subsequent event if they take oral HRT.

D. R. Mishell, Jr, MD

Estrogen Replacement Therapy and Ovarian Cancer Mortality in a Large Prospective Study of US Women

Rodriguez C, Patel AV, Calle EE, et al (American Cancer Society, Atlanta, Ga)
JAMA 285:1460-1465, 2001
14–19

Background.—The use of postmenopausal estrogen has been associated with an increased risk for 2 hormone-related cancers, endometrial and breast cancer. However, the effect of postmenopausal estrogen use on ovarian cancer is unclear.

Methods.—Data were obtained from the American Cancer Society's Cancer Prevention Study II, a prospective study following up a cohort of 211,581 postmenopausal women from 1982 to 1996. At study enrollment, the women had no history of cancer, hysterectomy, or ovarian surgery. Baseline information was obtained by questionnaire.

Findings.—Nine hundred forty-four women died from ovarian cancer during the 14-year follow-up. Compared with women who never used estrogen replacement therapy (ERT), women using ERT at baseline had greater death rates from ovarian cancer, with a rate ratio (RR) of 1.51. Risk among former estrogen users was slightly but nonsignificantly increased, with an RR of 1.16. Duration of use correlated with increased risk in baseline and former users. The RR in baseline users with 10 or more years of use was 2.2. In former users with 10 or more years of use, the RR was 1.59. The annual age-adjusted ovarian cancer death rates per 100,000 women were 64.4 for baseline users of 10 or more years' duration, 38.3 for former users with 10 or more years' duration, and 26.4 for never users. The risk among former users with 10 or more years' duration declined with time since last use reported at study entry.

Conclusion.—Postmenopausal estrogen use lasting 10 years or longer was associated with an increased risk for ovarian cancer mortality. This risk persisted for up to 29 years after discontinuation of estrogen.

▶ The results of this large, prospective study suggest that postmenopausal ERT used for 10 or more years, but not for a shorter duration, may slightly increase the risk for death from ovarian cancer. However, the results are based upon a single questionnaire administered in 1982 and many women were excluded from the subsequent mortality analysis, including all those who had a hysterectomy. A recent meta-analysis of 15 case-control studies investigating the risk of epithelial ovarian cancer with ERT found the cumulative odds ratio to be 1.1 (confidence intervals, 0.9-1.3) with all but 1 of the individual reports showing no significant change in risk. Thus, the body of epidemiologic evidence fails to confirm a link between ERT use and ovarian cancer, despite the findings of this single study. Clinicians should inform their patients that consistency of results of several observational epidemiologic studies are needed to determine whether a causal relation actually exists and that nearly all of the other published studies have failed to confirm a relation between ERT use and an increased risk for ovarian cancer.

D. R. Mishell, Jr, MD

Risk of Ovarian Cancer in Relation to Estrogen and Progestin Dose and Use Characteristics of Oral Contraceptives

Ness RB, and the SHARE Study Group (Univ of Pittsburgh, Pa; et al)
Am J Epidemiol 152:233-241, 2000   14–20

Introduction.—Oral contraceptives (OCs) are considered to be the most powerful known chemopreventive agents for ovarian cancer. Earlier trials have demonstrated that an OC with 50 µg or more of estrogen diminishes the risk of ovarian cancer. It is not known whether the newer, lower-dose formulations have this same protective effect. Reported are findings of a population-based, case-control trial designed to address the impact of dose of OC on its association with ovarian cancer.

Methods.—All patients were women 20 to 69 years of age in whom epithelial ovarian cancer was diagnosed within the 6 months before interview. There were 767 completed case interviews between May 1994 and July 1998 from 39 hospitals; these were compared with 1367 community controls who were aged 65 years or younger. Controls were ascertained by random digit dialing (through Health Care Financing Administration lists) and were frequency matched by 5-year age groups and 3-digit telephone exchanges. Standardized 1.5-hour interviews were conducted by trained interviewers in the homes of participants. Contraceptive use, including type, frequency, and duration of use, was recorded. Pills containing less than 100 µg of mestranol or less than 50 µg of ethinyl estradiol were considered low-dose formulations; those containing 100 µg or more of mestranol or 50 µg or more of ethinyl estradiol were considered high dose. Progestins were considered low dose if their relative potency was below 0.5 mg norgestrel; high dose was 0.5 mg norgestrel or more.

Results.—Compared with never-users, the adjusted risk of ovarian cancer was decreased by 40% for OC users overall. Longer duration of use provided greater protection, independent of age at initiation. The dose of estrogens and progestins in OC formulations did not markedly affect the decrease in ovarian cancer risk (Table 2). The impact of OC use was not variable by invasiveness of tumor or by histologic type. The ovarian cancer risk reduction was similar for women who began OC before 1972, when high-dose pills dominated the market; between 1972 and 1980; and after 1980, when newer, lower-dose OC dominated. After adjustment for duration of OC use, the odds ratio for low-estrogen/low-progestin compared with high-estrogen/high progestin pills was identical.

TABLE 2.—Oral Contraceptive Use Characteristics, Including Estrogen and Progestin Dose, Among Ovarian Cancer Cases and Controls, Delaware Valley Area, May 1994 to June 1998

Variable	Cases (n = 767)	Controls (n = 1,367)	Crude OR	95% CI	Adjusted OR*	95% CI
Oral contraceptive use						
Never	341	426	1.0		1.0	
Ever	426	940	0.6	0.5, 0.7	0.6	0.5, 0.8
Oral contraceptive duration (years)						
Never	341	426	1.0		1.0	
<1	141	266	0.7	0.5, 0.8	0.7	0.6, 1.0
1-4	162	362	0.6	0.4, 0.7	0.7	0.5, 0.9
5-9	88	189	0.6	0.4, 0.8	0.6	0.5, 0.9
≥10	32	120	0.3	0.2, 0.5	0.3	0.2, 0.5
Time since last oral contraceptive use (years)						
Never	341	426	1.0		1.0	
<10	82	231	0.4	0.3, 0.6	0.4	0.3, 0.6
10-19	110	248	0.5	0.4, 0.7	0.6	0.4, 0.8
20-29	181	382	0.6	0.5, 0.7	0.6	0.5, 0.8
≥30	50	76	0.8	0.6, 1.2	1.0	0.6, 1.4
Age at first oral contraceptive use (years)						
Never	341	426	1.0		1.0	
<20	119	311	0.5	0.4, 0.6	0.6	0.4, 0.8
20-24	180	364	0.6	0.5, 0.8	0.6	0.5, 0.8
25-29	61	146	0.5	0.4, 0.7	0.5	0.4, 0.8
30-34	37	70	0.7	0.4, 1.0	0.8	0.5, 1.2
≥35	26	48	0.7	0.4, 1.1	0.8	0.4, 1.3
Calendar year of oral contraceptive initiation						
Never	341	426	1.0		1.0	
Before 1972	264	533	0.6	0.5, 0.8	0.7	0.5, 0.8
1972-1980	106	277	0.5	0.4, 0.6	0.5	0.4, 0.7
After 1980	56	130	0.5	0.4, 0.8	0.6	0.4, 0.9
Estrogen/progestin dose†						
Never	338	426	1.0		1.0	
High estrogen/high progestin	49	135	0.5	0.3, 0.7	0.5	0.3, 0.7
High estrogen/low progestin	8	14	0.7	0.3, 1.7	0.7	0.3, 1.8
Low estrogen/high progestin	9	24	0.5	0.2, 1.0	0.6	0.3, 1.3
Low estrogen/low progestin	140	377	0.5	0.4, 0.6	0.5	0.3, 0.6

*Adjusted for age, number of pregnancies, family history of ovarian cancer, and race.
†For combination oral contraceptives of known dose, based on vacuolization test.
Abbreviation: OR, Odds ratio.
(Courtesy of Ness RB, and the SHARE Study Group: Risk of ovarian cancer in relation to estrogen and progestin dose and use characteristics of oral contraceptives. *Am J Epidemiol* 152:233-241, 2000, by permission of Oxford University Press.)

Conclusion.—The protection provided by OC against ovarian cancer seems to be independent of the dose of estrogen or progestin. The diminished risk of ovarian cancer from OC use continues for 30 or more years after discontinuation of the OC and is protective after relatively short durations of exposure (1 to 4 years).

▶ Many case-control and cohort studies have consistently shown that use of OCs reduces the risk of epithelial ovarian cancer. The protective effect persists for decades after the use of OCs has ceased. In this large population-based case-control study, a significant protection against development of ovarian cancer persisted for as long as 30 years after discontinuation of OC use and protection occurred with as little as 1 to 4 years' total duration of OC use. With 10 or more years of OC use, there was a 70% reduction in development of ovarian cancer. Most of the earlier studies reported that reduction in ovarian cancer risk occurred with higher OC dose formulations than those currently used. In this study, a similar amount of protection occurred with the lower-dose OC formulations currently being used. In this study, as well as others, there is no information about the relation of formulations containing only 20 mg of ethinyl estradiol and the subsequent risk of developing ovarian cancer.

D. R. Mishell, Jr, MD

Breast Cancer Survival and Hormone Replacement Therapy: A Cohort Analysis
DiSaia PJ, Brewster WR, Ziogas A, et al (Univ of California, Irvine; Chao Family Comprehensive Cancer Center, Orange, Calif)
Am J Clin Oncol 23:541-545, 2000   14–21

Introduction.—The use of hormone replacement therapy (HRT) after a diagnosis of breast cancer is 1 of the most emotionally charged issues in the field of oncology. Breast cancer survivors are the largest group of former cancer patients in the United States, so there is ample reason to examine this controversy. A matched cohort analysis was performed to examine the impact of HRT on mortality rate in breast cancer survivors.

Methods.—Survivors of breast cancer who elected to receive HRT after diagnosis of breast cancer (cases) and controls from a regional cancer registry were identified. All women with an intact uterus received either the hormonal therapy prescribed before breast cancer diagnosis or combination therapy with oral estrogen and progestin. Women who underwent previous hysterectomy received estrogen replacement therapy alone. Con trols were matched according to disease stage, year of diagnosis of breast cancer, and age at diagnosis of breast cancer. Survival and life tables were calculated.

Results.—There were 125 HRT users and 362 controls. Ninety-eight percent of the HRT users (123/125) received systemic estrogen and 72% (90/125) also received a progestational agent. Mean interval between diagnosis of breast cancer and start of HRT was 46 months (range, 0-401 months). Median age 51.9 years for cases and 52.1 years for controls. There was a survival advantage for breast cancer survivors who received HRT versus controls at 15 years after the diagnosis of breast cancer (88% vs 63%; P = .003). A similar survival analysis, which included only patients with a known breast cancer stage and their matched controls (107 and 313 patients, respectively), showed a similar significant survival of cases versus controls at 15 years after diagnosis of breast cancer (85% vs 56%; P = .01). When the entire cohort was considered, there was an almost 70% decrease in the risk of death among HRT users compared with controls.

Conclusion.—This analysis does not indicate that HRT use is associated with compromised survival. In fact, a survival advantage was observed for breast cancer survivors who elected HRT.

▶ About 175,000 women are initially diagnosed with breast cancer each year in the United States. About 70% of these women are still alive 5 years after their diagnosis. A great deal of controversy and uncertainty exist as to whether to treat these women with estrogen replacement when they become postmenopausal, especially when vasomotor symptoms, atrophic vaginitis, or both develop. There have been no prospective randomized controlled trials to determine the effect of giving estrogen to postmenopausal breast cancer survivors compared with withholding therapy. This matched-cohort analysis gives clinicians and women some reassurance that administration of estrogen to women with a history of breast cancer does not increase their overall mortality rate. In fact, in this analysis, the women who took estrogen had a higher rate of survival. This information should be presented to women with a history of breast cancer to aid in their decision-making process regarding the use of exogenous estrogen.

D. R. Mishell, Jr, MD

Estrogen Replacement Therapy and Gallbladder Disease in Postmenopausal Women

Uhler ML, Marks JW, Judd HL (Loyola Univ, Maywood, Ill; Univ of California Los Angeles)
Menopause 7:162-167, 2000   14–22

Background.—Estrogen replacement therapy (ERT) has numerous benefits for postmenopausal women. However, some evidence indicates that ERT increases the incidence of gallbladder disease, presumably because of estrogen's effects on hepatic lipid metabolism. The English language literature from 1970 to the present was systematically reviewed to examine the association between ERT and gallbladder disease in postmenopausal women.

Biological basis for effect of ERT on gallstone formation.—Most gallstones (80%) are composed of cholesterol (pure or mixed with pigment, mucoglycoprotein, or calcium carbonate). Three processes are believed to be required for cholesterol gallstone formation: the supersaturation of bile with cholesterol, the rapid nucleation of cholesterol crystals in bile, and the growth of cholesterol crystals into larger and larger gallstones. Estrogen increases cholesterol saturation in bile and alters the composition of biliary acids by increasing levels of cholate and decreasing levels of chenodeoxycholate. Estrogen may also decrease bile flow, which would presumably promote cholesterol precipitation into crystals.

Results of studies evaluating the effect of estrogen on gallstone formation.—The authors reviewed the results of 7 studies (2 cohort studies, 2 cross-sectional studies, and 3 case-control studies). Specifically, 3 of the 5 retrospective observational studies found that postmenopausal women using ERT had an increased incidence of gallbladder disease (relative risks, 1.02-3.72). In a large prospective cohort study of almost 55,000 postmenopausal nurses, those using ERT were twice as likely to require cholecystectomy as women who had never used hormones. Two clinical studies prospectively evaluated the risk of gallbladder disease associated with the use of ERT in postmenopausal women. One of these studies was a 3-year trial of 875 postmenopausal women who were given placebo or conjugated equine estrogens (0.625 mg/d) and 3 groups who were given a combination of equine estrogens and cyclic or continuous progestins. Gallbladder disease developed in 2 women in the placebo group, 2 women in the estrogen only group, and 4 to 5 women in each of the 3 groups given estrogen plus progestin. However, the incidence of gallbladder disease did not differ significantly between groups, probably because of the small group sizes and the relatively brief treatment period.

The other prospective clinical trials included 2763 postmenopausal women with coronary heart disease who were given either placebo or conjugated equine estrogen (0.625 mg/d) plus medroxyprogesterone acetate (2.5 mg/d). During an average follow-up of 4 years, gallbladder disease developed in significantly more women in the ERT group (84 of 1380, or 60.8%) than women receiving placebo (62 of 1383, or 23.1%) (relative hazard, 1.38).

The route of estrogen administration has different effects on hepatic and nonhepatic markers of estrogen's actions. Hepatic first-pass metabolism after oral dosing enhances the effect of estrogen on lipid and protein synthesis. Thus, it has been hypothesized that nonoral administration of estrogen may reduce its effects on bile composition. Nonetheless, 1 study showed that oral or transdermal estrogen administration both cause significant increases in the biliary cholesterol saturation index and levels of arachidonic acid and prostaglandin E_2 and significant decreases in nucleation time. Each of these factors would increase the likelihood of gallstone formation.

▶ Some, but not all, observational epidemiologic studies—including the large, prospective Nurses' Health Study—indicate that when exogenous estrogen is given to postmenopausal women, there is a significantly increased risk of the development of gallbladder disease. There is a biological basis for this effect of estrogen, and women should be counseled about this possible deleterious effect of taking ERT.

D. R. Mishell, Jr, MD

15 Infertility

Body Mass Index and Delayed Conception: A European Multicenter Study on Infertility and Subfecundity
Bolúmar F, and the European Study Group on Infertility and Subfecundity
(Univ Miguel Hernández, Alicante, Spain; et al)
Am J Epidemiol 151:1072-1079, 2000   15–1

Introduction.—Obesity is a common health problem in developed countries. Few trials have examined the effect of obesity on subfertility, which is defined as the inability to conceive after 9.5 months of unprotected intercourse. The effect of body mass index (BMI) on time to pregnancy was examined in a population-based sample of pregnant women from 5 European countries.

Methods.—The European Study on Infertility and Subfecundity was conducted between February and December 1992. Pregnant women were recruited after a minimum of 20 weeks' gestation during prenatal visits or when giving birth at a hospital or clinic. BMI was calculated. The time to pregnancy was categorized in months and was used to estimate a couple's fecundability.

Results.—Of 4035 women recruited, the 2587 with planned pregnancies were followed up. About 12% were overweight (BMI greater than 25 kg/m²) and just over 3% were obese (BMI 30 kg/m² or greater). There was a significant correlation between obesity and delayed conception (odds ratio [OR], 11.54; 95% confidence interval [CI], 3.68-36.15). An increased risk of delayed conception was also observed among women whose BMI was less than 20 kg/m² (OR, 1.70; 95% CI, 1.01-2.83).

The same analysis conducted among female nonsmokers showed no correlation between either obesity (OR, 0.79) or leanness (OR, 1.10) and delay in conception. In lean women, those who smoked over 15 cigarettes daily had a higher risk for delayed conception, compared with normal weight women who were nonsmokers (OR, 3.43; 95% CI, 1.43-8.24). Obese women had a significantly higher risk for delayed conception at any level of tobacco use. The adjusted fecundability ratio was 0.52 for female smokers whose BMI was 30 kg/m² or greater. After adjustment for risk factors, 47% of women who were obese and 19% of lean women needed over 12 months to conceive, compared with 12% of normal-weight women (Fig 2).

"

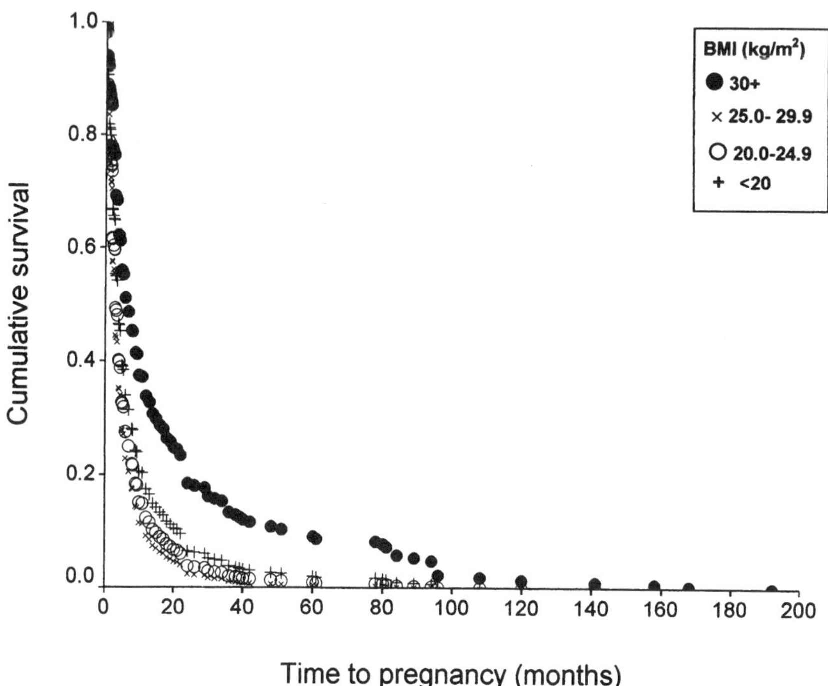

FIGURE 2.—Adjusted distribution of waiting time to pregnancy, according to body mass index (*BMI*) at the beginning of the waiting time to pregnancy, for European women smokers whose pregnancies were planned. (Courtesy of Bolúmar F, and the European Study Group on Infertility and Subfecundity: Body mass index and delayed contraception: A European multicenter study on infertility and subfecundity. *Am J Epidemiol* 151:1072-1079, 2000, by permission of Oxford University Press.)

Conclusion.—There is a strong correlation between obesity and delayed conception in pregnant women who plan their pregnancies.

▶ This study found that obese and underweight women who smoked ciga-rettes and eventually conceived required a longer time until conception occurred than smokers of normal body weight. A similar delay in time to conception for obese or lean women was not observed in nonsmokers. Other studies have shown that there is an association between obesity and anovulation which could cause women not to conceive. Smoking also results in a delay in the time to conception. Infertile women who smoke should be counseled to stop smoking, and infertile obese women who fail to ovulate regularly should be counseled to lose weight.

D. R. Mishell, Jr, MD

Prediction of Ovulation by Urinary Hormone Measurements With the Home Use ClearPlan® Fertility Monitor: Comparison With Transvaginal Ultrasound Scans and Serum Hormone Measurements

Behre HM, Kuhlage J, Gaβner C, et al (Inst of Reproductive Medicine of the Univ, Münster, Germany)
Hum Reprod 15:2478-2482, 2000

15–2

Background.—Practical methods for determining ovulation in consecutive cycles in individuals are needed. The home use performance of the ClearPlan Fertility Monitor (CPFM) (Unipath Diagnostics Co, Princeton, NJ) to predict ovulation was assessed against transvaginal US and serum hormone measures.

Methods.—Fifty-three women, aged 18 to 39 years, were included in the study. All had a normal uterus and at least 1 ovary, had a cycle length of 21 to 42 days, and were free of medication interfering with ovarian function. Data on a total of 149 cycles were analyzed.

Findings.—One hundred thirty-five cycles had a monitor luteinizing hormone (LH) surge and US-confirmed ovulation. During the 2 days of CPFM peak fertility, ovulation was detected in 91.1% of the cycles (Fig 1). Ovulation was noted in 51.1% and 43.2% of cycles 1 and 2 days, respectively, after the serum LH surge. In none of the cycles did ovulation occur before CPFM peak fertility or the serum LH surge day.

Conclusion.—Home use of the CPFM is helpful for timing intercourse for conception. It may also have potential as a diagnostic tool and for monitoring infertility treatment.

▶ The home urinary test to predict ovulation described in this report measures both estrone glucuronide and LH. Detection of high levels of estrone glucuronide is indicative of the change from low to high fertility while detection of high levels of LH is an indication of peak fertility. Ovulation, as determined by US, occurred on the first day of peak fertility in 21% of ovulatory cycles and on the second day of peak fertility in 76% of ovulatory cycles. The optimal time to have sexual intercourse in order to have conception occur is the day before ovulation, with the next best chance of conception occurring with intercourse occurring on the day of ovulation or 2 days before ovulation. Therefore, it remains to be determined whether women using the test described in this report will have a greater chance of a successful pregnancy than with a test that only measures LH on a random or first morning urine sample.

D. R. Mishell, Jr, MD

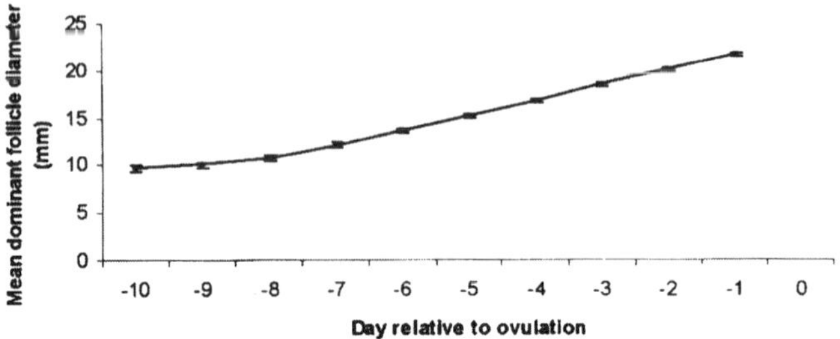

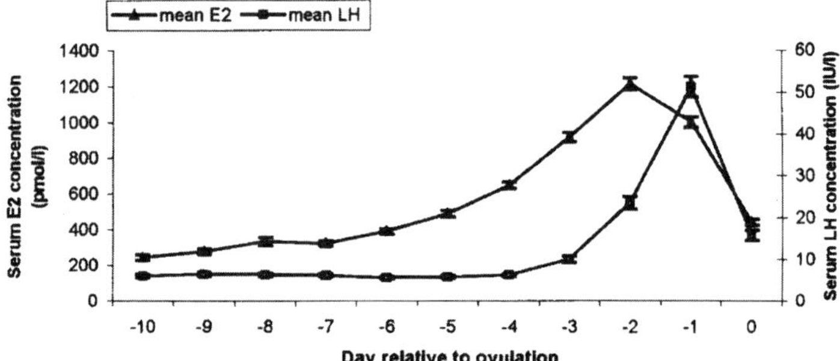

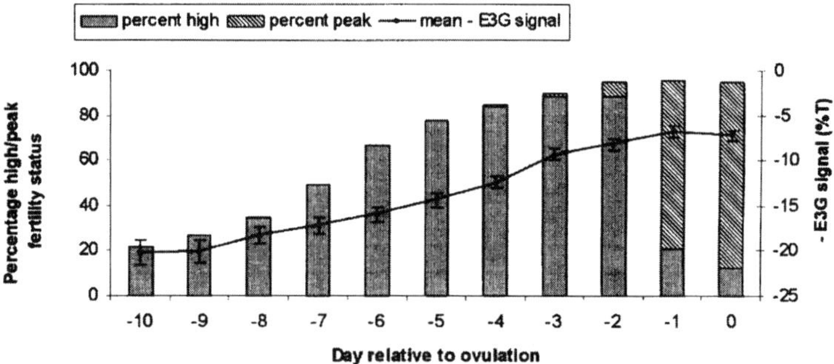

FIGURE 1.—Dominant follicle diameter (mean ± SEM) (**upper panel**), serum concentrations of estradiol (*E2*) and luteinizing hormone (LH) (**middle panel**), and urinary estrone-3-glucuronide (*E3G*) signal and percentage of high/peak fertility status (**lower panel**) relative to day of ovulation (day 0). According to the study design, not all women had transvaginal US and hormone measurement on each day displayed. *Abbreviation:* % *T*, Percentage transmission units. (Courtesy of Behre HM, Kuhlage J, Gaβner C, et al: Prediction of ovulation by urinary hormone measurements with the home use ClearPlan® fertility monitor: Comparison with transvaginal ultrasound scans and serum hormone measurements. *Hum Reprod* 15:2478-2482, 2000. Copyright, European Society for Human Reproduction and Embryology, by permission of Oxford University Press.)

Air-Contrast Sonohysterography as a First Step Assessment of Tubal Patency

Jeanty P, Besnard S, Arnold A, et al (Women's Health Alliance, Nashville, Tenn)
J Ultrasound Med 19:519-527, 2000   15–3

Background.—Hysterosalpingography is often used to assess tubal patency in infertile women, but newer methods are gaining in popularity. The use of air as a sonographic contrast agent (air-contrast sonohysterography) was described.

Methods.—Air-contrast sonohysterography was performed to assess tubal patency in 114 women with infertility and 1 woman after tubal ligation. None of the patients was given prophylactic antibiotics. Patients initially underwent conventional pelvic US, then they underwent air-contrast sonohysterography. In brief, the procedure for air-contrast sonohysterography is similar to that for conventional sonohysterography, except as follows: A balloon catheter is introduced into the uterus and filled with 1.5 mL air. Saline solution (5-10 mL) is injected into the uterine cavity, then the balloon is carefully withdrawn against the internal os until a seal is created. The syringe is disconnected and filled with 5 to 10 mL of air, and the passage of air bubbles into the fallopian tubes is imaged starting from the level of the cornu. In some cases, the release of air into the peritoneal cavity can be visualized. After both tubes have been assessed, the balloon is deflated and the uterine cavity is imaged with saline solution.

Results.—Cervical stenosis prevented introduction of the balloon catheter in 5 patients (4.3%); their data were excluded from analyses. Air-contrast sonohysterography successfully imaged a total of 217 tubes (3 tubes had been surgically removed) in the remaining 110 patients. On average, air-contrast sonohysterography took 5 minutes 22 seconds, with insonation used for 2 to 3 minutes. Average air volumes for imaging the left and right fallopian tubes were 11.8 and 12.2 mL, respectively. Air-contrast sonohysterography indicated that 177 of the 217 tubes (81.5%) were definitely patent and 12 tubes (5.5%) were probably patent; 28 tubes (13%) were nonvisualized. Additionally, 3 cases of synechiae, 9 cases of polyps, and 2 cases of submucosal fibroids were identified during the examination. During follow-up from 2 weeks to 21 months, 27 patients (24.5%) became pregnant at a mean of 25 weeks after the procedure. Among the 83 patients who did not conceive during follow-up, 15 patients (29 tubes) underwent laparoscopy with chromopertubation.

Air contrast sonohysterographic and laparoscopic assessments of tubal patency agreed in 17 patent tubes and in 6 closed or nonvisualized tubes (79.4% agreement). Of the 6 discrepancies, 5 tubes were considered patent by laparoscopy alone and 1 tube was considered patent by air-contrast sonohysterography alone. The sensitivity, specificity, positive predictive value, and negative predictive value of air-contrast sonohysterography for open tubes were 85.7%, 77.2%, 54.5%, and 94.4%, respectively; corresponding values for closed tubes were 87.5%, 80.9%, 63.6%, and 94.4%.

Complications were experienced by 36.3% of patients, and were generally mild; the most common complication was cramping while the uterus was distended with saline solution.

Conclusion.—Air-contrast sonohysterography is a comfortable, safe, rapid, and accurate first-line procedure for assessing tubal patency in women with infertility. The procedure was comfortable even for patients with closed tubes, as the air simply refluxed around the balloon catheter. (With hysterosalpingography, the resistance to pushing the piston of the syringe is greatly increased when tubes are closed, and this increased pressure is painful.) Additionally, air-contrast sonohysterography can identify other uterine abnormalities, such as synechiae, polyps, and endoluminal fibroids.

Three-Dimensional Hysterosalpingo-Contrast Sonography (3D-HyCoSy) as an Outpatient Procedure to Assess Infertile Women: A Pilot Study

Kiyokawa K, Masuda H, Fuyuki T, et al (Keiyu Hosp, Yokohama, Japan)
Ultrasound Obstet Gynecol 16:648-654, 2000   15–4

Background.—Because of its accuracy, minimal invasiveness, and cost effectiveness, hysterosalpingo-contrast sonography (HyCoSy) has been widely used to assess tubal patency in infertile women. Two-dimensional HyCoSy has a few drawbacks, however, including the fact that the full contour of the uterine cavity is rarely depicted in a single scanning plane. The effectiveness of 3-dimensional (3D) HyCoSy as an outpatient procedure for investigating tubal patency was evaluated.

Methods.—The subjects were 25 infertile women 27 to 40 years of age (mean, 32.6 years) who underwent tubal insufflation followed by 3D-HyCoSy with saline as a contrast agent and, 3 hours later, x-ray hysterosalpingography (XHSG). Patients received prophylactic antibiotics, but no sedation or anesthesia was used during the procedures. None of the patients had pelvic pathology according to results of transvaginal US. During tubal insufflation, carbon dioxide gas was pumped into the uterine cavity and intrauterine pressures were recorded. Immediately thereafter, sterile saline solution was continuously instilled via a balloon catheter, and 3D-HyCoSy was performed transvaginally.

The scanning plane was selected to include the entire length of both fallopian tubes and the uterine cavity. The acquisition of volume data of color Doppler flow signals took about 13 seconds per scan, and the acquisition of volume data of the uterine cavity took about 3 seconds per scan. XHSG was performed by physicians blinded to the results of 3D-HyCoSy.

Results.—Of the 50 tubes examined, XHSG identified 46 patent tubes and 4 occluded ones. 3D-HyCoSy identified 38 patent tubes and 12 occluded ones. Thus, results of 3D-HyCoSy and XHSG agreed in 68% of cases. In all 8 discordant cases, 3D-HyCoSy showed unilateral occlusion but XHSG subsequently confirmed patency. Compared with XHSG, the specificity, sensitivity, positive predictive value, and negative predictive value of 3D-HyCoSy were 100%, 84.4%, 100%, and 33.3%, respectively. 3D-HyCoSy was significantly superior to XHSG in depicting the full contour of the uterine cavity (96% vs 64% of cases). Nine patients (36%) reported abdominal pain during saline solution injection or balloon catheter insertion; only 1 required pain medication.

Conclusion.—The efficacy of 3D-HyCoSy in the outpatient assessment of tubal patency compares well with that of conventional XHSG. 3D-HyCoSy is superior, however, in its imaging of the uterine cavity. It also appears to be better tolerated in that the procedure is less invasive than XHSG; none of the patients required prophylactic sedation or anesthesia, and only 1 required pain medication after the procedure. Images with 3D-HyCoSy were acquired quickly, and saline solution is less expensive than the contrast agents used with XHSG. Thus, 3D-HyCoSy has several advantages over XHSG in the outpatient assessment of infertile women.

Three-Dimensional Power Doppler Imaging in the Assessment of Fallopian Tube Patency

Sladkevicius P, Ojha K, Campbell S, et al (St George's Hosp Med School, London)
Ultrasound Obstet Gynecol 16:644-647, 2000
15–5

Background.—Hysterosalpingo-contrast sonography (HyCoSy) is often performed with the use of echo-positive contrast agents such as Echovist. Echovist (Schering AG, Germany) consists of galactose microparticles suspended in an aqueous galactose solution. This agent loses its contrast properties in 10 minutes, so the HyCoSy procedure must be completed within 10 minutes. This is difficult to do when performing standard 2-dimensional (2D) HyCoSy, in part because the entire fallopian tube is rarely visualized in 1 scanning plane, and thus the transvaginal probe must be manipulated to visualize different parts of the tube. The efficacy of 2D-HyCoSy was compared with that of 3-dimensional power Doppler scanning (3D-PDI) in the evaluation of tubal patency.

Methods.—The subjects were 67 infertile women whose tubal patency was being assessed. All patients underwent 2D US and color Doppler imaging to evaluate the uterus and ovaries. Then 5 to 10 mL of sterile saline solution was injected to identify any intracavitary abnormalities. Echovist-200 was injected and conventional gray-scale 2D-HyCoSy of the tubes was performed to identify the presence of contrast. Subsequently, additional contrast agent was injected continuously, and color-coded 3D-PDI was performed to identify the flow of medium through the tube.

Results.—The entire length of the fallopian tube could be visualized with 3D-PDI. Neither 2D-HyCoSy nor 3D-PDI identified proximal filling in 9 tubes. Of the remaining 125 tubes, 2D-HyCoSy showed free spillage of the contrast medium from the distal end in 58 tubes (46%), while

3D-PDI showed free spillage in 114 tubes (91%). The duration of the procedure was significantly shorter with 3D-PDI compared with 2D-HyCoSy (mean, 5-7 vs 10 minutes). However, because the operator required about 6 minutes to analyze the stored information, operator time for the 2 procedures was similar. 3D-PDI also required significantly less contrast medium than 2D-HyCoSy (mean, 5.9 vs 11.2 mL).

Conclusion.—Color-coded 3D-PDI with surface rendering enabled the entire length of the fallopian tube to be visualized, and free spillage of contrast agent into the peritoneal cavity was seen in more than 90% of patent tubes. Because scanning time was less with 3D-PDI than with 2D-HyCoSy, less contrast agent was required. The success of 2D-HyCoSy appears to depend more on the scanning operator's skills in manipulating the probe to image the entire fallopian tube, while the success of 3D-PDI depends more on the settings of the US equipment.

▶ Several new sonographic techniques have been utilized to determine whether the oviducts of infertile women are patent. Use of these techniques can be performed more rapidly and cause less discomfort than conventional hysterosalpingography. They also avoid the use of ionizing radiation and appear to reduce the risk of pelvic infection. Any sonographic technique that utilizes fluid as a contrast agent is called hysterocontrast sonography, which is abbreviated as HyCoSo. These 3 studies (Abstracts 15–3, 15–4, and 15–5) report findings of the use of air contrast sonohysterosalpingy and 3D Doppler HyCoSo techniques to assess tubal patency. It is likely that some type of 3D Doppler HyCoSo will replace hysterosalpingography as a diagnostic technique for demonstrating the presence or absence of tubal patency when evaluating the female partner of the infertile couple.

D. R. Mishell, Jr, MD

Transvaginal Power Doppler Findings in Laparoscopically Proven Acute Pelvic Inflammatory Disease

Molander P, Sjöberg J, Paavonen J, et al (Univ of Helsinki)
Ultrasound Obstet Gynecol 17:233-238, 2001   15–6

Background.—The clinical diagnosis of pelvic inflammatory disease (PID) can be inaccurate. The value of power Doppler transvaginal sonography (TVS) for diagnosing PID was investigated.

Methods.—Thirty women hospitalized for suspected acute PID were included in the study. Conventional and power Doppler TVS were performed in these patients as well as in a control group of 20 women with proved hydrosalpinx formation. The patients with suspected acute PID also underwent laparoscopy.

Findings.—Laparoscopy confirmed PID diagnosis in 20 of the 30 women with clinically suspected PID. Specific TVS findings differentiating the PID group from the control group were wall thickness exceeding 5 mm, cogwheel sign, incomplete septa, and the presence of cul-de-sac fluid.

Power Doppler TVS showed hyperemia in all women with acute PID but in only 2 women with hydrosalpinx. Pulsatility indexes were significantly lower in the PID group than in the control group, with mean values of 0.84 and 1.5, respectively.

Conclusion.—The overall accuracy of power Doppler TVS in the diagnosis of PID was 93% in this series. The sensitivity and specificity of this modality were 100% and 80%, respectively. Specific TVS findings augment the clinical diagnosis of PID, enabling simple classification of disease severity.

▶ When pelvic laparoscopy is routinely performed in women with the clinical diagnosis of acute salpingitis, it has been reported that many of them have another etiology as the cause of their symptoms. In order to diagnose acute salpingitis with greater accuracy than clinical examination, the results of this study show that power Doppler TVS is an extremely sensitive method for improving the accuracy of the diagnosis of acute salpingitis.

D. R. Mishell, Jr, MD

Prognostic Value of Baseline Serum Oestradiol in Controlled Ovarian Hyperstimulation of Women With Unexplained Infertility
Costello MF, Hughes GJ, Garrett DK, et al (Univ of New South Wales, Sydney, Australia; Royal Hosp for Women, Sydney, Australia)
Aust N Z J Obstet Gynaecol 41:69-74, 2001   15–7

Background.—Predicting outcomes for couples undergoing assisted reproductive treatments is important. The prognostic value of baseline serum estradiol (E_2) level on cycle pregnancy rate (PR) in women with unexplained inferility (UI) treated by controlled ovarian hyperstimulation (COH) was investigated.

Methods.—Data were obtained on 374 cycles of COH in 145 women younger than 42 years. All women had UI and were treated between 1992 and 1995. Treatment consisted of human menopausal gonadotrophin alone or human menopausal gonadotrophin plus clomiphene citrate. Outcomes were determined as cycle pregnancy rate (PR) according to the cycle day 1 level of E_2.

Findings.—Patients with an E_2 level greater than 150 pmol/L on cycle day 1 of COH had a significantly lower PR than those with E_2 concentrations of 150 pmol/L or less, the rates being 4% and 13%, respectively. In a logistic regression analysis, women with day 1 E_2 concentrations of less than 150 pmol/L were 3.2 times more likely to conceive than those with day 1 E_2 levels exceeding 150 pmol/L. In addition, the effects of day 1 E_2 concentrations on the chances of pregnancy were unrelated to day 1 serum levels of follicle-stimulating hormone.

Conclusion.—Women with UI undergoing COH with a baseline serum E_2 level exceeding 150 pmol/L appear to have a significantly lower PR than those with an E$_2$ level of 150 pmol/l or less. Such women should be counseled on the reduced likelihood of pregnancy.

▶ Women with UI, defined as ovulatory women with patent oviducts whose partner has a normal semen analysis, are increasingly being treated with COH with either clomiphene citrate or human menopausal gonadotropin followed by intrauterine insemination. Per cycle pregnancy rates with this therapy are about 15%. In this study, when COH was followed by timed natural intercourse, the per cycle pregnancy rate was 13.2% in women with day 1 E$_2$ levels of less than 150 pml/L (equivalent to 50 pg/mL). However, women with higher day 1 E$_2$ levels had a much lower pregnancy rate. The results of this study need to be confirmed in other clinics. However, clinicians may wish to measure a day 1 E$_2$ level when treating patients with UI with COH and intrauterine insemination in order to help counsel them about their chances of success.

D. R. Mishell, Jr, MD

Effect of the Total Motile Sperm Count on the Efficacy and Cost-Effectiveness of Intrauterine Insemination and in Vitro Fertilization

Van Voorhis BJ, Barnett M, Sparks AET, et al (Univ of Iowa, Iowa City)
Fertil Steril 75:661-668, 2001

15–8

Background.—The severity of male-factor infertility may be an important variable in the success of intrauterine insemination (IUI). The prognostic factors for achieving pregnancy with IUI and in vitro fertilization (IVF) were investigated.

Methods.—Data on 1039 infertile couples undergoing a total of 3479 IUI cycles and on 424 infertile couples undergoing a total of 551 IVF cycles were analyzed. The importance of several factors to the prognosis was assessed, including the woman's age, gravidity, duration of infertility, diagnoses, use of ovulation induction, and sperm parameters. The relative efficacy and cost effectiveness of IUI and IVF were determined based on sperm count findings.

Findings.—Independent predictors of pregnancy after IUI were female age, gravidity, and use of ovulation induction. The mean total sperm count in the ejaculate, with a threshold ejaculate of 10 million, was also an important variable. For IVF, female age was the only significant predictor for clinical and ongoing pregnancy. When the mean total motile sperm count was less than 10 million, IVF with intracytoplasmic sperm injection was more cost effective than IUI.

Conclusion.—A mean total motile sperm count of 10 million appears to be a useful threshold value for deciding on IUI or IVF for the treatment of infertile couples. In this study, IVF with intracytoplasmic sperm injection was more cost effective than IUI when the mean total motile sperm count was less than 10 million.

▶ The results of this study suggest that if the average total motile sperm count in the ejaculate of the male partner of an infertile couple is more than 10 million and the woman is ovulating with at least 1 patent oviduct, it is more cost effective to treat the couple with controlled ovarian hyperstimulation and IUI than with IVF. If the total motile sperm count in the ejaculate is less than 10 million, it is better to perform IVF with intracytoplasmic sperm injection than IUI with controlled ovarian hyperstimulation.

D. R. Mishell, Jr, MD

Homologous Intrauterine Insemination: An Evaluation of Prognostic Factors Based on a Review of 2473 Cycles

Khalil MR, Rasmussen PE, Erb K, et al (Odense Univ, Denmark)
Acta Obstet Gynecol Scand 80:74-81, 2001   15–9

Background.—Homologous intrauterine insemination (IUI-H), involving the deposition of purified motile spermatozoa directly into the uterine cavity at ovulation, has been used for a variety of indications, often preceding the more rigorous and costly in vitro fertilization. Factors influencing the outcome of IUI-H were reported.

Methods and Findings.—Data on 893 couples undergoing a total of 2473 IUI-H treatment cycles during 9 years were included in the retrospective analysis. The overall clinical pregnancy rate per IUI-H cycle was 11.9%, increasing significantly from 8.7% in 1990 to 14.8% in 1998. Eighteen percent of the women had multiple births. The birth rate per couple was 27.2% after an average of 2.8 treatment cycles. Pregnancy rates were greatest in the first treatment cycle. After the fourth treatment cycle, the birth rate increased only slightly. Factors positively and significantly associated with successful IUI-H outcomes were first treatment cycle; up to 5 mature follicles; use of CClhMG-FSH compared with clomiphene citrate only for ovarian stimulation; number of motile sperms inseminated of more than 5 million; time of insemination, preferably between day 13 and 16 of the cycle; and anovulatory or idiopathic infertility.

Conclusion.—IUI-H is a simple, cost-effective treatment yielding acceptable pregnancy rates for up to 4 treatment cycles when at least 3 or 4 mature follicles have developed at the time of insemination. Success also relies on the use of hormonal ovarian stimulation and induction of ovulation, insemination between cycle day 13 and 16, and the availability of at least 5 million motile spermatozoa for insemination. Couples with tubal abnormalities or with less than 5 million motile spermatozoa should be referred directly for in vitro fertilization.

▶ This large series of infertile couples treated with controlled ovarian hyperstimulation (COH) and IUI-H had a per cycle pregnancy rate of about 12%. This rate is consistent with the 10% to 15% pregnancy rate reported by other investigators using this therapy to treat infertile couples with unexplained infertility. In this series, the per cycle pregnancy rate of couples with unexplained infertility treated with COH and IUI was 14%. These investigators reported that if the number of motile sperm inseminated was less than 5 million, the per cycle pregnancy rate fell to 5%. Others have reported that satisfactory pregnancy rates were achieved if at least 1 million motile sperm were inseminated. Thus, COH plus IUI-H can be performed for a few cycles for couples with unexplained infertility as well as mild types of male factor infertility with a certain amount of motile spermatozoa, as shown in this and the previous study (Abstract 15–8).

D. R. Mishell, Jr, MD

Vaginal Misoprostol Enhances Intrauterine Insemination

Brown SE, Toner JP, Schnorr JA, et al (Eastern Virginia Med School, Norfolk; Hôpital de Nyon, Switzerland; Univ Hosp Geneva)
Hum Reprod 16:96-101, 2001

15–10

Introduction.—There may be a link between prostaglandins (PGs) and fertility inasmuch as lower concentrations of PG have been found in the seminal fluid of men from infertile couples. Misoprostol is a commercially available synthetic PG that is structurally related to PGE_1, one of the most dominant PGs in human ejaculate. The usefulness of vaginally placed misoprostol as adjunctive therapy at the time of intrauterine insemination (IUI) was assessed, along with its tolerability and effects on clinical pregnancy rates.

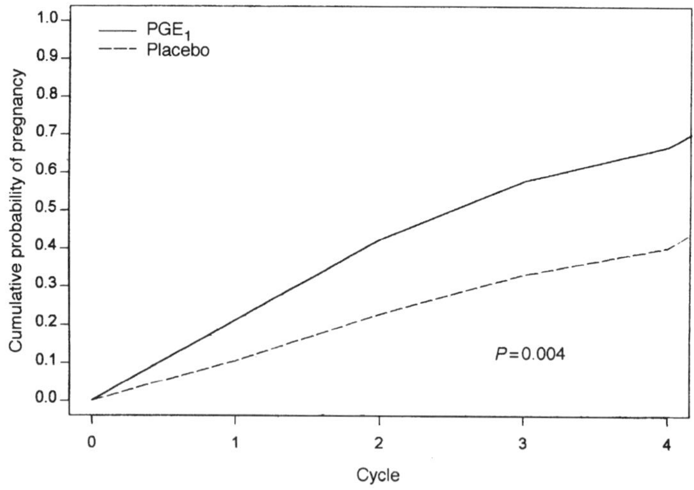

FIGURE 1.—PGE_1 and placebo cumulative pregnancy rates for all cycles. (Courtesy of Brown SE, Toner JP, Schnorr JA, et al: Vaginal misoprostol enhances intrauterine insemination. *Hum Reprod* 16:96-101, 2001. Copyright European Society for Human Reproduction and Embryology, by permission of Oxford University Press.)

Methods.—Two hundred seventy-four women were assessed during 494 IUI cycles that resulted in 64 pregnancies (13% per cycle) in a prospective, placebo-controlled, randomized, and double-blind trial. For treatment of infertility, all women underwent either natural cycle, clomiphene citrate, gonadotropin, or clomiphene/gonadotropin stimulation. Before speculum removal after IUI, an opaque white suppository was placed in the posterior vaginal fornix and contained either placebo or 400 μg of misoprostol. Pregnancy rates for PGE_1 and placebo cycles were calculated.

Results.—Of 241 misoprostol cycles, 43 resulted in pregnancy (17% per cycle). For placebo, 241 cycles resulted in 21 pregnancies (9% per cycle). The cumulative pregnancy rate with misoprostol was significantly higher than with placebo ($P = .004$) (Fig 1). The pregnancy rate in clomiphene-stimulated misoprostol-treated cycles was significantly higher than for placebo ($P = .006$). For gonadotropin (FSH)-stimulated misoprostol cycles, the pregnancy rate was higher than for placebo. The difference was of borderline significance. The active treatment and placebo cycles had similar rates of subjective side effects, complications, and pain variables.

Conclusion.—The use of vaginal misoprostol may improve the chance of pregnancy in women having IUI in a wide variety of cycle types.

▶ Controlled ovarian hyperstimulation (COH) with clomiphene citrate or gonadotrophins followed by IUI of sperm separated from seminal fluid is frequently used to treat couples with unexplained infertility. The results of this randomized controlled trial with misoprostol indicate that when this prostaglandin E1 analogue was placed in the vagina shortly after IUI, the pregnancy rate per cycle was significantly increased compared with that achieved with placebo (17% per cycle vs 9% per cycle). Since the use of misoprostol was not accompanied by an increase in side effects, clinicians performing COH and IUI may wish to place 2 200-mg tablets of misoprostol in the vagina after the IUI procedure in an attempt to improve the rate of conception.

D. R. Mishell, Jr, MD

Assisted Reproductive Technology in the United States: 1997 Results Generated From the American Society for Reproductive Medicine/Society for Assisted Reproductive Technology Registry
Society for Assisted Reproductive Technology and American Society for Reproductive Medicine (Birmingham, Ala)
Fertil Steril 74:641-653, 2000   15–11

Background.—The Society for Assisted Reproductive Technology (SART) has been collecting data on assisted reproductive technology (ART) since 1988. The results of ART procedures performed in 1997 were analyzed using SART data.

Methods.—Three hundred thirty-five programs submitted data on procedures conducted in 1997. The data analysis was done after November 1998 to determine pregnancy outcomes.

Findings.—A total of 73,069 cycles of ART were initiated. In vitro fertilization, with or without micromanipulation, was involved in 51,344 cycles, yielding a delivery rate per retrieval of 27.9%. Another 1943 cycles involved gamete intrafallopian transfer, which yielded a delivery rate per retrieval of 30%. The 1104 cycles done with zygote intrafallopian transfer were associated with a 28% delivery rate per retrieval. The delivery rate per transfer of 4616 donor oocyte cycles was 40%; of 10,181 frozen embryo transfer procedures, it was 18.8%; of 1584 frozen embryo transfers using donated oocytes, it was 22.2%; and of 600 cycles involving a host uterus, it was 34.6%. In addition, 1173 cycles were reported as combination treatments: 40 as research, 258 as embryo banking, and 226 as other. Overall, 17,311 pregnancies resulted in 25,059 infants.

Conclusion.—More programs reported ART treatment in 1997 than in 1996. The number of reported cycles increased by 10.9%, a significant difference from 1996. Deliveries per retrieval in comparable cycle types improved by 1.8%, a 6.9% increase in the 1996 success rate.

▶ In vitro fertilization, with or without intracytoplasmic sperm injection, is being increasingly used to treat all infertile couples in the United States, despite the fact that the cost is infrequently reimbursed by insurance providers or HMOs. The number of cycles reported to this registry increased more than 10% in 1997, compared with 1996. The comments by the investigators from the Centers for Disease Control and Prevention, which follow this 1997 report, state that rates of birth defects and neonatal deaths in this report are most likely erroneously low because of bias. These investigators believed that the techniques used to determine the rates of pregnancy outcome by the ART centers were incomplete and unreliable. Thus concern still exists that in vitro fertilization procedures, and intracytoplasmic sperm injection in particular, may be associated with an increased risk for genetic abnormalities in the fetuses conceived after these techniques than occurs with normal procreation.

D. R. Mishell, Jr, MD

Cumulative Probability of Achieving an Ongoing Pregnancy After Invitro Fertilization and Intracytoplasmic Sperm Injection According to a Woman's Age, Subfertility Diagnosis and Primary or Secondary Subfertility

Stolwijk AM, Wetzels AMM, Braat DDM (Univ of Nijmegen, The Netherlands)

Hum Reprod 15:203-209, 2000   15–12

Background.—Couples considering additional in vitro fertilization (IVF) procedures need to know the probability of success after several such

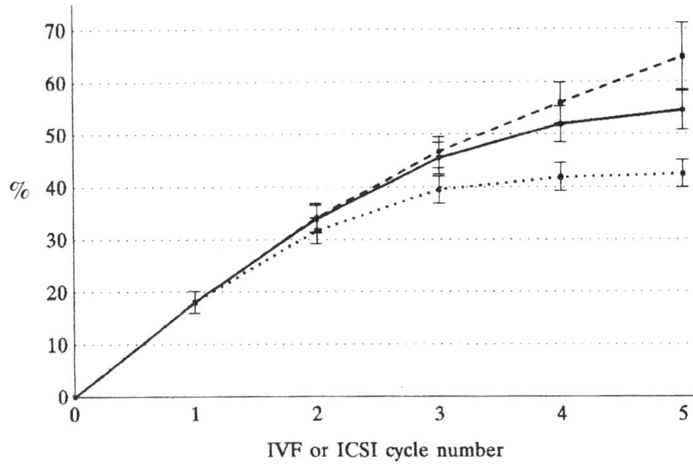

FIGURE 1.—Cumulative probability of achieving an ongoing pregnancy after in vitro fertilization (IVF) or intracytoplasmic sperm injection (ICSI) cycles with 95% confidence interval for the total population. *Dashed line* indicates optimistic, *solid line* indicates realistic, and *dotted line* indicates pessimistic cumulative probability. (Courtesy of Stolwijk AM, Wetzels AMM, Braat DDM: Cumulative probability of achieving an ongoing pregnancy after in-vitro fertilization and intracytoplasmic sperm injection according to a woman's age, subfertility diagnosis and primary or secondary subfertility. *Hum Reprod* 15:203-209, 2000. Copyright, European Society for Human Reproduction and Embryology, by permission of Oxford University Press.)

treatments. The cumulative probabilities of achieving ongoing pregnancy after successive IVF cycles were determined based on the woman's age, subfertility diagnosis, and the presence of primary or secondary subfertility.

Methods.—Between 1991 and 1998, 1315 couples underwent a total of 2984 IVF intracytoplasmic sperm injection (ICSI) cycles. "Realistic" cumulative probabilities of achieving ongoing pregnancy were analyzed.

Findings.—After 5 consecutive IVF/ICSI cycles, the "realistic" cumulative probability of attaining ongoing pregnancy was 54.5%, about 10% lower than the optimistic probability determined by life-table analysis and about 10% higher than the most pessimistic estimate (Fig 1). Women aged 35 years or younger had a greater probability of achieving ongoing pregnancy than did older women. Because ICSI is now an option, no obvious differences were noted between subfertility diagnosis subgroups. After the first 2 cycles, the cumulative probability of ongoing pregnancy was greater in women with secondary subfertility than in those with primary subfertility, but this advantage disappeared after further treatments.

Conclusion.—These data can be used to counsel couples considering multiple IVF treatments, but they will not be valid for all IVF centers. However, the presence or absence of differences in trends between subgroups are clear indicators of relevant qualitative difference between subgroups at any center.

▶ This epidemiologic analysis of treatment of infertility with IVF and ICSI provides very useful information for counseling infertile couples about their likelihood of having a clinical pregnancy that advances beyond 12 weeks gestation after initiating ovarian stimulation. The cumulative pregnancy rate, using these criteria of success, was 54% after 5 cycles of IVF, with or without ICSI. Results will vary in different centers. Therefore, infertile couples should obtain information about pregnancy success in the clinic they are attending for IVF, with or without ICSI, not only for the first cycle of treatment but also for the cumulative rate of success after several cycles of therapy.

D. R. Mishell, Jr, MD

Intracytoplasmic Sperm Injection Increased Fertilization and Good-Quality Embryo Formation in Patients With Non–Male Factor Indications for In Vitro Fertilization: A Prospective Randomized Study
Khamsi F, Yavas Y, Roberge S, et al (Toronto Fertility Sterility Inst)
Fertil Steril 75:342-347, 2001

15–13

Introduction.—Intracytoplasmic sperm injection (ICSI) provides an acceptable pregnancy rate in couples with male factor infertility. Some investigators believe that patients in in vitro fertilization (IVF) programs should be informed that a certain percentage of couples will have no fertilization with standard IVF and that performance of ICSI on some of the retrieved oocytes will ensure some fertilization of good-quality embryos. The fertilization rate and formation of good-quality embryos were compared between conventional IVF and ICSI in patients with non–male factor infertility in a prospective, controlled investigation.

Methods.—Thirty-five women with non–male factor infertility were enrolled. Cultured oocytes were inseminated 5 to 8 hours after being retrieved, then randomly assigned to either standard IVF or ICSI. Fertilization was verified by detection of 2 pronuclei at 14 to 18 hours after IVF insemination or ICSI. Two days later, embryos were evaluated and graded as good or poor quality. Good quality embryos were transferred on day 3 in all except 3 patients, who underwent embryo transfer on day 2.

Results.—On the basis of the number of oocytes assigned to ICSI, regardless of whether they were subsequently injected with sperm, the fertilization rate was 71.3%; for standard IVF, this rate was 57.2% (P = .005). Four women had no fertilization, and 7 had low fertilization (10% to 33%) with standard IVF insemination. Fairly normal fertilization (50% to 100%) occurred among sibling oocytes that underwent ICSI. Of 187 oocytes that underwent standard IVF insemination, 88 developed good-quality embryos (47.1%). In the remaining 188 sibling oocytes that underwent ICSI, 121 formed good-quality embryos (64.4%) (P = .001).

Conclusion.—The rate of formation of good-quality embryos per fertilized oocyte was 82% and 90%, respectively, for IVF and ICSI (P = NS). This suggests that ICSI does not improve or reduce the formation of good embryos. The difference between IVF and ICSI in good embryo formation per oocyte was related to the better fertilization rate observed with ICSI.

The success of IVF was more certain when half of the oocytes were subjected to ICSI. Patients undergoing IVF should be counseled regarding the benefit of ICSI in some oocytes.

▶ The use of ICSI to accomplish IVF has greatly increased the pregnancy rates of couples with male factor infertility. The results of this study suggest that fertilization rates and development of good-quality embryos in couples with causes of infertility other than male factor who undergo IVF are also increased when ICSI is performed on half the ova retrieved. It remains to be determined whether use of ICSI for IVF in infertile couples who do not have male factor infertility or who fail to ovulate after routine IVF enhances pregnancy rates per treatment cycle and is cost-effective.

D. R. Mishell, Jr, MD

Reducing the Risk of High-Order Multiple Pregnancy After Ovarian Stimulation With Gonadotropins

Gleicher N, Oleske DM, Tur-Kaspa I, et al (Ctr for Human Reproduction-Illinois, Chicago; Ctr for Human Reproduction-New York; Found for Reproductive Medicine, Chicago; et al)
N Engl J Med 343:2-7, 2000

15–14

Background.—Infertile women undergoing ovulation induction by gonadotropins have an especially high incidence of multiple gestation. Whether the number of high-order multiple pregnancies (defined as 3 or more fetuses) can be decreased is unknown.

Methods and Findings.—Data on 3347 consecutive treatment cycles in 1494 infertile women were analyzed. Four hundred forty-one treatments resulted in pregnancy, including 314 with singletons, 88 with twins, 22 with triplets, 10 with quadruplets, 5 with quintuplets, and 2 with sextuplets. The incidence of high-order multiple pregnancy was unrelated to number of follicles 16 mm or greater or to peak serum estradiol levels greater than 2000 or 2500 pg/mL. However, increasing total numbers of follicles as well as peak serum estradiol levels were significantly associated with an increasing risk of high-order multiple pregnancy. Younger age was also significantly associated with risk of high-order multiple pregnancy. This risk was also increased in women with a peak serum estradiol level of 1385 pg/mL or greater and with 7 or more follicles on the day of ovulation induction.

Conclusion.—Less intensive gonadotropin simulation may decrease the incidence of high-order multiple pregnancy in infertile women. However, lessening the intensity of such treatment reduces this risk only to a limited extent and to the detriment of overall pregnancy rates.

▶ When ovulation induction in anovulatory women or controlled ovarian hyperstimulation (COH) in infertile ovulatory women is performed with gonadotropins, there is a high incidence of multiple births with many gestations resulting in triplets or a higher-order number of fetuses. The use of clomiphene citrate instead of gonadotropins is associated with a much lower incidence of twins, and it is uncommon for triplets or higher-order pregnancies to occur when this agent is used for ovulation induction or COH. Therefore, when treating unexplained infertility, it is probably better to initiate COH with clomiphene citrate instead of gonadotropins followed by intrauterine insemination. If pregnancy does not occur after 4 to 6 cycles of this therapy, it is probably better to proceed directly to in vitro fertilization instead of using COH with gonadotropins to lower the risk of development of pregnancies with multiple gestations.

D. R. Mishell, Jr, MD

Blastocyst Transfer: A Useful Tool for Reduction of High-Order Multiple Gestations in a Human Assisted Reproduction Program
Toledo AA, Wright G, Jones AE, et al (Reproductive Biology Associates, Atlanta, Ga)
Am J Obstet Gynecol 183:377-382, 2000

15–15

Introduction.—High-order multiple gestations are becoming more common as the result of assisted reproductive technologies. These pregnancies are exceptional risks and are accompanied by considerable perinatal and maternal morbidity. The main reason for multiple pregnancies after in vitro fertilization (IVF) is the standard practice of transferring 3 or more cleavage-state embryos.

Implantation rates after transfer of cleavage-stage embryos are 10% to 20%, compared with 35% after blastocyst transfer. A sequential culture system was used to compare pregnancy, implantation, and multiple gestations in patients who received a day 3 transfer of cleavage-stage embryos versus a day 5 transfer of expanded blastocysts.

Methods.—All patients undergoing an IVF procedure between October 1998 and September 1999 were given the option of having either a day 3 or a day 5 transfer. Ongoing pregnancy rates, implantation rates (determined by the total number of visualized gestational sacs), and multiple pregnancy rates were calculated and compared.

Results.—There were 656 patients who had an IVF procedure during the evaluation period. Of these, 218 had three 8-cell embryos on the morning of day 3 and had the option of a day 3 or day 5 transfer. Ninety-two patients chose to have a day 3 transfer of cleaved embryos and 126 chose to undergo extended culture with a day 5 transfer of blastocysts.

The average numbers of embryos transferred were 3.1 and 2.0, respectively, for the day 3 group and the day 5 group. Implantation rates were 33% for the day 3 group and 35% for the day 5 group ($P = 5.9$). For the day 3 group, there were 47 singleton, 22 twin, 8 triplet, and 1 quadruplet ongoing gestations. For the day 5 group, there were 41 singleton and 24 twin ongoing gestations.

Conclusion.—The transfer of cleaved embryos on day 3 and blastocysts on day 5 had similar pregnancy and implantation rates in patients with similar day 3 embryo quality. There were no triplets or higher gestations in the blastocyst transfer group versus 8 sets of triplets and 1 set of quadruplets in the cleaved embryo transfer group.

▶ Although this was not a randomized trial, the observational data provide an indication that the transfer of a mean of 2-day 5 blastocysts instead of 3-day 3 zygotes resulted in similar implantation and pregnancy rates and prevented the occurrence of triplet and quadruplet gestation. With the use of sequential culture for IVF, it appears preferable to transfer only 1 or 2 five-day blastocysts rather than 3 or more 3-day embryos if the recipient is less than age 40 to reduce the incidence of high-order multiple gestations with their multiple adverse consequences.

D. R. Mishell, Jr, MD

Bleeding and Spontaneous Abortion After Therapy for Infertility
Pezeshki K, Feldman J, Stein DE, et al (Maimonides Med Ctr, Brooklyn, NY; State Univ of New York, Brooklyn)
Fertil Steril 74:504-508, 2000
15–16

Background.—Spontaneous abortion (SAB) is especially troubling to patients with previous infertility. Such patients often question whether the treatment leading to pregnancy was associated with the adverse outcome. The incidence of early pregnancy bleeding after various infertility treatments, the incidence of such bleeding after naturally occurring pregnancy, and whether such bleeding is related to SAB were investigated.

Methods.—Four hundred eighteen women with 500 consecutive clinical pregnancies were included. Methods of conception included ovulation induction, in vitro fertilization, and interventions not requiring ovulation induction, such as surgery and insemination. Women conceiving naturally composed a control group.

Findings.—The treatment groups had comparable rates of SAB. SAB was significantly more prevalent after bleeding than when bleeding did not occur; those rates were 30.8% and 19.8%, respectively. Bleeding predicted SAB only in women younger than 35 years.

Conclusion.—The risk of SAB is not greater in infertile women conceiving after reproductive treatments than in women conceiving naturally. Neither previous diagnosis nor treatment appears to be related to the occurrence of SAB in infertile women. Bleeding carries a twofold relative risk of SAB.

▶ In this study, about one fourth of all infertile women who conceived after various types of infertility therapy and had a gestational sac observed sonographically had a subsequent SAB. Interestingly, this high rate of SAB was similar in couples with different causes of infertility and different therapies.

If infertile women who conceive had evidence of uterine bleeding in early gestation, the rate of SAB significantly increased to 31%, compared with the 20% incidence of SAB in women who did not have uterine bleeding. These data can be used to inform infertile women who have uterine bleeding in early pregnancy with a viable fetus that they have about a 70% chance of not having a miscarriage.

D. R. Mishell, Jr, MD

16 Contraception

Clinical Breast and Pelvic Examination Requirements for Hormonal Contraception: Current Practice vs Evidence
Stewart FH, Harper CC, Ellertson CE, et al (Univ of California, San Francisco; Population Council, Mexico City; Family Health Internatl, Research Triangle Park, NC; et al)
JAMA 285:2232-2239, 2001   16–1

Background.—Clinical breast and pelvic examinations are commonly performed before hormonal contraceptives are prescribed. However, these examinations are unnecessary and may be a barrier to access to such contraception. Publications and recommendations from professional organizations on the role of these examinations in the provision of hormonal contraception were reviewed.

Review.—Clinicians can safely prescribe hormonal contraception based on careful medical history and blood pressure measurement. Breast and pelvic examinations and screening for cervical cancer and sexually transmitted infections are important, but they are not necessary for providing hormonal contraception. Because screening for sexually transmitted infections and cervical and breast cancer are essential components of family planning and reproductive health care, all women, especially those who are older, should be advised to have these breast and pelvic examinations. Eliminating the clinical and pelvic examination requirement before hormonal contraceptive prescription may prevent delays in achieving effective contraceptive protection. It may also help organizations develop innovative outreach programs. Continued study will be needed to determine the impact of such a change on women's health.

▶ The authors of this review present compelling evidence to support the decision not to require a breast and/or pelvic examination prior to initiating hormonal contraception. Requiring these examinations, especially for teenagers, creates a barrier to the use of these effective methods of avoiding pregnancy.

D. R. Mishell, Jr, MD

Oral Contraceptive Use and Glucose Metabolism in a National Sample of Women in the United States

Troisi RJ, Cowie CC, Harris MI (Social and Scientific Systems, Inc, Bethesda, Md; Natl Inst of Diabetes and Digestive and Kidney Diseases, Bethesda, Md)
Am J Obstet Gynecol 183:389-395, 2000   16–2

Background.—Glucose metabolism abnormalities have long been associated with oral contraceptive (OC) use. Whether OC users in a nationally representative population of US women had increased measures of glucose metabolism was investigated.

Methods.—As part of the Third National Health and Nutrition Examination Survey, conducted from 1988 to 1994 in 89 randomly selected US locations, 5482 women, aged 17 to 44 years, participated in a home interview. Most current OC users took low-dose estrogen formulations. The most commonly used preparations were a triphasic formulation containing 0.035 mg ethinyl estradiol and 0.5, 0.75, and 1 mg norethindrone (23.9%) and a monophasic formulation containing 0.035 ethinyl estradiol and 1 mg norethindrone (20.7%).

Findings.—Current OC users had no increases in glucose metabolism measures. Hemoglobin A_{1c}, fasting glucose, insulin, and C-peptide concentrations were unassociated with current use duration, age at initiation of OC, or major formulation type. Among former OC users, women who had recently stopped OC use had no evidence of higher values (Fig 1).

Conclusion.—Current OC use does not appear to be associated with increased measures of glucose and insulin metabolism. These findings are consistent with reports of no adverse effects of these formulations.

▶ The older, higher-dose OCs impaired glucose metabolism, resulting in higher circulatory glucose levels. The results of this large study indicate that the formulations in use today, with lower amounts of estrogen and progestin, do not adversely affect glucose metabolism. Therefore, these agents can be administered to women with a history of gestational diabetes or the presence of diabetes mellitus, as long as there is no evidence of vascular disease.

D. R. Mishell, Jr, MD

FIGURE 1

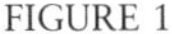

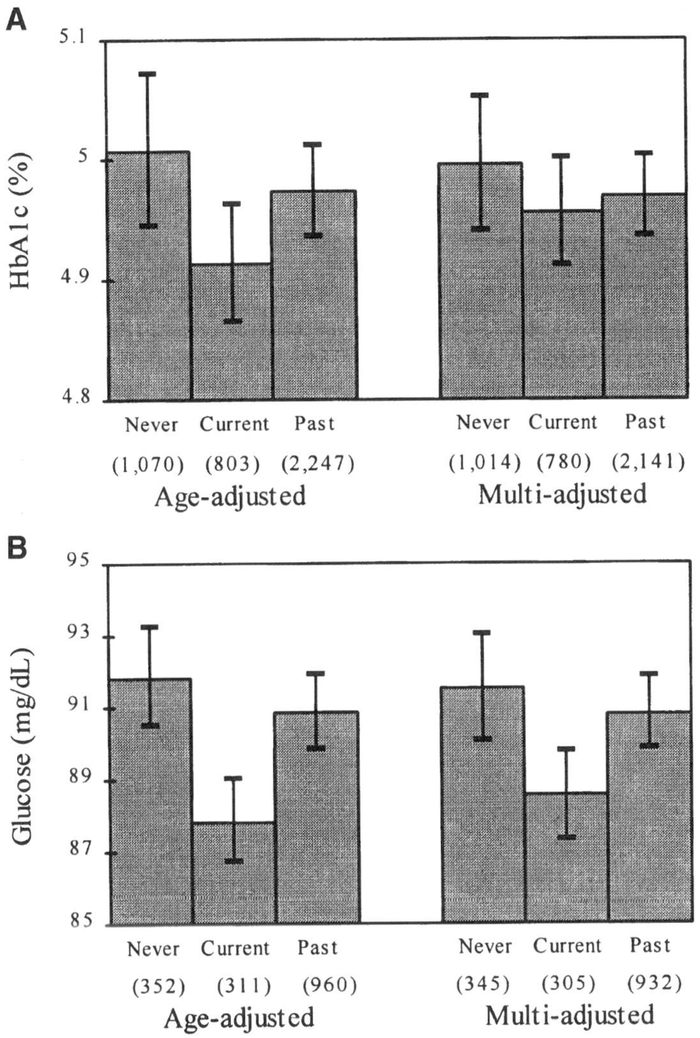

A

B

(Continued)

FIGURE 1 (cont.)

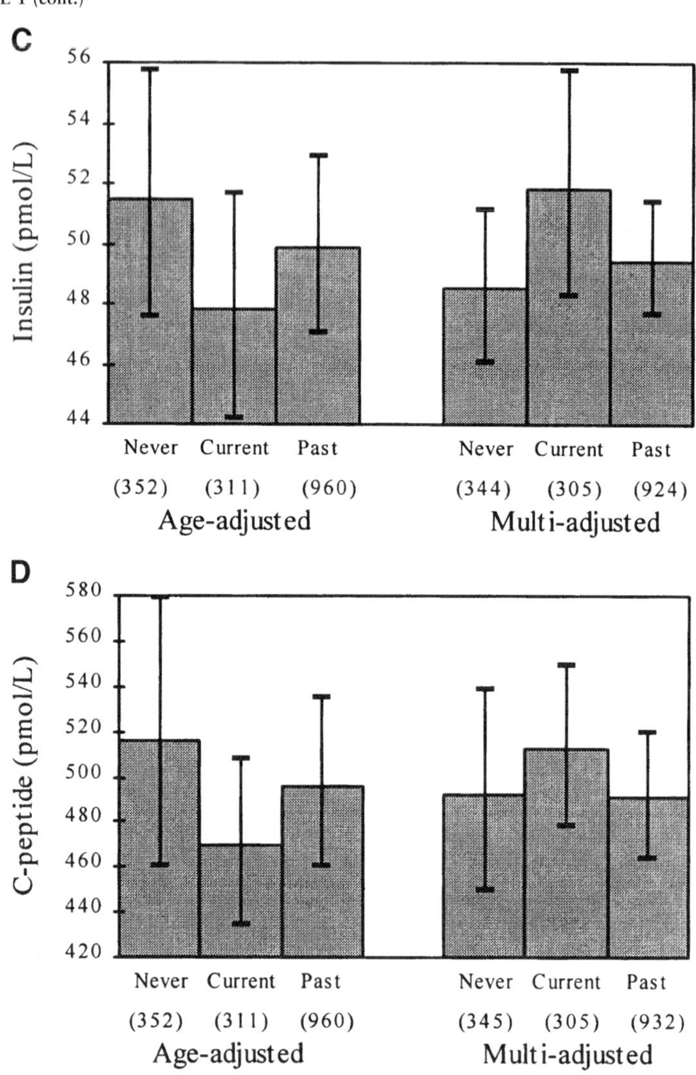

FIGURE 1.—Age-adjusted and multivariate-adjusted means for levels of hemoglobin A (HBA$_{1c}$). (**A**), fasting glucose (**B**), fasting insulin (**C**), and fasting C-peptide (**D**) according to oral contraceptive use among women without a medical history of diabetes. *Numbers in parentheses* indicate number of subjects; numbers vary according to study sample used in analysis and missing values for covariates included in regression models. $P > .2$, all comparisons except age-adjusted HbA$_{1c}$ level for current users versus those who had never used oral contraceptives ($P = .002$); age-adjusted fasting glucose level for current users versus never users ($P < .0001$) and former users (*Past*) ($P = .0004$) of oral contraceptives; and multivariate-adjusted fasting glucose for current users versus never users ($P = .002$) and former users ($P = .004$) of oral contraceptives. (Courtesy of Troisi RJ, Cowie CC, Harris MI, et al: Oral contraceptive use and glucose metabolism in a national sample of women in the United States. *Am J Obstet Gynecol* 183:389-395, 2000.)

Short-term Effects of a Progestational Contraceptive Drug on Food Intake, Resting Energy Expenditure, and Body Weight in Young Women
Pelkman CL, Chow M, Heinbach RA, et al (Pennsylvania State Univ, University Park)
Am J Clin Nutr 73:19-26, 2001   16–3

Background.—The hormonal fluctuations that occur during the menstrual cycle have been found to affect energy intake and expenditure. The possible effects on body weight regulation that may occur when these cyclic changes are suppressed by hormonal contraceptives have not been determined.

Methods.—Twenty women with normal weight were enrolled in a single-blind, placebo-controlled experiment. Body weight, resting energy expenditure (REE), and 3-day food intake were measured in the follicular and luteal phases of 2 menstrual cycles. A single injection of depot medroxyprogesterone or saline solution was then given, and measurements were repeated.

Findings.—Before injection, the menstrual cycle phase affected energy intake as well as REE. The women consumed more energy and expended more energy at rest in the luteal phase than in the follicular phase. Treatment with the contraceptive agent did not significantly affect energy intake, REE, or body weight.

Conclusion.—Menstrual cycle phases affected energy intake and REE. However, depot medroxyprogesterone acetate (DMPA) did not affect energy intake or expenditure, nor did it cause weight gain.

▶ It is widely believed by women that exogenous administration of contraceptive hormones and postmenopausal hormones cause an increase in body weight. However, in randomized trials of hormone replacement and observational studies of oral contraceptives, either type of exogenous sex steroid has been shown to not increase body weight. It has been stated that injection of 150 mg of DMPA causes an increase in appetite and weight gain. However, the result of this meticulous randomized trial, in which women were allowed to ingest as much food and beverage as they wished, a single injection of DMPA was shown to not increase appetite or body weight. Women should be counseled that administration of DMPA will not cause weight gain or a need for caloric restriction.

D. R. Mishell, Jr, MD

Decreased Urinary Calcium Loss and Lower Bone Turnover in Young Oral Contraceptive Users
Zittermann A (Univ of Bonn, Germany)
Metabolism 49:1078-1082, 2000   16–4

Introduction.—The effect of oral contraceptives (OCs) on bone health has not been determined. Trials conflict regarding the impact of OC use on

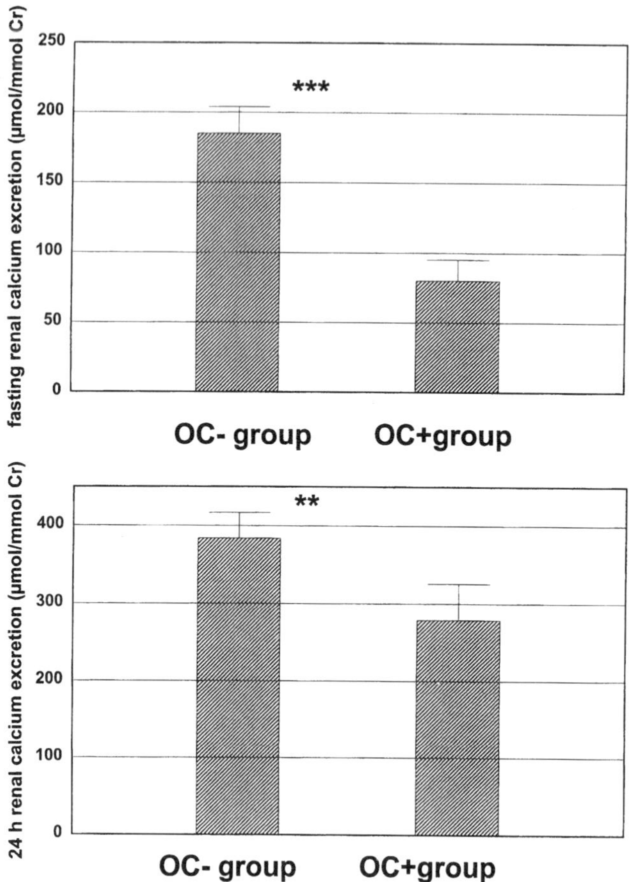

FIGURE 1.—Fasting renal calcium excretion and 24-hour renal calcium excretion (mean ± SEM) in OC+ and OC− groups. Data are based on 36 samples from 12 OC+ and 57 samples from 19 OC− subjects. *Double asterisk* indicates $P < .01$; *triple asterisk* indicates $P < 001$. *Abbreviation*: OC, Oral contraceptive. (Courtesy of Zitterman A: Decreased urinary calcium loss and lower bone turnover in young oral contraceptive users. *Metabolism* 49:1078-1082, 2000.)

bone mineral density, calcium (Ca) and bone metabolism, and bone mass. The effects of OC on various indexes of skeletal metabolism were examined in 31 young women.

Methods.—Twelve OC users (OC+ group; mean age, 24.8 years) and 19 eumenorrheic nonusers (OC− group; mean age, 25.5 years) underwent measurement of Ca and bone metabolism. Urine samples (fasting 2-hour and 24-hour specimens) were collected at 3 different time points: baseline, day 28, and day 56. Three blood samples were obtained at 28-day intervals during an 8-week evaluation period for estradiol, sex hormone–binding globulin, insulin, and propeptide of type I procollagen (PICP).

Results.—Both groups were similar in measures of energy, nutrient intake (7-day food record), body mass index, and serum 25-hydroxyvitamin D levels. Serum levels of estradiol and sex hormone–binding globulin mirrored the use and nonuse of OC. The 2-hour fasting renal Ca excretion for the OC+ group was 43% of that for the OC− group. Also, 24-hour renal Ca excretion was lower in the OC+ group versus the OC− group (Fig 1). Compared with the OC+ group, the excess daily Ca excretion was 1.38 mmol (55.2 mg) for the OC− group. The OC− group had a 19.2% higher PICP concentration and a 26.6% higher fasting renal hydroxyproline excretion rate, compared with the OC+ group.

Conclusion.—Oral contraceptive use reduces urinary Ca loss and diminishes the rate of bone turnover in young women.

▶ When endogenous estrogen levels decline postmenopausally, there is an increased rate of bone resorption and urinary Ca excretion, resulting in osteoporosis in many women. The rate of bone resorption is reduced by administration of exogenous estrogen. The results of this study indicate that when pharmacologic doses of exogenous estrogen are administered to reproductive-age women, there is also decreased Ca excretion, reflecting a lower rate of bone resorption. This effect results in greater bone mass among OC users compared with age-matched nonusers. One study has shown that women who ingest OCs have less postmenopausal hip fractures than women who do not use OCs.

D. R. Mishell, Jr, MD

Low-Dose Oral Contraceptive Use and the Risk of Myocardial Infarction
Rosenberg L, Palmer JR, Rao RS, et al (Boston Univ; Brookline, Mass; Columbia Univ, New York)
Arch Intern Med 161:1065-1070, 2001

16–5

Background.—Oral contraceptives (OCs) containing 50 µg of estrogen or more appear to increase the risk for myocardial infarction (MI) among current users, especially heavy smokers. Whether the newer lower-dose OCs also increase MI risk was investigated.

Methods.—Data on women seen between 1985 and 1999 in 75 hospitals in the northeastern United States were analyzed in this case-control study. Six hundred twenty-seven women with a nonfatal first MI and 2947 hospitalized women younger than 45 years (controls) provided information on OC use and MI risk factors.

Findings.—Compared with never use, current use was associated with a 1.3 overall odds ratio (OR). The OR was 2.5 among heavy smokers, 1.0 among lighter smokers, and 1.3 among nonsmokers. Compared with OC nonuse and nonsmoking, women currently using OCs who smoked heavily had a 32 OR, markedly higher than the OR for smoking alone, which was 12. Neither formulation type nor estrogen dose affected ORs. Past OC use was not associated with MI risk.

Conclusion.—Current use of low-dose OCs among nonsmokers and light smokers does not appear to carry an increased risk for MI. However, women who smoke heavily while using such contraception may be at a greatly increased risk for MI.

▶ The results of this large case-control study provide confirmatory data that use of the currently marketed formulations of OCs by nonsmoking women without hypertension does not increase the risk of MI. Although smoking less than 25 cigarettes per day increased the risk of MI about fivefold compared with that of nonsmokers, the risk was no greater among OC users who smoked less than 25 cigarettes per day than it was among non–OC users. Women who smoked more than 25 cigarettes per day and also used OCs had a 32-fold greater risk for having an MI than did nonsmoking women not using OCs which was greater than the 12-fold increased risk for heavy smokers not using OCs. Clinicians should strongly advise women who are heavy smokers to use other methods of contraception instead of combination OCs.

D. R. Mishell, Jr, MD

Oral Contraceptives and Benign Ovarian Tumors
Westhoff C, Britton JA, Gammon MD, et al (Columbia Univ, New York; Mount Sinai School of Medicine, New York; Univ of North Carolina, Chapel Hill; et al)
Am J Epidemiol 152:242-246, 2000   16–6

Introduction.—The use of oral contraceptives (OCs) is associated with decreased risk of ovarian cancer. Its effect on benign ovarian tumors is not known. The relationship between OC use and benign ovarian tumors was examined in a case-control investigation.

Methods.—The cohort comprised patients with surgically confirmed benign ovarian tumors diagnosed between January 1, 1992, and December 31, 1993. Benign tumors included serous cystadenomas, mucinous cystadenomas, endometriomas (or ovarian endometriosis), teratomas, Brenner tumors, and fibroma-thecomas. Controls were identified by random digit dialing. A total of 1259 women with 1460 confirmed tumors were identified. Women with a concurrent diagnosis of cancer were excluded. Controls were approximately frequency matched to patients with benign tumors by 10-year age groups. Eighty-eight percent of the participants completed a structured questionnaire administered in person, usually in the participant's home. Telephone interviews were used when needed.

Results.—Tumors included 196 serous adenomas, 176 teratomas, 311 endometriomas, and 65 mucinous adenomas. Ever use of OCs was correlated with a modest reduction in the risk of benign ovarian tumors (age- and hospital-adjusted odds ratio = 0.79). A strong trend of diminishing risk with duration of use was observed for all tumor types (P = .006 for months of OC use evaluated as a continuous variable); all of this trend seemed to be due to the reduced risk seen in women with endometriomas (P = .001). Most OC users had discontinued OC use for a minimum of 5 years before the reference date. These women had a reduced risk of all benign tumor subtypes. Nearly all recent users had been exposed only to low-estrogen-dose OCs.

Conclusion.—The use of OCs was correlated with a modest and long-lasting reduced risk of benign ovarian tumors. Current and past users of OCs had fewer benign ovarian tumors than never-users. Long-term OC users had a lower risk than short-term users. Women with endometriomas had the greatest reduced risk.

▶ Several studies have shown that OC use decreases the risk of developing functional ovarian cysts, and many studies have shown that OC use decreases the risk of developing epithelial ovarian cancer. The result of this study indicates that OC use may also reduce the risk of developing benign ovarian neoplasms as well as endometriomas. The reduction in the risk of developing these neoplasms persists after OC use is discontinued. The decreased risk of developing these benign ovarian neoplasms with OC use is an additional noncontraceptive health benefit of OCs.

D. R. Mishell, Jr, MD

Oral Contraceptives and Colorectal Cancer Risk: A Meta-analysis

Fernandez E, La Vecchia C, Balducci A, et al (Institut Català d'Oncologia, Barcelona; Istituto di Ricerche Farmacologiche "Mario Negri," Milan, Italy; Università degli Studi di Milano, Milan, Italy; et al)

Br J Cancer 84:722-727, 2001　　　　　　　　　　　　　　　　16–7

Background.—The use of combined oral contraceptives (OCs) and the risk of colorectal cancer have been found to be associated inversely. A meta-analysis of published studies was presented.

Methods and Findings.—Epidemiologic studies published as full articles in English up to June 2000, which included quantitative data on OC use, were included in the analysis. In the 8 case-control studies, the pooled relative risks of colorectal cancer for women who had ever used OCs was 0.81 (Fig 1). The pooled estimate from the 4 cohort studies was 0.84. When all studies were combined, the estimate was 8.2, with no apparent heterogeneity. Duration of use was uncorrelated with a risk reduction; the apparent protection seemed to be greater for women who had more recently used OCs.

Conclusion.—OC use is correlated inversely to the risk of colorectal cancer. Further research is needed to better define the risk profile according to duration and recency of use.

▶ There is a growing body of epidemiologic evidence, as summarized by this meta-analysis, that the use of OCs when young is associated with about a 20% risk of development of both colon cancer and rectal cancer when women become older. The mean age of the women in these studies was 55 to 60 years. Unlike the protection of OCs against both ovarian and endome-

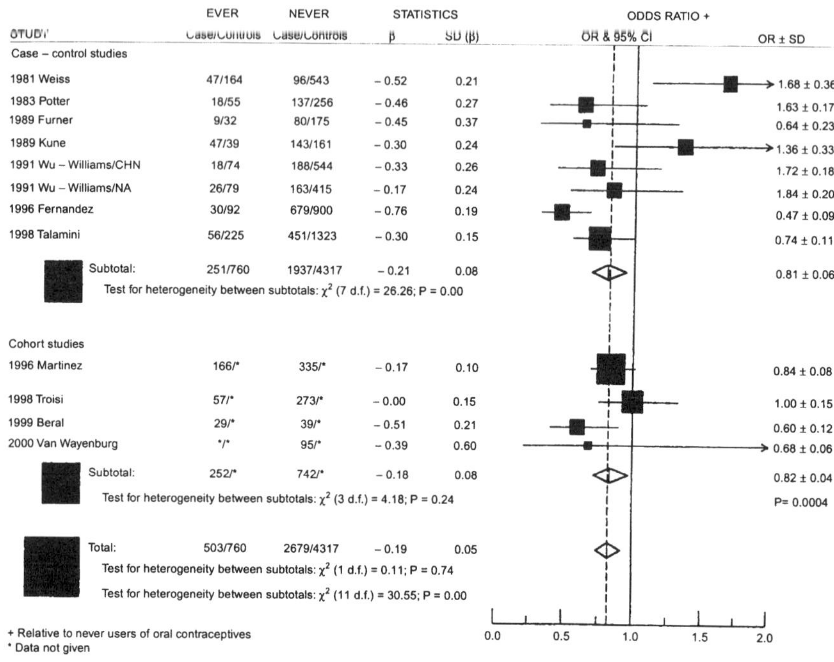

FIGURE 1.—Summary of relative risk estimates of colorectal cancer for ever versus never use of oral contraceptives from case-control and cohort studies. *Abbreviations: SD*, Standard deviation; *OR*, odds ratio; *CI*, confidence interval. (Courtesy of Fernandez E, La Vecchia C, Balducci A, et al: Oral contraceptive and colorectal cancer risk: A meta-analysis. *Br J Cancer* 84:722-727, 2001.)

trial cancer, a longer duration of OC use was not found to be associated with greater reduction in risk of colorectal cancer development than was short duration of use. Thus, a causal relationship of a protective effect of OCs remains to be established. However, support for the belief that estrogen causes a reduction in colorectal cancer is provided by the data showing that postmenopausal estrogen use has also been associated with a lower risk of colon cancer.

D. R. Mishell, Jr, MD

Risk of Breast Cancer With Oral Contraceptive Use in Women With a Family History of Breast Cancer

Grabrick DM, Hartmann LC, Cerhan JR, et al (Mayo Clinic and Mayo Clinic Cancer Ctr, Rochester, Minn; Univ of Minnesota, Minneapolis)
JAMA 284:1791-1798, 2000

Background.—Studies of women in the general population suggest a weak association between oral contraceptive (OC) use and breast cancer. However, the effects of OC use on risk in women with a family history of breast cancer are unknown. The relationship between OC use and breast cancer risk was assessed in a large cohort of families with a history of breast cancer.

Methods.—The analysis included 426 families of women given a diagnosis of breast cancer at a university tumor clinic between 1944 and 1952. In telephone interviews, follow-up data were collected from relatives of the probands, including 394 daughters and sisters and 3002 granddaughters and nieces. Information was also gathered from 2754 women who married into the probands' families. The breast cancer risk associated with OC use was calculated in terms of relationship to the probands.

Results.—In sisters and daughters of probands, there was a significant relationship between ever-use of OCs and increased breast cancer risk (relative risk [RR], 3.3; 95% confidence interval [CI], 1.6-6.7) after adjustment for age and birth cohort. No such relationship was evident for granddaughters and nieces of probands, nor for women who married into the families. The association was little changed with adjustment for other variables, including parity, age at first birth, age at menarche, age at menopause, oophorectomy, smoking, and education. The risk was strongest (RR, 3.3; 95% CI, 1.5-7.2) for women who took OCs during or before 1975, when OCs contained higher dosages of estrogen and progestin. There were only 2 cases of breast cancer among first-degree relatives of probands who used OCs after 1975, making it difficult to assess risk in this group.

Conclusion.—In families with breast cancer, the use of older formulations of OCs is associated with a significantly increased risk of breast cancer. Women who used OCs in 1975 or before and have a first-degree relative with breast cancer may therefore be at particularly high risk. The relationship between use of current OC formulations and breast cancer risk among women with a family history of the disease remains to be determined.

▶ Several other large epidemiologic studies—including the Nurses Health Study, The Cancer and Steroid Hormone Study, and the Collaborative Group Reanalysis—have reported that among women with a family history of breast cancer there is no significantly different risk of breast cancer between OC users and nonusers. This study found that the risk of breast cancer was higher among first, but not second, degree relatives of women with breast cancer who used high–estrogen dose OCs, but not the low–estrogen dose OCs that are used currently. A major problem of this study is that OC use was characterized only for relatives who were still alive at the time of follow-up. Thus, most sisters and older daughters, particularly those with breast cancer, were already deceased and could not contribute information about OC use. Women with a family history of breast cancer should be counseled that their risk of breast cancer development is not increased with low–estrogen dose OCs—the formulations being used today.

D. R. Mishell, Jr, MD

Oral Contraception and Ear Disease: Findings in a Large Cohort Study

Vessey M, Painter R (Inst of Health Sciences, Oxford, England)
Contraception 63:61-63, 2001

Background.—Numerous researchers have found that the use of oral contraceptives (OCs) may increase the risk of certain ear diseases, particularly otosclerosis and vestibular disorders. However, the amount of published data is limited. The association between OCs and ear disease was further investigated in a large cohort study.

Methods and Findings.—Data on 17,032 women, aged 25 to 39 years, were obtained from the Oxford-Family Planning Association contraceptive study. The women had been followed up for up to 26 years. The association between first hospital referral for each ear condition and the possible confounding variables of age, parity, social class, smoking status, height, weight, and body mass index was determined. After adjustment for these possible confounders, no relationship was found between OC use and ear disease.

Conclusion.—This analysis showed no relationship between OC use and the risk of ear disease. However, data for some conditions, especially otosclerosis, were sparse, suggesting the need for further research.

▶ A few case reports have suggested that OC use may be related to the development of otosclerosis. It has also been postulated that OC use may be related to vertigo and altered vestibular function. This large, prospective study initiated between 1968 and 1974 when women were using high steroid–dose OCs, found no evidence that OC use was associated with any type of ear disease.

D. R. Mishell, Jr, MD

A Prospective Study on the Effects of Depot Medroxyprogesterone Acetate on Trabecular and Cortical Bone After Attainment of Peak Bone Mass

Merki-Feld GS, Neff M, Keller PJ (Univ Hosp, Zürich, Switzerland; Centre for Osteoporosis, Zürich, Switzerland)
Br J Obstet Gynaecol 107:863-869, 2000

Background.—Depot medroxyprogesterone acetate (DMPA) is used for contraception worldwide. Bone mass changes in women aged 30 to 45 years taking DMPA were evaluated to determine whether bone mass depends on the duration of DMPA use or estradiol level.

Methods.—Thirty-six DMPA users were enrolled in the prospective longitudinal study. Every 12 weeks, 150 mg of DMPA was injected. Peripheral quantitative CT was used to measure bone mass at the distal radius.

Findings.—The mean annual changes were 1.6% in trabecular bone mass and −0.26% in cortical bone mass. The reduction in cortical bone mass was nonsignificant. Neither the duration of DMPA use nor estradiol concentrations correlated with bone parameters.

Conclusion.—DMPA did not adversely affect bone mass in women aged 30 to 45 years. Further research is warranted.

▶ The results of this prospective study indicate that the use of DMPA by women of late reproductive age has little effect upon bone mineral density. In young adolescent women, this long-acting progestin contraceptive decreases bone mineral density. To date, there are no data regarding fracture risk in women who have used DMPA and few data regarding changes in bone density after DMPA is discontinued.

D. R. Mishell, Jr, MD

Evaluation of Contraceptive Efficacy and Cycle Control of a Transdermal Contraceptive Patch vs an Oral Contraceptive: A Randomized Controlled Trial
Creasy GW, for the ORTHO EVRA/EVRA 004 Study Group (Centre Médical de Halles de Ste-Foy, Quebec; et al)
JAMA 285:2347-2354, 2001   16–11

Background.—Poor compliance reduces the efficacy of oral contraception (OC). The efficacy, cycle control, and safety of and compliance with a transdermal contraceptive patch were compared with those of OC.

Methods.—Forty-five US and Canadian clinics enrolled 1417 healthy women in the randomized, open-label, parallel group study between October 1997 and June 1999. Eight hundred twelve women received a transdermal contraceptive patch and 605 received OC for 6 or 13 cycles. Patch treatment involved the application of 3 consecutive 7-day patches followed by 1 patch-free week.

Findings.—Overall and method-failure Pearl indexes (number of pregnancies per 100 person-years of use) were lower in the patch group than in the OC group but not significantly. The patch group had a significantly greater incidence of breakthrough bleeding or spotting in the first 2 cycles. In all cycles, however, the incidence of breakthrough bleeding alone was similar in the 2 groups. Perfect compliance was achieved in 88.2% of cycles in the patch group and 77.7% of the cycles in the OC group. The rate of complete patch detachment was 1.8%. Both forms of contraception were well tolerated. However, women in the patch group had significantly more application site reactions, breast discomfort, and dysmenorrhea than those in the OC group.

Conclusion.—The efficacy and cycle control of the contraceptive patch is comparable to a combination OC. Compliance with the patch was better than that with OC.

▶ Delivery of a progestin and estrogen transdermally was found to be an effective means of contraception, with failure rates slightly lower than with use of an OC. For some women, applying a skin patch once a week may bo preferable to ingesting a pill every day. In this study, about 1 in 5 women did not consistently take the OC as directed, but only 1 in 10 women did not consistently apply the skin patch as directed. It is therefore probable that once a week dosing of contraceptive steroid results in better compliance than daily dosing and may result in higher contraceptive effectiveness.

D. R. Mishell, Jr, MD

Efficacy, Tolerability and Acceptability of a Novel Contraceptive Vaginal Ring Releasing Etonogestrel and Ethinyl Oestradiol

Roumen FJME, Apter D, Mulders TMT, et al (Atrium Medisch Centrum, Heerlen, The Netherlands; Väestöliitto, Helsinki; NV Organon, Oss, The Netherlands)
Hum Reprod 16:469-475, 2001

16–12

Background.—The hormonal activity of a progestogen and an estrogen is the basis for combined oral contraceptive (COC) agents. COCs, in combination with good cycle control, can provide highly effective and reversible protection against pregnancy, but daily intake of tablets is required. Efforts in the development of new COCs have been directed toward the use of regimens that would contain the lowest suitable dose of both the progestogen and the estrogen, so that steroid-associated adverse events can be minimized. However, when the daily dose of estrogen has been reduced to less than 20 µg of ethinyl estradiol (EE), cycle control has sometimes been compromised. The NuvaRing, a novel contraceptive vaginal ring, has been developed to address this issue. The NuvaRing is a flexible, soft, transparent ring that will release both a progestogen and an estrogen at nearly constant rates over 3 consecutive weeks. In a pharma-

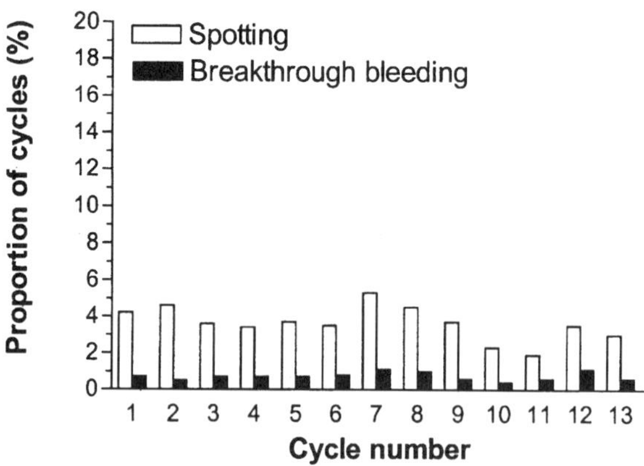

FIGURE 2.—Incidence of irregular bleeding in the intent-to-treat population. (Courtesy of Roumen FJME, Apter D, Mulders TMT, et al: Efficacy, tolerability and acceptability of a novel contraceptive vaginal ring releasing etonogestrel and ethinyl oestradiol. *Hum Reprod* 16:469-475, 2001. Copyright European Society for Human Reproduction and Embryology, by permission of Oxford University Press.)

TABLE 3.—Incidences (Percentages) of Bleeding as a Proportion of
Intention-to-Treat Assessable Cycles*

Irregular bleeding (breakthrough bleeding/spotting):	2.6-6.4
Withdrawal bleeding	
Absence	0.6-2.1
Early	5.4-7.7
Early with spotting only	2.8-5.4
Late	20.4-27.3
Late with spotting only	16.5-21.4

*Percentages apply to cycles 1-12 or incidences of late withdrawal bleeding, and to cycles 1-13 otherwise.

(Courtesy of Roumen FJME, Apter D, Mulders TMT, et al: Efficacy, tolerability and acceptability of a novel contraceptive vaginal ring releasing etonogestrel and ethinyl estradiol. *Hum Reprod* 16:469-475, 2001. Copyright European Society for Human Reproduction and Embryology, by permission of Oxford University Press.)

---

codynamic study, NuvaRing was associated with complete inhibition of ovulation and ovarian suppression that was comparable to a COC of 150 µg desogestrel 30 µg EE. The results of the first large-scale study of the efficacy of NuvaRing are presented.

Methods.—A total of 1145 women were treated with NuvaRing in a year-long, multicenter study in which the contraceptive efficacy, cycle control, tolerability, and acceptability were assessed. Each ring was used for 1 cycle, which comprised 3 weeks of ring use followed by a ring-free period of 1 week. A total of 12,109 cycles (928 woman-years) were evaluated.

Results.—There were 6 pregnancies among 1145 women in the treatment period, for a Pearl Index of 0.65. Good cycle control was obtained, and irregular bleeding was rare (Fig 2). Withdrawal bleeding occurred in 97.9% to 99.4% of assessable cycles (Table 3). There was a high level of compliance with the prescribed regimen, and criteria were fulfilled in 90.85% of cycles. NuvaRing was well-tolerated in all patients.

Conclusions.—NuvaRing was found to be an effective and convenient method for hormonal contraception. The majority of women in the large-scale trial found NuvaRing easy to use, and the ring was well-tolerated.

Use of the Novel Combined Contraceptive Vaginal Ring NuvaRing for Ovulation Inhibition

Mulders TMT, Dieben TOM (NV Organon, Oss, The Netherlands)
Fertil Steril 75:865-870, 2001   16–13

Background.—A novel combined-contraceptive vaginal ring (Nuva-Ring), which contains etonogestrel and ethinyl estradiol (EE) was evaluated. Etonogestrel is the biologically active metabolite of desogestrel. Both desogestrel and EE are steroids that have been used in a variety of established contraceptive products. The flexible, colorless NuvaRing has an outer diameter of 54 mm and a cross-sectional diameter of 4 mm. An

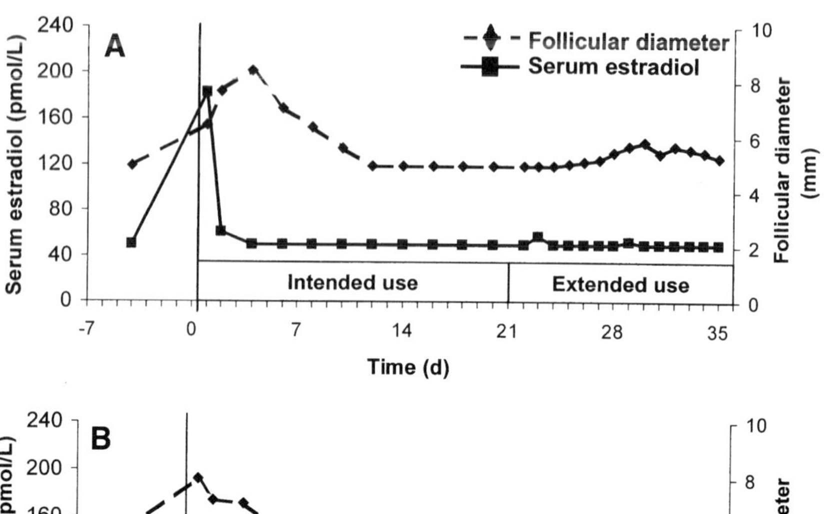

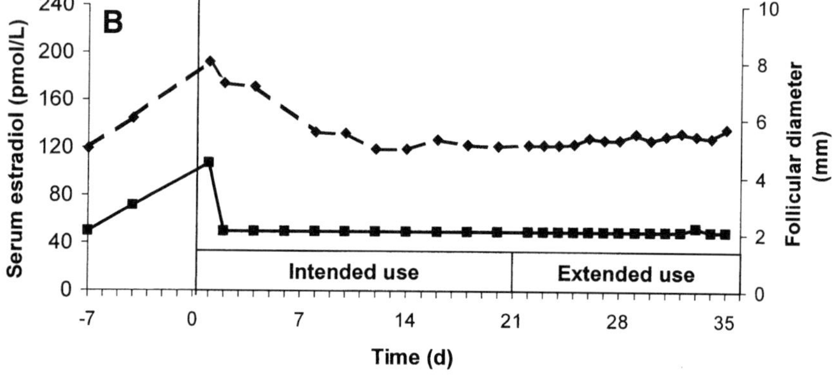

FIGURE 1.—Median follicular diameter (in millimeters) and serum 17β-estradiol concentrations (in picomoles per liter) for (**A**) group 1 (n = 8) and (**B**) group 2 (n = 8) during treatment with NuvaRing (days 1-35). Median values have been calculated for the diameter of the largest follicle and the peak serum hormone level per research subject per day. (Reprinted by permission from the American Society for Reproductive Medicine, from Mulders TMT, Dieben TOM: Use of the novel combined contraceptive vaginal ring NuvaRing for ovulation inhibition. *Fertil Steril* 75:865-870, 2001.)

average of 120 µg of etonogestrel and 15 µg of EE per day are released by the NuvaRing. The effects of the vaginal ring on the functioning of the ovaries were assessed.

Methods.—A randomized, open-label, crossover study was conducted in a clinical pharmacology unit and involved 16 healthy female volunteers. In group 1, volunteers were administered 1 cycle of combined oral contraceptive (COC) containing desogestrel (150 µg) and EE (30 µg), followed by a 3-week period of treatment with NuvaRing. In group 2, the Nuva-Ring treatment period was followed by a cycle of COC in the form of desogestrel–EE. The main outcome measures were follicular diameter, serum hormone concentrations (follicle-stimulating hormone, 17β estradiol, luteinizing hormone, and progesterone), and endometrial thickness.

Results.—The use of NuvaRing for the recommended 3 weeks resulted in complete inhibition of ovulation, as determined by vaginal US (follicular diameter) and by concentrations of serum luteinizing hormone and progesterone (Fig 1). The inhibition of ovulation was maintained for an additional 2 weeks of NuvaRing use. There was a comparable degree of ovarian suppression between the 2 groups. In addition, ovarian suppression after 3 weeks of NuvaRing treatment was comparable to ovarian suppression on day 21 of desogestrol–EE intake. NuvaRing was well tolerated by all patients.

Conclusions.—Treatment with NuvaRing was found to completely inhibit ovulation throughout the normal 3-week period as well as an extended period of use. Ovarian suppression was found to be comparable to that provided by the desogestrel–EE COC.

▶ Steroids inserted into the vagina are absorbed through the vaginal epithelium at a relatively constant rate. Thus, circulating levels of the steroids remain relatively stable while they are being released from the vaginal ring, unlike the fluctuating levels that occur after oral intake of steroid contraceptive pills. In addition, because the steroids are absorbed directly into the circulation, the first-pass effect through the liver that occurs after ingestion is avoided. For this reason, the daily release of both the estrogen and progestin component of the contraceptive ring is less than the amount ingested in oral contraceptive (OC) pills. However, as reported in the article by Mulders et al (Abstract 16–13), ovulation is completely inhibited for up to 5 weeks of ring use. Despite the lower dose of steroids absorbed, the contraceptive efficacy is as good and bleeding control seems better than that which occurs with low-dose OCs. The prolonged duration of use of the ring avoids the necessity of daily pill taking, and it is more convenient for the woman to insert and remove the ring after 3 weeks than it is to take a pill every day. Forgetting to take an OC pill each day results in a typical use-failure rate of OCs that has been reported to be about 5% in the first year of use. When the contraceptive ring is approved by regulatory agencies, it will allow women to have access to an additional effective, reversible, safe method of contraception, and it is hoped that it will reduce the high incidence of unwanted pregnancies that now occurs in US women.

D. R. Mishell, Jr, MD

Safety and Efficacy of Levonorgestrel Implant, Intrauterine Device, and Sterilization
Meirik O, for the International Collaborative Post-Marketing Surveillance of Norplant (Geneva, Switzerland; et al)
Obstet Gynecol 97:539-547, 2001   16–14

Introduction.—Norplant implants continuously release levonorgestrel at low concentrations and provide effective contraception for 5 years. The safety and efficacy of levonorgestrel-releasing contraceptive implants, intrauterine devices (IUDs), and sterilization were assessed in developing countries using controlled cohort methodology.

Methods.—Thirty-two family planning clinics in 8 countries offered Norplant, 30 offered IUDs, and 17 offered sterilization. Participants were women aged 20 to 40. All agreed to attend the clinic for 6 weeks after enrolling, then semiannually for 5 years, regardless of change of contraceptive methods. Incidence rate ratios of health events were estimated for beginning and current method use.

Results.—There were 7977 women in the Norplant group, 6625 in the IUD group, and 1419 in the sterilization group. Overall follow-up for 78,323 woman-years of observation was 94.6%. The pregnancy rates for all 3 contraceptive methods were less than 1 per 100 woman-years. Compared with control subjects, only 2 women in the Norplant group had significant excess risk of serious morbidity. The rate of gallbladder disease was higher among women who initiated Norplant use than among control subjects (rate ratio, 1.52). The incidence of hypertension and borderline hypertension was also higher in Norplant users compared with control subjects (rate ratio, 1.81). New findings were increased risks of respiratory diseases and reduced risks of inflammatory diseases of the genital tract in Norplant users compared with IUD users and sterilized women.

Conclusion.—During a follow-up period of 5 years, Norplant users had higher rates of gallbladder disease, higher blood pressure, and lower rates of acute pelvic infection than IUD users and sterilized women (rate ratios, 1.52, 1.81, and .34, respectively).

▶ This large postmarketing surveillance study provides useful information about the effectiveness and adverse effects of levonorgestrel-releasing contraceptive implants (Norplant). At the end of 5 years, the cumulative pregnancy rate was 1.5 per 100 women compared with 0.7 per 100 women who chose sterilization. About two thirds of women who chose Norplant were continuing to use it after 5 years. The major health risks associated with Norplant were a slight increase in gallbladder disease and higher blood pressure. Unlike the effect in users of combined oral contraceptives, deep vein thrombophlebitis was not significantly increased with Norplant.

D. R. Mishell, Jr, MD

Return of Fertility in Nulliparous Women After Discontinuation of the Intrauterine Device: Comparison With Women Discontinuing Other Methods of Contraception

Doll H, Vessey M, Painter R (Univ of Oxford, England)
Br J Obstet Gynaecol 108:304-314, 2001   16–15

Background.—Many researchers have studied return to fertility after discontinuation of an intrauterine device (IUD). However, most women included in such previous studies were parous. The effects of IUD use on fertility in nulliparous women were investigated.

Methods.—Data on 558 married women recruited from 1982 to 1985 and followed up annually until 1994 at 17 family planning clinics in England and Scotland were analyzed. Ages ranged from 18 to 40.

Findings.—Conception occurred most quickly in women who had been using a barrier method of birth control. Fifty-four percent of these women gave birth within 1 year, compared with 39% of IUD users and 32% of oral contraceptive (OC) users. Fertility was not associated with duration of OC use. Women using IUDs for less than 42 months had more-favorable fertility patterns than those stopping OCs, with an increasing length of IUD use associated with declining fertility. Among women who had used an IUD for 78 months or longer, only 28% gave birth within a year of discontinuation. By 36 months, 79% of long-term IUD users and 91% of short-term IUD users had given birth. This correlation persisted after adjustment for potential confounding factors such as maternal age, husband's social class, and history of gynecologic illnesses.

Conclusions.—In nulliparous women, long-term use of an IUD appears to increase the risk of infertility. Such devices should be used sparingly in nulliparous women. Use for many years should especially be avoided.

▶ IUDs are most often used by multiparous women. Several studies have reported that their use by these women does not impair future fertility. The data in this study suggest that when IUDs are used by nulliparous women for 6 years or more, future fertility may be impaired. Since the study was initiated in 1982 and terminated in 1994 and used types of IUDs no longer marketed, its results may not be relevant to use of currently marketed IUDs, particularly the levonorgestrel-releasing device.

D. R. Mishell, Jr, MD

The Risk of Menstrual Abnormalities After Tubal Sterilization
Peterson HB, for the US Collaborative Review of Sterilization Working Group (Ctrs for Disease Control and Prevention, Atlanta, Ga)
N Engl J Med 343:1681-1687, 2000   16–16

Background.—Tubal sterilization has become the most used method of contraception in the United States. This method is highly effective and safe, but the existence of a post–tubal ligation syndrome of menstrual abnormalities has been debated since the early 1950s. A resolution of the debate regarding menstrual abnormalities after tubal sterilization is important for safeguarding women's health. Whether there is a greater likelihood of persistent menstrual abnormalities among women who have undergone tubal sterilization compared with women who have not undergone this procedure was determined by a review of data from the US Collaborative Review of Sterilization.

Methods.—In a multicenter, prospective cohort study, a total of 9514 women who underwent tubal sterilization and 573 women whose partners underwent vasectomies were followed up for up to 5 years by annual telephone interviews. All women were asked identical questions regarding 6 characteristics of their menstrual cycles in the presterilization and follow-up interviews. The risk of persistent menstrual changes was assessed by multiple logistic-regression analysis.

Results.—No greater likelihood was found for the reporting of persistent changes in intermenstrual bleeding or in the length of the menstrual cycle among women who had undergone sterilizations compared with women who did not. Women who underwent tubal sterilization were more likely to have experienced a decrease in the number of days of bleeding, the amount of bleeding, and menstrual pain and to have experienced an increase in cycle irregularity. In the group of women who had reported very heavy bleeding at baseline, women who underwent sterilization were more likely to report decreased bleeding than were women who did not undergo tubal sterilization.

Conclusions.—The incidence of menstrual abnormalities did not seem to be any greater for women who underwent tubal ligation than for women who did not undergo the procedure.

▶ Controversy exists as to whether tubal sterilization increases the risk of abnormal uterine bleeding and whether a post–tubal-ligation syndrome exists. Results from this very large prospective Collaborative Review of Sterilization study in which the menstrual patterns of women who underwent tubal sterilizations were compared with those of age- and ethnic-matched control subjects whose partners had vasectomies indicate few differences in menstrual patterns before and after the sterilization procedures. Women who had tubal sterilizations were more likely to have less bleeding, fewer days of bleeding, and less pain with menses after the procedure than that which occurred in women whose partners had vasectomies; however, the former group had greater cycle irregularity than the latter group. The results of this study dispel the belief that there is a post–tubal-ligation syndrome that results in greater amounts or increased days of uterine bleeding or both.

D. R. Mishell, Jr, MD

Effectiveness of Emergency Contraceptive Pills Between 72 and 120 Hours After Unprotected Sexual Intercourse
Rodrigues I, Grou F, Joly J (Univ of Montreal)
Am J Obstet Gynecol 184:531-537, 2001   16–17

Background.—The Yuzpe and Lancee emergency contraceptive pill consists of estrogen and progestin and is used within 72 hours of unprotected sexual intercourse. The efficacy of this pill when administered between 72 and 120 hours after unprotected intercourse was investigated.

Methods.—In this observational study, 2 groups of women were compared. One hundred thirty-one sought consultation within 72 hours of unprotected intercourse, and 169 sought care 72 to 120 hours after such intercourse.

Findings.—Pregnancy rates for the within-72-hours group and the 72- to 130-hour group were 0.8% and 1.8%, respectively. Efficacy varied from 87% to 90% in those receiving the contraception within 72 hours and from 72% to 87% for those receiving it between 72 and 120 hours.

Emergency contraception significantly decreased the risk of pregnancy in both groups.

Conclusion.—Women should be encouraged to seek consultation as soon as possible after unprotected sexual intercourse; however, emergency contraceptive pills can be recommended from 72 to 120 hours after unprotected intercourse. Emergency contraception administered 72 to 120 hours after intercourse significantly lowers the pregnancy rate.

▶ The use of emergency contraception with either levonorgestrel or a combination of levonorgestrel and ethinyl estradiol is currently advised for women who have had a single act of unprotected sexual intercourse within the previous 72 hours. The results of this study suggest that the use of emergency contraception may also be effective when coitus has occurred between 72 and 120 hours previously. These results need to be confirmed by additional studies with a larger number of women.

D. R. Mishell, Jr, MD

Mifepristone as a Late Post-coital Contraceptive

Ashok PW, Wagaarachchi PT, Flett GM, et al (Univ of Aberdeen, Scotland; Grampian Healthcare NHS Trust, Aberdeen, Scotland)
Hum Reprod 16:72-75, 2001   16–18

Background.—Mifepristone, given in a singe dose of 600 mg within 72 hours of unprotected sexual intercourse, is a highly effective postcoital contraceptive. Currently, the only method of emergency contraception for women seen after 72 hours but within 5 days of unprotected intercourse is the intrauterine contraceptive device (IUCD), which is unacceptable to many women requesting emergency contraception, most of whom are young and nulliparous. The efficacy of mifepristone given 72 hours to 5 days after unprotected intercourse in women declining the IUCD was investigated.

Methods.—Two hundred nineteen consecutive women seen over a 2-year period and meeting inclusion criteria were offered a choice of IUCD or mifepristone. Fifteen women chose the IUCD, and 204 chose mifepristone, given in 200 mg dose. In 1 woman, the IUCD could not be fitted, and mifepristone was administered. Women preferring mifepristone were younger and more likely to be nulliparous than those choosing the IUCD. One hundred fifty-five women given mifepristone and all 14 fitted with the IUCD coil were followed up.

Findings.—No treatment failures occurred in either group. One woman given mifepristone became pregnant after having unprotected intercourse shortly after treatment. Thus, the crude pregnancy rate was 0.65%. In the mifepristone group, 85% of expected pregnancies were prevented.

Conclusion.—These findings suggest that mifepristone is safe and effective when given between 72 hours and 5 days after unprotected intercourse. Mifepristone can be offered as an alternative to women declining the IUCD.

▶ Currently, more women in the United States are becoming aware of the existence and effectiveness of emergency contraception than occurred in the past. The effectiveness of both the Yuzpe regimen and levonorgestrel methods of emergency contraception declines with increasing time after unprotected intercourse. Use of these methods is not recommended more than 72 hours after unprotected coitus. Ingestion of mifepristone has been shown to be an effective method of emergency contraception, even when given in a single 10-mg dose. The results of this pilot study demonstrate that a single dose of 200 mg of mifepristone is an effective emergency contraception when it is given between 72 hours and 5 days after unprotected intercourse. Women who wish emergency contraception in this time frame should be offered mifepristone if it is available.

D. R. Mishell, Jr, MD

17 Abortion

Posttraumatic Stress Disorder After Pregnancy Loss
Engelhard IM, van den Hout MA, Arntz A (Maastricht Univ, The Netherlands)
Gen Hosp Psychiatry 23:62-66, 2001   17–1

Background.—Pregnancy loss is a stressful life event. The prevalence of posttraumatic stress disorder (PTSD) in response to pregnancy loss was investigated.

Methods.—About 1370 women were recruited in the first 12 weeks of pregnancy and completed baseline questionnaires on personality, social support, previous life events, and psychological symptoms. Short surveys were sent periodically throughout pregnancy. Women experiencing pregnancy loss were sent questionnaires at 1 and 4 months after the loss to assess possible PTSD and depression.

Findings.—One hundred thirteen women had a pregnancy loss, most within 20 weeks. The prevalence of PTSD at 1 month was 25%. The symptom severity was comparable to that of other traumatized populations. The risk of depression was increased in women with PTSD; the prevalence was 34% in the PTSD group and 5% in the non-PTSD group. Seven percent of women experiencing pregnancy loss met PTSD criteria at 4 months. Half of these cases were chronic. Depression rates did not decrease over 4 months.

Conclusion.—Pregnancy loss puts women at risk for PTSD. In most affected women, the disorder begins immediately after the loss and persists for several months.

▶ Because miscarriage is a common event, clinicians frequently do not realize the potential severe adverse psychological effects that may occur after early pregnancy loss. Women need emotional support and counseling after they have a miscarriage. If severe depression or PTSD occur, psychiatric care may be indicated.

D. R. Mishell, Jr, MD

"

A Prospective Randomized Control Trial Comparing Medical and Surgical Treatment for Early Pregnancy Failure

Demetroulis C, Saridogan E, Kunde D, et al (Newham Gen Hosp, London)
Hum Reprod 16:365-369, 2001   17–2

Background.—The most common gynecologic emergency is miscarriage. About 15% of recognized pregnancies abort spontaneously in the first trimester. The efficacy of a single dose of 800 µg misoprostol given intravaginally compared with surgical evacuation for treating early pregnancy failure was investigated.

Methods and Findings.—Eighty women with early fetal loss were assigned randomly to vaginal misoprostol or surgical curettage. Intravaginal misoprostol was effective in 82.5%. None of the women undergoing surgical curettage needed repeat evacuation. The 2 groups were comparable in significant abdominal pain after treatment. Pain duration was shorter in the surgery group, but these women needed more analgesics than those in the misoprostol group. The 2 groups did not differ in number of patients with significant vaginal bleeding, duration of bleeding, or severity of bleeding. All 33 women in whom medical treatment was successful reported satisfaction with their treatment, compared with only 58% of the surgical group.

Conclusion.—The administration of 800 µg of misoprostol intravaginally is safe and effective for the treatment of missed, incomplete, and anembryonic miscarriages. Larger studies are needed to verify these findings.

▶ Vaginal insertion of misoprostol is more effective than oral administration for both elective pregnancy termination and treatment of incomplete abortion or anembryonic gestation and embryonic death (missed abortion). It is much less expensive to treat incomplete abortion with misoprostol than to perform a surgical procedure. Side effects, patient satisfaction, and amount of uterine bleeding are not increased when the abnormal pregnancy is evacuated with the use of vaginal misoprostol instead of by curettage. Therefore, additional clinical trials with this regimen of medical management of incomplete abortion are encouraged.

D. R. Mishell, Jr, MD

The Treatment of Incomplete Miscarriage With Oral Misoprostol

Pandian Z, Ashok P, Templeton A (Univ of Aberdeen, Scotland)
Br J Obstet Gynaecol 108:213-214, 2001   17–3

Introduction.—Most published reports indicate that the ideal treatment of incomplete miscarriage has yet to be determined. The effectiveness of 3 sequential oral doses of misoprostol for treatment of incomplete miscarriage was assessed in a retrospective evaluation of 112 women.

Methods.—All participants underwent medical treatment for incomplete miscarriage between 6 and 13 weeks from January 1998 to July 1999. Successful treatment was considered complete uterine evacuation without the need for surgical curettage. Women who chose medical treatment over surgical treatment received 600 µg of oral misoprostol, followed by 2 additional oral doses of 400 µg at 2-hour intervals. Oral analgesia or parenteral analgesia was administered every 4 to 6 hours as needed. A further course of misoprostol was offered when products of conception were not passed, unless the patient requested surgical evacuation.

Results.—Ninety-five of 112 women (85%) experienced complete uterine evaluation without the need for surgical evacuation. Seventeen women (15%) underwent surgical evacuation. Ninety-seven women (87%) received 1 to 3 doses of misoprostol; the regimen was repeated in 15 women (13%). Of 5 women (4%) readmitted, 3 had suspected pelvic infection, 1 underwent diagnostic laparoscopy to exclude ectopic pregnancy, and 1 with a molar pregnancy underwent surgical evacuation of the uterus.

Conclusion.—Misoprostol was effective in the evacuation of the uterus in women with incomplete miscarriage. The unique aspect of this trial was the use of 3 oral doses of 600, 400, and 400 µg of misoprostol at 2-hour intervals, with the regimen repeated if necessary.

▶ Misoprostol is a prostaglandin E1 analogue that is effective for the treatment of early pregnancy failure as well as for elective termination of early pregnancy. The standard therapy for incomplete abortion is curettage, which can usually be performed rapidly with the use of local anesthesia. As reported in this study, administration of multiple doses of oral misoprostol to treat incomplete abortion has a high rate of success but necessitates hospitalization for 6 hours or more. In certain locations, clinicians may wish to use misoprostol instead of curettage if misoprostol reduces the cost of treating incomplete abortion.

D. R. Mishell, Jr, MD

Vaginal Misoprostol Administered 1, 2, or 3 Days After Mifepristone for Early Medical Abortion: A Randomized Trial
Schaff EA, Fielding SL, Westhoff C, et al (Univ of Rochester, NY; Columbia Univ, New York; Population Council of New York)
JAMA 284:1948-1953, 2000   17–4

Introduction.—The conventional timing of misoprostol administration after mifepristone is 2 days for patients undergoing medical abortion. More flexible intervals, which could make the regimen more convenient, have not been examined. Women who were no more than 56 days pregnant and desired an abortion of a confirmed intrauterine pregnancy were evaluated in a prospective, open-labeled, randomized, multicenter trial to ascertain whether 800 µg of vaginal misoprostol could be administered 1, 2, or 3 days after 200 mg of mifepristone without diminishing the safety and efficacy of the standard 2-day protocol for women seeking early abortion.

Methods.—There were 2295 healthy women aged 18 years or older from 16 primary care and referral abortion facilities. Forty patients (1.7%) were lost to follow-up. Patients received 200 mg oral mifepristone and were randomly assigned to self-administration of 800 µg of vaginal misoprostol at home 1, 2, or 3 days later (745, 778, and 772 patients, respectively). Patients were asked to return to the clinic up to 8 days after mifepristone administration for US. A second dose of misoprostol was given if the abortion was not complete. Patients with continued pregnancy, excessive bleeding, or retained pregnancy tissue 5 weeks later underwent aspiration curettage. Patients in all 3 groups were followed up for effectiveness of the procedure (including a complete medical abortion without surgical intervention), adverse events, acceptability of the procedure as revealed on patient questionnaires, reasons for surgical intervention, and adverse outcomes.

Results.—Of the 2255 women who completed follow-up, complete medical abortion rates were 98%, 98%, and 96%, respectively, among patients using misoprostol 1, 2, and 3 days after mifepristone administration. Fifty-five women aborted before misoprostol administration, 9 underwent early surgery, and 103 did not take misoprostol on their assigned day. No blood transfusions were required. The most frequently reported adverse effects were cramping and nausea; similar percentages of patients in all 3 groups reported these effects. There were 13 unexpected or serious adverse effects—6, 4, and 3, respectively, in patients using misoprostol on days 1, 2, and 3, respectively. The procedure was reported to be acceptable by more than 90% of the cohort.

Conclusion.—Vaginal misoprostol, 800 µg, may be used from days 1 to 3 after mifepristone, 200 mg, is administered for early medical abortion. It does not need to be administered exactly 48 hours after administration of mifepristone.

▶ Mifepristone (RU-486) followed by misoprostol has now been approved for marketing in the United States. Product labeling states that ingestion of 600 mg of mifepristone, 3 200-mg tablets, should be followed 48 hours later by oral administration of 400 mg of misoprostol in an office setting to terminate pregnancies of 49 days' gestation or less. The results of this very large randomized trial confirm results of previous studies, which reported that 200 mg of mifepristone followed by 800 mg of vaginally administered misoprostol is extremely effective for terminating pregnancies of 56 days' gestation or less. In this study, intravaginal insertion of misoprostol by the woman at home, 1, 2, or 3 days after ingestion of mifepristone, resulted in similar high rates of effectiveness. This regimen reduces the cost of medical abortion because only 1 200-mg tablet of mifepristone is used and 1 office visit is avoided.

D. R. Mishell, Jr, MD

Early Medical Abortion With Methotrexate and Misoprostol

Borgatta L, Burnhill MS, Tyson J, et al (Planned Parenthood Federation of America Inc, New York; Planned Parenthood of Northern New England Inc, Williston, Vt; Planned Parenthood of Wisconsin Inc, Milwaukee; et al)

Obstet Gynecol 97:11-16, 2001   17–5

Introduction.—Planned Parenthood sites that already offer surgical abortion services were invited to take part in an investigation of medical abortion using methotrexate (MTX) and misoprostol. Introduction of an early medical abortion program with MTX and misoprostol was evaluated with the use of a standardized protocol.

Methods.—Thirty-four sites enrolled 1973 women between October 1996 and July 1998. US was performed on site to verify gestational age of less than 49 days from the first day of the last menstrual period. MTX, 50 mg/m^2 of body surface area, was administered on day 1. Patients were asked to insert misoprostol 800 µg vaginally on day 5, 6, or 7. They were advised to undergo suction curettage if the pregnancy seemed viable 2 weeks after MTX or if any gestational sac persisted 4 weeks after MTX administration. Main outcomes were complete medical abortion and suction curettage.

Results.—A complete abortion was experienced by 1659 women (84.1%); 257 (13.0%) had suction curettage. The most frequent reason for curettage was patient option (8.9%). At 2 weeks after MTX administration, 1.4% of the women underwent curettage because of a persistent but nonviable pregnancy; 1.6% of them had curettage because of persistent, nonviable pregnancy at 4 weeks. One percent of the women underwent curettage on a physician's recommendation, usually because of bleeding. Suction curettage rates dropped with site experience ($P < .006$) and were lower at earlier gestational ages ($P < .004$) and in nulliparous women ($P < .004$).

Conclusion.—Medical abortion with MTX and misoprostol was safe and effective up to 7 weeks of gestation. These findings offer support for the introduction of this approach to community settings.

► The use of mifepristone and misoprostol is now approved for medical abortion in the United States and other countries for pregnancies of less than 7 weeks' gestation. MTX and misoprostol is less expensive than mifepristone and misoprostol, but the time until abortion occurs is longer with MTX than with mifepristone. One reason for this prolonged length of time is the difference in treatment protocols. With the MTX protocol, the misoprostol is given 5 to 7 days after MTX. With mifepristone, the misoprostol is given 2 days later. Another problem with this and other methods of medical abortion is the mean duration of bleeding, which in this study was nearly 12 days. It will be of interest to observe whether MTX will still be used before misoprostol now that mifepristone has received regulatory approval for inducing early abortion in many countries, including the United States.

D. R. Mishell, Jr, MD

Karyotype of the Abortus in Recurrent Miscarriage

Carp H, Toder V, Aviram A, et al (Sheba Med Ctr, Tel Hashomer, Israel)
Fertil Steril 75:678-682, 2001   17–6

Objective.—The incidence of chromosomal aberrations in recurrent spontaneous abortions is reported to be as high as 60%, but only 2 studies have examined this association. The incidence and type of chromosomal anomalies in the abortus after recurrent miscarriages, the prognosis for a live birth after a euploid or aneuploid abortion, the different incidence of chromosomal anomalies in primary aborters and secondary aborters, and the incidence of chromosomal anomalies correlated to maternal age were investigated in a 5-year study at 1 medical center.

Methods.—Between 1994 and 1999, 167 women, aged 20 to 45 years, with histories of 3 or more consecutive miscarriages, miscarried again. Chromosomal analyses were attempted on all abortuses using standard G-banding methods. The karyotypes of both parents were determined, and an analysis of glucose tolerance, toxoplasmosis serologic type, uterine anomalies, thyroid function, serum prolactin level, luteal phase, antinuclear factor level, and anticardiolipin antibody level was undertaken.

Results.—Karyotyping was performed successfully in 125 abortuses: 36 (29%) were abnormal and included 5 with monosomy (45XO), 24 with trisomy, 5 with triploidy, and 2 with unbalanced translocation. Chromosomal trisomy was the most common aberration, occurring in 5 of 24 trisomies. In 17 patients who had a second abortus karyotyped, 5 had an aberrant initial karyotype, and 1 had an abortus whose tissue did not grow on culturing. All 5 women who miscarried an aberrant initial karyotype embryo subsequently miscarried again. Three embryos were euploid, and 2 had a repeat chromosomal anomaly. All 11 patients with a normal embryonic karyotype miscarried a euploid embryo in the second abortion. Patients aborting an aneuploid embryo were nonsignificantly more likely to have a subsequent live birth than women aborting a euploid embryo. Maternal age affected the incidence of trisomy but not that of translocation.

Conclusion.—The majority of recurrent miscarriages appear to be caused by something other than chromosomal aberrations. Fetal karyotyping is a valuable tool for assessing the risk of future miscarriages.

▶ It is probably of benefit for a woman with a history of unexplained recurrent abortions to have a karyotype of the fetal tissue if she aborts again. If the karyotype of the aborted tissue is abnormal, the prognosis for a subsequent viable pregnancy is better than if the karotype is normal. In addition, if the karotype is normal, the cause of the abortion is more likely to be due to some problem in the parents than in the fetus, and an appropriate diagnostic evaluation should be performed.

D. R. Mishell, Jr, MD

Factor V Leiden and Acquired Activated Protein C Resistance Among 1000 Women With Recurrent Miscarriage
Rai R, Shlebak A, Cohen H, et al (Imperial College, London; St Mary's Hosp, London; Univ College London Hosps Trust)
Hum Reprod 16:961-965, 2001   17–7

Background.—Both the congenital and acquired forms of activated protein C (APC) resistance are important risk factors for systemic venous thrombosis. The prevalence of APC resistance in women with a history of recurrent early miscarriage or with a history of 1 or more late miscarriages was investigated.

Methods.—Nine hundred four women with 3 or more consecutive fetal losses before 12 weeks' gestation and 207 women with 1 or more fetal losses after 12 weeks' gestation were studied. One hundred fifty parous women with no previous adverse pregnancy outcomes composed a control group. All women were white.

Findings.—Acquired APC resistance was significantly more common in women with early and women with late fetal losses, at 8.8% and 8.7%, respectively, compared with the control group, at 3.3%. The frequency of the factor V Leiden allele was comparable in all 3 groups, with prevalences of 3.3%, 3.9%, and 4%, respectively.

Conclusion.—Acquired APC resistance appears to be an important cause of pregnancy loss. The mechanism underlying this probably involves thrombosis of the placental vasculature.

▶ Controversy exists regarding what causal effect, if any, APC resistance has upon early pregnancy loss. In this large study the incidence of the factor V Leiden genetic mutation was similar in women with recurrent early abortion, those with at least 1 second-trimester loss, and the control population. However the incidence of acquired APC resistance, as determined by a shortened clotting time, in women without the factor V Leiden mutation, was nearly 3 times higher among women with recent early miscarriage and late miscarriage than among controls. It remains to be determined whether treatment with heparin and aspirin of women with recurrent pregnancy loss and acquired APC resistance will improve the rates of viable pregnancies.

D. R. Mishell, Jr, MD

Primary Habitual Abortions Are Associated With High Frequency of Factor V Leiden Mutation
Wramsby ML, Sten-Linder M, Bremme K (Karolinska Inst, Stockholm)
Fertil Steril 74:987-991, 2000   17–8

Background.—The etiology of spontaneous abortion is multifactorial. Established risk factors include chromosomal aberrations, anatomical malformations, hormonal imbalance, and phospholipid antibodies. Inherited abnormalities of the coagulation system, associated with a predisposition to thromboembolic complications and recurrent fetal loss, have recently been of interest. This study determined the prevalence of the mutation G1691A in factor V gene (Leiden mutation), of mutation C677T in the methylenetetrahydrofolate reductase (MTHFR) gene, and of polymorphism in G20210A in the prothrombin gene in women with recurrent fetal loss.

Methods.—Eighty-four women with a history of 3 or more consecutive miscarriages and 69 healthy women were included in the prospective, case-control analysis. Polymerase chain reactions were conducted to detect mutations and the polymorphism in the prothrombin gene.

Findings.—Twenty-eight percent of women with recurrent fetal loss carried the Leiden mutation. The 2 groups did not differ in the prevalence of mutation C677T in the MTHFR gene or in polymorphism G20210A in the prothrombin gene.

Conclusion.—The Leiden mutation may have an important role in primary recurrent fetal loss. This mutation induces a hypercoagulable state. Thus, microthrombosis in the placenta may explain recurrent abortions.

▶ In contrast to the previous report (Abstract 17–7) (which found that the incidence of the factor V Leiden mutation in Bristish women with recurrent spontaneous abortion was not increased compared with controls) in this study of Swedish women, the incidence of the mutation was much greater than in normal controls. It is possible that the factor V mutation increases the risk of miscarriage only in certain ethnic groups, but this appears unlikely. At present, it appears better to determine the presence of activated protein C resistance in women with recurrent spontaneous absortion by performing clotting tests instead of tests to detect the genetic marker.

D. R. Mishell, Jr, MD

Hypercoagulable Thrombophilic Defects and Hyperhomocysteinemia in Patients With Recurrent Pregnancy Loss

Raziel A, Kornberg Y, Friedler S, et al (Assad-Harofeh Med Ctr, Zerifin, Israel; Sheba Med Ctr, Tel Hashomer, Israel)
Am J Reprod Immunol 45:65-71, 2001   17–9

Background.—Increased thrombosis may compromise placental perfusion, resulting in complications and recurrent pregnancy loss. Heritable thrombophilic defects and hyperhomocysteinemia are associated with increased thrombosis. Thus, their prevalnce in women with recurrent pregnancy loss was investigated.

Methods and Findings.—Thirty-six nonpregnant women with recurrent pregnancy loss and 40 parous women were assessed for protein S, protein C, and anti-thrombin III deficiency, and mutations for factor V Leiden, methylenetetrahydrofolate reducatse (MTHFR), and prothrombin gene, as well as hyperhomocysteinemia and combinations of these pathologies. Women with recurrent pregnancy loss had a relatively high prevalence of plasma coagulation protein deficiencies compared with parous women. The former also had an increase in factor V Leiden mutation, but it was nonsignificant. Thirty-one percent of women with RPL had hyperhomocysteinemia, and 16% had MTHFR mutation homozygosity. Combinations of hyperhomocysteinemia and MTHFR mutation were noted in 3 patients, with folate deficiency in 2 and B_{12} deficiency in 3.

Conclusion.—Combinations of gene mutations, plasma protein deficiencies, and hyperhomocysteinemia appear to be more prevalent in women with recurrent pregnancy loss than in parous women. Such conditions are associated with an increased risk of thrombosis. Further large-scale studies are needed to determine causality.

▶ In this group of 36 women with unexplained recurrent spontaneous abortion about one third had hyperhomocysteinemia and about 40% had evidence of an inheritable thrombophilic defect. The diagnostic evaluation of women with recurrent spontaneous abortion should include measurement of serum homocysteine as well as tests to measure protein C, protein S, antithrombotin, and activated protein C resistance. Therapy of elevated homocysteine levels includes oral administration of vitamin B_6 and folate and monthly injections of vitamin B_{12}. If a hereditary thrombophilic defect is found, therapy with heparin and aspirin can be tried. No study has demonstrated that in women with inherited thrombophilia, such therapy for the treatment of recurrent spontaneous abortion is more effective than placebo or aspirin alone.

D. R. Mishell, Jr, MD

Antiphospholipid and Antiprotein Syndromes in Non-thrombotic, Non-autoimmune Women With Unexplained Recurrent Primary Early Foetal Loss: The Nîmes Obstetricians and Haematologists Study–NOHA

Gris J-C, Quéré I, Sanmarco M, et al (Faculté de Pharmacie, Montpellier, France; Centre Hospitalier Universitaire, Nîmes, France; EAMENRT "Dynamique des incohérences cardio-vasculaires," Nîmes, France; et al)
Thromb Haemost 84:228-236, 2000   17–10

Background.—In the absence of any habitual etiology, recurrent early fetal loss has been thought to be related to various antiphospholipid or antiprotein antibodies. A hospital-based case-control study of women with no antecedent of thromboembolic or autoimmune disease was reported.

Methods.—Three groups of 518 women each were studied. Group 1 had unexplained primary recurrent early fetal loss; group 2 had explained episodes of such loss; and group 3 had successful pregnancies with no previous obstetric accident. The groups were matched based on age, number of pregnancies, and time since the end of the last pregnancy. Significant biological markers were assessed prospectively.

Findings.—The various antibodies depended on parity and the presence of previous fetal loss. Cutoff values were determined by using data from women with explained accidents and adjusted for parity. The only independent, retrospective risk factors for unexplained early fetal loss were anti-phosphatidylethanolamine IgM, anti–β2-glycoprotein I IgG, anti-annexin V IgG antibodies, and lupus anticoagulant. During the subsequent pregnancy, these markers were associated with a significant risk of fetal loss, despite low-dose aspirin treatment.

Conclusion.—Among nonthrombotic, nonautoimmune women with unexplained primary recurrent early fetal loss, subgroups can be identified with positive anti-phosphatidylethanolamine IgM antibodies, positive anti–β2-glycoprotein I IgG antibodies, positive anti-annexin V IgG antibodies, or lupus anticoagulant. Particularizing these subgroups will allow therapeutic trials to be done in well-defined populations.

▶ Others have reported that the presence of lupus anticoagulant and anti-cardiolipin antibodies, but not other antiphospholipid antibodies, are associated with recurrent early pregnancy loss. Treatment with heparin and aspirin for women with recurrent miscarriage who have lupus anticoagulant or anticardiolipin antibodies results in higher viable pregnancy rates than treatment with placebo or aspirin alone. The results of this study indicate that other antiphospholipid antibodies may also have an etiologic role in causing early pregnancy loss. Randomized controlled trials should be performed to determine whether treating women with recurrent early pregnancy loss and these other antiphospholipid antibodies with heparin and aspirin improves the incidence of viable birth.

D. R. Mishell, Jr, MD

Prospective Pregnancy Outcome in Untreated Recurrent Miscarriers With Thyroid Autoantibodies
Rushworth FH, Backos M, Rai R, et al (Imperial College School of Medicine, London)
Hum Reprod 15:1637-1639, 2000   17–11

Background.—Women who carry thyroid antibodies are at greatly increased risk of miscarriage. Thyroid antibodies do not appear to be correlated with antiphospholipid antibodies, but they may be an independent predictor of poor reproductive outcome. The prevalence of thyroid antibodies among women with recurrent miscarriages was evaluated, as were their correlation with antiphospholipid antibodies and predictive value for future pregnancies.

Methods.—The study included 870 consecutive, nonpregnant women seen at a recurrent miscarriage clinic. The patients (median age, 34 years) all had a history of at least 3 consecutive miscarriages. Only karyotypically normal couples were included. The prevalence and associations of thyroglobulin antibodies (TgAb) and thyroid microsomal antibodies (TmAb) were assessed.

Findings.—Overall, 19% of women had thyroid antibodies. Only 5% had TgAb, while 60% had TmAb; 35% had both TgAb and TmAb. A history of thyroid disease was noted in 13 patients and thyroid function abnormalities in another 15. Pregnancy outcomes were evaluated in 98 tested women with normal thyroid-stimulating hormone. In 24 untreated pregnancies of women confirmed as being euthyroid, the live-birth rate was 58%. A live-birth rate of 58% was also observed in 81 untreated pregnancies in 710 women who tested negative for thyroid antibodies.

Conclusion.—For women with recurrent miscarriages, the presence of thyroid antibodies cannot predict the outcomes of future pregnancies. Routine thyroid antibody screening does not appear indicated in the workup of women with unexplained miscarriage.

▶ Women with unexplained recurrent spontaneous abortion are more likely to have antithyroid antibodies than is the general antenatal population. Other studies have reported that the presence of antithyroid antibodies in euthyroid women is a risk marker for recurrent spontaneous abortion (RSA). It has been recommended that women with antithyroid antibodies be treated with IV immunoglobulin, as the presence of the antibodies are a marker of altered immune function. The results of this study differ from earlier reports, as the incidences of live births were similar in a group of women with unexplained RSA with and without antithyroid antibodies. Therefore, clinicians need more information before deciding that IV immunoglobulin therapy is truly beneficial in the treatment of unexplained RSA in women with thyroid antibodies.

D. R. Mishell, Jr, MD

Does Aspirin Have a Role in Improving Pregnancy Outcome for Women With the Antiphospholipid Syndrome? A Randomized Controlled Trial
Pattison NS, Chamley LW, Birdsall M, et al (Univ of Auckland, New Zealand; Natl Women's Hosp, Auckland, New Zealand)
Am J Obstet Gynecol 183:1008-1012, 2000   17–12

Background.—For many women with antiphospholipid syndrome and recurrent fetal loss, antiphospholipid antibodies are the only identifiable abnormality. The antibodies are often present at a low level. Previous trials have included women with divergent clinical presentations grouped together and not stratified by clinical presentation or antibody type or level. The efficacy of low-dose aspirin therapy in women with antiphospholipid antibodies in whom recurrent miscarriage is the only sequela was investigated in a pilot study.

Methods.—Fifty women with a history of 3 or more miscarriages and antiphospholipid antibodies were enrolled in the double-blind, randomized, placebo-controlled study. The women received aspirin, 75 mg daily, or placebo.

Findings.—Eighty-five percent of placebo recipients and 80% of aspirin recipients gave birth to live infants. This difference was nonsignificant. In addition, the groups did not differ in antenatal complications or neonatal morbidity.

Conclusion.—Low-dose aspirin is not beneficial for women with recurrent early fetal loss as the only sequela of the antiphospholipid syndrome. A large, controlled, randomized trial is needed to identify the best treatment for this patient population.

▶ The results of this study in women with recurrent spontaneous abortion and the antiphospholipid syndrome, without a prior history of thrombosis or lupus erythematosus, found a high rate of viable births (85%) in women receiving a placebo and intensive supportive care. This viable pregnancy rate was not further increased with the use of aspirin. The results of this study raise questions about the need for prednisone, heparin, or IV immunoglobulin therapy for women with recurrent spontaneous abortion and the antiphospholipid syndrome if they receive intensive supportive care. Additional large randomized, placebo-controlled trials are necessary to determine whether there is benefit in any pharmaceutical therapy for the treatment of recurrent spontaneous abortion and the antiphospholipid syndrome.

D. R. Mishell, Jr, MD

Pregnancy Outcome in Recurrent Spontaneous Abortion Associated With Antiphospholipid Antibodies: A Comparative Study of Intravenous Immunoglobulin Versus Prednisone Plus Low-Dose Aspirin
Vaquero E, Lazzarin N, Valensise H, et al (Univ of Rome "For Vergata"; Fatebenefratelli Hosp, Rome)
Am J Reprod Immunol 45:174-179, 2001   17–13

Background.—Antinuclear antibodies, antithyroid antibodies, and antiphospholipid antibodies (aPLs) have been associated with recurrent spontaneous abortion. The use of IV immunoglobulin (IVIG) was compared with prednisone plus low-dose aspirin (LDA) in pregnant women with a history of recurrent fetal loss and aPL syndrome.

Methods.—Eighty-two women with recurrent fetal loss and aPL syndrome were enrolled in the prospective, 2-center trial. Twenty-nine received prednisone plus LDA at 1 center, and 53 received IVIG at the other center.

Findings.—The live-birth rates were 78% in the IVIG group and 76% in the prednisone plus LDA group. The mean birth weight was greater in the IVIG group (Fig 1). Women given prednisone plus LDA had significantly greater incidences of hypertension and gestational diabetes (14% each) than did women given IVIG (5% each).

Conclusion.—Pregnancy outcomes were better with IVIG treatment than with prednisone plus LDA in these patients with aPL syndrome. In addition, the pregnancy complications rates associated with IVIG were lower than with prednisone plus LDA.

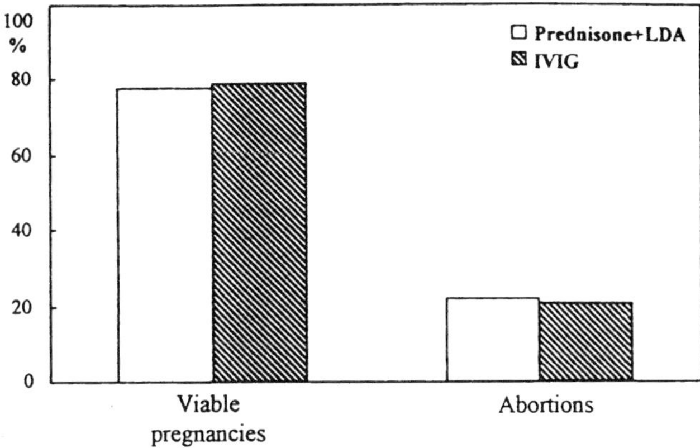

FIGURE 1.—Pregnancy outcome in patients with antiphospholipid antibodies treated with IV immunoglobulin (*IVIG*) and prednisone plus low-dose aspirin (*LDA*). (Courtesy of Vaquero E, Lazzarin N, Valensise H, et al: Pregnancy outcome in recurrent spontaneous abortion associated with antiphospholipid antibodies: A comparative study of intravenous immunoglobulin versus prednisone plus low-dose aspirin. *Am J Reprod Immunol* 45:174-179. Copyright 2001, by Munksgaard International Publishers Ltd. Copenhagen, Denmark.)

▶ Three types of therapy have been successfully used for women with recurrent spontaneous abortion having aPLs. These therapies are prednisone with LDA, heparin with aspirin, and IVIG. The viable birth rate with each of these therapies is about 80%, significantly better than treatment with aspirin alone. Since prednisone plus LDA is associated with a greater risk of pregnancy complications than heparin plus aspirin, the latter therapy has replaced the former. Many centers are treating all women with unexplained recurrent spontaneous abortion, as well as that associated with aPLs, with periodic administration of IVIG throughout pregnancy. The results of this nonrandomized clinical trial indicate that IVIG has a similar level of effectiveness as prednisone and LDA but has a lower rate of pregnancy complications. Until a randomized trial shows that IVIG is superior to heparin and aspirin, the latter therapy should be given to women with recurrent spontaneous abortion who have aPLs since it is much less expensive than IVIG.

D. R. Mishell, Jr, MD

Vitamin B$_{12}$ Deficiency, Infertility and Recurrent Fetal Loss

Bennett M (Ha'Emek Med Ctr, Afula, Israel)
J Reprod Med 46:209-212, 2001   17–14

Background.—Infertility has been associated with vitamin B$_{12}$ deficiency. Pregnancy occurring in women with this deficiency may result in recurrent early fetal loss. The relationship between infertility and recurrent fetal loss in vitamin B$_{12}$–deficient patients was investigated.

Methods and Findings.—Fourteen women seen with 15 episodes of vitamin B$_{12}$ deficiency were included in the study. Four episodes of infertility (duration, 2-12 years) had occurred in this group. Eleven women had had recurrent fetal loss. In 6 episodes, recurrent fetal loss was followed by infertility of more than 1 year in duration.

Conclusion.—When vitamin B_{12} deficiency first develops, hypercoagulability resulting from increased homocysteine levels may lead to fetal loss. A more prolonged deficiency leads to infertility through changes in ovulation, the development of the ovum, or defective implantation.

▶ Vitamin B_{12} deficiency is an uncommon condition, but this case series suggests that when it is present, it may be a cause of infertility as well as recurrent spontaneous abortion. It appears reasonable to measure homocysteine levels in all women with recurrent miscarriage as a deficiency of vitamin B_{12} can result in increased serum homocysteine levels, which can cause thrombophillia and pregnancy loss. It may also be beneficial to measure circulating B_{12} levels in women with infertility as well as recurrent miscarriage.

D. R. Mishell, Jr, MD

Recurrent Miscarriage—An Aspirin a Day?
Rai R, Backos M, Baxter N, et al (Imperial College, London)
Hum Reprod 15:2220-2223, 2000   17–15

Introduction.—Pregnancy is a hypercoagulable state because of the fact that (1) microthrombi are common in the placental vasculature of women with recurrent miscarriage, (2) placental thrombosis has been found in association with individual thrombophilic defects, and (3) there is an increased incidence of both congenital and acquired thrombophilic defects among women with adverse pregnancy outcomes at all gestational ages. The value of low-dose aspirin in improving the subsequent live birth rate among women with either unexplained recurrent early miscarriage or unexplained late pregnancy loss was examined in an observational investigation of the prospective pregnancy of 1055 women.

Methods.—In this study, recurrent early miscarriage was defined as less than 13 weeks' gestation (805 women) or unexplained late pregnancy loss (250 women). Participants were placed in 1 of 2 groups: those who chose to take low-dose aspirin, 75 mg daily, and those who did not take aspirin. Aspirin consumption was initiated within 5 weeks of amenorrhea and continued until delivery. All participants took folic acid, 400 µg daily, until 14 weeks' gestation for prophylaxis against neural tube defects. None of the women took heparin.

Results.—Among women with recurrent early miscarriages, there was no significant difference in the live birth rate for those who did (251 of 367; 68.4%) and did not take aspirin (278 of 438; 63.5%; odds ratio 1.24). This association was independent of the number of previous early miscarriages (Fig 1). Women with a previous late miscarriage who took aspirin has a significantly higher live birth rate (122 of 189; 64.6%),

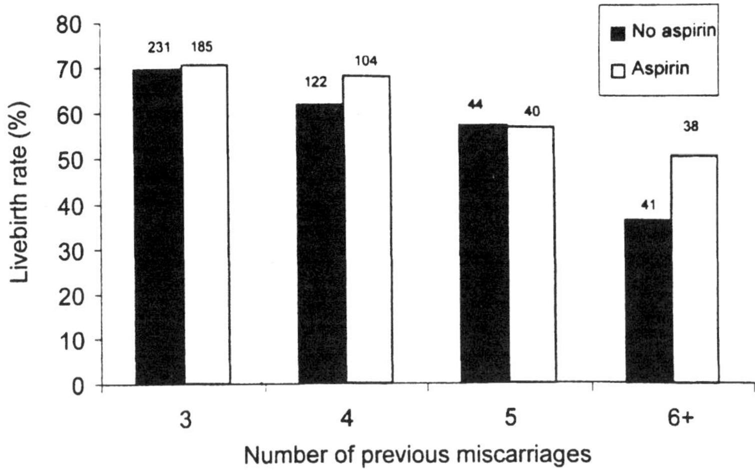

FIGURE 1.—Prospective pregnancy outcome among women with unexplained recurrent early miscarriage. *Values above each bar* are the number of patients in each group. (Courtesy of Rai R, Backos M, Baxter N, et al: Recurrent miscarriage—An aspirin a day? *Hum Reprod* 15:2220-2223, 2000. Copyright, European Society for Human Reproduction and Embryology, by permission of Oxford University Press.)

compared with those who did not take aspirin (30 of 61; 49.2%; odds ratio, 1.88).

Conclusion.—The empirical use of low-dose aspirin in women with unexplained recurrent early miscarriage is not justified.

▶ The results of this observational study indicate that daily ingestion of 75 mg of aspirin throughout pregnancy may be of benefit to women with a history of unexplained miscarriage whose gestation had advanced beyond 13 gestational weeks before abortion occurred. However, the use of low-dose aspirin was of no benefit to a group of women who had a history of 3 or more abortions during the first 13 gestational weeks. Whether or not low-dose aspirin is of true benefit in treating unexplained second trimester abortion needs to be determined by a randomized, controlled trial. Until such a study is completed, clinicians may wish to treat women with unexplained second trimester abortion with low-dose aspirin since its use in pregnancy does not appear harmful.

D. R. Mishell, Jr, MD

Obstetric and Neonatal Outcome in Women With a History of Recurrent Miscarriage: A Cohort Study

Jivraj S, Anstie B, Cheong Y-C, et al (Sheffield Hallam Univ, Sheffield, England)
Hum Reprod 16:102-106, 2001   17–16

Introduction.—Recurrent miscarriage is usually considered to be the loss of 3 or more consecutive pregnancies. The risk of miscarriage for a subsequent pregnancy is well documented. The obstetric and neonatal outcomes of pregnancy that has progressed beyond 24 weeks are not well defined. The obstetric and neonatal outcomes of 162 pregnancies that progressed beyond 24 weeks in women with a history of recurrent miscarriages were compared with a control population between January 1, 1992, and June 30, 1998.

Methods.—The hospital numbers of patients who attended the recurrent miscarriage clinic during the evaluation period were identified, and the hospital computer system was reviewed for any antenatal or labor ward admissions of these patients after 24 weeks of gestation. Controls consisted of all deliveries in the same hospital within the evaluation period.

Results.—Among the 162 pregnancies that progressed beyond 24 weeks in women with a history of recurrent miscarriages, there were 4 perinatal deaths; 16 infants were admitted to the special care baby unit. Compared with controls, the rates were significantly higher in the recurrent miscarriage group for preterm delivery (13% vs 3.9%), small-for-gestational-age (13% vs 2.1%), perinatal loss (2.5% vs 1%), and cesarean section (36% vs 16.7%). The ratio of male to female infants was equal between groups. Groups were similar in the rate of hypertension and diabetes.

Conclusion.—Patients with recurrent miscarriages are at high risk of obstetric problems and require close surveillance in the antenatal period.

▶ Women with a history of recurrent miscarriage should be considered to be at high risk of obstetric problems, and their pregnancies should be managed accordingly. After their pregnancies reach 24 weeks' gestation, careful monitoring of fetal growth and activity is important because of the increased risk of perinatal death, including intrauterine death, as well as preterm delivery and small-for-gestational-age infants.

D. R. Mishell, Jr, MD

18 Ectopic Pregnancy

Diagnosing Ectopic Pregnancy: Decision Analysis Comparing Six Strategies
Gracia CR, Barnhart KT (Univ of Pennsylvania, Philadelphia)
Obstet Gynecol 97:464-470, 2001   18–1

Background.—A major cause of morbidity and mortality in women of reproductive age is ectopic pregnancies, which have been shown to account for 9% of pregnancy-related deaths in the first trimester. The incidence of ectopic pregnancies has increased, but the mortality rate associated with ectopic pregnancies has fallen dramatically as diagnostic methods have improved. The only clinical signs and symptoms of an ectopic pregnancy are abdominal pain or vaginal bleeding in the first trimester, but these signs are not sensitive or specific. The majority of women with these symptoms have normal intrauterine pregnancies, so a timely and accurate diagnosis of the ectopic pregnancy is necessary with methods that will not interrupt viable uterine pregnancies. Although several diagnostic protocols for ectopic pregnancies have been published, no approach has been determined to be superior to others. Six published methods of diagnosing an ectopic pregnancy were compared.

Methods.—In a decision analysis, 6 diagnostic algorithms were compared. The algorithms involved combinations of the following diagnostic strategies: clinical examination, transvaginal US, measurement of serum progesterone level, measurement of serum human chorionic gonadotropin (hCG) level, and dilatation and curettage. The study group was composed of hemodynamically stable women who were seen at a tertiary care university emergency department with abdominal pain or bleeding in their first trimesters. The outcome measures for the study included the number of missed ectopic pregnancies, potentially interrupted intrauterine pregnancies, surgical and diagnostic procedures, time until diagnosis, and cost.

Results.—The most favorable outcomes were obtained with US followed by measurement of serum hCG level in women with nondiagnostic scans (Table 2). No ectopic pregnancy was missed in these women, only 1% of all potential intrauterine pregnancies were interrupted, and the time to diagnosis averaged 1.46 days. Quantitative measurement of the hCG level followed by US only in women whose hCG levels were above the discriminatory zone was optimal only when the sensitivity of US for the diagnosis of an intrauterine pregnancy was less than 93%. Measurement

421

TABLE 2.—Outcomes for Each Diagnostic Strategy

Strategy	Missed EP/10,000	Interrupted IUP/10,000	LS/10,000	DC/10,000	US/10,000	H/10,000	Days to Diagnosis/ Patient	Blood Draws/ 10,000	*Total Charge/ Patient
US→hCG	0	70	940	2581	10,250	0	1.46	5227	$1958
hCG→US	0	122	940	2463	8276	0	1.66	14,375	$1842
P→US→hCG	24	25	916	3547	3272	0	1.25	12,108	$1692
P→hCG→US	24	39	916	3191	2555	0	1.26	15,003	$1569
US→US	0	121	940	3319	11,760	1760	1.21	0	$2486
Clinical Examination	940	0	0	0	0	0	1.0	0	0

*Excluding the emergency department clinical examination fee.

Abbreviations: EP, ectopic pregnancy; *IUP*, intrauterine pregnancy; *P*, progesterone; *LS*, laparoscopy; *H*, hospitalization; *hCG*, human chorionic gonadotropin; *DC*, dilatation and curettage.
(Reprinted with permission from The American College of Obstetricians and Gynecologists, from Gracia CR, Barnhart KT: Diagnosing ectopic pregnancy: Decision analysis comparing six strategies. *Obstet Gynecol* 97(3):464-470, 2001.)

of the serum progesterone level was associated with missed ectopic pregnancies and was thus not favored (2.6%).

Conclusions.—With the current accuracy of tests for the diagnosis of an ectopic pregnancy, the best outcomes were obtained with algorithms that combined US and measurement of hCG level. In this study, the most efficient and accurate method of diagnosing ectopic pregnancies was found to be the use of US as the first step.

► Currently, the 3 most common tests used for the diagnosis of unruptured ectopic pregnancies in women with pelvic pain and/or uterine bleeding in early pregnancy are transvaginal pelvic US and measurement of serum hCG and serum progesterone levels. With the use of this decision analysis, it was found that pelvic US followed by measurement of serum hCG levels resulted in the best decision making. With this strategy, no ectopic pregnancy was missed and fewer intrauterine pregnancies were interrupted than with other strategies that failed to diagnose ectopic pregnancies.

D. R. Mishell, Jr, MD

The Utility of Maternal Creatine Kinase in the Evaluation of Ectopic Pregnancy
Birkhahn RH, Gaeta TJ, Leo PJ, et al (New York Methodist Hosp, Brooklyn)
Am J Emerg Med 18:695-697, 2000   18–2

Background.—The incidence of ectopic pregnancy (EP) has increased 4-fold since 1970. This increase is partially artifactual, as advances in diagnostic strategies have improved the likelihood of identifying ectopic gestations before spontaneous tubal abortion. However, other factors have also contributed to the increase in EP, including the increasing incidence of pelvic inflammatory disease, fertility drugs, and pelvic surgery. The diagnosis of EP in the hemodynamically stable patient is dependent on a suggestive clinical history, linked with the availability of 2-dimensional US and quantitative serum levels of human chorionic gonadotropin, beta subunit (B-hCG). The lack of availability of these diagnostic modalities can present a challenge to the emergency physician who must determine how best to evaluate a patient in the first trimester of pregnancy with abdominal pain and/or vaginal bleeding. The utility of a maternal creatine phosphokinase (CPK) assay in the prediction of the presence of an EP in an emergency department setting was evaluated.

Methods.—An observational study was conducted in the emergency department of a teaching hospital. The patient group included women with first-trimester pregnancies seen with lower abdominal pain and/or vaginal bleeding between March 1996 and March 1997. A total of 21 patients were randomly matched with pregnant patients in whom EP was found not to be the diagnosis later. The serum CPK values at presentation were compared between these 2 groups by means of 2-tailed analysis of variance. Odds ratios and frequency tables were generated on the basis of

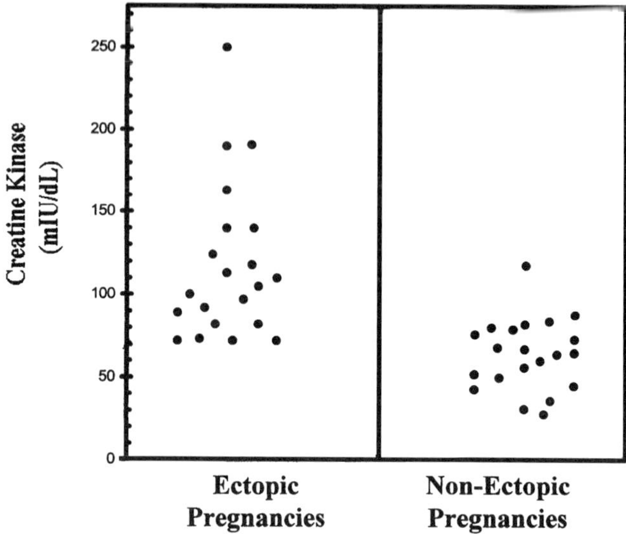

FIGURE 1.—Absolute values of maternal creatine kinase ranged from 72 to 250 mIU/dL in patients with ectopic pregnancies and from 31 to 118 mIU/dL in patients without ectopic pregnancies. (Courtesy of Birkhahn RH, Gaeta TJ, Leo PJ, et al: The utility of maternal creatine kinase in the evaluation of ectopic pregnancy. *Am J Emerg Med* 18:695-697, 2000.)

the a priori hypothesis that a serum CPK value of more than 70 mIU/dL might be useful as a predictor of EP.

Results.—The mean serum CPK level for the EP group was 118 mIU/dL compared with 64 mIU/dL in the non-EP group (Fig 1). The serum CPK level as a predictor of EP was found to have a sensitivity of 100%, a specificity of 69.1%, a positive predictive value of 72.4%, and a negative predictive value of 100%.

Conclusions.—A CPK level of more than 70 mIU/dL is an important adjuvant diagnostic tool for eliminating EP as a diagnosis.

▶ The results of this small study suggest that measurement of serum CPK levels may be of use in women with symptoms consistent with the diagnosis of an unruptured EP when pelvic US and quantitative hCG measurement fail to confirm the diagnosis. In this study, no woman with an EP had a CPK level less than 70 mIU/dL. A prospective study with a large number of women with symptoms of unruptured EPs should be performed to confirm the clinical value of measuring the CPK level in women suspected of having unruptured EPs.

D. R. Mishell, Jr, MD

A Randomised Trial Comparing Single Dose Systemic Methotrexate and Laparoscopic Surgery for the Treatment of Unruptured Tubal Pregnancy
Sowter MC, Farquhar CM, Petrie KJ, et al (Natl Women's Hosp, Auckland, New Zealand; Univ of Auckland, New Zealand)
Br J Obstet Gynaecol 108:192-203, 2001   18–3

Introduction.—Despite reported high levels of success with methotrexate (MTX) for treatment of ectopic pregnancy, few centers currently use MTX with any frequency. If effective and well-tolerated, a single IM dose of MTX administered without prior diagnostic laparoscopy could allow management of ectopic pregnancy entirely within the outpatient setting and considerably reduce treatment cost and disruption to the lives of women undergoing treatment. Single-dose systemic MTX, 50 mg/m^2, was compared with laparoscopic surgery for treatment of women with unruptured tubal pregnancy in an open, pragmatic, prospective randomized trial.

Methods.—Clinically stable women with unruptured tubal pregnancy diagnosed by transvaginal US and quantitative serum β-hCG measurement were recruited between July 28, 1997, and September 27, 1998. Inclusion criteria included serum β-hCG concentration below 5000 IU/L and a tubal pregnancy less than 3.5 cm in diameter. The primary outcome measures were treatment success, physical and psychological functioning, side effects, and subsequent ipsilateral tubal patency.

Results.—Of 218 women with ectopic pregnancies seen at 3 hospitals, 79 (36% eligibility rate) were eligible for trial entry and 62 (78% recruitment rate) were recruited. Twenty-six of the 28 women (93%) who were randomly assigned to laparoscopic surgery needed no further treatment, compared with 22 of the 34 women (65%) who were randomly assigned to MTX ($P < .01$). Two women (7%) in the laparoscopic surgery group experienced persistent trophoblast. Nine women (26%) in the MTX group needed more than 1 dose of MTX, and 5 (15%) underwent laparoscopy during follow-up. In the laparoscopic surgery group, 3 women (11%) had negative laparoscopies and 2 (7%) had a ruptured fallopian tube at the time of surgery. Women treated with MTX had significantly better physical functioning scores. Groups had similar psychological outcomes. Women in the MTX treatment group had significantly greater and more prolonged vaginal bleeding. The possibility of MTX treatment failure was higher at higher serum β-hCG concentrations. Ipsilateral tubal patency rates were similar for both treatment groups.

Conclusion.—Treatment of tubal pregnancy with single-dose systemic MTX was less effective than treatment with laparoscopic salpingotomy. This approach was well tolerated, but it should be offered only as an alternative to surgery to women with mild symptoms and low serum β-hCG concentrations.

▶ For women with small unruptured ectopic pregnancies, a single dose of MTX can be used for therapy instead of laparoscopic surgery. Even though the success rate of laparoscopic surgery is higher than that of MTX if a woman has a small unruptured ectopic pregnancy with low levels of hCG, she should be informed about the benefits and risks of MTX therapy. The information obtained in this randomized trial can be used to enhance the pretreatment counseling of women with small unruptured tubal pregnancies.

D. R. Mishell, Jr, MD

An Economic Evaluation of Single Dose Systemic Methotrexate and Laparoscopic Surgery for the Treatment of Unruptured Ectopic Pregnancy

Sowter MC, Farquhar CM, Gudex G (Natl Women's Hosp, Auckland, New Zealand)

Br J Obstet Gynaecol 108:204-212, 2001

18–4

Objective.—Ectopic pregnancies account for 1% to 2% of all pregnancies in developed countries. Methotrexate (MTX) allows treatment on an ambulatory basis and laparoscopy can be avoided, but no economic evaluations have compared single-dose MTX treatment with surgery. The direct and indirect costs of a single dose of MTX were compared with laparoscopic surgery for the treatment of unruptured ectopic pregnancies.

Methods.—An economic evaluation was conducted alongside a randomized trial to determine the costs of treating ectopic pregnancies in 62 women randomly allocated to receive single-dose MTX (n = 34) or laparoscopy (n = 28). Costs of initial and follow-up visits, all drugs, surgery and anesthesia, in-patient hotel, and additional treatments and complications were tallied.

Results.—Single-dose MTX was successful in 22 women (65%). Nine women (26%) required more than 1 dose. Eight (24%) were readmitted, and 4 underwent surgery. Laparoscopy was performed in 28 women. Seventeen had a salpingotomy or tubal abortion and required weekly serum β-human chorionic gonadotropin (β-hCG) measurements. Eleven women having salpingotomies required no follow-up. Two women had persistent trophoblasts, and 1 required another laparoscopy. Indirect costs were calculated for all 62 women. Indirect costs were determined for 32 women randomly assigned to MTX and for 26 women randomly assigned to laparoscopy. Average total direct costs were a significant 52% lower for the MTX group ($NZ1470) compared with the laparoscopy group ($NZ3083). Indirect costs were also a significant 40% lower in the MTX group ($NZ1141) compared with the laparoscopy group ($NZ1899). Most of the difference was accounted for by the reduced number of lost working days for the women treated with MTX. Direct cost differences were greatest at serum β-hCG concentrations of less than 1500 IU/L. There were no differences in indirect costs above β-hCG concentrations of 1500 IU/L. If all 218 eligible women had been treated with MTX, the direct cost savings per woman would have been $NZ580. If upper pretreatment serum β-hCG levels had been limited to 1500 and 1000 IU/L, only 24% and 20% of women would have received MTX, and direct costs would have been decreased to $NZ422 and $NZ386 per woman; the respective reduction in indirect costs would have been $NZ273, $NZ264, and $NZ248 for each scenario.

Conclusion.—MTX use reduced direct and indirect costs by 52% and 40%, respectively, compared with laparoscopy for women with ectopic pregnancies. Approximately 20% to 25% of women could be treated with MTX.

▶ This study of the costs of treatment of early unruptured ectopic pregnancy demonstrated that the use of MTX is much less expensive than treatment with laparoscopic surgery if the initial β-hCG level is less than 1500 IU/L. Women treated with MTX also had less time away from work, which also resulted in indirect cost savings. Single-dose MTX therapy is an effective, relatively inexpensive method for the treatment of early unruptured ectopic pregnancies.

D. R. Mishell, Jr, MD

Survival Analysis of Fertility After Ectopic Pregnancy
Ego A, Subtil D, Cosson M, et al (Centre Hospitalier Régional Universitaire de Lille, France)
Fertil Steril 75:560-566, 2001

18–5

Background.—Earlier reports indicate that between 20% and 60% of women are infertile after an ectopic pregnancy. However, in recent years, we have seen great advances in the diagnosis and management of ectopic pregnancy. The effects of these advances on future fertility were evaluated, and risk factors associated with future infertility were identified.

Methods.—The subjects were 328 women 18 to 42 years of age (mean age, 28.5 years) who experienced an ectopic pregnancy between April 1994 and March 1997 and who were subsequently trying to achieve a spontaneous pregnancy. None of the subjects had been using an intrauterine contraceptive device at the time of the ectopic pregnancy. Subjects were interviewed by telephone every 6 months for 2 years and every year thereafter to determine whether they had become pregnant. Subjects who became pregnant were asked how long it took them to become pregnant, any medical treatment required, and the outcome.

Results.—At the time of the index ectopic pregnancy, 123 of the 328 subjects (39%) smoked, 21 (6%) had had a prior ectopic pregnancy, and 100 (31%) reported being infertile for 1 year or longer. Additionally, 57 subjects (17%) had fallopian tube damage caused by previous ectopic pregnancy, pelvic inflammatory disease, or tubal surgery. The ectopic pregnancy had ruptured in 55 subjects (17%); overall, 55% had undergone conservative management for the ectopic pregnancy and 45% had undergone radical treatment. Seventeen subjects (5%) underwent in vitro

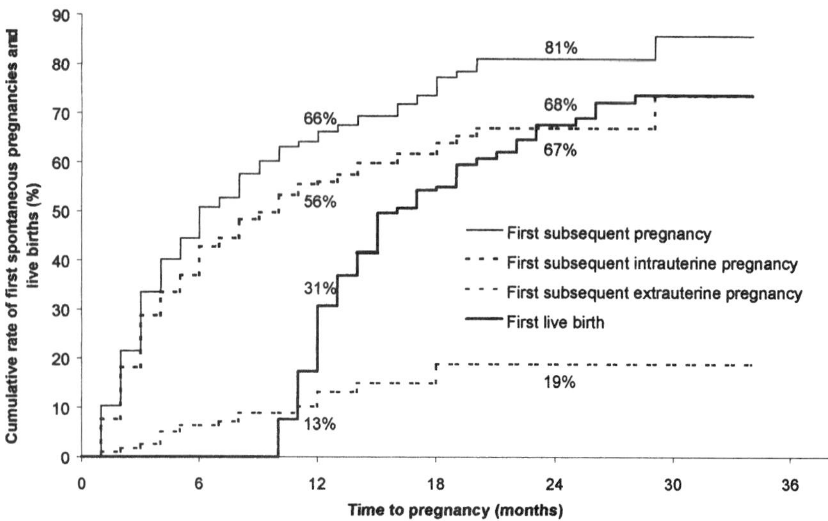

FIGURE 2.—Cumulative rate of first spontaneous pregnancies and live birth. (Reprinted with permission from the American Society for Reproductive Medicine courtesy of Ego A, Subtil D, Cosson M, et al: Survival analysis of fertility after ectopic pregnancy. *Fertil Steril* 75:560-566, 2001.)

fertilization after a mean of 10 months. Overall, 215 subjects (65.6%) became pregnant at a mean of 5.2 months after the ectopic pregnancy. Most of these pregnancies (182, or 84.7%) were intrauterine (27 of which ended in miscarriage). However, 22 subjects (10.2%) experienced a recurrent ectopic pregnancy at a mean of 6.1 months after the index event. (It was too early to identify the site of implantation in 11 pregnancies.) The cumulative pregnancy rates at 1 and 2 years were 66% and 81%, respectively (Fig 2), while the cumulative ectopic pregnancy rates at 1 and 2 years were 13% and 19%. Cumulative intrauterine pregnancy rates at 1 and 2 years were 56% and 67%, respectively, and the cumulative live birth rates at 1 and 2 years were 31% and 68%.

Regression analyses identified 3 factors independently and significantly associated with a decreased likelihood of an intrauterine pregnancy: age greater than 35 years (adjusted odds ratio [OR], 0.53 compared with women 35 years of age or younger), previous tubal damage (adjusted OR, 0.46), and a history of infertility (adjusted OR, 0.69). Neither smoking status, lifestyle factors, previous ectopic pregnancy, the presence of adhesions, nor the type of treatment used for the index event was significantly associated with subsequent fertility.

Conclusion.—Of these 328 women who did not have an intrauterine contraceptive device in place at the time of their index ectopic pregnancy, 81% became pregnant within 2 years and 68% had a live birth. Having a previous ectopic pregnancy per se was not a risk factor for subsequent infertility. Factors that decreased the likelihood of subsequent spontaneous intrauterine pregnancy were age greater than 35 years, previous tubal damage, and a history of infertility.

▶ The data obtained in this follow-up study of a large number of women with ectopic pregnancy provide useful information for clinicians counseling of women with an ectopic pregnancy who desire future fertility. As ectopic pregnancy is now being frequently diagnosed earlier in gestation and prior to tubal rupture, the prognosis for a future intrauterine pregnancy has improved. In this study, 2 years after an ectopic pregnancy had occurred, about 80% of women wishing to conceive had done so. About one fifth of the women had another ectopic pregnancy and two thirds had an intrauterine pregnancy. The chances of conceiving again were significantly reduced if the woman was older than 35, had a history of infertility, or had evidence of prior tubal damage.

D. R. Mishell, Jr, MD

Fertility After Ectopic Pregnancy: Effects of Surgery and Expectant Management
Strobelt N, Mariani E, Ferrari L, et al (Univ of Milan-Biocca, Monza, Italy; Georgetown Univ, Washington, DC)
J Reprod Med 45:803-807, 2000   18–6

Background.—Greater options now exist for treating ectopic pregnancy. They not only save the patient's life but preserve fertility. Fertility rates among women undergoing expectant management were compared with those of women undergoing surgery.

Methods.—One hundred eighty consecutive patients with a diagnosis of ectopic pregnancy between 1988 and 1995 were included. A history of sterility, infertility, use of intrauterine devices, endometriosis, pelvic inflammatory disease or pelvic surgery before ectopic pregnancy, and type of treatment for ectopic pregnancy were included in the statistical analysis.

Findings.—Ninety-seven of the 180 women wished to conceive. Intrauterine contraception rates were 63% in those treated with expectant management and 51% in those treated by primary surgery. Successfully completing expectant treatment was associated with subsequent intrauterine pregnancy rates similar to those of surgical treatment. The rates of subsequent intrauterine conception in women undergoing delayed surgery after failure of expectant management were comparable with those of primary surgery. Anamnestic factors significantly adversely affecting reproductive outcome were a history of infertility, a history of ectopic pregnancy, and previous pelvic surgery.

Conclusion.—Subsequent intrauterine contraception rates are comparable after expectant and surgical treatment of ectopic pregnancy, even when expectant management fails and secondary surgery is necessary. A subgroup of patients at greater risk for poor reproductive outcomes can be identified by gynecologic history.

▶ The duration of follow-up was not stated in this study and the data were not calculated by survival analysis. Nevertheless, it is reassuring to observe that expectant management of an early, unruptured ectopic pregnancy in women desiring future fertility was associated with similar rates of subsequent intrauterine pregnancy (about 60%) and ectopic pregnancy (about 10%) as for women who had surgical excision of their ectopic pregnancy.

D. R. Mishell, Jr, MD

Fertility Following Radical, Conservative-Surgical or Medical Treatment for Tubal Pregnancy: A Population-Based Study

Bouyer J, Job-Spira N, Pouly JL, et al (Hosp Hôtel-Dieu, Clermont-Ferrad, France; Hosp Antoine Béclère, Clamart, France)
Br J Obstet Gynaecol 107:714-721, 2000   18–7

Introduction.—Improvements in the diagnosis and management of ectopic pregnancies have shifted concerns from the immediate health of the woman to preservation of her subsequent fertility. Conservative treatments have a tendency to increase the recurrence rate of ectopic pregnancy because they leave the fallopian tube damaged. The subsequent fertility of women who experienced ectopic pregnancy was compared according to type of treatment received, taking into account the factors influencing the choice of treatment.

Methods.—A population-based trial was conducted to examine 835 ectopic pregnancies registered between 1992 and 1996 in the Auvergne (France) Ectopic Pregnancy Register. Cohort members were between 15 and 44 years of age, and all were treated by either surgical or medical procedures for an ectopic pregnancy. Treatments were considered to be either radical (salpingectomy), conservative-surgical (salpingotomy), or medical (methotrexate injection). Of 476 women with tubal ectopic pregnancy who were not using contraception at the time of conception, subsequent fertility was assessed for the 291 women who attempted to conceive again. Reproductive outcomes were compared according to ectopic pregnancy treatment. The primary outcome measures of fertility were recurrence of ectopic pregnancy and spontaneous intrauterine pregnancy.

Results.—The initial treatment was considered radical for 178 women (37%), conservative-surgical for 262 (55%), and medical for 25 (8%); treatment failure rates were 1%, 5%, and 36%, respectively. The 2-year cumulative recurrence rate was 27%, with no significant between-group differences. For women with previous infertility factors (particularly diseased contralateral tube), treatments differed significantly. The rate of intrauterine pregnancy was lower for radical treatment and higher for medical treatment than for conservative-surgical treatment. In women with no infertility factor, treatment groups did not differ significantly.

Conclusion.—Conservative procedures seem to best preserve subsequent fertility in women with previous infertility factors, especially those with diseased contralateral tubes. For women with no infertility factor, there was no significant difference among treatment approaches, although medical treatment seemed to be the most effective in conserving fertility.

▶ The results of this follow-up study of a large number of women with ectopic pregnancies provide useful information for clinicians. A woman with an unruptured tubal pregnancy who wishes future fertility can be treated by conservative surgery (salpingostomy or salpingotomy), by radical surgery (salpingectomy), or, when appropriate, by medical therapy with methotrexate. Unfortunately, there are no long-term results of fertility when the initial treatment is performed as part of a randomized trial. The results of this study indicate that conservative surgical or medical therapy is followed by higher intrauterine pregnancy rates than radical surgery in women with prior infertility or an abnormal contralateral oviduct. Thus, if future fertilization is desired in women with either of these conditions, it would be best not to perform salpingectomy if possible. There was no significant difference in subsequent intrauterine pregnancy rates after any of the 3 treatment modalities in women without prior infertility and a normal-appearing contralateral oviduct, but conservative surgery is still advisable because the contralateral oviduct may have abnormalities that are not grossly visible.

D. R. Mishell, Jr, MD

19 Premenstrual Syndrome

Efficacy of Selective Serotonin-Reuptake Inhibitors in Premenstrual Syndrome: A Systematic Review
Dimmock PW, Wyatt KM, Jones PW, et al (Keele Univ, Stoke-on-Trent, England)
Lancet 356:1131-1136, 2000
19–1

Background.—Evidence for the importance of serotonin in the pathogenesis of premenstrual syndrome (PMS) has continued to build. In light of this increasing evidence, the use of selective serotonin-reuptake inhibitors (SSRIs) has been on the increase as first-line therapy. The efficacy of SSRIs in the management of severe PMS was evaluated in this meta-analysis.

Methods.—Medical and scientific databases were searched for reports of published clinical trials of SSRIs in the management of PMS. Pharmaceutical companies were also approached for data, and citations of relevant articles were reviewed; 29 studies of the use of SSRIs in the treatment of PMS were identified. After exclusion of 14 studies for the lack of a placebo group, a preliminary report of the included trial, or inadequate quality, 15 randomized, placebo-controlled studies were included in the final analysis. Data included in the meta-analysis were information on study design, participants, drugs and dosing regimens used, outcome measures, side effects, and sources of funding. The standardized mean differences between the treatment and placebo groups were determined for an overall estimate of efficacy. A reduction in the overall symptoms of PMS was used as the primary outcome measure.

Results.—A total of 904 women were included in the primary analysis. An overall standardized mean difference of –1.066 was identified, which corresponded to an odds ratio of 6.91 (95% CI, 3.90-12.2) in favor of SSRIs (Fig 3). SSRIs were found to be effective in the treatment of physical and behavioral symptoms. No significant difference in symptom reduction was found between continuous and intermittent dosing or between trials that were independently funded and those funded by pharmaceutical companies. Withdrawal from a study as a result of side effects was 2.5 times more likely in the active-treatment group than in the placebo group.

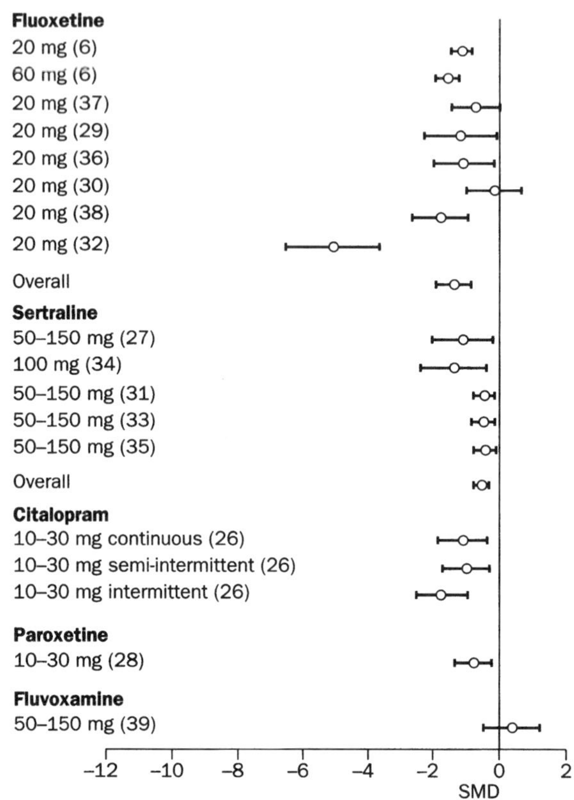

FIGURE 3.—Standardized mean differences (SMD) for proportion of patients who showed improvement in overall premenstrual symptoms by individual selective serotonin-reuptake inhibitors and dose used. (Courtesy of Dimmock PW, Wyatt KM, Jones PW, et al: Efficacy of selective serotonin-reuptake inhibitors in premenstrual syndrome: A systematic review. *Lancet* 356(9236):1131-1136, copyright by The Lancet Ltd. 2000.)

Conclusions.—This meta-analysis indicates that SSRIs are effective in use as first-line therapy for patients with severe PMS. The safety of these agents has been established in trials of affective disorder, and the side effects of SSRIs at low doses have been found to be acceptable.

▶ This review of published randomized placebo-controlled trials of the use of SSRIs confirms their benefit in the management of premenstrual symptoms. Because a similar benefit was found with both intermittent and continuous therapy, it would seem best to use one of these agents only during the luteal phase so that the side effects of the drug could be decreased. Administration of 20 mg fluoxetine daily was the most studied agent.

D. R. Mishell, Jr, MD

The Efficacy of Fluoxetine in Improving Physical Symptoms Associated With Premenstrual Dysphoric Disorder

Steiner M, Romano SJ, Babcock S, et al (McMaster Univ, Hamilton, Canada; Eli Lilly Co, Indianapolis, Ind; St Mary's Hosp, Montreal; et al)
Br J Obstet Gynaecol 108:462-468, 2001   19–2

Background.—Premenstrual dysphoric disorder (PDD), a severe variant of premenstrual syndrome, affects 3% to 8% of women of reproductive age. The efficacy of fluoxetine, a specific serotonergic re-uptake inhibitor, in the treatment of PDD was investigated.

Methods.—Four hundred five women were included in the randomized, double-blind, placebo-controlled, parallel study. Three hundred twenty women had prospectively diagnosed PDD. Women received fluoxetine, 20 or 60 mg/d, or placebo. The physical symptoms of PDD were assessed on visual analogue scales and on self-rated and observer premenstrual tension syndrome scales.

Findings.—Fluoxetine was superior to placebo in reducing the symptoms of breast tenderness and bloating but not headache. The 2 dosages of fluoxetine did not differ in their effects on physical symptoms.

Conclusion.—Daily fluoxetine treatment is more effective than placebo in improving the most common physical symptoms of PDD. The efficacy of a 20 mg/day dose is comparable to that of 60 mg/day.

▶ This is another well-done study which shows that administration of fluoxetine improves the physical as well as the emotional symptoms of the premenstrual syndrome. A dose of 20 mg/day was as effective as 60 mg/day, and the lower dose was better tolerated. This serotonin reuptake inhibitor is effective therapy for the premenstrual syndrome.

D. R. Mishell, Jr, MD

Rizatriptan in the Treatment of Menstrual Migraine

Silberstein SD, Massiou H, Le Jeunne C, et al (Thomas Jefferson Univ, Philadelphia; Merck & Co Inc, West Point, Pa; Hôpital Lariboisière, Paris; et al)
Obstet Gynecol 96:237-242, 2000   19–3

Background.—Migraine attacks associated with menstruation are more severe and difficult to treat than attacks not associated with menstruation. The efficacy of oral rizatriptan, 5 or 10 mg, in the treatment of menstrually associated migraine attacks was investigated in a retrospective analysis of data from 2 large clinical trials.

Methods and Findings.—The studies were randomized, double-blinded, placebo-controlled trials with a 2-period, crossover design. A subgroup of 335 women had menstrually associated migraine. Two hours after dosing, 68% of 139 women taking rizatriptan, 10 mg, and 70% of 115 women taking rizatriptan, 5 mg, reported pain relief, compared with 44% of those taking placebo. Rizatriptan was effective in both menstrual and nonmenstrual migraine in all women.

Conclusion.—Rizatriptan, 5 or 10 mg, effectively relieves menstrually associated migraine attacks. Associated migraine symptoms, functional disability, and the need for escape medications were reduced in these series.

▶ This randomized trial found that the use of rizatriptan, a serotonic receptor agonist, relieved the pain in about two thirds of women with migraine attacks associated with the onset of menstruation, significantly better than the 44% of patients relieved of pain with placebo. The headache recurred within 24 hours in about one third of the patients who initially had pain relief with rizatriptan. Recurrence can also be treated with rizatriptan, but at least 2 hours should elapse between doses. In this study, rizatriptan had a similar level of effectiveness when treating women with menstrual migraine as on women with headaches not associated with menses. Other serotonic receptor agonists, such as sumatriptan and zolmitriptan, have also been shown to be effective therapies for treating menstrual migraine.

D. R. Mishell, Jr, MD

20 Sexuality

Bupropion Sustained Release (SR) for the Treatment of Hypoactive Sexual Desire Disorder (HSDD) in Nondepressed Women
Segraves RT, Croft H, Kavoussi R, et al (Case Western Reserve Univ, Cleveland, Ohio; Harry Croft MD and Associates, San Antonio, Tex; MCP-Hahnemann School of Medicine, Philadelphia, et al)
J Sex Marital Ther 27:303-316, 2001   20–1

Introduction.—The cause of hypoactive sexual desire disorder (HSDD) in women remains unknown in many cases. In some women, however, dopaminergic dysregulation may be involved. Among individuals with depression, bupropion improved sexual functioning when this agent was substituted for other antidepressants. This article describes initial results of bupropion sustained release (SR) in nondepressed women with HSDD.

Methods.—Women eligible for the study had a primary diagnosis of HSDD and were not affected by relationship disorder or acute life stress. Excluded were women with sexual dysfunction related to an organic cause and those with conditions that might interfere with response to treatment. The 3-phase study consisted of a screening phase, a placebo phase, and an active treatment phase. Participants who did not respond to placebo were eligible to enter an 8-week, single-blind active treatment in which they received bupropion SR. Improvement in HSDD was assessed biweekly from day 14 to day 84.

Results.—Fifty-one of the 55 women who entered the 8-week active treatment phase had evaluable data. The mean age of this group was 42. Most were white, premenopausal, and were not using oral contraceptives or hormone replacement therapy. The mean duration of HSDD before study entry was 6 years. During treatment, the mean dose of bupropion SR was 287 mg/day. Fifteen (29%) women were treatment responders, with results seen as early as 2 weeks after initiation of bupropion SR. Significant increases were reported for interest in sexual activity, sexual arousal, and sexual fantasy, and 39% of the women reported satisfaction with sexual desire by the end of the treatment phase. Five patients had to discontinue treatment because of skin reactions. The only adverse events reported in at least 5% of women and occurring more often during treatment than in the placebo phase were insomnia, tremor, and rash. Overall, bupropion was well tolerated.

Conclusion.—This is the first report on the safety and efficacy of bupropion SR in the treatment of HSDD in nondepressed women. The positive sexual effects noted may be attributable to the drug's enhancement of dopaminergic neurotransmission.

▶ Bupropion is approved for the treatment of adult depression and smoking cessation. It is a norepinephrine and dopamine reuptake inhibitor. Dopaminergic activity has been reported to modulate the desire phase of the sexual response cycle. Women with hypoactive sexual desire disorder lack sexual thoughts and interest in sexual activity. Bupropion was well tolerated and resulted in a significant increase in sexual fantasy, arousal, and activity.

D. S. Miller, MD

A New Non-Pharmacological Vacuum Therapy for Female Sexual Dysfunction

Billups KL, Berman L, Berman J, et al (Edina, Minn)
J Sex Marital Ther 27:1-7, 2001   20–2

Introduction.—Difficulty in or inability to achieve clitoral tumescence may be related to and associated with female sexual dysfunction. The EROS-CTD™ (Clitoral Therapy Device, Urometrics, Inc.), is a therapeutic device designed to help achieve and maintain clitoral engorgement, increase blood flow to the clitoris, and ultimately enhance arousal and orgasm. After the EROS-CTD device is placed over the clitoris, the pump is activated to create a gentle vacuum over the clitoris, which causes increased blood flow and engorgement. The EROS-CTD device was used to evaluate whether engorgement of the clitoris is correlated with enhanced sensation, increased lubrication, and improved sexual arousal.

Methods.—Thirty-two patients with female sexual dysfunction were evaluated, many of whom had already failed earlier attempts at self-stimulation or vibrator usage. Of 32 patients, 9 were premenopausal and 11 were postmenopausal with complaints of female sexual dysfunction; an additional 10 were premenopausal and 2 were postmenopausal women with no sexual function complaints. Patients underwent complete physical evaluation, including a pelvic examination, determinations of serum estradiol and follicle-stimulating hormone levels in all postmenopausal women, and a brief psychosexual history. Patients were instructed in how to use the EROS-CTD device. Participants were asked to record any changes in sexual pleasure, including clitoral and labial engorgement orgasm, and vaginal lubrication. They also completed the Female Intervention Efficacy Index. A second office visit was required at completion of 6 at-home sessions and within 3 months of initiation of therapy.

Results.—None of the women with or without female sexual dysfunction reported any adverse clinical effects, including hypersensitization, skin irritation, hematoma, compromise of skin integrity, infection, or allergic response to materials. Genital examination at trial completion did not show any evidence of clitoral trauma, hematoma, or irritation. In women with female sexual dysfunction, 90% reported greater sensation using the device than without the device (P < .001). Among those with no sexual dysfunction, 58% reported increased sensation and 42% reported no change. Increased lubrication was reported in 80% of patients with dysfunction (P < .001) compared with 33% of those with no dysfunction. Increased ability to achieve orgasm was noted in 55% of patients with female sexual dysfunction compared with 42% of those with no complaints of sexual dysfunction. Increased sexual satisfaction was observed by 80% of patients with female sexual dysfunction compared with 25% of patients with no dysfunction (P < .001).

Conclusion.—The EROS-CTD therapy was effective in treating female sexual dysfunction, including symptoms of diminished genital sensation, reduced vaginal lubrication, decreased ability to achieve orgasm, and reduced sexual satisfaction. No adverse effects were reported and there was no evidence of clitoral trauma, bruising, or irritation.

▶ The EROS-CTD is the first FDA-approved device for the treatment of female sexual dysfunction. That approval was based on very modest data of which this study was pivotal. While clitoral erection may occur concomitantly with arousal and lubrication, the evidence is less compelling that it is necessary, sufficient, or critical for orgasm to occur. It is possible that much of the improvement seen was due not so much to the vacuum-facilitated clitoral erection as the effect of physician-prescribed manipulation that may free the patient from guilt arising from taboos existing in many aspects of society that discourage female self-pleasuring. Hopefully, this device will be prescribed after a careful psychosexual history and physical as it is unlikely to correct the most common causes of sexual dysfunction such as relationship problems or medication side effects.

D. S. Miller, MD

21 Upper Genital Tract

Adnexa

Adnexal Masses in Pregnancy: A Review of 130 Cases Undergoing Surgical Management

Whitecar P, Turner S, Higby K (Brooke Army Med Ctr, Ft Sam Houston; Univ of Texas, San Antonio)
Am J Obstet Gynecol 181:19-24, 1999
21–1

Objective.—Because of the increase in the number of pregnant women with diagnoses of adnexal masses, maternal and fetal outcomes in patients undergoing surgical management were reviewed in a multicenter study.

Methods.—Records were reviewed for all 130 pregnant women, aged 15 to 45 years, with diagnoses of adnexal masses requiring a laparotomy or aspiration between 1989 and 1994 at all US Army medical centers and between 1992 and 1994 at all US Army community hospitals. Adnexal masses that resolved or those found in association with ectopic pregnancies were excluded.

Results.—Laparotomies were performed in 86 patients, and extirpation of the mass during cesarean section was performed in 43. One patient has ultrasonically guided aspiration of an ovarian cyst. The incidence of adnexal masses requiring surgery was 1 of 1312 live births. There were 8 malignancies (6.1%; 1/21,322 live births). Ten patients were found to have leiomyomas on laparotomy. There were 58 nulliparous women. The average age of women with malignant tumors was 29 years. US results were incapable of distinguishing masses with low malignant potential from benign neoplasms and were incapable of distinguishing leiomyomas. There was 1 neonatal and 2 intrauterine deaths but no spontaneous abortions. Patients who had laparotomies before 23 weeks' gestation had significantly fewer adverse outcomes than those who had laparotomies after 23 weeks' gestation (odds ratio, 0.15).

Conclusion.—Although the incidence of adnexal masses during pregnancy agrees with results of previous studies, the percentage of malignant tumors or tumors with malignant potential was more than twice as great as previously reported. US was incapable of distinguishing tumors of low malignant potential from benign masses and incapable of identifying the source of the mass in patients with leiomyomas. MRI should be considered for these patients.

▶ This is a multicenter report on the outcomes of 130 pregnant women who underwent laparotomy for diagnosis and treatment of adnexal masses or who were found to have incidental adnexal pathologic conditions at cesarean delivery. In this population, 6% of the adnexal masses evaluated were found to be either malignant or ovarian tumors of low malignant potential. The investigators found that surgeries performed earlier in gestation (< 23 weeks), were not likely to be associated with prematurity, whereas half of the surgeries performed in the third trimester were associated with premature delivery. Sonographic evaluation failed to identify tumors of low malignant potential or exclude leiomyomas. The authors would tend to agree with the accepted custom of operating on the pregnant woman with a persistent adnexal mass greater than 6 cm. MRI may be useful when the mass is thought to be a leiomyoma.

R. D. Arias, MD

Torsion of the Uterine Adnexa: Pathologic Correlations and Current Management Trends
Argenta PA, Yeagley TJ, Ott G, et al (Mount Sinai School of Medicine, New York; Univ of Pennsylvania, Philadelphia)
J Reprod Med 45:831-836, 2000   21–2

Introduction.—Torsion of the uterine adnexa is a rare condition, and in many patients an inaccurate diagnosis is made preoperatively. Cases of ovarian or adnexal torsion were reviewed to evaluate the clinical and pathologic correlates of specimens removed for the diagnosis of adnexal torsion and to examine trends in management of the condition.

Methods.—Cases were obtained from the records of 3 Philadelphia area hospitals for the period from January 1987 to March 1998. Those cases eligible for review had evidence of torsion of the ovary, tube, or entire adnexa at the time of definitive surgical evaluation. To assess the impact of increasing use of laparoscopy, surgical data were analyzed in 2 subsets: 1987 to 1992 and 1992 to 1998.

Results.—A preoperative or postoperative diagnosis of torsion was identified in 115 cases, 104 of which had surgically confirmed adnexal torsion. The median age of the patients was 32.5 years, and the median period from onset of symptoms to surgical diagnosis was 2 days. Most patients reported intermittent, lateralizing low abdominal pain of less than 2 weeks' duration and nausea. Adnexal torsion was included in the preoperative diagnosis in 38% of the patients. The most common conditions associated with adnexal torsion were previous abdominal surgery (35%) and concomitant pregnancy (16%); in 45% of patients, however, no risk factors were identified. Treatments varied from very conservative to very aggressive. Laparoscopy was employed initially in 47 patients, 28 of whom required conversion to laparotomy. In the earlier period (1987 to 1992), 62% of laparoscopies were converted, but only 38% were converted in more recent years (1992 to 1998). Neoplastic and functional tumors of the ovary accounted for more than 90% of diagnoses at microscopic evaluation, with cancer diagnosed in fewer than 1% of cases.

Conclusion.—Most cases of adnexal torsion are associated with a benign process. The more traditional treatment, salpingo-oophorectomy, is slowly being replaced by more conservative, adnexa-sparing procedures. A laparoscopic approach is recommended initially, because many cases of adnexal torsion can be managed with these procedures.

▶ Intermittent, lateralizing, lower abdominal pain and nausea in association with a pelvic mass should raise suspicion of adnexal torsion. Women in the early reproductive age group have the most to gain from early surgical intervention. In this group, the potential to salvage ovarian function, both reproductive and endocrinologic, is greatest. The risks associated with untwisting seem low. When cystectomy with ovarian preservation would otherwise be the preferred management, the additional finding of torsion should not necessarily lead the surgeon to adnexectomy. It is interesting to note that preoperative evaluation with Doppler US had a positive predictive value of only 37% in this series.

R. D. Arias, MD

Torsion of the Previously Normal Uterine Adnexa: Evaluation of the Correlation Between the Pathological Changes and the Clinical Characteristics
Chen M, Chen C-D, Yang Y-S (Natl Taiwan Univ, Taipei)
Acta Obstet Gynecol Scand 80:58-61, 2001   21–3

Introduction.—Adnexal torsion rarely involves ovarian cancer, but treatment remains a clinical dilemma when preservation of fertility is desired. A retrospective study was conducted to determine the feasibility of adnexal preservation in patients with torsion of a previously normal adnexa and to examine the correlation between severity of pathologic changes and clinical characteristics.

Methods.—A review of the charts of patients in whom adnexal torsion was diagnosed at the study institution between 1984 and 1998 yielded 70 cases, 69 of which had pathology reports. Data obtained included age, symptoms, duration of time from symptom onset to surgery, type of surgical procedure, operative findings, and complications. Thirteen of 69 patients had pathologic diagnoses of torsion of the previously normal adnexa. Pathologic slides from these 13 cases were examined for severity of changes: congestion and hemorrhage only, hemorrhagic necrosis, thrombus formation, and the presence of residual ovarian tissue.

Results.—Patients ranged in age from 10 to 44 years; duration of ischemia ranged from 6 hours to 288 hours. In all 13 patients, the affected adnexa was described as cyanotic and ischemic. Congestion and swelling caused the twisted adnexa to range from 4 cm to 15 cm in diameter. Pathologic findings were congestion, hemorrhage, and hemorrhagic necrosis of varying severity. Thrombus formation was identified in 2 patients with lengthy duration of torsion (48 and 288 hours) and in 1 patient with a shorter duration of torsion (18 hours). No residual ovarian cortex remained in all cases with prolonged ovarian or combined tubal and ovarian torsion (torsion duration, 48 hours or more).

Conclusion.—The likelihood of preserving normal ovarian tissue decreases as the time between symptoms onset and surgery increases. Local thrombus, however, correlated poorly with duration of torsion. Because the 13 patients included in the review had previously normal adnexa, torsion alone can lead to thrombus.

▶ Prompt surgical intervention in patients suspected of adnexal torsion improves the chances of preserving reproductive and endocrine function in the involved ovary. Duration of symptoms seems to be only a rough approximation of degree of torsion, but more than 48 hours of symptoms correlated with a greater amount of necrosis on pathologic evaluation. The importance of local thrombus formation (if any) remains obscure, and its presence was not predicted by increased duration of symptoms or number of twists. Fear of thrombosis should not prevent the surgeon from untwisting adnexa for either of these reasons.

R. D. Arias, MD

Endometrium

Effect of Adjuvant Tamoxifen on the Endometrium in Women With Breast Cancer: A Prospective Study Using Office Endometrial Biopsy
Barakat RR, Gilewski TA, Almadrones L, et al (Mem Sloan-Kettering Cancer Ctr, New York)
J Clin Oncol 18:3459-3463, 2000   21–4

Introduction.—The National Surgical Adjuvant Breast and Bowel Project, a randomized trial of tamoxifen versus placebo in women with estrogen-positive breast cancer confined to the breast with negative nodes showed a 7.5-fold increase in the risk for developing endometrial cancer in the tamoxifen-treated group. A case-controlled trial using surveillance, epidemiology, and end-result data reported a 4-fold increased risk of endometrial cancer in women with breast cancer with over 5 years of tamoxifen use compared with nonusers. The frequency of developing abnormal pathologic changes in the endometria was examined in tamoxifen-treated women to characterize the type of pathologic changes involved.

Methods.—Between October 1991 and September 1998, 159 patients starting tamoxifen therapy for breast cancer confined to the breast and axillary lymph nodes were enrolled in a prospective trial. Office endometrial biopsies (EMBs) were acquired at start of tamoxifen and at 6-month intervals for 2 years. Three subsequent annual EMBs were performed for each patient, amounting to a 5-year surveillance.

Results.—Median patient age was 50 years. Patients were able to be evaluated if EMBs were performed a minimum of 1 year after the start of tamoxifen treatment. There were 9 (5.7%) patients with protocol violations. There were 635 EMBs performed in 111 assessable patients (mean, 5.8 EMBs). Median surveillance time was 36 months. Eighty-two (12.9%) of 635 biopsy specimens yielded insufficient tissue for diagnosis. Fourteen patients (12.6%) underwent dilation and curettage (D&C) because of an abnormal EMB, persistent bleeding, or for examination of adnexal masses at the time of laparoscopy. The D&C findings included: 1 complex hyperplasia, 1 abnormal histiocytes, 2 simple hyperplasia, 4 polyps, 1 endocervical polyp, and 2 decidualization. Three of the D&Cs were negative. Hysterectomy was performed in 3 patients.

Conclusion.—The endometrial cavity was able to be evaluated with EMB in 95% of patients. The protocol led to an increase in the number of surgical procedures (14 patients required D&C). Because the annual risk of endometrial cancer is 2 per 1000 women, in this population and about 15% of these cancers result in patient's death, annual screening could potentially decrease mortality in only about 0.03% of all tamoxifen-treated patients.

▶ The reporting of a disproportionate number of endometrial cancers developing in women on the "antiestrogen" tamoxifen was a source of considerable alarm especially for our breast chemotherapy colleagues. Despite that most of the cancers reported were accompanied by bleeding and there was little evidence to support screening of asymptomatic patients for endometrial cancer, a study was undertaken. Many patients were biopsied but only 1 cancer was found. Thus, the recommendations of the American College of Obstetricians and Gynecologists of merely evaluating patients with symptoms are reaffirmed.

D. S. Miller, MD

Reference

1. American College of Obstetricians and Gynecologists: *Tamoxifen and endometrial cancer.* ACOG Committee Opinion #232. Washington, DC: ACOG; April 2000.

Quality of Life and Cost-Effectiveness of Levonorgestrel-Releasing Intrauterine System Versus Hysterectomy for Treatment of Menorrhagia: A Randomised Trial
Hurskainen R, Teperi J, Rissanen P, et al (Univ Hosp Helsinki; STAKES, Finland; Univ Hosps of Turku, Finland; et al)
Lancet 357:273-277, 2001   21–5

Introduction.—Hysterectomy has been the usual treatment for excessive menstrual blood loss, but medical treatment with the levonorgestrel-releasing intrauterine system (IUS) avoids the morbidity and risk of complications associated with surgery. Hysterectomy and IUS for menorrhagia were compared in terms of quality of life and cost-effectiveness.

Methods.—Study participants were referred to 5 university hospitals in Finland between November 1994 and November 1997. Eligible women ranged in age from 35 to 49 years, were menstruating, had completed their families, and were eligible for hysterectomy. From a total of 598 women screened, 228 were randomly selected and analyzed for the primary end point (116 assigned to levonorgestrel-releasing IUS and 112 to hysterectomy). The IUS releases 20 µg levonorgestrel over 24 hours for at least 5 years from a polydimethylsiloxane reservoir. Questionnaires were completed by patients and gynecologists at follow-up visits 6 and 12 months after treatment.

Results.—At 6 months, the IUS was in situ in 97 women (82%); in 10 the IUS was removed, and 9 underwent hysterectomy. At 12-month follow-up, the IUS was in situ in 81 (68%) women and 24 women (20%) had undergone hysterectomy. Among the women with the IUS in situ at 12 months, 41 (53%) reported amenorrhea or oligomenorrhea and 26 (32%) reported intermenstrual bleeding. Hysterectomy was performed vaginally in 30 patients, abdominally in 21, and laparoscopically in 56. The most common postoperative complications were wound infection (12), infected pelvic hematoma (6), and urinary retention (4). At 12-month follow-up, both IUS and hysterectomy groups showed significant improvement in health-related quality-of-life measures and in psychological well-being. Women who underwent hysterectomy had less pain than those treated with IUS. Both direct cost per woman and productivity losses (absence from work) per woman were significantly lower in the IUS group.

Conclusion.—Both hysterectomy and IUS significantly improve health-related quality of life in women with menorrhagia. Hysterectomy is more expensive, but the treatment effect is permanent and there is less pain than with IUS.

▶ There are many potential uses for a long-acting progestin-releasing intrauterine device. While providing effective, reversible contraception, it offers the potential advantage of decreasing menstrual blood loss as well as dysfunctional uterine bleeding. For women in the perimenopause, a potent local uterine progestin might permit the use of unopposed systemic estrogen or a specific estrogen receptor modulator, while reducing the risk of endometrial hyperplasia. These women might also be expected to have a better chance for an amenorrheic transition to menopause despite fluctuating gonadotropins and serum estrogens. The treatment of menorrhagia with the levonorgestrel-releasing IUS was compared with hysterectomy in this study. It would appear to offer an acceptable alternative for many women.

R. D. Arias, MD

Gestational Trophoblastic Disease

Gestational Trophoblastic Disease: A Study of Mode of Evacuation and Subsequent Need for Treatment With Chemotherapy

Tidy JA, Gillespie AM, Bright N, et al (Univ of Sheffield, England; Weston Park Hosp, Sheffield, England)
Gynecol Oncol 78:309-312, 2000

21–6

Introduction.—Many gynecologists now use pharmacologic methods to evacuate the uterus for pregnancy termination and management of early pregnancy loss. The optimal method of uterine evacuation for gestational trophoblastic disease (GTD) is uncertain, and an association between medical methods to evacuate a molar pregnancy and an increased need for chemotherapy has been reported. The question of whether the mode of evacuation influenced the subsequent need for chemotherapy in patients with GTD was investigated in a retrospective study.

Methods.—The United Kingdom has a national screening program for GTD. All cases are registered at 3 centers, one of which is Weston Park Hospital in Sheffield. A review of registration and case note records from Weston Park Hospital for 1986 to 1996 yielded 4257 cases of GTD. The method of uterine evacuation was classified as spontaneous, suction curettage, sharp curettage, medical, or other (hysterotomy, hysterectomy, other, and unknown). Evacuation methods were analyzed for 2 periods (1986-1989 and 1990-1996) to identify changes in practice over time.

Results.—During the period of review, suction curettage was used as the primary mode of evacuation. The rates of spontaneous evacuation, sharp curettage, and medical evacuation all decreased. A total of 231 women (5.4% of those registered) required chemotherapy for persistent GTD. The mode of evacuation was significant in determining the subsequent need for chemotherapy (Table 2). Women who underwent medical evacuation more frequently required chemotherapy (women managed by hysterectomy were excluded from the analysis because GTD was generally atypical). Of

TABLE 2.—Mode of Evacuation and Need for Chemotherapy

Mode of Evacuation	Cases Registered	Cases Treated	Cases Treated (Percentage of Cases Registered)
Spontaneous	129	3	2.3
Suction curettage	2886	169	5.9
Sharp curettage	1100	42	3.8
Medical evacuation	77	7	9.1
Hysterotomy	2	0	0
Hysterectomy	13	5	38.5
Other	40	4	10
Unknown	10	1	10
Total	4257	231	5.4

(Courtesy of Tidy JA, Gillespie AM, Bright N, et al: Gestational trophoblastic disease: A study of mode of evacuation and subsequent need for treatment with chemotherapy. *Gynecol Oncol* 78:309-312, 2000.)

the 77 women who underwent medical evacuation (usually with prostaglandin), 20 (26%) subsequently required further evacuation of the uterus.

Conclusion.—Suction curettage is a safe and increasingly employed method of uterine evacuation in GTD. The use of medical methods of uterine evacuation has increased rates of incomplete evacuation and of the need for treatment with chemotherapy.

▶ With the advances in the pharmacopeia (ie, misoprostol, mifepristone) available for the elective or indicated termination of pregnancy or induction of labor, it is appropriate to revisit past experience to consider the potential role for these therapies in treatment of hydatidiform mole. The nonsurgical evacuation of hydatidiform mole may be an appealing concept. However, past experience has shown that these methods are associated with a higher risk of developing gestational trophoblastic tumor and requiring treatment with chemotherapy, presumably caused by the deportation of trophoblastic cells from uterine contractions. This was the authors' experience, where 26% of the patients undergoing medical evacuation required a subsequent surgical procedure with 9% requiring chemotherapy, nearly twice the rate seen in patients treated by curettage only. Hysterectomy, which in other studies has been shown to be the most effective treatment of hydatidiform mole, was only occasionally used for atypical cases, of which 38% required chemotherapy.

D. S. Miller, MD

Choriocarcinoma and Partial Hydatidiform Moles

Seckl MJ, Fisher RA, Salerno G, et al (Imperial College, London)
Lancet 356:36-39, 2000   21–7

Objective.—Although complete hydatidiform moles (CMs) occur in 1 of 1000 pregnancies and partial hydatidiform moles (PMs) occur in 3 of 1000 pregnancies, the risk of development of gestational trophoblastic tumor (GTT) is 15% for a CM and 0.5% for a PM. Gestational choriocarcinoma has occurred after as many as 3% of CMs but has never been proved to occur after a PM. Because of the relative rarity of subsequent GTT, some have advocated discontinuing human chorionic gonadotropin (hCG) follow-up. If PMs can transform, such discontinuation could risk lives. Whether PMs can transform into choriocarcinomas was reviewed.

Methods.—A search of the Charing Cross Hospital gestational trophoblastic disease database identified 5 of 15 patients with PMs who subsequently were given diagnoses of choriocarcinoma. Flow cytometry was performed on formalin-fixed paraffin-embedded tissue. DNA was prepared from 2 patients and their partners and amplified using polymerase chain reaction to identify microsatellite polymorphisms.

Case 1.—Woman, 27, with vaginal bleeding after 7 weeks of amenorrhea, had a positive pregnancy but no viable fetus. She had a dilatation and curettage (D&C), began to take oral contraceptives, but was admitted 7 months later for bleeding. She had 2 more D&Cs but continued to bleed. The fourth D&C revealed trophoblastic hyperplasia. She had an acute abdomen and a bulky, bleeding, and perforated uterus. She had a hysterectomy, and tumor deposits were seen on the bladder and pelvic side wall. She had lung metastases but no CNS disease. She received chemotherapy. Her first D&C showed a triploid PM on reexamination. Subsequent D&Cs revealed choriocarcinoma that contained a single maternal and 2 paternal alleles at several independent loci. The PM also contained those alleles.

Cases 2 and 3.—Two women, with first trimester bleeding, had molar pregnancies, which were terminated and identified as PMs. The second patient had bleeding several months later and was given a diagnosis of choriocarcinoma. Both patients had chemotherapy. Both had PMs and choriocarcinomas that were triploid and had 1 maternal and 2 paternal contributions.

Conclusion.—The risk that a PM will develop into choriocarcinoma is at least 20% in patients with PM who develop GTT.

▶ Since PMs were described in 1978, it has been assumed that this entity only rarely persisted after evacuation to manifest as GTT. Histologically, these were almost all invasive moles, and choriocarcinoma was not thought to develop. The group from Charing Cross and Hammersmith Hospitals in London, England have confronted this assumption with this early report. Although only 0.5% of PMs followed by the authors' center developed into GTTs, 20% of those were identified histologically as choriocarcinoma. Thus, patients who have posttrophoblastic tumors after a PM should receive careful staging of their tumors.

D. S. Miller, MD

22 Cervical Disease

Cost Effective Screening

Setting the Target for a Better Cervical Screening Test: Characteristics of a Cost-Effective Test for Cervical Neoplasia Screening
Myers ER, McCrory DC, Subramanian S, et al (Duke Univ, Durham, NC; Health Economics Research Inc, Boston)
Obstet Gynecol 96:645-652, 2000

22–1

Background.—One of the most common malignant conditions in women is carcinoma of the cervix. As a result of improved screening, there has been a steady decline in both the incidence and mortality rate associated with cervical carcinoma in the United States. Reduction of 43% in incidence and 46% in mortality rate from 1973 to 1995 has been achieved in the United States, but reductions of this magnitude have not occurred in countries in which cytologic screening is not widely available. In recent years, several adjunctive technologies for reduction of the incidence of false-negative results of conventional smears have been approved by the US Food and Drug Administration. In recent studies, it has been found that the cost effectiveness of these technologies is directly related to the frequency of screening. The potential effects on costs and outcomes of changes in sensitivity and specificity with new screening methods for cervical cancer were evaluated.

Methods.—The effects of sensitivity, specificity, and screening frequency on cost effectiveness of screening methods were estimated with a Markov model of the natural history of cervical cancer. A meta-analysis was used to obtain estimates of conventional Papanicolau test sensitivity of 51% and specificity of 97%. For this test the clinicians estimated the effect of reducing false-negative rates from 40% to 90% and increasing false-positive rates by up to 20%, both independently and jointly. The marginal cost of improving sensitivity varied from $0 to $15.

Results.—Life expectancy and costs were increased when specificity was held constant and sensitivity of the Papanicolau test was increased. When sensitivity was held constant, decreasing specificity resulted in increased costs for Papanicolau tests; this effect was more dramatic at more frequent intervals. There was a significant effect of decreased specificity on the cost effectiveness of improved sensitivity on Papanicolau tests. Most of these effects were found to be related to the cost of evaluation and treatment of low-grade lesions.

Conclusions.—Overall costs were increased with the use of policies or technologies that increased the sensitivity of cervical cytologic screening, even when the cost of the technology was identical to the cost of conventional Papanicolau tests. The relatively high prevalence of low-grade lesions would appear to be the cause of these effects, which were magnified at increasing screening intervals. Methods that provide increased ability for the detection of lesions that are most likely to become cancerous are needed to improve the efficiency of screening for cervical cancer.

▶ Following the approval by the Food and Drug Administration of several new technologies related to cervical cancer screening (PAPNET, AUTOPAP, and THINPREP), the American College of Obstetricians and Gynecologists commissioned the Agency for Health Care Policy and Research to conduct an evidence-based review of cervical cytology.[1] That meta-analysis showed that conventional Papanicolaou test screening had a sensitivity of 51% (not 80% as has traditionally been taught) and a specificity of 97%. These new technologies have been shown to increase sensitivity but have minimal impact on specificity. Thus, these new, more sensitive technologies will be cost effective compared with conventional Papanicolaou smear screening only if they are associated with improved specificity, permit decreased screening frequency, or allow use of less expensive treatments for low-grade abnormalities. Increased test sensitivity alone is not sufficient to allow wholesale abandonment of the traditional Papanicolaou smear.

D. S. Miller, MD

Reference

1. McCrory D, Matchar DB, Bastian L, et al: Evaluation of cervical cytology. Evidence report/technology assessment no. 5. AHCPR publication no 99-E010. Rockville, (MD): Agency for Health Care Policy and Research, 1999.

Impact of Increasing Papanicolaou Test Sensitivity and Compliance: A Modeled Cost and Outcome Analysis

Montz FJ, Farber FL, Bristow RE, et al (John Hopkins Hosp, Baltimore, Md)
Obstet Gynecol 97:781-788, 2001   22–2

Introduction.—Widespread use of the Papanicolaou smear for cervical cancer screening has led to a significant reduction in the incidence of and mortality rate from the disease. However, in certain subpopulations, including black and Hispanic women, incidence rates of cervical cancer continue to be high. Black women have increased their compliance with regular Papanicolaou smear screening, but their incidence and mortality rates of cervical cancer remain elevated. Liquid-based cytology, recently approved by the US Food and Drug Administration, is reported to lower the false-negative rate compared with the traditional Papanicolaou smear.

A theoretical model was used to determine the cost-effectiveness of liquid-based cytology.

Methods.—An adaptation of a time-varying Markov model was used to follow a theoretic cohort of 100,000 women from ages 20 through 80. Three specific and different populations were evaluated: all women, white women, and black women. Separate analyses were performed with the use of 3 compliance rates (self-reported, Healthy People 2000, and Healthy People 2010) and 2 Papanicolaou test sensitivities (conventional smear and liquid-based cytology). The baseline value for false-negative rates was estimated to be 49% for the conventional smear and 27% for liquid-based cytology.

Results.—With current compliance patterns, use of a liquid-based cytology test could reduce cervical cancer incidence by approximately 32% for all subpopulations. Increasing compliance to Healthy People 2001 goals resulted in 23%, 21.7%, and 17% reductions in cervical cancer incidence for all women, white women, and black women, respectively. Liquid-based cytology would be cost effective if implemented in any of the 3 populations, and the cost-effectiveness ratio improves as the risk profile of the screened population increases. With liquid-based cytology yielding a 20% false-negative rate (a 60% improvement over the conventional Papanicolaou smear), the cost-effectiveness ratio is less than $20,000 per life year saved for all populations and less than $10,000 per life year saved for black women.

Conclusion.—Liquid-based cytology for detection of cervical cancer would be cost-effective in improving outcomes in all populations studied. This new technology may represent the most cost-effective approach in high-risk populations, including elderly women whose risk is high and whose compliance with screening guidelines is low.

▶ Most of the advances in cervical cancer screening technology come with a price, usually an increased price. The concern is that the diversion of resources required to implement the new technology will result in fewer patients being screened. This computer modeling study reports that the use of liquid-based cytology techniques should result in a greater reduction in cervical cancer incidence than improving screening compliance with a traditional Papanicolaou smear to the goals set by the Healthy People 2000 project. The projected cost per year of life saved was well below the $50,000 "cost-effective" threshold. However, does a Thin Prep really cost $19.50? And have black women really already achieved the screening goals of the Healthy People 2000 project?

D. S. Miller, MD

HPV Testing

Is Human Papillomavirus Testing of Value in Clinical Practice?
Kaufman RH, Adam E (Baylor College of Medicine, Houston)
Am J Obstet Gynecol 180:1049-1053, 1999

22–3

Objective.—Because high-risk human papilloma virus (HPV) has been implicated in the development of cervical intraepithelial and invasive carcinomas, screening infected patients might be a useful way to identify those most likely to have a high-grade lesion (grade 2 or 3 cervical intraepithelial neoplasia [CIN]) or invasive carcinoma. However, in the classification of Papanicolaou smears, atypical squamous cells of undetermined significance (ASCUS) have been variously interpreted by cytopathologists so that the reported frequency of ASCUS is highly variable. Results of a review of cytology studies, as well as the current opinion of the authors relative to the value of HPV testing in clinical practice, are discussed.

Discussion.—In a population with a high prevalence of infection, many may not have and never will have CIN. Therefore, a test that improves detection by 10% to 15% does not provide a meaningful improvement. Most women with ASCUS findings will not have significant disease of the cervix. However, because the frequency of low- and high-grade CIN may be as high as 40% when the incidence of grade 2 or 3 10% or greater, a finding of ASCUS cannot be ignored. With the HPV file and Hybrid Capture tests, the sensitivity for detecting grade 2 or 3 CIN varied from 56% to 93%, had a positive predictive value ranging from 17% to 28%, and had a specificity varying between 24.2% and 66.8%. With use of the polymerase chain reaction, the results were 48% to 95%, 22% to 93%, and 40% to 95% for sensitivity, positive predictive value, and specificity, respectively.

Conclusion.—Current HPV testing methods are of little clinical value in detecting high-grade lesions or invasive cervical carcinoma.

▶ The quest has intensified to improve the accuracy of traditional methods for screening for cervical disease. The refinement of our ability to identify ever-smaller fragments of nuclear material has led to a search for clinical applications. The prospect of improving the current methods of screening for cervical disease is certainly laudable, but, as this article suggests, the goal remains elusive. Finite resources demand prudence before the wholesale adoption of promising, but unproven, techniques.

R. D. Arias, MD

Comparison of Self-Collected Vaginal, Vulvar and Urine Samples With Physician-Collected Cervical Samples for Human Papillomavirus Testing to Detect High-Grade Squamous Intraepithelial Lesions

Sellors JW, Lorincz AT, Mahony JB, et al (St Joseph's Hosp, Hamilton, Ontario; McMaster Univ, Hamilton; Digene Corp, Silver Spring, Md; et al)
Can Med Assoc J 163:513-518, 2000   22–4

Background.—The development of squamous intraepithelial lesions (SIL) and invasive cervical carcinoma have been strongly correlated with certain types of human papillomavirus (HPV) in cervical samples. The test characteristics of HPV assessment were determined with samples obtained by both patients and their physicians.

Methods.—Women referred to a colposcopy clinic because of cervical cytologic screening abnormalities were studied. Two hundred women collected vulvar, vaginal, and urine samples for HPV testing. The physician then obtained cervical samples for HPV testing. Colposcopy was performed, with biopsy as indicated.

Findings.—Twenty-nine percent of the women had high-grade SIL. In this group, carcinogenic types of HPV were detected in 86% of the self-collected vaginal samples, in 62% of the self-collected vulvar samples, and in 45% of the self-collected urine samples. Carcinogenic types of HPV were found in 98% of the cervical samples obtained by physicians. The sensitivity of self-collected samples ranged from 45% to 86%, and the specificity ranged from 53% to 70%. Physician-collected samples had a sensitivity and specificity of 98% and 52%, respectively.

Conclusions.—Self-collection of samples for HPV testing warrants further evaluation as a possible screening test for cervical cancer prevention programs. Most women in the series found the self-collection of urine, vulvar, and vaginal samples to be acceptable.

▶ Cytology-based screening programs to prevent deaths caused by cervical cancer have been very successful in most developed countries. Their application in developing countries has been more problematic because the need for laboratory facilities and trained cytotechnologists and cytopathologists is difficult to meet in resource-poor areas. Thus, a test that requires fewer resources and less technology to support it may be feasible. The ideal scenario for this would be patient-collected specimens that could be analyzed by resource-minimal methodology but would reliably identify women who would benefit from intervention. Other studies have shown that patient-collected samples can be gathered in resource-poor areas.[1] This study showed the validity of the test in a colposcopy clinic population where most of the patients' results were confirmed by biopsy. The sensitivity of the test was good. However, the positive predictive value left something to be desired in that the test generated at least 1 false-positive result for each true-positive in all types of specimens collected.

D. S. Miller, MD

Reference

1. Wright TC, Denny L, Kuhn L, et al: HPV DNA testing of self-collected vaginal samples compared with cytologic screening to detect cervical cancer. *JAMA* 283:81-86, 2000.

Evaluation of a Human Papillomavirus Assay in Cervical Screening in Zimbabwe

Womack SD, Chirenje ZM, Blumenthal PD, et al (Johns Hopkins School of Hygiene and Public Health, Baltimore, Md; Univ of Zimbabwe, Harare; Johns Hopkins School of Medicine, Baltimore, Md; et al)
Br J Obstet Gynaecol 107:33-38, 2000   22–5

Objective.—The highest rates of cervical cancer are in developing countries, and the lowest rates are in industrialized countries. Because certain types of human papillomavirus (HPV) are linked to invasive cervical cancer, an HPV assay may be useful as a screening method. An HPV assay for primary cervical screening was evaluated in Zimbabwe, where the cervical cancer incidence between 1990 and 1992 was as high as 47.6/100,000.

Methods.—Women (n = 2206), aged 25 to 55 years, attending primary care clinics in 2 areas of Zimbabwe, were screened by cytologic examination, visual inspection with acetic acid, and colposcopy. Complete data were available for 2140 women. Genital tract specimens were sent to Baltimore, Md, and tested by using a second-generation microtiter Hybrid Capture II (HC II) assay. Women with abnormal colposcopy results underwent biopsy. There were 150 biopsy-proven high-grade squamous intraepithelial lesions and 213 cases of biopsy-proven low-grade lesions.

Results.—Final results showed 73.8% normal results, 16.2% low-grade lesions, and 10% high-grade lesions. The HPV prevalence increased with disease severity. HIV prevalence was 42.7%, which decreased significantly from 48.5% in women aged 25 to 34 years to 25.6% in women aged 45 to 56 years. The sensitivity and specificity for screening high-grade lesions were 81% and 62%, respectively. Sensitivity and specificity estimates were similar for HC II and visual inspection. Biopsy-proven diagnoses were obtained for 70% with high-grade lesions and for 62% with low-grade lesions. The prevalence of HPV was 35% in women with normal results, primarily because of concurrent HIV infection. In women with HIV antibody data (23%), more than half were HIV-seropositive. The HPV prevalence decreased with age.

Conclusion.—Because of its low specificity, the HC II assay at a cutoff value of 1 pg/mL is not a suitable screening test for HPV infection.

▶ Although cytology-based cervical cancer screening programs have been very successful in western industrialized countries, this has not been the case in developing countries because of lack of cytology facilities, colposcopists, and resources. Cervical cancer remains the most common cancer in women in many developing countries. Screening strategies that require less technology, less personnel, and less resources might be capable of having an effect on this problem. Because many intraepithelial neoplasia lesions of the cervix will eventually clear without treatment, a better marker for lesions likely to progress to cancer is needed. Some believe that the HC II HPV assay may be such a test. This study was conducted in a high-prevalence population in Zimbabwe and included cytologic examination and colposcopy of all patients. There was a good correlation between high-risk HPV prevalence and high-grade intraepithelial lesions, which also correlated with viral load. Unfortunately, the positive predictive value was low: 19% for high-grade lesions and 39% for low-grade lesions. These results are confounded by the fact that more than half of the patients tested were also HIV positive, clearly a more grim public health problem in that part of the world.

D. S. Miller, MD

Comparison of Three Management Strategies for Patients With Atypical Squamous Cells of Undetermined Significance: Baseline Results From a Randomized Trial

Solomon D, for the ALTS Group (Natl Cancer Inst, Bethesda, Md)
J Natl Cancer Inst 93:293-299, 2001   22–6

Background.—More than 5% of an estimated 50 million Papanicolaou tests performed annually in the United States have abnormal findings, and more than 2 million women receive an equivocal cervical cytologic diagnosis (atypical squamous cells of undetermined significance [ASCUS]) each year. Identification of the minority of women with clinically significant disease while avoiding excessive follow-up evaluation of other women is dependent on the development of effective colposcopy triage strategies. The results of the ASCUS/LSIL (low-grade squamous intraepithelial lesion) Triage Study (ALTS) are presented. The ALTS was conducted as a randomized, multicenter clinical trial of the management of women with low-grade and equivocal cervical cytologic abnormalities.

Methods.—The ALTS compared the sensitivity and specificity of 3 management strategies for the detection of cervical intraepithelial neoplasia grade 3 (CIN3): immediate colposcopy (considered to be the reference standard), triage to colposcopy based on human papillomavirus (HPV) results from Hybrid Capture 2 (HC 2) and thin-layer cytologic results, or triage based solely on cytologic results. The cross-sectional enrollment results for 3488 women with referral diagnoses of ASCUS were presented.

Results.—The underlying prevalence of histologically confirmed CINIII was 5%. The sensitivity for detection of CINIII or above by testing for cancer-associated HPV DNA was 96%; 56% of women were referred for colposcopy. The sensitivity of a single repeated cytologic evaluation with a triage threshold of high-grade SIL or above was found to be 44%; 7% of patients were referred for colposcopy. The sensitivity of a lower cytologic triage threshold of ASCUS or above was 85%; 59% of patients were referred for colposcopy.

Conclusions.—These findings indicate that HC 2 testing for cancer-associated HPV DNA can be useful in the management of women with diagnoses of ASCUS. HC 2 was found to have greater sensitivity for the detection of CIN3 or above, and its specificity was comparable to a single additional cytologic test indicative of ASCUS or above.

▶ In spite of the stunning success of Papanicolaou test screening in decreasing the incidence of and deaths caused by cervical cancer in the United States over the last 50 years, it was believed by some that there was a problem with Papanicolaou test nomenclature. In 1988, the National Cancer Institute convened a group of cytologists and a few gynecologists who proposed the Bethesda System, a previously untested, much less validated classification system. They presented a new management dilemma to gynecologists: ASCUS. Fortunately, most Papanicolaou tests with ASCUS findings do not indicate a premalignant cervical problem because only 5% to 15% will be CINIII or worse. However, 10% to 40% of CINIII diagnoses are preceded by a finding of ASCUS on Papanicolaou testing. Obviously, the cost of performing colposcopy on the 2 million women whose Papanicolaou test findings will return as ASCUS is cost prohibitive. A preliminary management strategy was suggested.[1] To help us deal with this new dilemma, another test was introduced—one that detects high-risk HPV, the HC 2 (Digene). A large randomized trial was undertaken. The ALTS trial has been completed, and the results are beginning to emerge. A modification of one of the previously recommended strategies, Papanicolaou test follow-up, was one of the experimental arms in this study.[1] Using HC 2 to trigger subsequent colposcopy was more sensitive and specific for detecting CIN3 or worse than was a follow-up Papanicolaou test with a finding of high-grade SIL. However, HC 2 was only subtly better than was a follow-up Papanicolaou test with a finding of ASCUS or worse as the colposcopy indicator. Several more important issues remain to be addressed, including cost-effectiveness and the role of the subclassification of ASCUS (ie, reparative vs favoring dysplasia) in the treatment algorithms.

D. S. Miller, MD

Reference

1. Kurman RJ, Henson DE, Herbst AL, et al: Interim guidelines for management of abnormal cervical cytology. The 1992 National Cancer Institute Workshop. *JAMA* 271:1866-1869, 1994.

When to Screen

Frequency of Cervical Smear Abnormalities Within 3 Years of Normal Cytology

Sawaya GF, Kerlikowske K, Lee NC, et al (Univ of California, San Francisco; Veterans Affairs Med Ctr, San Francisco; Ctrs for Disease Control and Prevention, Atlanta, Ga)
Obstet Gynecol 96:219-223, 2000
22–7

Introduction.—Most of the findings from nearly 50 million Papanicolaou tests performed annually in the United States are normal. Cervical screening outcomes associated with age and 3 screening intervals (1, 2, and 3 years) were prospectively examined in 128,805 females screened in community-based clinics throughout the United States within 3 years of normal test results through the National Breast and Cervical Cancer Early Detection Program.

Methods.—Participants had findings from their first Papanicolaou tests reported as normal between 1991 and 1998 and at least 1 additional subsequent test within the next 36 months. Females with second tests that showed glandular cell abnormalities were excluded. Tests read as high-grade squamous intraepithelial lesions (SIL) and suggestive of squamous cell cancer were considered high-grade SIL or worse.

Results.—The average age of the rescreened cohort was 48.9 years (range, 12-96 years). The mean time to a second test was 15.7 months (range, 9-36 months). Most second test results (94.1%) were either normal or interpreted as infections, inflammations, or reactive changes. More than 40% of the cohort was not white. The highest incidence of cytologic abnormalities was among females younger than 30 years. With increasing age, the incidence of atypical squamous cells of undetermined significance, low-grade SIL, and high-grade SIL or worse diminished markedly ($P <$ .001 for each category). Age-adjusted incidence rates of high-grade SIL or worse were similar among females screened at 9 to 12 months, 13 to 24 months, and 25 to 36 months (25, 29, and 33 of 10,000, respectively; $P =$ .46) after normal test results. The age-adjusted incidence rates of atypical squamous cells of undetermined significance were unchanged ($P =$ .36). The incidence of tests interpreted as low-grade SIL rose as time from the normal test result increased ($P =$ .01).

Conclusion.—Within 3 years after normal cytologic results, cervical smear results interpreted as high-grade SIL or worse were rare. The incidence rate was unrelated to the time since the last normal cervical smear result. Optimal screening strategies for females with recent normal cytologic findings need to be based on comprehensive modeling trials that incorporate the true risks and benefits of repetitive screening.

▶ As recommended by the American College of Obstetricians and Gynecologists, the standard of care for the frequency of Papanicolaou test screening for most women has been annually.[1] Other organizations, including the American Cancer Society and the US Preventive Services Task Force, have suggested that longer intervals may be allowed.[2,3] The data to support this more relaxed guideline are derived and certainly not supported by any randomized controlled trials. This study used data from the National Breast and Cervical Cancer Early Detection Program. It may provide reassurance to gynecologists that longer intervals between Papanicolaou tests are safe, in that age-adjusted incidence rates for high-grade SIL or worse are similar for women screened 9 to 36 months after a previous normal cytologic result. Follow-up of this study as well as further studies will be required because only 20% of the patients screened returned and were eligible, and intervals longer than 36 months were not evaluated.

D. S. Miller, MD

References

1. American College of Obstetricians and Gynecologists: *Routine Cancer Screening. ACOG Committee Opinion No. 185.* Washington, DC, American College of Obstetricians and Gynecologists, 1997.
2. Smith RA, Von Eschenbach AC, Wender R, et al: American Cancer Society guidelines for the early detection of cancer: Update of early detection guidelines for prostate, colorectal, and endometrial cancers. *CA Cancer J Clin* 51:38-75, 2001.
3. US Preventive Services Task Force: Guide to clinical preventive services: An assessment of the effectiveness of 169 interventions, in *Report of the U.S. Preventive Services Task Force.* Baltimore, Md, Williams & Wilkins, 1996.

The Positive Predictive Value of Cervical Smears in Previously Screened Postmenopausal Women: The Heart and Estrogen/Progestin Replacement Study (HERS)
Sawaya GF, for the Heart and Estrogen/Progestin Replacement Study (HERS) Research Group (Univ of California, San Francisco; et al)
Ann Intern Med 133:942-950, 2000   22–8

Introduction.—The use of topical estrogen creams in postmenopausal women with atypical squamous cells of undetermined significance (ASCUS) is supported in a report from the National Cancer Institute. Up to 3.5% of all cervical smears show ASCUS, and over 70% of cytological abnormalities in women over age 50 years are caused by ASCUS. Women over 55 years of age are 3 times more likely than their younger counterparts to use hormone replacement therapy. The independent effect of hormone replacement therapy on the development of cytologic abnormalities is not known.

The positive predictive value of cervical smears in previously screened postmenopausal women was examined. The effect of oral estrogen plus progestin on incident cervical cytologic abnormalities was examined in a prospective cohort trial (incidence) and multicenter, randomized, double-blind, placebo-controlled trial (hormone therapy).

Methods.—A total of 2561 women with a uterus, normal cytologic characteristics at baseline, and coronary artery disease were randomly assigned to treatment with either oral conjugated equine estrogens, 0.625 mg/d, plus medroxyprogesterone acetate, 2.5 mg/d, or placebo. Smears performed in the first 2 years of the 4-year trial were assessed to allow at least 2 years for a final diagnosis to be determined. The most important histologic outcomes were high-grade cervical intraepithelial neoplasia (grades II to III) and invasive cervical cancer. This Heart and Estrogen/progestin Replacement Study was designed and performed by co-investigators and was funded by Wyeth-Ayerst Research.

Results.—The mean age of the subjects was 66.7 years. Patients were followed for an average of 4.1 years. Most abnormalities were reported as ASCUS (21.0%). Repeated smears were the most frequent initial procedure performed in women with ASCUS (92%) and atypical glandular cells of undetermined significance (65%). The incidence of new cytologic abnormalities in the 2 years after a normal smear was 110 per 4895 person-years (23 per 1000 person-years [95% confidence interval, 18-27 per 1000 person-years]).

Results of most final diagnoses (94 of 110 or 85%) were normal. The positive predictive value of any smear abnormality observed 1 year after a normal smear was 0%; for 2 years, it was 0.9%. In hormone-treated versus non–hormone treated women, the incidence of cytologic abnormalities was nonsignificantly higher, mostly because of a nonsignificant 58% greater incidence of ASCUS.

Women who had 5 or more offspring were at a higher risk for all cytologic abnormalities (relative risk, 1.56; confidence interval, 1.02-2.37). The mean patient age at first intercourse was 20.1 years; 38% reported first intercourse before age 18 years. Nearly half had been sexually active within the past 5 years; 31% had been sexually active within the past year, and 3% reported having a new male partner within the past 5 years.

Conclusion.—Because of poor predictive value, cervical smears should not be performed within 2 years of normal cytologic results in postmenopausal women. These findings are generalized to postmenopausal women with a cervix who have had a recent normal cervical smear and should not be applied to postmenopausal women who have never been screened or those who have not been screened recently.

▶ This study provides support for the recommendation of the US Preventive Services Task Force for decreasing or eliminating Papanicolaou smears in previously well-screened but now postmenopausal women, especially in view of the 1% positive predictive value of an abnormal smear reported. However, the nature of the population in the HERS trial may preclude the generalization of its conclusions since these were patients with established coronary artery disease whose medical problems may have limited their interest and/or ability in acquiring new partners and/or risk factors, in that only 31% had been sexually active within the past year, and only 3% had had a new male partner within the past 5 years. Since the average age of these patients was 67 years, the results are likely more generalizable to a geriatric, as opposed to a postmenopausal, population.

D. S. Miller, MD

Reference

1. Guide to Clinical Preventive Services: Report of the US Preventive Services Task Force, ed 2. Baltimore, Williams & Wilkins, 1996.

Routine Vaginal Cuff Smear Testing in Post-Hysterectomy Patients With Benign Uterine Conditions: When Is It Indicated?

Videlefsky A, Grossl N, Denniston M, et al (Emory Univ, Atlanta, Ga; Grady Mem Hosp, Atlanta, Ga; St Marks Hosp, Salt Lake City, Utah; et al)
J Am Board Fam Pract 13:233-238, 2000   22–9

Background.—About 85% of hysterectomies in American women are done for benign disease. The cytologic findings from vaginal cuff smears in women undergoing hysterectomy for benign conditions were reported.

Methods.—Two hundred twenty randomly selected women with 1 or more vaginal cuff smears were studied. All had undergone hysterectomy for benign uterine disease and were followed up for a mean of 89 months.

Findings.—Ninety-seven percent had no cytologic abnormalities on vaginal cuff smears. No invasive carcinomas were identified cytologically. Three percent of the patients had dysplastic lesions. Seventy percent had 1 or more infections, including bacterial vaginosis, trichomoniasis, candidiasis, koilocytosis suggesting human papillomavirus, and cytopathic effects of herpes. Patients with dysplasia had a much higher prevalence of koilocytosis.

Conclusion.—Most routine vaginal cuff cytology screening testing appears to be unnecessary for women undergoing hysterectomy for benign disease. These data are consistent with previous reports concluding that such testing is not needed in this patient population.

▶ There are few data regarding the utility of posthysterectomy vaginal cuff smears. The American College of Obstetricians and Gynecologists, in its Committee Opinion No. 152, nonetheless recommends periodic cytologic evaluation when risk factors for dysplasia exist.[1] The interval between such tests is not specified. In this observational study of 220 women and 1211 vaginal cuff smears, 2 women were found to have severe vaginal dysplasia. In 1 of these, dysplasia developed 26 months after hysterectomy for leiomyoma; the patient had a previously normal pap smear. The other woman had preexisting cervical dysplasia. When the high-risk nature of this population is considered, these results are especially reassuring. Certainly the low-risk woman who has a hysterectomy for benign reasons can be counseled that pap smears are not required if her examination is normal.

R. D. Arias, MD

Reference

1. ACOG Committee on Gynecologic Practice "Recommendations on Frequency of Pap Test Screening," Committee Opinion Number 152, March 1995.

Glandular Lesions

Clinical Evaluation of Atypical Glandular Cells of Undetermined Significance

Geier CS, Wilson M, Creasman W (Med Univ of South Carolina, Charleston)
Am J Obstet Gynecol 184:64-69, 2001   22–10

Introduction.—The only atypical glandular cells of undetermined significance (AGUS) guidelines published to date are the recent recommendations of the American Society of Colposcopy and Cervical Pathology. These guidelines advocate cervical and vaginal colposcopy and endocervical curettage. The clinical importance of AGUS was examined retrospectively, along with risk factors for serious pathologic conditions.

Methods.—A computerized database was used to identify all females with cervical cytologic specimens with a cytologic diagnosis of AGUS who were seen between January 1992 and June 1997. Medical records were reviewed for patient demographic characteristics and for determination of the presence or absence of associated pathologic conditions of the cervix and endometrium.

Results.—A total of 492 patients had cytologic results reported as AGUS. For 224 patients, AGUS was the only cytologic diagnosis. Two hundred and sixty-eight patients had both AGUS and an additional squamous abnormality, including atypical squamous cells of undetermined significance and cervical intraepithelial neoplasia I, II, or III. Two patients were excluded because of histories of endometrial cancer. A histologic examination was obtained within 1 year in 353 patients. Among these 353 patients who underwent histologic examination, 227 (64%) had benign cervical and endometrial findings. Eighteen glandular lesions (5%) were identified, including complex hyperplasia with atypia, adenocarcinoma in situ of the cervix, and adenocarcinoma of the endometrium. A squamous lesion was observed in 108 patients (31%). Most squamous lesions (81%) were identified in patients with AGUS associated with a squamous abnormality; only 19% were seen in patients with AGUS as the only diagnosis. Females who were younger than 35 years had a significantly higher rate of histologic abnormalities compared with women older than 50 years ($P <$ .0001), and most lesions were squamous. Women older than 50 years had a notably higher rate of glandular histologic abnormalities ($P <$ .001) (Fig 2).

Conclusion.—More than one third of females with Papanicolaou tests showing AGUS have histologic abnormalities. Females younger than 35 years with a cytologic evaluation of AGUS have a higher rate of histopathologic findings, and most are squamous lesions. Women 50 years or older with a cytologic evaluation of AGUS have more glandular lesions

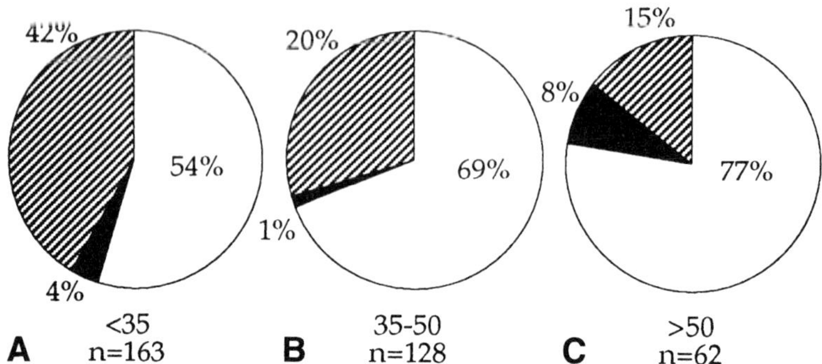

FIGURE 2.—Distribution of histopathologic conditions among women younger than 35 years (**A**), 35 to 50 years (**B**), and older than 50 years (**C**). *White areas*, benign findings; *black areas*, glandular pathologic findings; *striped areas*, squamous pathologic findings. (Courtesy of Geier CS, Wilson M, Creasman W: Clinical evaluation of atypical glandular cells of undetermined significance. *Am J Obstet Gynecol* 184:64-69, 2001.)

than their younger counterparts. The term *AGUS* is a misnomer because it represents a marker for serious pathologic processes.

▶ The glandular conundrum left to us by the Bethesda System revolves around the term *AGUS*, atypical glandular cells of uncertain significance, which accounts for less than 1% of Papanicolaou tests. These authors confirm the findings of others[1]—that the significance of AGUS is not quite so uncertain, in that 30% of them will have "significant abnormalities" that, in fact, are not glandular but that are usually squamous. Fortunately, less than 1% of these were cancer. Squamous lesions were more commonly found after a Papanicolaou test with AGUS findings in younger women, and the glandular lesions were more commonly seen in postmenopausal women (Fig 2). These findings support the guidelines of the American Society of Colposcopy and Cervical Pathology, which recommend a cervical and vaginal colposcopy with endocervical curettage as evaluation of an AGUS Papanicolaou test. In my own practice, if that evaluation does not adequately explain the finding of AGUS, then I will often also perform an endometrial biopsy.

D. S. Miller, MD

Reference

1. Cox JT: ASCCP practice guidelines: Management of glandular abnormalities in the cervical smear. *J Lower Genital Tract Dis* 1:41-45, 1997.

Conservative Management of Adenocarcinoma in Situ of the Cervix

Shin CH, Schorge JO, Lee KR, et al (Brigham and Women's Hosp, Boston)
Gynecol Oncol 79:6-10, 2000

22–11

Introduction.—Adenocarcinoma in situ (AIS) of the cervix is considered the precursor lesion of most cases of invasive adenocarcinoma, and hysterectomy has been the recommended treatment. But for younger women who desire to maintain fertility, conservative management with cone biopsy alone may be considered. In a study of women treated with cone biopsy for cervical AIS, investigators examined outcome during a median follow-up of 30 months.

Methods.—The records of all patients who underwent cone biopsy for AIS at Brigham and Women's Hospital between December 1987 and September 1999 were retrospectively reviewed. Data were gathered from hospital charts, cytology and pathology reports, and operative records.

Results.—During the study period, 133 patients received a diagnosis of AIS and 132 were treated with an initial cone biopsy. Of these 132, 95 (72%) were managed conservatively with a cold knife cone or loop electrical excisional procedure, thereby preserving the uterus. Hysterectomy was performed in the remaining 37 women (28%). Patients managed conservatively were significantly younger and less parous than patients who underwent hysterectomy. Negative margins were obtained in 92 (97%) of 95 conservatively managed women. Nine women subsequently required evaluation for abnormalities after cone biopsy with negative margins, but none had pathologic evidence of recurrent AIS. Twenty-three infants were delivered during follow-up, and 6 women who were treated with cone biopsy during pregnancy had successful pregnancy outcomes. Among the 37 women who had a hysterectomy, 32 elected to have the procedure, 4 had persistently positive cone biopsy margins, and 1 had endometrial hyperplasia. No patient had invasive adenocarcinoma in a hysterectomy specimen.

Discussion.—The outcomes of conservatively managed patients in this series were better than might have been expected from the current literature on cervical AIS. Favorable results were attributed to negative cone margin status, recurrence defined as pathologic confirmation of AIS, exclusion of invasive cancer cases, and a young patient population. Conservative management of AIS by cone biopsy with negative margins is a feasible treatment option when preservation of fertility is desired.

▶ This study is the largest report in the literature on the management of adenocarcinoma in situ. The authors retrospectively reviewed the method of treatment and outcome of 132 patients; 95 (72%) were followed conservatively after conization and the vast majority of them, 92, had negative margins. The median age of this highly motivated, conservatively managed group was 29 years, and 74% were nulliparous. Ten women were evaluated for cytopathologic abnormalities during a median follow-up of 30 months; 1 had pathologic evidence for adenocarcinoma in situ and underwent hysterectomy. As a result of conservative management, 23 infants were delivered of the 95 women. The authors provide the most compelling evidence to date that younger women with cervical adenocarcinoma in situ may be effectively treated with cone biopsy alone if negative margins can be achieved.

D. S. Miller, MD

23 Operative Gynecology

Anatomy

The Distribution of Pelvic Organ Support in a Population of Female Subjects Seen for Routine Gynecologic Health Care
Swift SE (Med Univ of South Carolina, Charleston)
Am J Obstet Gynecol 183:277-285, 2000   23–1

Background.—The incidence of specific symptoms often associated with pelvic organ prolapse has been described, but previous studies have not correlated these symptoms with the degree of prolapse as determined by physical examination. The goal of this study was a description of the distribution of pelvic organ support stages in a group of women who were seen at several outpatient gynecologic clinics for routine gynecologic health care.

Methods.—An observational study was conducted involving 497 women seen for routine gynecologic health care at 4 outpatient gynecology clinics. The average age of the participants was 44 years (range, 18 to 82 years). General biographic data were collected from each woman regarding obstetric history, medical history, and any prior surgery. A pelvic examination was then administered to each woman. Pelvic organ support was determined and described on the basis of the pelvic organ prolapse quantification system. The stages of support (0 to 4) were evaluated by variable for trends with Pearson χ^2 statistics.

Results.—The overall distribution of pelvic organ prolapse quantification system stages was stage 0, 6.4%; stage 1, 43.3%; stage 2, 47.7%; and stage 3, 2.6%. There were no cases of stage 4 pelvic organ prolapse in any of the participants examined. Several variables with a statistically significant trend toward increased pelvic organ prolapse quantification system stage were noted, including advancing age, increased gravidity and parity, an increasing number of vaginal births, delivery of a macrosomic infant, a history of hysterectomy or pelvic organ prolapse operations, postmenopausal status, and the presence of hypertension.

Conclusions.—The distribution of the pelvic organ prolapse quantification system stages was described as a bell-shaped curve, with most study participants having stage 1 or stage 2 support. There were no participants with stage 0 support and very few with stage 3 support. Women with many of the commonly cited etiologic factors for development of pelvic organ prolapse were found to have a statistically significant increase in pelvic organ quantification system stage of support.

▶ This author describes the distribution of pelvic organ prolapse in a heterogeneous North American population. These were adult women seeking routine gynecologic care. As expected, gravity, parity, and a history of a macrosomic infant delivery were associated with a loss of pelvic support. Women with a history of surgery for prolapse were also at increased risk. The prevalence of pelvic organ prolapse with advancing age was also noted. The lack of standardized terminology to describe pelvic organ support has previously hampered our understanding of risk factors as well as the natural history of pelvic support. This contribution is a good first step toward clarification.

R. D. Arias, MD

Location of the Ureters in Relation to the Uterine Cervix by Computed Tomography

Hurd WW, Chee SS, Gallagher KL, et al (Indiana Univ, Indianapolis; Univ of Michigan, Ann Arbor)
Am J Obstet Gynecol 184:336-339, 2001

23–2

Background.—Ureteral injury is a serious complication of hysterectomy. It reportedly occurrs in 0.1% to 2.5% of all gynecologic surgeries. Because both the cervix and the ureters can be visualized on CT, this study determined the location of the ureter in relation to the uterine cervix on clinically indicated CT studies, as well as whether patient age or weight affects this relationship.

Methods and Findings.—Fifty-two women were studied. The mean distance from ureter to cervical margin at the most dorsal reflection of the ureter was 2.3 cm. Although this value was uncorrelated with age, a linear relationship between this distance and body mass index was noted. In heavier women, the ureter was slightly more proximal to the cervical margin.

Conclusion.—In women with apparently normal pelvic anatomy, the mean distance between ureter and cervix was 2.3 cm. In 12%, this distance was less than 0.5 cm, which may explain the relatively common occurrence of ureteral injury during hysterectomy.

▶ Gynecologists performing hysterectomy for benign indications rely on good technique and the fact that the ureter follows an established course. This study of the relationship between the ureter and the cervix found this distance to be unexpectedly close (less than 0.5 cm) in 12% of the women studied. At least 1 woman had a cervix-to-ureter interval of 0.1 cm. This is particularly alarming since these CT measurements were obtained in women with little or no known pelvic pathology. A trend toward medial displacement of the ureter in obese women was also noted. This information should reinforce the need for meticulous technique—especially at the level of the cardinal ligaments.

R. D. Arias, MD

Cervical Procedures

Comparison of Endocervical Curettage and Endocervical Brushing
Klam S, Arseneau J, Mansour N, et al (McGill Univ, Montreal; Sir Mortimer B Davis–Jewish Gen Hosp, Montreal; Royal Victoria Hosp, Montreal)
Obstet Gynecol 96:90-94, 2000   23–3

Background.—Many clinicians have argued against the routine use of endocervical curettage (ECC) for a number of reasons, including patient discomfort, relatively high cost, and false-positive and false-negative results. In recent years, therefore, many clinicians have been using less painful methods, such as endocervical brushing for sampling of the canal. However, in previous studies of endocervical brushing, false-positive rates of 63% to 75% have been obtained. One possible result of these high rates is an increase in the number of unnecessary excisional procedures. If it could be determined that endocervical brushing was as accurate in terms of diagnostic yield as ECC with less patient discomfort, the brush technique could be considered an attractive alternative to ECC in evaluation of the endocervical canal. The 2 methods were compared with respect to diagnostic yield by histology and patient discomfort.

Methods.—A total of 315 nonpregnant women who were referred for colposcopy after abnormal Papanicolau test results were randomly assigned to endocervical sampling with either a metal curette (ECC) (157 patients) or an endocervical brush (158 patients). All the women underwent extensive endocervical canal brushing, and the samples were submitted for histologic study. Of these 315 patients, 147 also underwent electroconization. The results were evaluated in a masked fashion against the histologic findings in electroconization specimens. Melzack's Present Pain Intensity Scale was used to record the pain scores.

Results.—The false-positive rate for endocervical brushing was 29% compared with a false-positive rate of 31% for ECC. False-positive results were attributed to contamination of the endocervical sample by lesional epithelium near the external os. The proportion of scanty specimens was higher for endocervical brushing (8%) than for ECC (2%). None of the samples obtained by ECC was insufficient for diagnosis, whereas one sample obtained by brushing was insufficient for diagnosis. No statistically significant differences in the median pain scores of the 2 groups were noted.

Conclusions.—Endocervical brushing and ECC were found to be similar in diagnostic yield and patient discomfort. The false-positive rates for endocervical brushing were lower in this study than in other reports in the literature for cytologic analysis. ECC has remained the procedure of choice in the evaluation of the endocervical canal, but endocervical brushing was shown to be an acceptable alternative.

▶ Most colposcopists have been taught to perform ECC at the time of colposcopy. This concept has been called into question over the years because of the high false-positive rate for ECC and the consequent interventions the patients must endure. Others have shown that most of these false-positive results are caused by contamination of the curettage on the external lesion.[1] Prior studies have shown that endocervical brushing cytology can be comparable to ECC in terms of diagnostic accuracy but has been reported to be more comfortable. This study evaluated endocervical brush histology compared with ECC histology and found those methods to be equivalent. They were even equivalent in terms of operator or patient perceived discomfort.

D. S. Miller, MD

Reference

1. Spirtos NM, Schlaerth JB, d'Ablaing G III, et al: A critical evaluation of the endocervical curettage. *Obstet Gynecol* 70:729-733, 1987.

Risk Factors for Cervical Stenosis After Loop Electrocautery Excision Procedure
Suh-Burgmann EJ, Whall-Strojwas D, Chang Y, et al (Massachusetts Gen Hosp, Boston)
Obstet Gynecol 96:657-660, 2000

23–4

Introduction.—See-and-treat strategies that use loop excision in women with cervical dysplasia on initial evaluation is gaining favor because of its cost effectiveness and patient preference. The negative approaches for this procedure have not been examined extensively. Bleeding is the most common complication immediately after loop excision. Cervical stenosis and cervical incompetence are the primary long-term consequences of this procedure. Knowing the risk factors for cervical stenosis after loop excision would be useful to clinicians and allow patients to better understand their risk of developing long-term sequelae. The frequency of and risk factors for the development of cervical stenosis after loop electrosurgical excision procedure (LEEP) was examined retrospectively.

Methods.—Outpatient medical records were reviewed for women treated by loop excision for cervical dysplasia between August 1996 and January 1998. During follow-up, 164 women were evaluated for cervical stenosis. Stenosis was considered to be present if manual dilation was needed to allow endocervical sampling with the use an endocervical curette 3 mm wide. Multivariate analysis with stepwise logistic regression was used to assess: age, parity, tobacco use, hormonal status, use of oral contraceptives, pathology, previous loop excision, and dimensions of excision specimens as predictors of cervical stenosis.

Results.—Average patient age was 32 years. Ten of the 164 (6%) women evaluated had cervical stenosis. The only independent predictors of stenosis were previous loop excision and volume of excision specimen.

Conclusion.—There was a correlation between cervical stenosis and history of loop excision and volume of tissue removed, indicating that women who undergo second excisions or large excisions should be counseled that they may be at increased risk for stenosis.

▶ It is expected that a surgical procedure performed for a disease will have a risk of complications. The benefits of that procedure should exceed the risk. This risk-benefit analysis should be carefully considered when a surgical procedure is used in patients who may not have the disease as is performed in the so-called "see-and-treat" strategies that involve applying LEEP to patients who have a suspicious colposcopy but not yet histologically proved disease.[1] Whether cervical stenosis is a significant complication is debatable because the authors don't provide us with the long-term reproductive follow-up for these patients. Does it result in obstructed labor and increase the risk of cesarean section? It is also not well studied whether any of the excisional or destructive treatments of cervical intraepithelial neoplasia may increase the risk of incompetent cervix or prematurity.

D. S. Miller, MD

Reference

1. Burger RA, Monk BJ, van Nostrand KM, et al: Single-visit program for cervical cancer prevention in a high-risk population. *Obstet Gynecol* 86:491, 1995.

Hysteroscopy

Vaginal Misoprostol for Cervical Priming Before Operative Hysteroscopy: A Randomized Controlled Trial
Preutthipan S, Herabutya Y (Mahidol Univ, Bangkok, Thailand)
Obstet Gynecol 96:890-894, 2000   23–5

Introduction.—Most of the common complications encountered during operative hysteroscopy are related to the difficulty of cervical dilation. In a recent study, the authors showed that vaginal misoprostol, a prostaglandin E_1 analog, facilitates cervical dilation and diagnostic hysteroscopy. This trial investigated the effectiveness of vaginal misoprostol for cervical priming before operative hysteroscopy.

Methods.—Study participants were drawn from a group of women suspected of having intrauterine abnormalities during routine investigation for infertility. From this group, 152 women with definite intrauterine lesions were randomly assigned to receive either 200 µg vaginal misoprostol or placebo. Hysteroscopy was performed mostly in the proliferative phase of the menstrual cycle, with the patient under general anesthesia and propofol used as a total IV anesthesia. Outcomes assessed included cervical width before hysteroscopy, need for cervical dilatation, combined time of cervical dilatation up to Hegar number 6 and 7-9 before inserting the operative instrument, duration of the operative hysteroscopy, and complications.

Results.—The misoprostol and placebo groups were similar in age, body weight, number of patients with previous cervical dilatation, and type of operative hysteroscopy. Cervical dilation before operative hysteroscopy was required by 75.3% of patients in the misoprostol group versus 94.9% of those in the placebo group. The mean cervical dilation estimated by Hegar dilator differed significantly between the treated (7.3 mm) and control (3.8 mm) groups. The treated group had a significantly shorter median time of cervical dilation to Hegar number 9 and mean operative time. Cervical tears occurred in 11.4% of patients in the placebo group, but in only 1.4% of the misoprostol group. There were 2 uterine perforations, both in the placebo group.

Conclusion.—The use of vaginal misoprostol applied before operative hysteroscopy resulted in increased baseline cervical dilatation and a reduction in mechanical dilation of the cervix. Cervical complications were fewer with misoprostol than with placebo, and the adverse effects of the drug were not serious (mild lower abdominal pain in 35.6% of patients and slight vaginal bleeding in 19.2%).

▶ The use of vaginal misoprostol 200 µg 9 to 10 hours before operative hysteroscopy was effective in reducing operative time—especially time devoted to mechanical cervical dilation. Cervical lacerations were also significantly reduced. Adverse effects included mild lower abdominal pain (36%) and vaginal spotting (9%). Misoprostol appears safe and effective in reducing difficulties associated with cervical dilation for operative hysteroscopy and may have special use in women with risk factors for cervical stenosis.

R. D. Arias, MD

Feasibility and Pain Control in Outpatient Hysteroscopy in Postmenopausal Women: A Randomized Trial
Giorda G, Scarabelli C, Franceschi S, et al (Istituto Nazionale dei Tumori, Aviano, Italy)
Acta Obstet Gynecol Scand 79:593-597, 2000
23–6

Introduction.—Because postmenopausal women are likely to have narrowing of the cervical canal, diagnostic hysteroscopy is often a painful procedure. Narrow-diameter hysteroscopes have been introduced, but large-diameter scopes are still widely used. Three types of CO_2 hysteroscopy were compared for discomfort and feasibility in a group of postmenopausal women.

Methods.—The study included 361 women, who were randomly assigned to 1 of 3 methods of diagnostic hysteroscopy as an outpatient procedure. The study was not blinded. Procedures were performed with a

5-mm diagnostic sheath without local anesthesia (group 1, n = 119), with a 5-mm diagnostic sheath with paracervical block (group 2, n = 121), and with a 3.5-mm diagnostic sheath without local anesthesia (group 3, n = 119). The 3 groups were similar in mean age, years after menopause, and number of vaginal deliveries. Paracervical block, performed at least 5 minutes before hysteroscopy, consisted of a 20-mL solution of 1% mepivacaine. Examinations were considered complete only if distention of the uterine cavity made the tubal ostia, fundus, and 4 endometrial surfaces clearly visible. Patients were asked to rate their pain on a visual numerical scale after the procedure.

Results.—Hysteroscopy was performed for abnormal uterine bleeding in 47.4%, surveillance of antiestrogen treatment in 30.5%, abnormal endometrial cytology or histology in 14.1%, and increased endometrial thickness at US in 8%. Hysteroscopy failed because of stenosis in 9% of group 1, 10% of group 2, and 0.4% of group 3 patients. Paracervical block itself was painful in 18.2% of patients, and 38.8% had bleeding from the injection site. Pain was judged intolerable by 17% of group 1 and 6% of group 2 patients, but by none of group 3 patients. Gas leakage caused hysteroscopy to be inconclusive in 16 group 3 patients and in 2 groups 1 and 2 patients.

Conclusion.—In postmenopausal women, paracervical block significantly reduces the pain associated with a large sheath hysteroscopy. The use of a narrow sheath is less painful, but gas leakage may not allow a complete examination. In such cases, however, the procedure can be completed by changing to a large sheath hysteroscope.

▶ A simple, safe, reliable and well-tolerated method of evaluating bleeding in menopausal women remains elusive. Pain control during office hysteroscopy is more often complicated by the presence of a stenotic cervix in this age-group. The use of a 3.5-mm sheath was the ideal preference of patients in this evaluation of tolerability. In the subset in which evaluation was incomplete secondary to technical difficulty associated with the small diameter, the option of advancing to a 5-mm sheath with a paracervical block was employed with success.

A significant proportion of patients in this study were tamoxifen users. The use of a smaller diameter sheath in this group may be especially useful, since the necessity of repeat evaluation during the 5-year course of prophylactic therapy is increased, and other methods of endometrial evaluation (especially US) are less reliable.

R. D. Arias, MD

Prediction of Endometrial Ablation Success According to Perioperative Findings

Shamonki MI, Ziegler WF, Badger GJ, et al (Univ of Vermont, Burlington)
Am J Obstet Gynecol 182:1005-1007, 2000   23-7

Objective.—Endometrial ablation is an alternative to hysterectomy for women with menorrhagia that does not respond to medical management, although the procedure fails in 10% to 33% of patients. What predisposes a woman to success or failure after endometrial ablation is not known. Endometrial ablation success was retrospectively correlated with preoperative symptoms, physical and ultrasonographic findings, and findings at the time of the operation to assist the clinician in counseling patients about the most appropriate treatment.

Methods.—Medical records of 120 women, aged 27 to 49 years, who underwent endometrial ablation with danazol (800 mg/d orally) or leuprolide (3.75 mg in 1 IM injection per month) between May 1987 and November 1996, were reviewed. Patients who required additional treatment were regarded as having ablation failures.

Results.—Ablation failure occurred in 44 women (37%) and was similar for Nd:YAG ablation (28%) and rollerball ablation (39%). There was no association between the presence (38%) or absence of a retroverted uterus (26%) and failed outcome. Failure rates were higher when intracavitary lesions were present (47%) rather than absent (29%), and a trend toward higher failure rates was found with preoperative (47%) rather than without preoperative (33%) intramural fibroid tumors. More patients who had ablation therapy failure were taking leuprolide (47%) rather than danazol (28%), particularly in women younger than 40 years. In women older than 40 years, there was no difference in ablation failure whether they were given leuprolide or danazol.

Conclusion.—Leuprolide treatment and intramural fibroid tumors were positive predictors of ablation failure, and a normal appearance of the cavity at ablation was a negative predictor of ablation failure. Patients at higher risk of ablation failure should be given other treatment options.

▶ With adequate preoperative hormonal preparation, well-selected cases, and an experienced operator, a success rate as high as 63% was achieved in this short-term study. Follow-up time was a little more than 9 months, on average. Other pertinent outcomes included the surprising increased risk of failure when ablation was associated with the loop excision of an intracavitary lesion. One might have expected that the complete resection of the lesion would have given this group an improved chance of success; the ablation would merely have provided additional insurance against excessive bleeding. Also interesting was the improved outcome with danazol in younger women when compared with the now more frequently used leuprolide acetate injection. It appears that perimenopausal women with normal endometrial cavities have the best chance of favorable short-term treatment outcomes with use of this modality.

R. D. Arias, MD

Hysterectomy

Cost-Effectiveness of Universal Cystoscopy to Identify Ureteral Injury at Hysterectomy
Visco AG, Taber KH, Weidner AC, et al (Duke Univ, Durham, NC)
Obstet Gynecol 97:685-692, 2001   23–8

Background.—The cost-effectiveness of routine cystoscopy during abdominal, vaginal, and laparoscopically assisted vaginal hysterectomy were evaluated in this study in terms of the cost per ureteral injury identified and treated.

Methods.—A hospital-based perspective was used in the construction of a decision-analysis model for the estimation of the outcomes and costs of cystoscopy or no cystoscopy performed during abdominal hysterectomy. A similar decision-analysis model was constructed for vaginal and laparoscopically assisted vaginal hysterectomy. Estimated costs were derived from the Duke University Medical Center and from average Medicare reimbursements for similar diagnostic related groups from the Health Care Financing Administration. A review of the literature was conducted to determine the incidence of ureteral injury. A number of variables were used in the sensitivity analysis, including ureteral rate, silent ureteral injury rate, cost of cystoscopy, and cost of therapeutic interventions. A silent renal death rate of 0% was assumed.

Results.—The performance of routine cystoscopy at abdominal hysterectomy was found to be cost saving above a threshold ureteral injury rate of 1.5%. At a rate of 0.2%, there was a slight increase in the cost of routine intraoperative cystoscopy of $108 per abdominal hysterectomy. There was an associated cost of $54,000 per ureteral injury identified. However, at a ureteral injury rate of 2%, routine cystoscopy was associated with a marginal cost savings of $44 per hysterectomy and a cost savings of $2200 per ureteral injury identified. In the model of vaginal hysterectomy and laparoscopically assisted vaginal hysterectomy, a threshold ureteral injury rate of 2%, above which routine cystoscopy was cost saving, was obtained. The variables with the greatest effect on cost-effectiveness in both models were the incidence of ureteral injury and the cost of readmission.

Conclusions.—The cost-effectiveness of routine intraoperative cystoscopy depends on the rate of ureteral injury independent of the route of hysterectomy. Routine intraoperative cystoscopy is cost effective when the rate of ureteral injury is in excess of 1.5% for abdominal hysterectomy and 2% for vaginal or laparoscopically assisted vaginal hysterectomy.

▶ Routine diagnostic cystoscopy does not appear to be warranted in uncomplicated hysterectomy by either the vaginal or abdominal route. If, however, the rate of ureteral injury is greater than 1.5% for a given procedure or service, universal cystoscopy appears to be not only prudent but cost effective. The cost savings presumes that the operating surgeon has the skills, training, and privileges to perform intraoperative cystoscopy. This study serves to highlight the importance of evaluating the rate of ureteral injury on gynecologic services. Although universal cystoscopy appears unwarranted for most gynecologic services, diagnostic cystoscopy remains an important tool for evaluating ureteral patency in high-risk cases.

R. D. Arias, MD

Recovery From Vaginal Hysterectomy Compared With Laparoscopy-Assisted Vaginal Hysterectomy: A Prospective, Randomized, Multicenter Study

Soriano D, Goldstein A, Lecuru F, et al (Hôpital Hôtel-Dieu de Paris)
Acta Obstet Gynecol Scand 80:337-341, 2001   23–9

Introduction.—Laparoscopic-assisted vaginal hysterectomy (LAVH) is considered a safe alternative to the standard abdominal hysterectomy for patients with benign uterine pathosis. One advantage attributed to LAVH is rapid recovery, but some studies have shown no difference in recovery times between LAVH and standard vaginal hysterectomy (VH). LAVH and VH were compared with respect to recovery during hospitalization.

Methods.—A total of 80 women participated in the trial; 40 were assigned to the LAVH group and 40 to the VH group. All patients had a uterine size greater than 280 g and were without a suspicious adnexal mass. To eliminate bias related to the anesthetic method, all procedures were performed with patients under endotracheal general anesthesia. Patients in the VH and LAVH groups were compared for operative time and recovery data, including analgesic requirements and duration of hospital stay.

Results.—The 2 groups were comparable in age, parity, premenopausal state, previous pelvic surgery, and indications for surgery. Myoma and adenomyosis were the most common pathologic diagnoses in each group. Three patients in the LAVH group were excluded from analysis because of laparoconversion, required because of inaccessibility to the uterine pedicle. Mean operative time was 108 minutes in the VH group and 160 minutes in the LAVH group, and the rate of complications was lower in the VH group (15% vs 32.5%). Analgesic requirements and mean hospital stay (5.3 days after VH and 5.7 days after LAVH) did not differ in the 2 groups.

Conclusion.—Standard VH is a shorter operation than LAVH, even in cases of enlarged uteri. In contrast with some previous reports, short-term recovery did not differ between the 2 surgical methods.

▶ LAVH may, appropriately, be used as an alternative to abdominal hysterectomy when a purely vaginal approach is precluded by adnexal pathosis or when the history or examination raises suspicion of pelvic adhesions. The use of laparoscopy in cases that may be addressed purely by the vaginal route merely adds to expense and operative time. The reported advantage of laparoscopic assistance found in a retrospective review were absent in this prospective trial. In addition, all cases of laparoconversion secondary to excessive bleeding occurred in the laparoscopic arm. The addition of laparoscopy to a VH does not necessarily make the case easier for either the patient or the surgeon.

R. D. Arias, MD

Vaginal Route as the Norm When Planning Hysterectomy for Benign Conditions: Change in Practice

Varma R, Tahseen S, Lokugamage AU, et al (Basildon & Thurrock Gen Hosps, England; Royal Free and Univ College London Med School)
Obstet Gynecol 97:613-616, 2001   23–10

Background.—No significant reduction has been found in the number of hysterectomies in the United Kingdom, despite improvements in medical therapy for menstrual disorders and the development of surgical techniques for endometrial ablation that require minimal access. The current ratio of abdominal hysterectomies to vaginal hysterectomies is 4:1 for the treatment of benign disease, although the vaginal route has mainly been restricted to the treatment of prolapses. The reverse should be the case because fewer perioperative complications are associated with the vaginal route, which allows earlier recovery and return to work. Vaginal hysterectomies have also been shown to be less expensive than either abdominal or laparoscopically assisted hysterectomies. However, a change in practice has not occurred, despite strong advocacy for the vaginal approach and guidelines for determining the route of the hysterectomy. These investigators studied whether a deliberate decision to perform as many hysterectomies as possible by the vaginal route could be effective in increasing the proportion of vaginal hysterectomies for treatment of benign conditions in the absence of a prolapse.

Methods.—The study group comprised all patients who underwent hysterectomies for benign conditions (with the exception of prolapse) at a general hospital in the United Kingdom; all procedures were performed by a single surgeon over 5 years. A total of 272 patients were included. The primary end point for the study was the change in the route of hysterectomies, and it was observed at yearly intervals.

Results.—The route of surgery at the initiation of the study was 68% abdominal and 32% vaginal. By the end of the fifth year, the pattern had been altered to 5% abdominal and 95% vaginal. Conversion from a vaginal to an abdominal hysterectomy occurred in only 2 patients during the study. No change in case mix occurred during this period. By the fifth year of study, most of the associated oophorectomies that were performed were also vaginal procedures. No increase in patient morbidity was noted.

Conclusions.—The attitude of the surgeon, not the clinical situation, was found to be a major determining factor in the route chosen for a hysterectomy. Vaginal hysterectomies can be performed without the need for extra training, special skills, or complex equipment.

▶ Nulliparity, previous cesarean section, desire for an oophorectomy, and lack of uterine descensus are common reasons to choose the abdominal over the vaginal route for a hysterectomy. This article evaluates the feasibility of a vaginal hysterectomy for every patient with a benign pathologic condition and a uterus less than 16 weeks' size. The importance of preoperative counseling and patient consent for conversion to an abdominal route or laparoscopic assistance is emphasized. The option of making the final assessment for the appropriate surgical route at the time of examination under anesthesia is another useful point. Given the advantages offered by vaginal surgery, it should be considered a primary option and only rejected when infeasible.

R. D. Arias, MD

Laparoscopy

Laparoscopy in Patients Following Transverse Rectus Abdominis Myocutaneous Flap Reconstruction
Muller CY, Coleman RL, Adams WP Jr, et al (Univ of Texas, Dallas)
Obstet Gynecol 96:132-135, 2000   23–11

Background.—The increase in the number of survivors of breast cancer has presented the gynecologist with many issues specific to this patient population. There may be a need for pelvic surgery for therapeutic or prophylactic indications years after a mastectomy with immediate reconstruction, which is the current standard of care for patients with breast cancer. Impressive cosmetic results in women undergoing mastectomies have been attainable thanks to advances in reconstructive surgery, including the use of the transverse rectus abdominus musculocutaneous (TRAM) flap. A technique for the performance of laparoscopic pelvic surgery in women who have undergone TRAM flap procedures is reviewed.

Technique.—In this technique, an examination under anesthesia is performed in the low lithotomy position parallel to the floor. The abdominal aorta is then palpated and outlined, and a pneumoperitoneum is created by umbilical or left upper-quadrant Veress needle placement. If the patient has an acceptable umbilical location, port placement is accomplished through the incision of the umbilical relocation. Other options for port placement have included left upper-quadrant or paramedian placement so that the ligamentum teres vessels can be avoided. Placement of lateral operative ports (5 mm) is performed with reference to the transverse incision present, the pelvic pathologic condition, and the location of the umbilicus. Electrocautery, intracorporeal and extracorporeal suturing and knot-tying, and clips are preferred for the minimization of the port size.

Results.—Laparoscopic-assisted vaginal hysterectomies and oophorectomies with use of the periumbilical incision or trocar placement were performed in 4 consecutive survivors of breast cancer after unilateral or bilateral TRAM reconstruction. The only complication was a superficial breakdown of skin from an adhesive allergy in 1 patient. The allergy required 6 weeks to completely resolve.

Conclusions.—Laparoscopic pelvic surgery in women who have undergone TRAM reconstruction seems feasible. An understanding of the anatomical and physiologic variations related to the TRAM procedure is required for the planning of a safe operation.

▶ Laparoscopic surgery after abdominal wall reconstruction requires special surgical consideration as well as preoperative counseling with regard to certain distinct points. The availability of the operative report is important, and special attention should be paid to the location of the vascular pedicle so that injury to the residual blood supply can be avoided. Limitations of distention as well as alterations in landmarks need to be considered when assessing the feasibility of this technique. The use of smaller trocars and careful attention to wound care and skin integrity are also recommended. The authors' experience with 4 patients undergoing operative laparoscopy after TRAM flap reconstruction provides a useful review of this increasingly common surgical challenge.

R. D. Arias, MD

Preventing Postoperative Pain by Local Anesthetic Instillation After Laparoscopic Gynecologic Surgery: A Placebo-Controlled Comparison of Bupivacaine and Ropivacaine

Goldstein A, Grimault P, Henique A, et al (Hotel-Dieu Hosp, Paris)
Anesth Analg 91:403-407, 2000   23 12

Introduction.—Postoperative pain is unpredictable, which underscores the need for systemic prevention of pain before wake-up from anesthesia. The fact that pain is composed of several components explains the need for multimodal analgesic techniques for effective postoperative analgesia. The effect of intraperitoneal instillation of local anesthetics on postoperative pain after laparoscopic gynecologic surgery was examined in a prospectively, double-blind, randomized, placebo-controlled trial of 180 patients.

Methods.—Patients were randomly assigned to receive an intraperitoneal instillation of 20 mL of either bupivacaine 0.5% (group B), ropivacaine 0.75% (group R), or saline (group S) at completion of surgery. Acetaminophen and ketaprofen were administered intravenously to all patients. Pain was evaluated with a 0 to 10 graded numerical scale (NS) every 5 minutes in the postanesthesia care unit. Intravenous morphine was given when NS was above 4. Pain evaluation continued every 4 hours on the ward; patients received subcutaneous morphine as needed to keep the NS score below 4. A 4-point scale was used to assess postoperative nausea and vomiting (PONV).

Results.—Morphine consumption at wake-up and during the first 24 hours was significantly lower ($P < .05$) in group B (mean, 0.92 mg at wake-up; 3.08 mg over 24 hours) and group R (mean, 0.25 mg at wake-up; 0.69 mg over 24 hours), compared with group S (mean, 4.18 mg at wake-up; 12.93 mg over 24 hours). The morphine-sparing effect of ropivacaine was significantly superior to that of bupivacaine. Both bupivacaine and ropivacaine were effective in the prevention of PONV.

Conclusion.—It is recommended that local anesthetics be instilled in all patients who undergo laparoscopic gynecologic procedures.

▶ Both ropivacaine and bupivacaine were effective in prevention of PONV after laparoscopic gynecologic surgery. Ropivacaine 0.75% was more effective than bupivacaine 0.5% in reducing the need for postoperative morphine. Given its safety and ease of instillation, local anesthetics, especailly ropivacaine, should be considered at the end of laparoscopic procedures.

R. D. Arias, MD

Additive Anti-emetic Efficacy of Prophylactic Ondansetron With Droperidol in Out-patient Gynecological Laparoscopy
Wu O, Belo SE, Koutsoukos G (Univ of Toronto)
Can J Anesth 47:529-536, 2000   23–13

Objective.—The incidence of postoperative nausea and vomiting (PONV) after gynecologic laparoscopy ranges from 40% to 77%. Because both ondansetron and droperidol have limited effectiveness in treating PONV, a randomized, double-blind study was conducted to determine prospectively whether prophylactic administration of either drug alone or in combination was effective in preventing PONV in outpatients undergoing gynecologic laparoscopy.

Methods.—Patients (n = 160), aged 16 to 65 years, were randomly allocated to receive IV treatment with saline, 4 mg ondansetron, 1.25 mg droperidol, or a combination of 4 mg ondansetron and 1.25 mg droperidol. Patients were assessed for nausea and vomiting at various times postoperatively. Each patient was called at 24 hours to record any PONV complaints.

Results.—Eight patients were excluded from the study. Before discharge, all 3 treatment groups had significantly less PONV than did the control group (71%). The combination group (23%) had less PONV than the ondansetron group (46%) and significantly less PONV than did the droperidol group (61%). The difference between the ondansetron and droperidol groups was not significant. After discharge, the PONV incidence for the ondansetron group and the droperidol group was similar to that of the placebo group. The combination group had significantly less PONV than the placebo group did. Pain scores on a visual analog scale were similar for all groups, but drowsiness scores on a visual analog scale were significantly higher in the droperidol group than in the other groups. The combination group had fewer requests for rescue medication than the other groups did.

Conclusion.—The combination of ondansetron and droperidol resulted in less PONV after outpatient gynecologic laparoscopy than either drug alone.

▶ Technological advances have greatly expanded the useful indications for pelvic laparoscopy. Unfortunately, PONV remains the rate-limiting step on the road to well-being for a large proportion of patients undergoing endoscopy. Here, the incidence of significant nausea and vomiting reached 75% in the placebo group. The dramatic reduction in symptoms associated with a combination of 4 mg ondansetron and 1.25 mg droperidol should encourage a reevaluation of prophylactic antiemetic programs used in our outpatient surgical suites.

R. D. Arias, MD

24 Ovarian Cancer

Diagnosis

Usefulness of Mass Screening for Ovarian Carcinoma Using Transvaginal Ultrasonography

Sato S, Yokoyama Y, Sakamoto T, et al (Hirosaki Univ, Japan)
Cancer 89:582-588, 2000

24–1

Objective.—Ovarian cancer has the worst prognosis of all gynecologic cancers. Ovarian cancer has a high cure rate if detected early, but early diagnosis is difficult. One institution has used transvaginal (TVS) as a screening modality in asymptomatic women since 1989. The prospective results of TVS mass screening over the course of 10 years were analyzed.

Methods.—The screening program consisted of primary and secondary screening and closer examination (Fig 1).

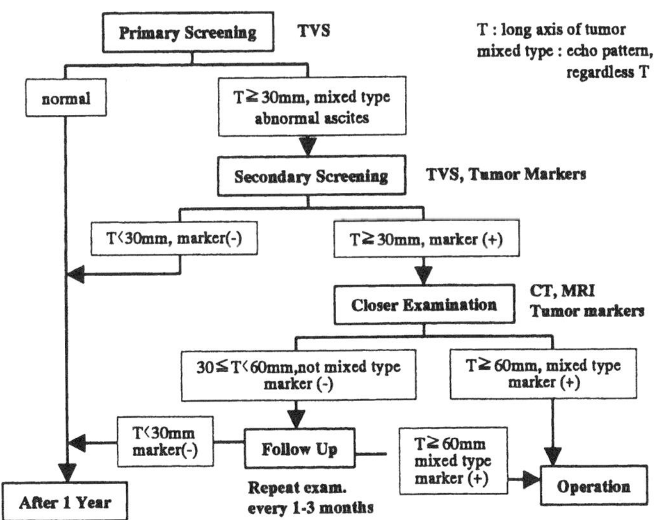

FIGURE 1.—Transvaginal ultrasonography (*TVS*) screening program. (Courtesy of Sato S, Yokoyama Y, Sakamoto T, et al: Usefulness of mass screening for ovarian carcinoma using transvaginal ultrasonography. *Cancer* 89(3):582-588, 2000. ©2000, American Cancer Society. Reprinted by permission of Wiley-Liss, Inc., a subsidiary of John Wiley & Sons, Inc.)

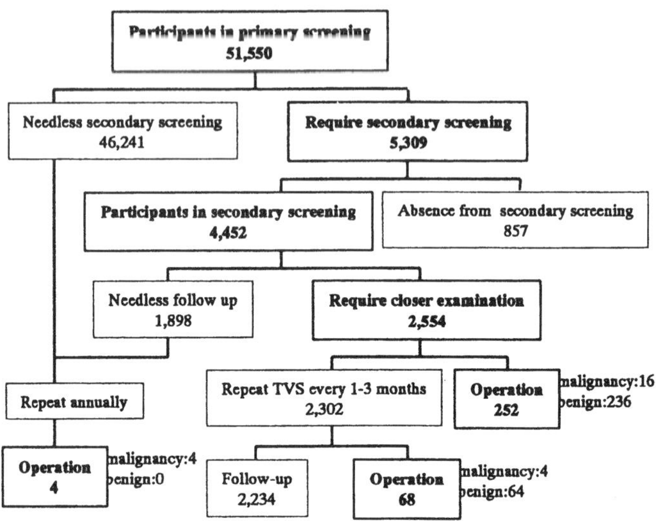

FIGURE 2.—Results of screening for ovarian carcinoma. *Abbreviation*: *TVS*, Transvaginal US. (Courtesy of Sato S, Yokoyama Y, Sakamoto T, et al: Usefulness of mass screening for ovarian carcinoma using transvaginal ultrasonography. *Cancer* 89(3):582-588, 2000. ©2000, American Cancer Society. Reprinted by permission of Wiley-Liss, Inc., a subsidiary of John Wiley & Sons, Inc.)

Results.—A total of 183,034 women entered the screening program; 51,550 were screened for the first time (Fig 2). Primary screening took about 1 minute per patient. Measuring the long axis of the ovaries using TVS took about 30 seconds. Of 324 women who underwent laparoscopy, 22 patients were given a diagnosis of ovarian cancer and 2 were found to have metastatic ovarian cancer, for a diagnostic rate of 0.047%. The 22 patients had stage I disease (17 patients), stage II disease (2 patients), stage III disease (2 patients), and stage IV disease (1 patient). Ten (45.5%) patients had a positive tumor marker, but only 5 (29.4%) of these patients had stage I tumors. Before screening, 56% of all patients were given a diagnosis of stage III and IV disease, whereas after screening, 58.8% of all patients were given a diagnosis of stage I disease. In Japan, the prevalence of ovarian cancer is 25% to 33% of that of uterine cervical cancer—a prevalence considerably lower than that in Europe or the United States. Of the 6 risk factors considered during screening, all 24 patients with a diagnosis of ovarian cancer had at least 1 factor.

Conclusion.—Screening TVS is a simple, quick, and reliable method that may be a valuable means of early detection of ovarian cancer.

▶ Most women with ovarian cancer will die of it because of the fact that most diagnoses are not made until the disease has metastasized. However, cure can be achieved if the malignancy can be detected and treated while still confined to the ovary. Several groups have sought to develop an effective screening strategy and, what is even more elusive, a cost-effective screening strategy.[1] The authors have conducted the largest study that I am aware of. It is differentiated from previous studies by the rapidity of its TVS examination. Over 50,000 patients were screened to find 17 early ovarian cancers. Typical of previous experience, 10 laparotomies had to be performed for each early ovarian cancer found. If these results can be reproduced, this appears to be the closest we have come to practical screening for ovarian cancer.

D. S. Miller, MD

Reference

1. van Nagell JR, DePriest PD, Reedy MD, et al: The efficacy of transvaginal sonographic screening in the asymptomatic women at risk for ovarian cancer. *Gynecol Oncol* 77:350-356, 2000

Ovarian Carcinoma Diagnosis: Results of a National Ovarian Cancer Survey
Goff BA, Mandel L, Muntz HG, et al (Univ of Washington, Seattle; Virginia Mason Med Ctr, Seattle, Wash; CONVERSATIONS!, Amarillo, Tex)
Cancer 89:2068-2075, 2000   24–2

Background.—Ovarian carcinoma is usually not detected until it has reached an advanced stage. Preoperative symptoms and factors that may contribute to delayed diagnosis for women with ovarian carcinoma were investigated.

Methods.—A 2-page survey was mailed to 1500 women who subscribed to a newsletter about ovarian carcinoma. Because some women copied the survey and gave it to additional patients, a total of 1725 surveys were returned. Forty-six states and 4 Canadian provinces were represented.

Findings.—Seventy percent of the respondents had stage III or IV disease. Overall, the median age of respondents was 52 years. Ninety-five percent of the women reported having symptoms before their diagnosis. Seventy-seven percent had abdominal symptoms; 70% had gastrointestinal symptoms; 58% had pain; 50% had constitutional symptoms; 34% had urinary problems; and 26% had pelvic symptoms. Women who ignored their symptoms were significantly more likely than those who did not to have a diagnosis of advanced disease. Length of time to diagnosis was less than 3 months for 55% but greater than 6 months for 26% and more than 1 year for 11%. Delay in diagnosis was associated significantly with lack of a pelvic examination at the first visit; existence of a multitude of symptoms; an initial diagnosis of no problem, depression, stress, irritable bowel, or gastritis; lack of US, CT, or CA 125 testing initially; and younger age at presentation.

Conclusions.—Most women with ovarian cancer have symptoms when they initially seek medical attention. Delays in diagnosis are common, ranging from more than 6 months to more than 1 year.

▶ It has long been assumed and taught that the reason that most ovarian cancer is not diagnosed until it is of advanced stage is that the disease is asymptomatic until late in its course. The authors evaluated these presumptions by going to the source, ovarian cancer survivors, and surveyed them about the events and symptoms that eventually led to their diagnoses. Some of our assumptions were confirmed: the symptoms are vague and not very specific, and patients who ignored their symptoms were more likely to have advanced disease. The diagnosis of early stage ovarian cancer was more likely to be made by gynecologists than by other primary care specialists. However, unexpectedly, most patients with stage I or II disease had symptoms, and the more physicians a patient saw, the more likely her diagnosis was delayed. Even though the prevalence of ovarian cancer is low, symptoms in women should be evaluated critically, nonspecific diagnoses should be made only occasionally, and pelvic examinations should be performed as a part of the complete examination of the female patient.

D. S. Miller, MD

Surgery

Pattern of Lymph Node Metastases in Clinically Unilateral Stage I Invasive Epithelial Ovarian Carcinomas

Cass I, Li AJ, Runowicz CD, et al (Univ of California, Los Angeles; Albert Einstein College of Medicine, Bronx, NY)
Gynecol Oncol 80:56-61, 2001   24–3

Introduction.—Lymphatic drainage of the ovary follows the gonadal blood supply. The dominant lymph channels coalesce in the infundibulopelvic ligament, then travel with the pampiniform plexus of the ovaries where they drain into the inferior pole of the kidney and move medially into the para-aortic and precaval lymph nodes (LNs). The pattern of lymphatic spread in unilateral stage I invasive ovarian carcinomas is under debate. The incidence and distribution of LN metastases in ovarian carcinomas were examined in disease clinically confined to 1 ovary.

Methods.—A retrospective review of medical records yielded 96 patients with disease visibly confined to 1 ovary. Pathology reports were examined to determine metastatic LN involvement, number of involved nodes, and location of involved nodes. Patients were excluded if they had gross disease in the pelvis or abdomen, as were those who had grossly positive LNs removed for debulking.

Results.—Fourteen (15%) patients had microscopically positive LNs on pathologic review. All 14 patients had grade 3 tumors. The upstaging of these 14 patients to stage IIIC disease was based on microscopic metastases alone. The grade 3 tumors were observed more frequently in patients who are LN-positive versus patients who are LN-negative ($P < .001$). Pelvic nodes were positive in 7 patients (50%), para-aortic nodes in 5 patients (36%), and both in 2 patients (14%). Of 2 patients who had LN sampling only on the side ipsilateral to the neoplastic ovary, 4 (10%) had LN metastases. Ten of 54 (19%) who had bilateral sampling had LN metastases. Five (50%), 3 (30%), and 2 (20%) of these 10 patients, respectively, had isolated ipsilateral LN metastases, isolated contralateral LN metastases, and bilateral metastases. Mean ovarian volumes were 550.7 cm^3 for ipsilateral LN metastases and 668.6 cm^3 for those with either bilateral or isolated contralateral LN metastases ($P = $ NS). Survival was similar for patients who were LN-positive and LN-negative.

Conclusion.—Bilateral LN sampling increased the detection of nodal metastases in patients with clinical stage I ovarian carcinoma with disease limited to 1 kidney. Disease may be understaged with ipsilateral sampling. Bilateral pelvic and para-aortic LN sampling is recommended for the accurate staging of ovarian carcinoma.

▶ This study illustrates the importance of complete surgical staging of patients who appear to have ovarian cancer confined to the ovary. Thirty percent of the patients were found to have disease spread beyond the ovaries, with 15% showing spread to the pelvic or para-aortic LNs. Of note, all these occult LN-positive patients had grade 3 cancers. The fact that some of these LN metastases were contralateral to the abnormal ovary reinforces the recommendation for bilateral LN sampling.

D. S. Miller, MD

Retroperitoneal Drainage After Complete Paraaortic Lymphadenectomy for Gynecologic Cancer: A Randomized Trial

Morice P, Lassau N, Pautier P, et al (Institut Gustave Roussy, Villejuif, France)
Obstet Gynecol 97:243-247, 2001   24–4

Background.—Lymphocysts are the most frequent complication of lymphadenectomy, which is an integral component in the surgical staging of gynecologic cancer. The customary practice for reduction of the risk of complications after lymphadenectomy has been drainage. However, several studies have suggested that drainage after lymphadenectomy is not effective in reducing morbidity. The relationship between retroperitoneal drainage after complete para-aortic lymphadenectomy for gynecologic cancer and subsequent development of lymphocysts was determined.

Methods.—A group of 80 women who underwent lymphadenectomy for cervical cancer (37 patients) or ovarian cancer (43 patients) were enrolled in this randomized trial. After undergoing complete para-aortic lymphadenectomy up to the level of the left renal vein, the women were randomly assigned to receive either drainage or no drainage of the para-aortic area. Most of the patients had pelvic drainage. The patients in both groups were assessed by abdominopelvic US at 8 to 12 days after surgery.

Focal points for the study included postoperative complications, duration of hospital stay, and characteristics of asymptomatic lymphocysts.

Results.—Forty-two women received para-aortic drainage, and 38 women received no para-aortic drainage. Complications occurred in 15 of 42 women (36%) who had drainage compared with 5 of 38 women (13%) who did not have drainage. Complications that were potentially related to drainage, including symptomatic lymphocysts or ascites, occurred in 3 patients (8%) in the undrained group compared with 11 patients (26%) in the drained group. The median duration of hospital stay was 9 days in the undrained group compared with 11 days in the drained group. Among patients in the undrained group there were 9 (24%) asymptomatic para-aortic lymphocysts detected during US compared with 2 (5%) in the drained group.

Conclusions.—In patients who did not undergo para-aortic drainage after complete para-aortic lymphadenectomy, the number of asymptomatic para-aortic lymphocysts was higher, but morbidity and the duration of hospitalization were increased in these patients. On the basis of these findings it is suggested that the practice of routine drainage of the retroperitoneum after para-aortic lymphadenectomy should be discontinued.

▶ Elimination of dead space has been an important principle of surgery dating back to Halsted. The application of this principle to the space left by pelvic lymphadenectomy has undergone evolution. Recent studies have shown that drainage of this space is not useful for reducing morbidity. The authors of this study do not appear to have benefited from that experience. While they undertook a randomized trial of drainage after para-aortic lymphadenectomy they, in fact, placed drains in the pelvis in all the patients. It is interesting to note that their incidence of pelvic lymphoceles was higher than their incidence of para-aortic lymphoceles in either the drained or the undrained group (Table 2 in the original article). The lesson to be learned from this and prior studies in regards to decreasing morbidity from pelvic or para-aortic lymphadenectomy is to not create a closed space in the lymphadenectomy bed. Rather, the lymphadenectomy lymph fluid should be allowed to vent into the peritoneal cavity where it then can be reabsorbed by the omentum and the under surfaces of the diaphragm.

D. S. Miller, MD

Splenectomy and Surgical Cytoreduction for Ovarian Cancer

Chen L-m, Leuchter RS, Lagasse LD, et al (Univ of California, Los Angeles)
Gynecol Oncol 77:362-368, 2000   24–5

Background.—Aggressive surgery for patients with ovarian cancer may include bowel resection and upper abdominal procedures, such as splenectomy. The role of splenectomy as a surrogate marker for aggressive tumor cytoreduction in this patient population and its effects on morbidity and survival were studied.

Methods and Findings.—Thirty-five patients with ovarian cancer undergoing splenectomy between 1986 and 1998 were included in the study. Splenic involvement was diagnosed before secondary surgery in 77%, of patients, compared with 15% before primary surgery. Parenchymal splenic involvement was observed at recurrence in 59% and initially in 23%. Major morbidity—including pneumonia, pulmonary embolism, sepsis, pancreatitis, and myocardial infarction—occurred in 23% of patients undergoing primary surgery and in 29% of those undergoing secondary surgery. Median progression-free intervals were 24 months and 14 months in primary and secondary surgery patients, respectively.

Conclusion.—Splenectomy can be performed at primary or secondary cytoreduction with acceptable morbidity in patients with ovarian cancer. Patients undergoing secondary cytoreduction may be selected preoperatively based on progression-free intervals, previous degree of cytoreduction, and macronodular tumor involvement on imaging.

▶ The gynecologic surgeon should always be able to differentiate that which can be done and that which should be done. These authors, as well as others before them, have shown that splenectomy at the time of primary or secondary ovarian tumor cytoreduction is feasible and not too morbid. The issue is when, or even if, splenectomy should be done. As the authors discuss (and I concur), splenectomy should be done for ovarian cancer not because it is possible, but only when it is the critical tumor burden that stands in the way of leaving the patient with no or minimal residual cancer. There is no advantage to the patient in adding 1 more billing code, leaving the patient without a spleen but with gross residual ovarian cancer.

D. S. Miller, MD

Chemotherapy

Phase III Trial of Standard-Dose Intravenous Cisplatin Plus Paclitaxel Versus Moderately High-Dose Carboplatin Followed by Intravenous Paclitaxel and Intraperitoneal Cisplatin in Small-Volume Stage III Ovarian Carcinoma: An Intergroup Study of the Gynecologic Oncology Group, Southwestern Oncology Group, and Eastern Cooperative Oncology Group

Markman M, Bundy BN, Alberts DS, et al (Cleveland Clinic Found, Ohio; Roswell Park Cancer Inst, Buffalo, NY; Albert Einstein College of Medicine, Bronx, NY; et al)

J Clin Oncol 19:1001-1007, 2001 24–6

Background.—Despite the value of combination chemotherapy, most women seen with advanced-stage ovarian cancer eventually die from disease. The efficacy of IV cisplatin and paclitaxel was compared with that of an experimental regimen of IV carboplatin followed by IV paclitaxel and intraperitoneal cisplatin.

Methods.—Five hundred twenty-three patients with small-volume stage III ovarian carcinoma were enrolled in the trial. By random assignment, they received IV paclitaxel, 135 mg/m², over 24 hours, followed by IV cisplatin, 75 mg/m², every 3 weeks for 6 courses, or IV carboplatin every 28 days for 2 courses, followed by IV paclitaxel, 135 mg/m², over 24 hours, then intraperitoneal (IP) cisplatin, 100 mg/m², every 3 weeks for 6 courses.

Findings.—Four hundred sixty-two patients were evaluable. Patients receiving the experimental treatment had greater levels of neutropenia, thrombocytopenia, and gastrointestinal and metabolic toxicities. This resulted in 18% of the patients receiving 2 or fewer courses of IP treatment. Median progression-free survival was 28 months in the experimental treatment group and 22 months in the standard treatment group. A borderline improvement in overall survival was associated with the experimental regimen.

Conclusion.—In patients with small-volume stage III ovarian carcinoma, treatment with moderately high-dose IV carboplatin, followed by IP paclitaxel and IV cisplatin, significantly improved progression-free survival compared with a standard regimen of IV cisplatin and paclitaxel. However, the improvement in overall survival was of borderline statistical significance, and the experimental treatment was associated with greater toxicity. Thus, it cannot be recommended for routine use.

▶ The concept of applying medicine directly to the offending disease dates back to antiquity. For ovarian cancer, this takes the form of the intraperitoneal application of chemotherapy. Since ovarian cancer is usually confined to the peritoneal surfaces of the abdominal cavity, very high concentrations of chemotherapy drugs can be deposited on the cancer, yet systemic drug levels will be much lower as, hopefully, also will be the systemic toxicity. Previous studies have suggested a small advantage for this route of treatment.[1] Unfortunately, this study did not clarify the issue, most likely because of the high-dose carboplatin that proceeded the intraperitoneal chemotherapy. Thus, we will have to await the results of the recently completed Gynecologic Oncology Group trial no. 172, which compared IV paclitaxel and cisplatin with intraperitoneal cisplatin and paclitaxel.

D. S. Miller, MD

Reference

1. Alberts DS, Liu PY, Hannigan EV, et al: Intraperitoneal cisplatin plus intravenous cyclophosphamide versus intravenous cisplatin plus intravenous cyclophosphamide for stage III ovarian cancer. *N Engl J Med* 334:1950, 1996.

Outpatient Taxol and Carboplatin Chemotherapy for Suboptimally Debulked Epithelial Carcinoma of the Ovary Results in Improved Quality of Life: An Eastern Cooperative Oncology Group Phase II Study (E2E93)
Schink JC, Weller E, Harris LS, et al (Univ of Wisconsin, Madison; Dana Farber Cancer Inst, Boston; Northwestern Univ, Chicago; et al)
Cancer J 7:155-164, 2001
24–7

Introduction.—Toxicity data and quality of life (QOL) evaluations help in developing future clinical trials in patients undergoing chemotherapy for suboptimally debulked epithelial carcinoma of the ovary. This Eastern Cooperative Oncology Group Phase II Study (E2E93) was performed to (1) examine the objective response rate and toxicities among patients with suboptimally debulked ovarian cancer treated with paclitaxel (3-hour infusion) and carboplatin, (2) assess the progression-free interval and overall survival, and (3) describe the changes in QOL over time in patients receiving paclitaxel and carboplatin.

Methods.—Women with International Federation of Gynecology and Obstetrics Stage II to IV epithelial ovarian cancer with suboptimal residual disease (more than 1 cm) were recruited. Patients underwent treatment with paclitaxel, 150 mg/m² over 3 hours, followed by carboplatin (area under the curve, 5) administered every 4 weeks for 6 cycles. The Functional Assessment of Cancer Therapy–Ovarian Cancer scale was used to examine QOL. Of 59 patients treated, 38 had measurable disease and 21 had evaluable disease.

Results.—The response rate, including complete and partial responses, was 72%. The progression-free interval in patients with measurable disease was 17.5 months; in those with evaluable disease, it was 11.1 months. Median survivals for measurable and evaluable disease were 30.1 months and 25.7 months, respectively.

The most frequently occurring grade 3 or higher toxicities were leukopenia (26%) and granulocytopenia (74%). The minimal toxicity of the regimen is evidenced by the high percentage of patients who completed therapy: 84% of patients with measurable disease and 71% of those who had nonmeasurable disease. None of the 10 patients who did not complete therapy stopped because of toxicity.

Patients experienced a significant improvement in QOL during ($P = .012$) and at completion of therapy ($P = .006$), compared with baseline. The physical well-being and functional well-being subscales were major contributors to improvements in QOL.

Conclusion.—This regimen is optimal therapy for most women with advanced ovarian cancer. It is convenient, well tolerated, and has response and survival rates comparable to more aggressive regimens. Most patients had significant improvements in QOL and physical well-being scores.

▶ The Gynecologic Oncology Group has presented, but not yet published, the results of its large randomized trial showing that an outpatient carboplatin and paclitaxel regimen is as effective as and more tolerable than its previous gold standard therapy of cisplatin and paclitaxel.[1] This study showed that a less-intense dose regimen could produce similar levels of activity against ovarian cancer. The authors are to be congratulated for not only measuring the usual response and survival rates, but also whether their treatment intervention actually improved the patient's life as measured by a validated QOL questionnaire, which showed a measurable improvement. While the baseline questionnaire was completed prior to the initiation of chemotherapy, it was done after surgery. Hopefully, this improvement is, in fact, attributable to the chemotherapy intervention as opposed to merely being a reflection of the recovery from surgery.

D. S. Miller, MD

Reference

1. Ozols RF, Bundy BN, Fowler J: Randomized phase III study of cisplatin (CIS)/paclitaxel (PAC) versus carboplatin (CARBO)/PAC in optimal stage III epithelial ovarian cancer (OC): A Gynecologic Oncology Group Trial (GOG 158). *Proc Am Soc Clin Oncol* 18:1373, 1999.

25 Uterine Corpus Malignancies

Adenocarcinoma

Malignant Potential of Positive Peritoneal Cytology in Endometrial Cancer

Hirai Y, Takeshima N, Kato T, et al (Cancer Inst Hosp, Tokyo)
Obstet Gynecol 97:725-728, 2001   25–1

Introduction.—There is controversy regarding the prognostic value of malignant cytology in peritoneal washings obtained from patients with endometrial cancer. The malignant potential of positive peritoneal cytology in endometrial cancer was investigated in a study of 50 patients with endometrial cancer.

Methods.—In a series of 448 patients with clinical stage I-II endometrial cancer treated between 1992 and 1999, 55 patients had peritoneal smears that were diagnosed as positive for malignant cells. In 50 of these patients a tube for cytologic analyses was inserted into the abdominal cavity, and washings were obtained through the tube 7 and 14 days after the operation. The standard operation was completed in all patients, and no residual macroscopic disease was found. No adjuvant therapy was administered until the cytologic collection was completed.

Results.—Washings from 5 patients (10%) showed persistence of positive peritoneal cytology. Included in this group were 4 of 7 patients with adnexal metastasis and 1 of 34 patients with disease confined to the uterus. No patient with nodal disease had positive peritoneal cytology. Overall, no malignant cells were found in 45 of the patients (90%) in any of the washings.

Conclusion.—Endometrial cancer cells found in the peritoneal cavity appear to disappear soon and to have a low malignant potential. In patients with adnexal metastasis, however, the cells may be capable of independent growth and may be associated with intraperitoneal recurrence.

▶ For decades there have been conflicting reports about the significance of peritoneal cytology for the prognostication of early endometrial cancer. Careful analysis has shown that recurrences seen after positive peritoneal cytology is associated with deep myometrial invasion or spread of disease beyond the uterus.[1] These authors finally provide us with a potentially plausible explanation of why peritoneal cytology may be significant in some but not most patients. Unfortunately, the long-term follow-up of these patients is not reported; it would be quite interesting to see whether the presence of persistent positive peritoneal cytology correlated with a worse prognosis.

D. S. Miller, MD

Reference

1. Lurain JR, Rumsey NK, Schink JC, et al: Prognostic significance of positive peritoneal cytology in clinical stage I adenocarcinoma of the endometrium. *Obstet Gynecol* 74:175, 1989.

Local Recurrence in High-Risk Node-Negative Stage I Endometrial Carcinoma Treated With Postoperative Vaginal Vault Brachytherapy
Ng TY, Perrin LC, Nicklin JL, et al (Royal Brisbane Hosp, Queensland, Australia)
Gynecol Oncol 79:490-494, 2000

25–2

Background.—The majority of women with endometrial cancer will have disease that is confined to the uterus; surgery alone will be successful in most of these women. However, some women with stage I disease are at risk for recurrence and might benefit from the use of postoperative adjuvant radiotherapy. The patterns of failure were evaluated after extended surgical staging and postoperative vaginal vault brachytherapy as the only adjuvant treatment in surgical patients with high-risk stage I endometrial carcinoma.

Methods.—In a retrospective evaluation, the records were examined for all patients with endometrial carcinoma who underwent vaginal vault brachytherapy as the only adjuvant treatment from January 1989 to December 1997. Of the total of 489 patients identified, 133 had extended surgical staging. For this report, the final study group consisted of 77 surgical stage I patients with substages IBG3 and any grade IC. Recurrences were recorded as occurring in the vagina, pelvis, or as distant.

Results.—In a mean follow-up interval of 45 months, 11 patients had recurrence (14%). The median time to recurrence was 15 months. The site of recurrence was the vagina in 7 patients and the pelvis in 1 patient, and distant recurrence was seen in 3 patients. Of the 7 vaginal recurrences, 5 occurred within 2 years. All the patients who had distant recurrence died from disease. Isolated recurrences in the vagina in 6 patients were successfully treated with radiotherapy with or without local excision. None of these patients had any evidence of disease at follow-up.

Conclusions.—The most common site of recurrence for patients with high-risk surgical stage I disease treated with postoperative vaginal vault brachytherapy is the vagina, and close follow-up in the first 2 years is critical to the detection of isolated vaginal recurrences. These isolated recurrences were found to be amenable to salvage treatment, with good disease-free survival.

▶ Two large randomized trials addressing the role of adjuvant radiation therapy in early stage endometrial cancer have recently been presented. The Gynecologic Oncology Group has reported but not yet published the results of its trial in completely surgically staged patients who were node negative.[1] The Post Operative Radiation Therapy in Endometrial Carcinoma study group has published its trial in patients with clinical stage 1 cancers who did not undergo lymphadenectomy.[2] Both studies showed that postoperative adjuvant external beam radiation therapy to the pelvis could decrease the risk of pelvic recurrence. However, it had minimal impact on overall survival. The reason for this lack of long-term benefit is obscure but likely relates to altered patterns of recurrence and a small but real number of patients who succumb to treatment complications. In spite of this, many still believe that external beam radiation should be offered. However, a well-informed patient should give pause before accepting this. The obvious conclusion of many is that other modes of adjuvant therapy should be considered, such as vaginal brachytherapy, which has a lower complication rate and excellent results, as seen in this study. Of note, even though a small number of patients did have disease recur in the vagina, most of them were salvaged by external radiation therapy. It has been suggested to our cooperative groups that the next study should have vaginal brachytherapy as the treatment arm.

D. S. Miller, MD

References

1. Roberts JA, Brunetto VL, Keys HM, et al: A phase III randomized study of surgery versus adjunctive radiation therapy in intermediate-risk endometrial carcinoma (GOG 99). *Gynecol Oncol* 68:135 [abstract], 1998.
2. Creutzberg CL, for the PORTEC study group: Surgery and postoperative radiotherapy versus surgery alone for patients with stage 1 endometrial carcinoma: Multicentre randomised trial. *Lancet* 335:1404-1411, 2000

Phase I Trial of Escalating Doses of Paclitaxel Combined With Fixed Doses of Cisplatin and Doxorubicin in Advanced Endometrial Cancer and Other Gynecologic Malignancies: A Gynecologic Oncology Group Study

Fleming GF, Fowler JM, Waggoner SE, et al (Univ of Chicago; Ohio State Univ, Columbus; James Cancer Hosp and Solove Res Inst, Columbus, OH; Univ of Washington, Seattle; et al)
J Clin Oncol 19:1021-1029, 2001   25–3

Introduction.—Paclitaxel, cisplatin, and doxorubicin (TAP combination) are drugs that have proven effective in achieving a response in patients with advanced endometrial cancer. Results are reported for a phase I trial designed to develop a tolerable regimen combining all 3 drugs, with or without granulocyte colony-stimulating factor (G-CSF), in patients with advanced endometrial and other gynecologic cancers.

Methods.—Patients eligible for the trial were chemotherapy naïve, but some had received pelvic radiation therapy (RT). All had a histologically confirmed recurrent or metastatic gynecologic malignancy (with the exception of epithelial ovarian cancer). Also included were patients with bladder cancer that was refractory to or inappropriate for local therapy. Doxorubicin was given as a brief infusion, whereas paclitaxel was administered for 3 hours and cisplatin for 60 minutes. Treatments were repeated every 3 weeks. Cisplatin and doxorubicin were fixed at most dose levels at 60 mg/m² and 45 mg/m², and paclitaxel was escalated in successive cohorts from 90 to 250 mg/m². For dose levels that included G-CSF, it was given as a daily subcutaneous injection at a dose of 5 µg/kg.

Results.—A total of 80 patients received 320 cycles of therapy. When G-CSF was not administered, myelosuppression prevented escalation beyond the starting dose for patients with or without a history of pelvic RT. Neurotoxicity became dose limiting for both groups when G-CSF was added to the regimen. There were major antitumor responses in 6 of 13 patients with measurable endometrial carcinoma and in 8 of 16 with measurable cervical carcinoma. Responses were observed at all dose levels.

Conclusion.—The TAP combination induces significant hematologic toxicity when growth factor support is not used. A marked escalation of the paclitaxel dose could be achieved, however, with addition of G-CSF. Peripheral neurotoxicity was dose limiting for the TAP regimen, but no cases of congestive heart failure were observed. The recommended phase II TAP regimen (paclitaxel 160 mg/m² for 3 hours, doxorubicin 45 mg/m² and cisplatin 60 mg/m², with G-CSF) is suitable for further testing in patients with high-risk, early-stage, and metastatic endometrial cancer.

▶ Until recently, cisplatin and doxorubicin was the gold standard first-line combination chemotherapy regimen for endometrial cancer.[1] Then paclitaxel was found to also have activity.[2] The Gynecologic Oncology Group then undertook this phase I trial in chemotherapy-naïve patients to determine if the 3 active drugs could be combined. This could only be done in therapeutic doses with growth factor support, which made the regimen tolerable and feasible. The response rate in patients with endometrial and cervical cancer were notable. This 3-drug combination was then compared to cisplatin and doxorubicin in the recently completed Gynecologic Oncology Group trial 177 and is now one arm of Gynecologic Oncology Group 189, where it is being compared with sequential megace and tamoxifen for advanced or recurrent endometrial cancer.

D. S. Miller, MD

References

1. Thigpen T, Blessing J, Homsley H, et al: Phase III trial of doxorubicin ± cisplatin in advanced or recurrent endometrial carcinoma: A Gynecologic Oncology Group (GOG) study. *Proc Am Soc Clin Oncol* 12:261 [abstract], 1993.
2. Ball HG, Blessing JA, Lentz SS, et al: A phase II trial of paclitaxel in patients with advanced or recurrent adenocarcinoma of the endometrium. A Gynecologic Oncology Group study. *Gynecol Oncol* 62:278-281, 1996.

Sarcomas

Pathologic Variables and Adjuvant Therapy as Predictors of Recurrence and Survival for Patients With Surgically Evaluated Carcinosarcoma of the Uterus

Yamada SD, Burger RA, Brewster WR, et al (Univ of California, Irvine, Orange)
Cancer 88:2782-2786, 2000   25–4

Objective.—Carcinosarcomas (CSs), the most common uterine sarcomas, have a very poor prognosis. Whether surgical staging provides useful prognostic information is unclear. Pathologic factors associated with extra-uterine disease, recurrence, and survival were retrospectively identified in patients believed to have disease confined to the uterus and who underwent a primary surgical staging procedure.

Methods.—Between 1974 and 1996, 62 patients with CS of the uterus were identified in tumor registries of 3 university hospitals in California and followed for a median of 22 months. Pelvic lymph node dissection was performed in 55 (89%) patients, para-aortic lymph node dissection in 26 (42%), and an omenectomy in 41 (62%). Kaplan-Meier life table analyses were performed to determine the effect of clinical and pathologic variables on recurrence and survival.

Results.—Metastatic disease was diagnosed in 19 (31%) patients who had pelvic lymph node dissection, in 4 (15%) patients who had para-aortic lymph node dissection, and in 8 (20%) of patients who had omenectomy. CS type (homologous or heterologous), carcinoma grade, and carcinoma histology (endometroid or nonendometroid) were not related to extra-uterine disease. During the follow-up period, 43 (55%) patients had a recurrence, 42% of which were extrapelvic. Disease-free and overall survival were significantly affected by the extent of disease. Adjuvant whole pelvic radiotherapy improved the overall survival rates but it did not decrease the risk of pelvic recurrence, nor did it confer a survival advantage on patients with disease confined to the uterine corpus and cervix. Multivariate analysis showed that only the presence of intraperitoneal disease was independently predictive of poor survival.

Conclusion.—Patients with CS pathologically confined to the uterine corpus have a 25% risk of recurrence and death from their disease. Optimal management and adjuvant therapy remain elusive.

▶ CS, also known as malignant mixed müllerian tumor, of the uterus is associated with a worse prognosis than adenocarcinoma of the endometrium. This study confirms the earlier and much larger report of the Gynecologic Oncology Group (GOG) that presumed that early CS shares many of the prognostic factors of adenocarcinoma of the endometrium,[1] but with a higher risk of metastasis. The fact that since 61% of the patients thought to have disease confined to the uterus in fact had metastases provides compelling support for the authors' recommendation of complete surgical staging of all patients with CS.

The higher than expected survival reported by the authors for their patients with disease confined to the uterus is more a testimony to their thorough staging than to better adjuvant therapy. No conclusion could be drawn in this study about adjuvant therapy. We await the results of the randomized GOG study (#150) comparing whole abdomen radiation therapy with ifosfamide and cisplatin combination chemotherapy in patients with completely resected disease.

D. S. Miller, MD

Reference

1. Major FJ, Blessing JA, Silverberg SG, et al: Prognostic factors in early-stage uterine sarcoma: A Gynecologic Oncology Group study. *Cancer* 71:1702, 1993.

Multimodality Therapy for Patients With Clinical Stage I and II Malignant Mixed Müllerian Tumors of the Uterus

Manolitsas TP, Wain GV, Williams KE, et al (Westmead Hosp, Australia; Royal Hosp of Women, Randwick, Australia)
Cancer 91:1437-1443, 2001   25–5

Background.—The value of adjuvant therapy in the treatment of malignant mixed Müllerian tumors (MMMT) of the uterus is still unclear. Outcomes of planned multimodality treatment for patients with apparent early-stage MMMT were reported.

Methods.—Thirty-eight patients with clinical stage I or II disease were offered treatment on a multimodality protocol. Treatment consisted of surgical removal of the uterus, fallopian tubes, and ovaries, plus surgical staging, followed by radiation therapy and chemotherapy with cisplatin and epirubicin.

Findings.—Overall survival was 74%, with a mean follow-up of 55 months. The average length of time to death from disease after diagnosis was 26 months. Patients completing the treatment according to protocol had a survival rate of 95%. Disease-free survival in this subgroup was 90%. Patients not receiving the recommended treatment for various reasons had an overall survival rate of 47%. Survival curve analysis demonstrated a significant survival advantage for patients completing the multimodality protocol.

Conclusion.—In this pilot study, patients receiving multimodality treatment for stage I or II MMMT had an excellent survival rate. A randomized, prospective study of this approach is warranted.

▶ It is expected that 50% of patients with MMMT which appear to be confined to the uterus will have recurrence and die of their malignancy. Adjuvant therapies after surgery given in the form of chemotherapy or radiation therapy have not had a significant impact on overall survival. The 74% overall survival rate (95% for those who completed the therapy) is very encouraging. The current Gynecologic Oncology Group study (No. 150) compares whole abdominal radiation therapy versus chemotherapy with ifosfamide and cisplatin in this group of patients. Not infrequently, cooperative groups are unable to reproduce the encouraging results reported from limited institutions' trials.

D. S. Miller, MD

A Phase III Trial of Ifosfamide With or Without Cisplatin in Carcinosarcoma of the Uterus: A Gynecologic Oncology Group Study

Sutton G, Brunetto VL, Kilgore L, et al (Indiana Univ, Indianapolis; Roswell Park Cancer Inst, Buffalo, NY; Univ of Alabama, Birmingham; et al)
Gynecol Oncol 79:147-153, 2000   25–6

Objective.—Single-agent response rates in the Gynecologic Oncology Group (GOG) phase II and phase III trials were 10% for doxorubicin, 17.9% for cisplatin, and 6.5% for etoposide. A GOG phase II trial reported a response rate of 34.8% for ifosfamide in 23 evaluable patients with uterine carcinosarcoma. The efficacy and toxicity of ifosfamide alone and in combination with cisplatin were evaluated in patients with carcinosarcoma of the uterus in a randomized, nonblinded study.

Methods.—Between February 1989 and July 1996, 102 evaluable patients were treated with ifosfamide (1.5 g/m²/d) and 92 received ifosfamide and cisplatin (20 mg/m²/d) for 5 days every 3 weeks for 8 courses.

Results.—Eighteen patients receiving combination therapy and 31 receiving ifosfamide completed all 8 courses of therapy. Two patients and 1 patient, respectively, received no therapy, 22 and 40 had disease progression, 10 and 5 died, 40 and 23 experienced toxicity or refused further treatment, and 2 and 3 did not complete the study for other reasons. Hematologic, central neurologic, and gastrointestinal effects were the most common adverse events reported by 191 patients. Adverse events were more common and more severe in the combination group. Six deaths may have been treatment-related in the combination group. In the ifosfamide group, 24% had a complete response and 12% had a partial response. The respective percentages in the combination group were 31%

and 23%. Total response depended on site of disease. For pelvis only, lung, and other, respective response rates were 47%, 21%, and 33% for ifosfamide and 61%, 54%, and 40% for the combination. The 5-year survival rate in patients with carcinosarcoma is typically in the range of 50%. Uterine sarcomas apparently have a differential sensitivity to drug therapy. In one study, 25% of patients with metastatic leiomyosarcoma but only 9.8% with carcinosarcoma responded to doxorubicin.

Conclusion.—Combination therapy with ifosfamide and cisplatin is more effective than ifosfamide alone in the treatment of uterine carcinosarcoma, even though most patients experience significant adverse reactions.

▶ The Gynecologic Oncology Group has studied multiple compounds in a phase II setting for activity against advanced carcinosarcoma. Unfortunately, few drugs are effective, with the most active being ifosfamide. Given the activity of ifosfamide-containing combinations against nongynecologic soft-tissue sarcomas, it was logical to combine it with the next-most-active drug, cisplatin, in this randomized trial. Unfortunately, this experience was not reduplicated for uterine carcinosarcomas. Thus, we await the results of further GOG phase II trials as well as the randomized trial of cisplatin with or without paclitaxel (GOG #161).

D. S. Miller, MD

26 Lower Genital Tract Cancers

Radical Hysterectomy

Class II Versus Class III Radical Hysterectomy in Stage IB-IIA Cervical Cancer: A Prospective Randomized Study

Landoni F, Maneo A, Cormio G, et al (Univ of Milan, Italy; Patologia Ostetrica Università di Bari, Italy; Istituto di Scienze Biomediche San Gerardo, Monza, Italy)
Gynecol Oncol 80:3-12, 2000　　　　　　　　　　　　　　　　　　26–1

Background.—Radical hysterectomy, the standard surgical treatment of cervical cancer confined clinically to the cervix and upper vagina in premenopausal patients, varies widely in its radicality among surgeons from different institutions. The impact of the extent of radicality in the surgical treatment of stage IB-IIA cervical carcinoma on survival, relapse pattern, and morbidity was studied.

Methods.—Two hundred forty-three patients with stage IB and IIA cervical cancer were enrolled in the prospective, randomized trial. Two types of radical hysterectomy were compared: class II and class III. Surgical procedures were performed between 1987 and 1993. Two hundred thirty-eight patients were evaluable.

Findings.—The 2 treatment groups were similar in complications unrelated to extent of dissection and in mean postoperative stay. However, late morbidity was 13% in the class II group and 28% in the class III group, a significant difference. Urologic morbidity was especially lower in the former than in the latter group. The recurrence rate and number of patients dying of disease did not differ significantly between the 2 groups. Overall survival rates at 5 years were 81% in the class II and 77% in the class III groups, respectively. Disease-free survival rates were 75% and 73%, respectively. Multivariate analysis confirmed that survival was not associated with type of surgery.

Conclusions.—Class II and class III radical hysterectomies appear to be equally effective in the treatment of stages IB and IIA cervical carcinoma. Class II surgery, however, carries a lower rate of late complications.

▶ The traditional surgical approach to cancer has involved resection of the affected organ with a wide margin of normal tissue and the draining lymph node bed. This approach can result in a primary cure for many but not all patients with organ-confined cancer and minimize the requirement for further treatment with radiation or chemotherapy. In the last century we surgical oncologists learned that more limited and less debilitating operations could still accomplish a successful outcome. This has been most vividly illustrated in those cancers arising from the breast and vulva. It has yet to be shown that this principle can be applied to cervical cancer. The authors are to be congratulated for attempting the first randomized study that addresses this issue. As expected, patients who underwent the less radical procedure had fewer complications. However, conclusions about survival are limited by the fact that more than half of the patients received radiation therapy for reasons not well described in the article. Obviously, the use of radiation therapy in the patients who had the less radical procedure could have obscured the advantage of the more radical procedure. It is well accepted and strongly recommended by our learned authorities that patients with local cervical cancer can be treated with either radical surgery or radical radiation but should not be treated with both because that significantly increases the rate of complications, as was also described here in this article.[1] Unfortunately, this article does not definitively put this issue to rest.

D. S. Miller, MD

Reference

1. Anonymous: National Institutes of Health Consensus Conference on Cervical Cancer. Bethesda, Maryland, April 1-3, 1996. *J Natl Cancer Inst Monogr* 21:1-148, 1996.

The Abandoned Radical Hysterectomy: A Gynecologic Oncology Group Study
Whitney CW, Stehman FB (Thomas Jefferson Univ, Philadelphia; Indiana Univ, Indianapolis)
Gynecol Oncol 79:350-356, 2000
26–2

Introduction.—Radical hysterectomy with pelvic lymphadenectomy is an established treatment for early-stage cervical cancer, but the procedure cannot be completed in some patients because of disease extent or other intraoperative findings. The records of patients for whom the planned radical operation was abandoned were reviewed to determine outcome in terms of recurrence-free interval and survival.

Methods.—Between 1981 and 1984, 33 institutions of the Gynecologic Oncology Group entered 1127 patients with stage IB carcinoma of the cervix in a prospective clinical trial. Eligible patients had invasion of 3 mm or more or lymphatic or capillary-vascular space involvement. Patients were scheduled to undergo laparotomy with radical hysterectomy and bilateral pelvic and para-aortic lymphadenectomy. Radical hysterectomy could be abandoned at operation, however, at the discretion of the treating gynecologic oncologist, who also selected postoperative therapy in such cases.

Results.—In 98 patients, (9%) the radical operation was not completed. Twenty-five of these patients had disease metastatic to para-aortic nodes, and 5 had disease metastatic to other sites. Pelvic extension was present in 26 patients. Sixty-three patients subsequently underwent pelvic radiation therapy and 1 or 2 intracavitary applications. Para-aortic fields were added for the 8 patients with positive para-aortic nodes. Four patients received chemotherapy alone, and 5 were treated with radiotherapy and chemotherapy. The median recurrence-free interval in the "abandoned-hysterectomy" group was only 19 months, versus 84 months or more for the completed-hysterectomy group. Median survival was 22 months for the abandoned-hysterectomy group and 113 months or more for the radical hysterectomy group. Among patients who did not undergo radical hysterectomy, survival was shortest for those with extrapelvic disease and longest for those with direct pelvic extension.

Conclusion.—In this prospective study of patients with stage IB cervical carcinoma, the Gynecologic Oncology Group found that planned radical hysterectomy had to be abandoned in 9% of all patients explored. These patients had a poorer outcome because of the unexpectedly greater extent of their disease.

▶ This study certainly confirms the belief of most gynecologic oncologists that patients whose disease precludes completion of radical hysterectomy have a worse prognosis. As the authors concede in their discussion, no treatment recommendations could be made from their analysis. The following important issues occasionally face the gynecologic oncologist intraoperatively: Should grossly involved lymph nodes be removed? And should the uterus and the cervix with its cancer be removed if the nodes are positive? It is currently our policy to attempt to resect grossly involved lymph nodes. If that can be accomplished, then an attempt is made to clear the primary cervical tumor mass. However, other reasonable practitioners believe that the procedure should be abandoned with the uterus left in situ to optimize radical radiation therapy. Whether the information residing in the Gynecology Oncology Group database can provide us with answers to these questions remains to be determined.

D. S. Miller, MD

Sentinel Lymph Node Mapping

Intraoperative Lymphatic Mapping in Cervix Cancer Patients Undergoing Radical Hysterectomy: A Pilot Study
O'Boyle JD, Coleman RL, Bernstein SG, et al (Univ of Texas, Dallas; Presbyterian Hosp, Dallas; Naval Med Ctr, Portsmouth, Va)
Gynecol Oncol 79:238-243, 2000   26–3

Background.—The feasibility of intraoperative lymphatic mapping and sentinel node identification (SLN) in the treatment of breast cancer and melanoma has been of increasing interest. The utility of these procedures in patients undergoing radical hysterectomy with pelvic lymphadenectomy for treating early cervical cancer was investigated.

Methods and Findings.—Twenty patients with normal-appearing lymph nodes had intracervical injection of isosulfan blue dye at planned radical hysterectomy and bilateral pelvic/low paraortic lymphadenectomy. Forty nodal basins were dissected. SLNs could be identified in 60% of the patients. A total of 23 SLNs were detected in 17 of the 40 dissected basins. Patients with tumors of greater than 4 cm had a lower likelihood of successful SLN identification than patients with tumors of 4 cm or smaller.

Conclusion.—In patients with cervical cancer undergoing radical hysterectomy, SLN identification and intraoperative lymphatic mapping are safe and feasible. In patients with larger tumors, lymphatic dye uptake appears to be less reliable.

▶ The concept that lymphatic flow from an early malignancy will drain to a "sentinel lymph node" which can be identified by a vital dye or radioactive colloid injected in or about the cancer has been substantiated in breast cancer and malignant melanoma. If this lymph node is involved by cancer, that "sentinel lymph node" will determine whether other nodes in the region might be involved and thus indicate a regional lymphadenectomy. If that node shows no cancer, then no further lymph node removal is required. For breast cancer and melanoma, this can result in a significant decrease in limb morbidity caused by chronic lymphadema and or lymphangitis. This concept is also becoming accepted for vulvar cancer where inguinal lymphadenectomy is associated with significant short- and long-term complications.[1]

This study shows that lymphatic mapping in cervical cancer patients undergoing radical hysterectomy is feasible and does not miss cancerous lymph nodes. The fact that it was more difficult to accomplish in larger tumors, which have a higher risk of lymph node metastases, is worrisome. If larger studies—especially with the addition or substitution of lymphoscintigraphy—are confirmatory, then this could lead to the laparoscopic identification of lymph node metastases and the appropriate triage of patients between radical surgery and radiation.[2]

R. D. Arias, MD

References

1. DeHullu JA, Hollema H, Piers DS, et al: Sentinel lymph node procedure is highly accurate in squamous cell carcinoma of the vulva. *J Clin Oncol* 18:2811, 2000.
2. Dargent D, Martin X, Mathevet P: Laparoscopic assessment of the sentinel lymph node in early stage cervical cancer. *Gynecol Oncol* 79:411, 2000.

Laparoscopic Assessment of the Sentinel Lymph Node in Early Stage Cervical Cancer

Dargent D, Martin X, Mathevet P (Université Claude Bernard, Lyon, France)
Gynecol Oncol 79:411-415, 2000   26–4

Introduction.—Systematic lymphadenectomy has long prevailed in the management of cervical cancer, but this procedure would not be required if the sentinel lymph node is determined to be negative. Preliminary results of a minimally invasive technique that allows the sentinel node to be identified in patients with early-stage cervical cancer were reported.

Methods.—The study enrolled 35 patients between October 1998 and January 2000. Disease stage was IA2 in 4 cases, IB1 in 22 cases, and IB2 or higher in 9 cases. Evaluation of the sentinel node was performed as the first step of the systematic pelvic lymphadenectomy. Patients with negative pelvic nodes had either a Schauta procedure (16 cases) or a radical trachelectomy (12 cases). A radical abdominal hysterectomy was performed if 1 or 2 pelvic nodes were involved (3 cases). The dose of patent blue violet (PBV) injected around the tumor was initially 2 mL but was increased to 4 mL because of a high failure rate. A 22-gauge spinal needle was used to administer the dye. When a blue-dyed lymph node (BDLN) was immediately obvious, this node was dissected and removed. Total results are based on 69 pelvic dissections, 68 performed by laparoscopy and 1 by laparotomy.

Results.—One or more BDLN was apparent in 59 of 69 dissections. The failure rate was related to quantity of injected blue dye; when 1.5 mL or less was injected the rate was 50%, but with injection of 4 mL, only 4 (10%) of 45 of BDLN were not identified. Fifty-three of 63 BDLN were located in contact with the external iliac vein, lateral to the inferior vesical artery and ventral to the origin of the uterine artery. The BDLN was likely to be the sentinel node. In the 48 cases with an uninvolved BDLN, the other nodes were uninvolved too. And in 11 cases with 1 or more lymph nodes involved, the BDLN was invariably involved.

Conclusion.—Use of PBV can dye the lymphatic fluid rising from the cervix into the vessels that drain into the lymph nodes in 89% of cases. A dose of at least 2 mL of injected PBV is required, and it is better to inject directly into the cervix than lateral to it. If additional studies confirm the sensitivity of the BDLN to be 100%, this laparoscopic approach could reduce the aggressiveness of local treatment.

▶ These authors describe the next step in sentinel lymph node approach to cervical cancer. The potential advantage of this technique in cervical cancer is not that the lymphadenectomy is particularly morbid, but that the sentinel lymph node procedure can identify patients with positive lymph nodes undetected by preoperative workup, and that identification does not require a laparotomy. Thus, the patient can be triaged to radiation therapy without the added morbidity of a laparotomy incision. Similar to the laparotomy, in these authors' experience, laparoscopic assessment of the sentinel lymph node was feasible and had a high sensitivity.

D. S. Miller, MD

Non Squamous Cervical Cancers

The Rising Incidence of Adenocarcinoma Relative to Squamous Cell Carcinoma of the Uterine Cervix in the United States—A 24-Year Population-based Study
Smith HO, Tiffany MF, Qualls CR, et al (Univ of New Mexico Health Sciences Ctr, Albuquerque)
Gynecol Oncol 78:97-105, 2000

26–5

Introduction.—Since the 1970s, the incidence of adenocarcinoma relative to squamous cell carcinoma of the uterine cervix has increased, although the incidence of all cervical cancer continues to decline. The SEER (Surveillance, Epidemiology, and End Results) Cancer Incidence database was used to compare the age-adjusted incidence and survival for invasive adenocarcinoma with the same factors for squamous cell carcinoma of the uterine cervix.

Methods.—Between 1973 and 1996, the SEER database recorded a total of 28,975 cases of invasive carcinoma of the uterine cervix, including 21,434 of squamous cell carcinoma and 4650 of adenocarcinoma. Within specified time periods, the age-adjusted incidence, absolute counts, and population of women at risk were extracted. Stage was defined as localized, regional, or distant.

Results.—During the 24-year period, the age-adjusted incidence rates per 100,000 for all invasive cervical cancers decreased by 36.9% (from 12.35 for 1973-1977 to 7.79 for 1993-1996). A similarly large decline (41.9%) was seen in the age-adjusted incidence rates for squamous cell carcinoma (from 9.45 for 1973-1977 to 5.49 for 1993-1996). But for adenocarcinoma, the age-adjusted incidence rates increased by 29.1% during the 2 periods (from 1.34 to 1.73). And the change in the percentage of adenocarcinoma relative to all cervical cancer increased from 10.8% between 1973 and 1997 to 22.4% between 1993 and 1996 (an increase of 107.4%). Thus, the proportion of adenocarcinoma increased relative to both total cases of invasive cervical cancer and for cases of squamous cell

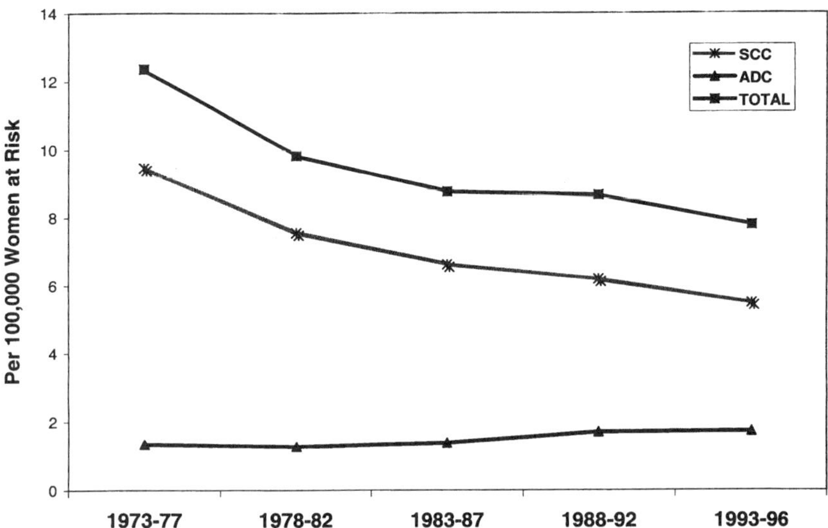

FIGURE 1.—The age-adjusted incidence rates (per 100,000) for invasive ADC (adenocarcinoma), SCC (squamous cell carcinoma), and total (all invasive cervical cancers inclusive of all histologic types) decreased 37% [12.35 (1973-1977) vs 7.7 (1993-1996)]; decreased 41.9% [9.45 (1973-1977) vs 5.49 (1993-1996)], and increased 29.1% [1.34 (1973-1977) vs 1.73 (1993-1996)], respectively. The proportion of ADC is increasing relative to total and SCC cases. (Courtesy of Smith HO, Tiffany MF, Qualls CR, et al: The rising incidence of adenocarcinoma relative to squamous cell carcinoma of the uterine cervix in the United States—A 24-year population-based study. *Gynecol Oncol* 78:97-105, 2000.)

carcinoma (Fig 1). The observed survival rates for adenocarcinoma compared with squamous cell carcinoma were poorer for regional disease.

Conclusion.—Although the incidence of all cervical cancer and squamous cell carcinoma continues to decline in the United States, the proportion of adenocarcinoma has doubled. Because of screening, carcinoma in situ is now more common than invasive cancer. But current screening practices may be insufficient to detect a significant proportion of adenocarcinoma precursor lesions.

▶ Over the last 30 years, we have seen a 40% decrease in the incidence of all invasive cervical cancers. This has been attributed to the widespread, but not universal, availability of Pap smears in developed countries. During this time, many authors have noted that as the number of cervical cancers decreased, the proportion of adenocarcinomas making up those seen has increased. It has been presumed that this is caused by the fact that the squamous precursor is much more easily detected by the Pap smear than the glandular precursor. The authors show that, in fact, there has been a 29% increase in the reported incidence of adenocarcinoma whereas the incidence of squamous cervical cancers and all cervical cancers has decreased. As seen in Fig 1, the absolute numbers are less alarming than the percentages. Press reports on this article suggest that this was caused by a defect in present Pap smear technology. That very well may be true, but no data are presented to substantiate or refute that assertion. It is probably just as likely that Pap smear screening allows for identification of squamous cell cancer precursors that can be successfully treated while preserving the cervix. Thus leaving more cervices at risk to develop adenocarcinomas. Another plausible explanation conceded by the authors in their discussion but with the data not shown, is that the increase in invasive adenocarcinomas "may also in part reflect an increase in the recognition (by pathologists) of cases with glandular elements as adenocarcinomas." Because the proportion of nonsquamous carcinomas was 23% in the 70s compared with 29% in the 90s, this article and others[1] illustrates the limitation of the data available on the SEER database.

D. S. Miller, MD

Reference

1. Fanning J, Gangestad A, Andrews SJ: National Cancer Data Base/Surveillance Epidemiology and End Results: Potential insensitive-measure bias. *Gynecol Oncol* 77(3):450-453, 2000.

Prospective Management of Stage IA$_1$ Cervical Adenocarcinoma by Conization Alone to Preserve Fertility: A Preliminary Report
Schorge JO, Lee KR, Sheets EE (Harvard Med School, Boston)
Gynecol Oncol 78:217-220, 2000   26–6

Objective.—Because evidence shows that an early invasive adenocarcinoma acts the same way as a squamous carcinoma, nonradical surgery may be an option for some patients with microinvasive disease. Preliminary experience with prospective treatment of stage IA$_1$ cervical adenocarcinomas in women who want to preserve their fertility is reported.

Methods.—Since 1998, at Brigham and Women's Hospital, women who wanted to preserve their fertility and who had a microscopic lesion ($\leq$3 mm invasive depth, $\leq$7 mm tumor width) and a conization specimen including the entire lesion with negative margins were eligible for cold knife conization (CKC) and surveillance.

Results.—Five women, aged 26 to 33 years, of 6 with stage IA cervical adenocarcinomas elected to undergo CKC. All had adenocarcinoma in situ, and none had lymph-vascular space invasion. One patient had 2 CKCs for adenocarcinoma in situ for persistently positive margins. One conization specimen showed deeply invasive adenocarcinoma. A second conization showed no residual disease. Three conization specimens had negative margins. None had recurrent disease during 6 to 20 months of follow-up.

Conclusion.—Patients with stage IA adenocarcinoma of the cervix may be safely treated by CKC and careful follow-up.

▶ A definition of microinvasive adenocarcinoma has been proposed.[1] Retrospective studies have shown that it rarely metastasizes or recurs.[2] As is done for squamous cancers, nonradical surgery has been proposed as a treatment option for the earliest detectable lesion. The authors from the Brigham and Women's Hospital in Boston prospectively treated 5 young women with International Federation of Gynecology and Obstetrics stage IA$_1$ cervical adenocarcinoma by conization alone. All strongly desired to preserve their fertility and were carefully followed up without evidence of disease recurrence for 6 to 20 months. This article supports the conservative treatment of highly motivated patients. However, a larger number of patients will be required to confirm the safety of this approach, preferably in a multicenter trial.

D. S. Miller, MD

References

1. Ostor A, Rome R, Quinn M: Microinvasive adenocarcinoma of the cervix: A clinicopathologic study of 77 women. *Obstet Gynecol* 89:88-93, 1997.
2. Schorge JO, Lee KR, Flynn CE, et al: Stage IA cervical adenocarcinoma: Definition and treatment. *Obstet Gynecol* 93:219, 1999.

Multimodality Therapy in Early-Stage Neuroendocrine Carcinoma of the Uterine Cervix

Boruta DM II, Schorge JO, Duska LA, et al (Brigham and Women's Hosp, Boston; Massachusetts Gen Hosp, Boston)
Gynecol Oncol 81:82-87, 2001   26–7

Background.—Mortality is high in patients with early-stage neuroendocrine cervical carcinoma (NECC), despite aggressive treatment. Because this tumor is rare, randomized, prospective studies cannot be conducted. One experience with NECC and a meta-analysis were reported.

Methods.—Eleven women underwent surgery and chemotherapy for NECC between 1978 and 1998 at the authors' center. In addition, 23 patients with early-stage NECC treated similarly and reported in the literature were identified. The median patient age was 37 years, and the median cervical tumor diameter was 3.2 cm.

Findings.—These 34 patients had an overall survival rate of 38% at 2 years. Women with lymph node metastases had a poor prognosis. Postoperative platinum and etoposide as well as vincristine, doxorubicin, and cyclophosphamide (VAC) therapy correlated with increased survival.

Conclusion.—Neuroendocrine cervical carcinoma is a very lethal form of cervical cancer. The most important prognostic factor appears to be lymph node metastasis. Postoperative chemotherapy with VAC or platinum and etoposide may improve a patient's chances for survival.

▶ NECC is a rare tumor with a very high mortality rate. The rarity of this problem precludes prospective clinical trials. Thus, the authors of this retrospective analysis have combined their own data with other published reports to identify prognostic factors and determine optimal multimodality therapy for early stage (IB-IIA) disease. The presence of lymph node metastasis was common in this population (52%) and was the sole prognostic factor iden-tified. Accordingly, the authors advocate complete pelvic and para-aortic node dissection and make a compelling argument for radical surgery fol-lowed by 4 to 6 cycles of adjuvant platinum and etoposide as optimal multimodality therapy for early-stage NECC, albeit based upon retrospective data.

D. S. Miller, MD

Prognostic Variables

Comparison of Clinical Outcome in Black and White Women Treated With Radiotherapy for Cervical Carcinoma
Grigsby PW, Hall-Daniels L, Baker S, et al (Washington Univ, St Louis)
Gynecol Oncol 79:354-361, 2000   26–8

Introduction.—The current United States mortality rate for cervical cancer in African-American women is twice that of white women, according to the American Cancer Society. The National Cancer Institute's Surveillance, Epidemiology, and End Result program reports a significant difference in cervical cancer survival for white versus African-American women. The American College of Surgeons has reported that the 8-year cumulative survival was poorer for African-American women versus white or Hispanic women. The significance of race on the cancer-specific survival outcome was examined in women treated with radiotherapy for advanced-stage cancer of the uterine cervix.

Methods.—Medical records of 922 women with cancer of the uterine cervix who were treated between 1959 and 1993 with radiotherapy were examined. The policy of the Mallinckrodt Institute of Radiology is to treat all patients, regardless of ability to pay. Women from all socioeconomic backgrounds were selected. There were 576 women with clinical stage II cancer and 346 with clinical stage III cancer. All women were treated by using standard medical care treatment policies according to disease stage. Data were examined by race and known treatment-related prognostic factors. Overall and cancer-specific survivals were calculated.

Results.—Five-year cancer-specific survivals for clinical stage II disease was 66% for white women and 61% for African-American women ($P = .56$). Corresponding 5-year overall survivals were 60% and 51%, respectively ($P = .02$). Five-year cancer-specific for clinical stage III disease were 38% and 47%, respectively ($P = .34$). Associated 5-year overall survivals were 32% and 40%, respectively ($P = .37$). No differences in treatment-related factors were observed. The only 2 independently significant variables were clinical disease stage and overall treatment time.

Conclusion.—Multivariate analysis showed that clinical stage and overall treatment time are significant variables impacting the control of tumor by radiotherapy in patients with stages II and III cervical carcinoma. Race was not an independent prognostic factor in this cohort. It is likely that African-American women had more advanced disease at diagnosis.

▶ Several large population-based cancer studies have previously reported that black women with cervical cancer have a worse mortality. These authors from the Mallinckrodt Institute of Radiology in St. Louis found that in a population where all patients were treated the same the outcome of black women compared with other races were equivalent in terms of cancer-specific survival. Likely the difference in overall survival between the patients seen in this and other studies had to do with more advanced stage at presentation and comorbidities. Similar results have also been recently reported from the United States Military Health Care System.[1]

D. S. Miller, MD

Reference

1. Farley JH. Hines JF, Taylor RR, et al: Equal care ensures equal survival for African-American women with cervical carcinoma. *Cancer* 91:869, 2001.

The Significance of Thrombocytosis in Patients With Locally Advanced Cervical Carcinoma: A Gynecologic Oncology Group Study

Hernandez E, Donohue KA, Anderson LL, et al (MCP-Hahnemann School of Medicine, Phildelphia; Gynecologic Oncology Group Statistical Office, Buffalo, NY; Indiana Univ, Indianapolis)
Gynecol Oncol 78:137-142, 2000

26–9

Background.—Thrombocytosis is detected at diagnosis in about one third of patients with cancer. Seventeen percent of patients with cervical carcinoma reportedly have thrombocytosis. The incidence of thrombocytosis and its impact on survival probability in women with locally advanced cervical carcinoma were studied.

Methods and Findings.—Two hundred ninety-four patients with stages IIB to IVA cervical carcinoma without periaortic node metastasis were treated with standardized radiation therapy and concurrent hydroxyurea or misonidazole. Thirty percent of the patients had thrombocytosis, defined as a platelet count exceeding 400×10^9/L. The chance of dying was 55% greater in patients without extrapelvic disease and with thrombocytosis than in those without thrombocytosis. Patients with thrombocytosis had larger tumors. In addition, bilateral parametrial involvement was more common in patients with thrombocytosis.

Conclusion.—Thrombocytosis is common among patients with advanced cervical carcinoma. It appears to be associated with tumor burden. Among patients with locally advanced cervical carcinoma and negative pelvic nodes, patients with thrombocytosis had a worse survival.

▶ It has been long recognized that thrombocytosis and thromboembolism can be harbingers of an occult cancer. This study and others have shown thrombocytosis to be a marker for tumor burden. However, thrombocytosis may also play a role in tumor growth or progression. Drugs which interfere with platelet activation such as aspirin, nonsteroidal anti-inflammatory drugs, and COX 2 inhibitors are being tested in colon cancer prevention trials. The interesting finding in this study is that thrombocytosis was more predictive in the patients with negative lymph nodes, suggesting a possible role for platelets in lymph node metastases.

D. S. Miller, MD

Cervical Cancer Chemotherapy

A Phase II Study of Topotecan in Patients With Squamous Cell Carcinoma of the Cervix: A Gynecologic Oncology Group Study
Muderspach LI, Blessing JA, Levenback C, et al (Univ of Southern California, Los Angeles; Roswell Park Cancer Inst, Buffalo, NY; Univ of Texas, Houston; et al)
Gynecol Oncol 81:213-215, 2001

26–10

Introduction.—The treatment of advanced cervical cancer with chemotherapeutic agents has achieved only limited success. Cisplatin is the most effective agent thus far, but other alternatives and combinations are needed. In a multicenter phase II study, the toxicity and activity of IV topotecan were assessed in patients with advanced, recurrent, or persistent squamous cell carcinoma of the uterine cervix.

Methods.—Forty-nine women were enrolled in the study during 1994 and 1995. All patients had not responded to primary surgical or radiation therapy, had not been treated with chemotherapy (aside from chemosensitizing agents used in conjunction with radiotherapy), and were not candidates for curative therapy. Intravenous topotecan was administered at 1.5 mg/m² per day for 5 consecutive days every 4 weeks, a regimen based on data from ovarian cancer studies. Dose levels were reduced for hematologic toxicity. Treatment was continued until disease progressed or adverse effects were intolerable.

Results.—Forty-three patients were evaluable for response. The median age of the group was 44 years, and most patients (88.4%) had previously received radiation therapy. A median of 2 courses (range, 1-14 cycles) was administered per patient. Three patients (7.0%) were complete responders and 5 (11.6%) partial responders. The median progression-free survival was 2.4 months; median overall survival was 6.4 months. Adverse effects included grade 4 neutropenia and grade 4 thrombocytopenia (68% and 18% of patients, respectively). Nonhematologic toxic effects were infrequent and not dose limiting.

Conclusion.—Topotecan could be administered with acceptable toxicity to patients with advanced, recurrent, or persistent squamous cell carcinoma of the cervix. The activity of topotecan in this setting was considered moderate, and the drug may be of potential use as a radiation sensitizing agent or in combination with cisplatin.

► As discussed last year, topotecan has shown modest but significant activity against advanced squamous cell carcinoma of the cervix in patients who have been previously treated with chemotherapy (see 2001 YEAR BOOK

OF OBSTETRICS, GYNECOLOGY, AND WOMEN'S HEALTH, pp 491-492). Thus, the next step was to evaluate topotecan in chemotherapy-naïve patients to determine its best role in advanced cervical cancer. As described here, even in the first-line setting, topotecan showed moderate activity that is of interest because topotecan may potentiate the activity of cisplatin through inhibition of DNA repair. Cisplatin is the most active drug yet identified against metastatic cervical carcinoma. Currently the Gynecologic Oncology Group is conducting a trial (#179) comparing topotecan and cisplatin versus cisplatin alone.

D. S. Miller, MD

Paclitaxel, an Active Agent in Nonsquamous Carcinomas of the Uterine Cervix: A Gynecologic Oncology Group Study
Curtin JP, Blessing JA, Webster KD, et al (Cornell Univ, New York; New York Univ; Roswell Park Cancer Inst, Buffalo, NY; et al)
J Clin Oncol 19:1275-1278, 2001   26–11

Introduction.—With improved drug supplies and broadening of phase II trials, interest has grown in the use of paclitaxel in patients with advanced or recurrent metastatic cancer of the cervix. A phase II trial was initiated in patients with advanced nonsquamous carcinoma of the cervix to determine its activity in patients who fail standard chemotherapy.

Methods.—All patients had at least 1 measurable lesion. The beginning dose of paclitaxel was 170 mg/m² (135 mg/m² in patients with prior pelvic radiation) administered as a 24-hour continuous IV infusion. Courses were repeated every 3 weeks. Dose escalations to 200 mg/m² and de-escalations to 110 mg/m² were adjusted as needed due to adverse effects.

Results.—Of 42 assessable patients, 4 had a complete response and 9 had a partial response (overall response rate was 31%). The main and dose-limiting toxicity was neutropenia.

Conclusion.—The response rate to paclitaxel is superior to that of other single agents in nonsquamous carcinoma of the cervix.

▶ Paclitaxel is approved by the Food and Drug Administration for the treatment of ovarian, breast and non-small cell lung cancer. It has also shown activity, against endometrial and squamous cancers of the cervix. Given that spectrum of activity, it was natural to test paclitaxel against nonsquamous cancers of the cervix that now account for more than 20% of cervical cancers. The 31% response rate is notable and better than that reported in the previous gynecologic oncology group experience. The next step should be combining paclitaxel with cisplatin in a phase II or III setting.

D. S. Miller, MD

Vulvar Cancers

Sentinel Lymph Node Procedure Is Highly Accurate in Squamous Cell Carcinoma of the Vulva

De Hullu JA, Hollema H, Piers DA, et al (Univ Hosp Groningen, The Netherlands; Vrije Universiteit, Amsterdam)
J Clin Oncol 18:2811-2816, 2000

26–12

Background.—Current standard treatment for early-stage squamous cell carcinoma of the vulva includes wide local excision and unilateral or bilateral inguinofemoral lymphadenectomy through different incisions. Inguinofemoral lymphadenectomy is generally considered beneficial for patients with nodes that clinically suggest metastasis, but it may not benefit those without clinically suggestive lymph nodes, of whom only about 20% will have lymph node metastasis. The diagnostic accuracy of the sentinel lymph node procedure in patients with squamous cell carcinoma of the vulva was investigated.

Methods.—Fifty-nine patients underwent a total of 107 inguinofemoral lymphadenectomies at the authors' center between 1996 and 1999. The combined technique used consisted of preoperative lymphoscintigraphy with ^{99m}Tc-labeled nanocolloid and intraoperative blue dye. Sentinel nodes that were negative at routine pathologic assessment were examined again with step sectioning and immunohistochemistry.

Findings.—Routine histopathologic evaluation identified lymph node metastases in 27 groins. The sentinel lymph node procedure identified all of these nodes. A negative sentinel lymph node had a negative predictive value of 100%. Step sectioning and immunohistochemistry detected another 4 metastases in 102 sentinel nodes judged to be negative on routine histopathology.

Conclusion.—Sentinel lymph node procedures using the combined technique accurately predict inguinofemoral node status in patients with early-stage cancer of the vulva. Step sectioning and immunohistochemistry slightly increase the sensitivity of this procedure.

▶ Vulvar cancer is the gynecologic malignancy best suited for the application of the sentinel lymph node biopsy technique. The draining lymph node bed is separate from the primary tumor. Metastases to lymph nodes are occasional. Thus, lymphadenectomy is not beneficial to most patients. The consequences of the lymphadenectomy may be quite morbid in terms of chronic lymphangitis and lymphedema. The avoidance of lymphadenectomy in patients whose groins are without cancer would offer a significant improvement in quality of life. The 100% negative predictive value is very encouraging. The Gynecologic Oncology Group has instituted a similar study, No. 173, which hopefully will confirm these results.

D. S. Miller, MD

Preoperative Chemo-Radiation for Carcinoma of the Vulva With N2/N3 Nodes: A Gynecologic Oncology Group Study
Montana GS, Thomas GM, Moore DH, et al (Duke Univ, Durham, NC; Univ of Toronto; Indiana Univ, Indianapolis; et al)
Int J Radiat Oncol Biol Phys 48:1007-1013, 2000   26–13

Background.—The extent of surgery done for advanced carcinoma of the vulva depends on disease extent at the primary site, adjacent organ involvement, and lymph node status. The efficacy of lymph node and primary tumor resection following chemoradiation was determined for patients with carcinoma of the vulva with N2/N3 lymph nodes.

Methods.—Forty-six patients underwent a split course of radiation, 4760 cGy, to the primary site and lymph nodes. Chemotherapy with cisplatin and 5-fluorouracil was given concurrently, and surgery followed.

Findings.—Eight patients did not complete all treatment. After chemoradiation, lymph node disease was resectable in 38 of 40 patients. Two patients did not have surgery because of pulmonary metastasis. Lymph node specimens were negative histologically in 15 of 37 patients. Recurrent or metastatic disease developed in 19 patients. Failure occurred in the primary area only in 9 patients, the lymph node area only in 1, and the primary area with distant metastasis in 1. Eight patients had distant metastases only. Local control of lymph node disease was achieved in 36 of 37 patients and in the primary area in 29 of 38 patients. Treatment-related complications were fatal for 2 patients.

Conclusion.—In these patients with vulvar carcinoma and N2/N3 nodes, preoperative chemoradiation yielded high rates of resectablity and local control of lymph nodes. Further research is needed to determine the best combination of chemotherapy, radiation therapy, and surgery for this patient population.

▶ The most frustrating challenge in vulvar cancer is that of delay. The average time from the onset of symptoms until diagnosis is over 1 year. Half the time that is the patient's doing and half the time a physician has contributed to the delay. Thus, it is not surprising that some patients will be seen with locally advanced disease accompanied by unresectable inguinal lymph nodes. The traditional approach with primary radical surgery has had little to offer these patients, and their outcome was dismal. The use of radiation or chemotherapy alone may have provoked a response but usually did not clear the groin of cancer. While the treatment reported here was morbid, it was tolerable. The treatment allowed for surgical resection of the tumor in most cases and a durable survival in a significant minority. Clearly, further evaluation of this treatment strategy is indicated. The Gynecologic Oncology Group is currently evaluating chemoradiation in the adjuvant setting for patients with positive inguinal nodes (GOG No. 185).

D. S. Miller, MD

27 Cancer Survivorship

Hormone Replacement

Estrogen Replacement Therapy in Endometrial Cancer Patients: A Matched Control Study

Suriano KA, McHale M, McLaren CE, et al (Kaiser Permanente-Anaheim Med Ctr, Calif; Chao Family Comprehensive Cancer Ctr, Orange, Calif; Univ of California, Orange; et al)
Obstet Gynecol 97:555-560, 2001

27–1

Introduction.—Clinicians have historically withheld hormone replacement therapy (HRT) in patients with endometrial cancer based on the theoretic risk that occult or quiescent foci of disease could be stimulated by administration of estrogen. No data support this practice. In fact, 3 retrospective series with a total of 53 patients have not demonstrated an increased incidence of recurrent disease among patients exposed to exog-

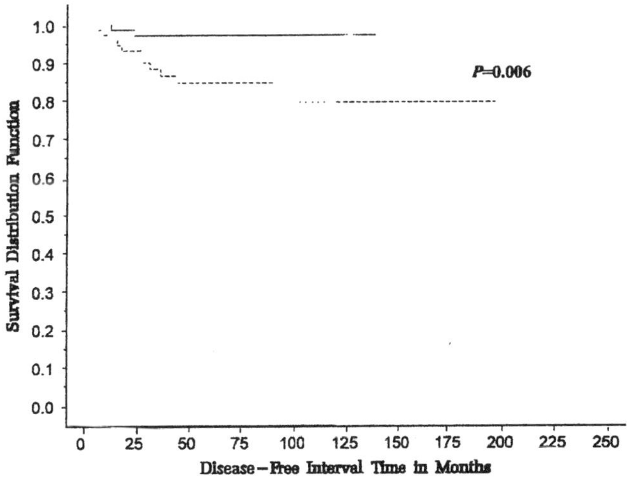

FIGURE 1.—Kaplan-Meier survival curve comparing the disease-free intervals of estrogen users and nonusers (N = 150). *Solid line* = estrogen users; *dotted line* = nonusers. (Courtesy of Suriano KA, McHale M, McLaren CE, et al: Estrogen replacement therapy in endometrial cancer patients: A matched control study. *Obstet Gynecol* 97:555-560, 2001, reprinted with permission from the American College of Obstetricians and Gynecologists.)

enous estrogen. The risk of recurrence and mortality was examined in a retrospective cohort of patients with a history of endometrial cancer.

Methods.—Among 249 women with surgical stage I, II, or III endometrial cancer treated from 1984 to 1998, 130 received HRT after primary cancer treatment; 49% received progesterone in addition to estrogen. Seventy-five matched treatment control pairs were identified in the cohort. The groups were matched using decade of age at diagnosis and disease stage. Groups were similar in parity, tumor grade, depth of invasion, histology, surgical treatment, lymph node status, postoperative radiation, and concurrent diseases. The cohorts were followed for number of recurrences and deaths from disease.

Results.—Patients in the HRT group were followed for a mean of 83 months, and control subjects were followed for a mean of 69 months. Two in 75 HRT users (1%) and 11/75 control subjects (14%) had recurrent disease. Hormone users versus nonusers had a significantly longer disease-free interval ($P = .006$) (Fig 1).

Conclusion.—Rates of recurrent disease and death do not seem to be increased among patients who have survived endometrial cancer.

▶ Controversy exists about treating postmenopausal women with a history of breast or endometrial cancer with HRT because the growth of both these tumors can be stimulated by estrogen. Clinical evidence of persistent endometrial cancer usually appears within a year or 2 after initial therapy. Therefore, if a woman treated for endometrial cancer has no evidence of disease 2 or more years after treatment, it appears that use of HRT has not been harmful. The results of this retrospective study suggest that initiation of HRT soon after treatment of endometrial cancer does not increase the rate of recurrence of disease. Clinicians can use the data from this study when they counsel women treated for endometrial cancer about the benefits and risks of HRT.

D. R. Mishell, Jr, MD

▶ This study, too, confronts dogma. While the link between hormones and breast cancer is controversial, it is more clearly evident with endometrial cancer. If that cancer is successfully treated, then will the estrogen replacement have an adverse effect? The concern is not so much that there would be an induction of a recurrence that would not normally happen, but that the time to an already destined recurrence would be accelerated. This was not seen. As these authors have shown in their case-control study, there appeared to be a benefit: an advantage for the patients who took estrogen replacement therapy. We obviously await confirmative trials. However, that may be some time, as the Gynecologic Oncology Group trial of hormone replacement therapy for endometrial cancer survivors is expected to accrue over 1000 patients and is several years from completion.

D. S. Miller, MD

Hormone Replacement Therapy After a Diagnosis of Breast Cancer in Relation to Recurrence and Mortality

O'Meara ES, Rossing MA, Daling JR, et al (Univ of Washington, Seattle)
J Natl Cancer Inst 93:754-762, 2001   27–2

Background.—Clinicians generally do not prescribe hormone replacement therapy (HRT) for women with a history of breast cancer out of concern that estrogen will stimulate recurrence. The impact of HRT on recurrence and mortality after breast cancer diagnosis was studied.

Methods.—Data on 2755 women, aged 35 to 74 years, enrolled in a large HMO were included in the analysis. All had been diagnosed as having incident invasive breast cancer between 1977 and 1994. Pharmacy records showed that 174 women used HRT after diagnosis. Each woman using HRT was matched to 4 randomly selected HRT nonusers by age, disease stage, and year of diagnosis. Women were recurrence free at the start of HRT or at the equivalent time since diagnosis.

Findings.—The breast cancer recurrence rate was 17 per 1000 person-years in HRT users after diagnosis and 30 per 1000 person-years in nonusers (Table 4). Rates of death from breast cancer were 5 per 1000 person-years in HRT users and 15 per 1000 person-years in nonusers. Total mortality rates were 16 and 30 per 1000 person-years in the HRT and non-HRT groups, respectively. Any type of HRT preparation was associated with relatively low rates of recurrence and death. Increased HRT dose was not associated with a trend toward lower relative risks.

Conclusion.—The risks of recurrence of and mortality from breast cancer were lower in women who used HRT after their cancer diagnosis than in those who did not. Such use of HRT did not adversely affect recurrence and mortality.

▶ The results of this large case-control study of women previously treated for breast cancer who were clinically free of recurrence suggest that the use of exogenous estrogen orally or vaginally has no adverse effect on the rate of recurrence or mortality from breast cancer. These results agree with those found in small case series and cohort comparison studies which also have shown no adverse effect of HRT upon the rate of breast cancer recurrence. No randomized control trials have been performed to more accurately study the effect of HRT upon women with a prior history of breast cancer. Therefore, clinicians should inform women that all the currently available data indicate that there is no evidence that use of estrogen by disease-free women with a prior history of breast cancer has an adverse effect upon the rate of recurrence of the disease.

D. R. Mishell, Jr, MD

▶ As discussed last year, the issue of offering HRT to survivors of cancers arising in endocrine organs or end organs is very controversial and associated with strong feelings, strong dogma, and few data (see 2001 YEAR BOOK OF OBSTETRICS, GYNECOLOGY, AND WOMEN'S HEALTH, pp 469). Fortunately, some

TABLE 4.—Recurrence of Breast Cancer in Relation to the Use of Hormone Replacement Therapy After a Diagnosis of Breast Cancer (Group Health Cooperative, 1977-1996)

	Person-Years	No. of Recurrences	Rate Per 1000 Person-Years* (95% CI)	Unadjusted Relative Risk† (95% CI)	Adjusted Relative Risk‡ (95% CI)
Any HRT					
Never	3356	101	30 (25 to 37)	1 (referent)	1 (referent)
Ever	916	16	17 (11 to 29)	0.58 (0.34 to 0.98)	0.50 (0.30 to 0.85)
Unopposed estrogens only§					
Never	2690	81	30 (24 to 37)	1 (referent)	1 (referent)
Ever	770	14	18 (11 to 31)	0.60 (0.34 to 1.07)	0.51 (0.28 to 0.93)
Estrogen with ≥ 1 cycle of progestogen§					
Never	475	15	32 (19 to 52)	1 (referent)	1 (referent)
Ever	121	2	17 (4 to 66)	0.53 (0.12 to 2.30)	0.42 (0.15 to 1.22)
Oral HRT‖					
Never	1750	46	26 (20 to 35)	1 (referent)	1 (referent)
Ever	453	8	18 (9 to 35)	0.67 (0.32 to 1.42)	0.57 (0.28 to 1.16)
Duration, mo¶					
0	1792	46	26 (19 to 34)	1 (referent)	1 (referent)
1-2	213	3	14 (5 to 44)	0.55 (0.17 to 1.77)	0.41 (0.14 to 1.23)
≥13	195	5	26 (11 to 62)	1.00 (0.40 to 2.52)	0.91 (0.37 to 2.23)
Dose, mg¶,**					
0	1792	46	26 (19 to 34)	1 (referent)	1 (referent)
>0-225	206	4	19 (7 to 52)	0.76 (0.27 to 2.10)	0.52 (0.21 to 1.31)
	201	4	20 (7 to 53)	0.78 (0.28 to 2.15)	0.76 (0.25 to 2.26)

Vaginal HRT only ††				
Never	1589	53	33 (25 to 44)	1 (referent)	1 (referent)
Ever	457	8	18 (9 to 35)	0.53 (0.25 to 1.10)	0.46 (0.21 to 1.01)
Tubes of cream					
2-4	229	3	13 (4 to 41)	0.39 (0.12 to 1.26)	0.29 (0.09 to 0.93)
≥5	228	5	22 (9 to 53)	0.66 (0.26 to 1.65)	0.70 (0.26 to 1.92)

*Rates were calculated from the reference date (ie, the date of hormone replacement therapy initiation in users or the equivalent date since diagnosis in matched nonusers.

†Relative risk (rate ratio) comparing users with nonusers. Users and nonusers were matched on age at diagnosis (35-44, 45-54, 55-64, and 65-74 years) year of diagnosis (1977-1982, 1983-1988, and 1989-1994), stage (I, II, and III), and time from diagnosis to the reference date (months).

‡Relative risk (hazard ratio) from Cox regression models. Adjusted for bilateral, oophorectomy, hysterectomy, mastectomy, tamoxifen, and matching.

§Analysis excluded 17 nonusers of hormone replacement therapy (with estrogens) who used progestins, ie, filled 2 or more prescriptions for a progestin within 6 months, some time after diagnosis and before any recurrence. Six hormone replacement therapy users who used progestins but did not receive progestins concurrently with an estrogen were also excluded, along with their matched nonusers.

‖Includes 98 users of oral hormone replacement therapy and their matched nonusers.

¶Cumulative use. Total person-years for the zero category differs from that for the "never" category because some oral users entered analysis having used only vaginal hormone replacement therapy to that time, whereas the time at risk among users in this analysis reflects oral use only. Person-years in the nonzero categories of use likewise reflect oral use only; thus, they do not sum to the total years in the "ever" category.

**Dose in conjugated-estrogen dose equivalents (Lobo RA: Clinical review 27: Effects of hormonal replacement on lipids and lipoproteins in postmenopausal women. *J Clin Endocrinal Metab* 73:925-930, 1991.

††Includes 75 users of vaginal, but not oral, hormone replacement therapy and their matched nonusers.

Abbreviations: CI, Confidence interval; *HRT,* hormone replacement therapy.

(Courtesy of O'Meara ES, Rossing MA, Daling JR, et al: Hormone replacement therapy after a diagnosis of breast cancer in relation to recurrence and mortality. *J Natl Cancer Inst* 93:754-762, 2001. By permission of Oxford University Press.)

light is being shed on this issue and dogma may be confronted. This study certainly provides reassurance to women and their doctors that the benefits may exceed the risks. The authors clearly show that the risk of recurrence of breast cancer in women who receive various types of HRT for varying durations of time was not adversely affected. In fact, those patients appear to be have done better. Clearly, we await the results of prospective trials, since this study was limited by the short follow-up (4 years) and the concerning finding that the risk of second primary contralateral breast cancers was higher in the patients who received HRT.

D. S. Miller, MD

Adjunctive Therapies

A Comparison of Complementary and Alternative Medicine Use by Gynecology and Gynecologic Oncology Patients

Von Gruenigen VE, White LJ, Kirven MS, et al (Akron Gen Med Ctr, Ohio; Twin Springs Med Ctr, Kidron, Ohio)
Int J Gynecol Cancer 11:205-209, 2001   27–3

Background.—There has been a continual increase in the use of complementary and alternative medicines (CAM) in the United States, with an increase in use of CAM from 34% in 1990 to 42% in 1997. Surveys have revealed that women and cancer patients are more likely to use CAM than are any other group, with CAM being used by 37% of advanced cancer patients. Similarly, breast cancer patients have been found to be more likely than the general public to use alternative therapies, including prayer, exercise, spiritual healing, and megavitamins. The CAM field has developed into a multibillion-dollar industry. The use of CAM in gynecology and gynecological oncology patients was described and compared.

Methods.—A questionnaire regarding CAM use was completed by 529 gynecology and gynecologic oncology patients who presented for care at 2 private outpatient gynecologic oncology offices in Ohio. The CAM categories assessed in the survey were drawn from the National Institutes of Health National Center for Complementary and Alternative Medicine (NCCAM) classification. Included in these classifications were diet and nutrition; mind-body techniques; bioelectromagnetics; traditional and folk remedies; pharmacological and biological treatments; manual healing methods; and herbal medicine.

Results.—Current use of some form of CAM was reported by 56% of gynecology and gynecologic oncology patients. The most frequently used CAM was nutritional supplementation (20%), followed by prayer as medical therapy (17%), exercise as medical therapy (12%), megavitamins (10%); and green tea (10%). Although 69% of patients reported that they believed CAM to be beneficial, only 32% of patients reported that they discussed these therapies with their physician. The women in this study spent a mean of $656.22 on CAM, with 32% receiving some reimbursement from insurers. Gynecologic oncology patients (66%) were significantly more likely to use CAM than were gynecology patients (52%), and to spend more money for CAM than gynecology patients. Among the 69 patients who were currently receiving modern medical treatment for cancer, 58% reported also using CAM, and 54% of these patients perceived some benefit from CAM.

Conclusions.—Cancer patients had a higher usage rate and expenditure for CAM in this study, particularly while they are also receiving medical therapy. Cancer patients in this study were also found to be more likely than patients without cancer to discuss the use of CAM with their physicians. CAM was perceived as beneficial by more than half of the cancer patients despite the lack of scientific data regarding its effectiveness.

▶ Until recently, most physicians, especially those who do not sell products in their offices, presumed that only the patients of others used alternative medicines. This study, among others, reminds us that a significant portion of our patients are seeking alternative solutions. This study is not so striking in that patients with gynecologic malignancies were using alternative medicines, but that patients without known cancer were frequently also using alternative medicines. While most of these therapies are inactive, many of these substances may have pharmacologic effects that may interact adversely with Food and Drug Administration approved medications.[1] When the physician is confronted by a patient using or seeking alternative medicines the practitioner should suppress the "fight or flight" response and attempt to deal rationally with the situation. I have found it very helpful to use and refer patients to the alternative medicines section of the American Cancer Society's Web site or to Quackwatch.com for an alternative view of these alternative therapies.

D. S. Miller, MD

Reference

1. Von Gruenigen VE, Hopkins MP. Alternative medicine in gynecologic oncology: A case report. *Gynecol Oncol* 77:190, 2000.

Bacteriology and Treatment of Malodorous Lower Reproductive Tract in Gynecologic Cancer Patients
Von Gruenigen VE, Coleman RL, Li AJ, et al (Univ of Texas, Dallas)
Obstet Gynecol 96:23-27, 2000

27–4

Background.—Necrotic gynecologic tumors may be accompanied by an offensive odor, which is disturbing not only to patients but also to their families and caregivers. This can present a reduction in care, as patients with malodorous tumors might receive suboptimal care when caregivers avoid entering a malodorous room. Malodorous cancers have a multifactorial etiology, but the interaction of specific types of bacteria or an overgrowth of normal vaginal organisms and tumor necrosis are important factors. The bacteriologic composition of lower genital tract cancers was determined so that rersearch on potential treatment modalities could be directed, and the impact of treatment of these odors on quality of life was determined.

Methods.—In a prospective case–cohort trial, Gram's stain, saline preparations, tumor pH determinations, and anaerobic and aerobic tumor cultures were obtained. The treatment group comprised 13 consecutive patients with malodorous gynecologic cancers, and the control group comprised 13 patients with nonmalodorous tumors. Patients in the malodorous group were treated with topical metronidazole for 7 days. Patients in the treatment group completed daily odor assessment questionnaires. A quality-of-life evaluation was accomplished by administration of the Functional Assessment of Cancer Therapy questionnaire before and after treatment.

Results.—The most common primary tumor site was cancer of the cervix, which accounted for 81% of malodorous gynecologic cancers. Among the 13 patients in the treatment group, 8 (62%) were found to have bacterial vaginosis compared with 4 of 13 (31%) in the control group. Isolation of aerobic and anaerobic bacteria from malodorous gynecologic cancers occurred with equal frequency. A graded improvement was noted on the odor assessment questionnaires with the use of topical antibiotic therapy. An improved quality of life after therapy was indicated on the Functional Assessment of Cancer Therapy questionnaire.

Conclusions.—Bacterial vaginosis was present in most patients with malodorous gynecologic tumors, and they experienced a decrease in the odor after treatment with topical metronidazole. These findings suggest the potential usefulness of this treatment for patients with malodorous pelvic tumors.

▶ The important role that the sense of smell plays in our lives is mostly overlooked by our very visual society. It is the loss of control over this powerful influence that adds silently to the misery of many patients with cancer. This article describes a simple intervention that produced a demonstrable effect on patient well-being. The social stigma associated with a serious disease, especially cancer, is compounded by the isolation brought about by an unpleasant odor. It is not surprising that this pervasive reminder of the diagnosis has a measurable effect on the quality of life of patients, their families, and caregivers.

R. D. Arias, MD

28 Breast Disease

Managing Menopausal Symptoms in Breast Cancer Survivors: Results of a Randomized Controlled Trial
Ganz PA, Greendale GA, Petersen L, et al (Univ of California, Los Angeles)
J Natl Cancer Inst 92:1054-1064, 2000
28–1

Background.—Many breast cancer survivors experience hot flashes, vaginal dryness, and stress urinary incontinence. Estrogen replacement therapy (ERT) is a common treatment for these symptoms of menopause, but it cannot be used in these patients. Furthermore, adjuvant therapy with tamoxifen or chemotherapy can exacerbate hot flashes in these women. A comprehensive menopausal assessment (CMA) intervention program was developed. Its efficacy in reducing menopausal symptoms in highly symptomatic breast cancer survivors was described.

Methods.—The subjects were 72 postmenopausal women (mean age, 54.5 years) who had received a diagnosis 8 months to 5 years earlier of stage I or II breast cancer and who had successfully undergone treatment. Any chemotherapy or radiation therapy had ended 4 months or more before their enrollment in this study, but 56% were taking tamoxifen. All patients had at least 1 moderate-to-severe target symptom; 97% had hot flashes, 71% had vaginal dryness, and 51% had stress urinary incontinence (Fig 2). Patients were randomly assigned to a usual care group (39 patients) or the CMA intervention group (33 patients). Before enrollment, both groups had completed daily symptom diary cards for 28 days and underwent thorough screening (including referral for counseling for psychosocial symptoms, if needed).

At baseline, patients in the intervention group received a structured, comprehensive evaluation of their target symptoms and an individualized plan of education, counseling, pharmacologic or behavioral interventions, psychosocial support, and referrals to help them manage their target symptoms. Two months after baseline, patients in the usual care group were telephoned to ask about any interventions or treatments they were using to help manage their symptoms, while patients in the intervention group had an in-person visit with a nurse to reevaluate their management strategy and modify it if necessary.

Three months after enrollment, both groups again completed daily symptom diary cards. Four months after enrollment, patients in the intervention group received a final interview, while patients in the usual care

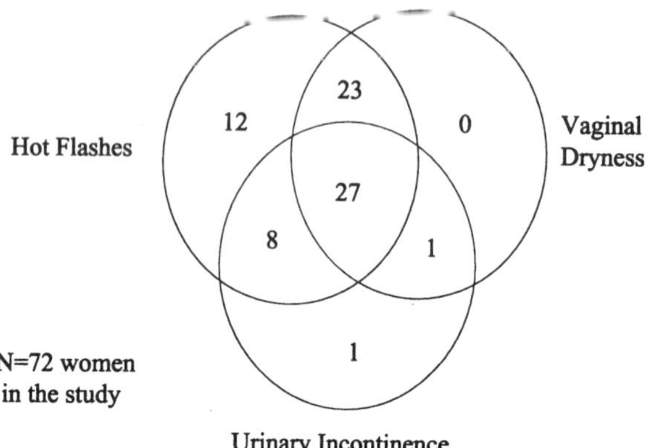

FIGURE 2.—Venn diagram showing distribution of individual menopausal symptoms (hot flashes, vaginal dryness, and urinary incontinence) and their overlap in the study sample of participants (72 patients) in the randomized trial of female breast cancer survivors with menopausal symptoms. (Courtesy of Ganz PA, Greendale GA, Petersen L, et al: Managing menopausal symptoms in breast cancer survivors: Results of a randomized controlled trial. *J Natl Cancer Inst* 92:1054-1064, 2000. By permission of Oxford University Press.)

group were offered the CMA intervention as a courtesy. The Menopausal Symptom Scale Score (a composite score), the Vitality Scale from the RAND Short Form Healthy Survey, and the Sexual Summary Scale from the Cancer Rehabilitation Evaluation System were used to assess changes between baseline and the end of the study (4 months) in both groups.

Results.—At the end of the study, outcome measures had not changed significantly in the usual care group (Fig 3). The Vitality Score did not

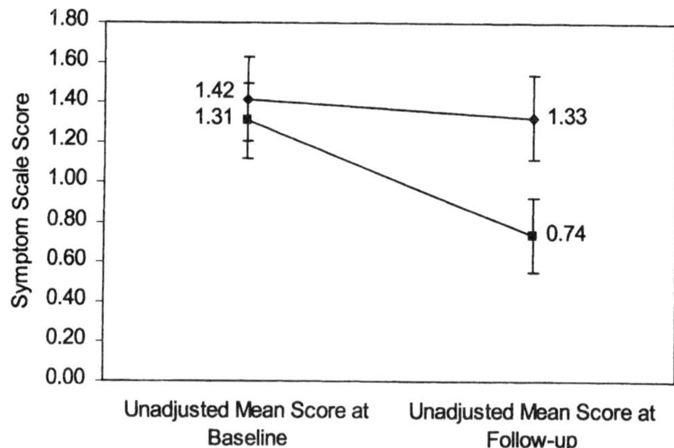

FIGURE 3.—Change in symptom scale score from baseline to follow-up in the intervention and usual-care groups (P = .0001) of the randomized study of breast cancer survivors. A lower score indicates a lesser severity of symptoms. *Ninety-five percent confidence intervals* are shown. The effect of group was also significant for an analysis adjusted for covariates (P = .001) (data not shown). *Closed diamonds* represent usual-care group; *closed squares* represent intervention group. (Courtesy of Ganz PA, Greendale GA, Petersen L, et al: Managing menopausal symptoms in breast cancer survivors: Results of a randomized controlled trial. *J Natl Cancer Inst* 92:1054-1064, 2000. By permission of Oxford University Press.)

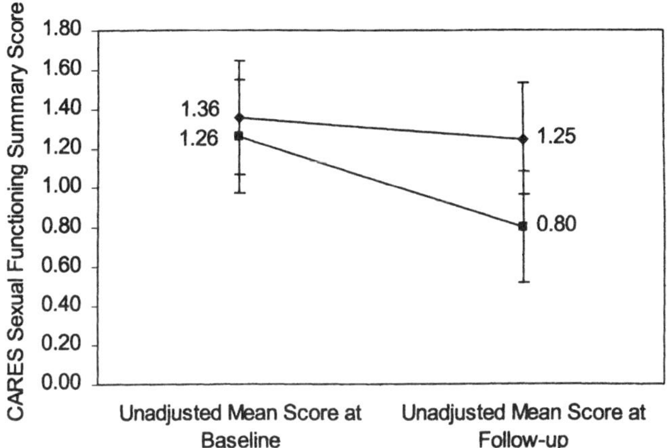

FIGURE 4.—Change in Cancer Rehabilitation Evaluation System (*CARES*) Sexual Functioning Summary Score from baseline to follow-up in the intervention and usual-care groups (*P* = .02) of the randomized study of breast cancer survivors. A lower score indicates a lesser severity of problems. *Ninety-five percent confidence intervals* are shown. The effect of group was also significant for an analysis adjusted for covariates (*P* = .01) (data not shown). *Closed diamonds* represent usual-care group; *closed squares* represent intervention group. (Courtesy of Ganz PA, Greendale GA, Petersen L, et al: Managing menopausal symptoms in breast cancer survivors: Results of a randomized controlled trial. *J Natl Cancer Inst* 92:1054-1064, 2000. By permission of Oxford University Press.)

significantly change in the intervention group. However, patients in the intervention group had significant improvement in the Menopausal Symptom Scale Score (unadjusted mean change in score, 0.57 in the intervention group vs 0.09 in the usual care group) and the Sexual Summary Scale (unadjusted mean change in score 0.46 vs 0.11, respectively) (Fig 4). While at least half of the patients in the intervention group used medications to treat hot flashes and vaginal dryness, 1 or 2 patients in the usual care group did so, too, and more than one third sought out information regarding the management of their symptoms. Additionally, patients in the usual care group often turned to alternative remedies, such as mind-body techniques (31%), vitamin therapy (31%), or a special diet (39%).

Conclusion.—Breast cancer survivors with moderate-to-severe menopausal symptoms can benefit from an education, counseling, and management plan to help manage their symptoms and improve sexual function. A thorough screening of target symptoms is key to individualizing the CMA intervention for each patient's main concerns. These patients are actively seeking treatments (both pharmacologic and alternative) to manage their menopausal symptoms, and clinicians must take an active role in addressing their symptoms and concerns.

▶ Most gynecologists have breast cancer patients with menopausal symptoms in their practice. The appropriate management is a dilemma. As this carefully structured and reported study states, ". . . most breast cancer survivors will be unwilling to consider ERT . . ." See also below.[1,2] The results achieved in this study are modest and the methods used are difficult to replicate in clinical practice, especially in a managed care setting. Thus, many women (breast cancer survivors) with menopausal/estrogen deficiency symptoms have turned to alternate complementary medications and methods.

Phytoestrogens have been particularly popular in spite of unproven effects on both the menopausal symptoms and breast cancer. Some rigorous studies are underway, but convincing scientific data that can be applied in clinical practice are lacking at this time. Several observational studies, both in Europe and the United States, have been published purporting to show little or no effect of ERT given for menopausal symptoms upon breast cancer disease-specific survival. Data from prospective, randomized clinical trials are not available.

Tibolone, a synthetic steroid structurally related to C-19 derivatives (noresthisterone) which is in clinical use in Europe and elsewhere, appears to be effective in controlling menopausal symptoms without any adverse effect on breast tissue.[3] In vivo and in vitro animal studies indicate that tibolone has an anti-estrogen tamoxifen-like effect on breast cells. However, no human data are currently available. The known common side effect is uterine bleeding (10% to 20% incidence)[4] which raises the question of the effect of tibolone on the endometrium. Clinical trials are needed.

W. H. Hindle, MD

References

1. Ganz PA, Greendale GA, Kahn B, et al: Are older breast carcinoma survivors willing to take hormone replacement therapy? *Cancer* 86:814-820, 1999.
2. Vassilopoulou-Sellin R, Klein MJ: Estrogen replacement therapy after treatment for localized breast carcinoma: Patient responses and opinions. *Cancer* 78:1043-1048, 1996.
3. Colacurci N, Mele D, De Franciscis P, et al: Effects of tibolone on the breast. *Eur J Obstet Reprod Biol* 80:235-238, 1998.
4. Rymer J, Fogelman I, Chapman MG: The incidence of vaginal bleeding with tibolone treatment. *Br J Obstet Gynaecol* 101:53-56, 1994.

SUGGESTED READING

Loprinzi CL, Kugler JW, Sloan JA, et al: Venlafaxine in management of hot flashes in survivors of breast cancer: A randomised controlled trial. *The Lancet* 356:2059-2063, 2000.

▶ Good news! This early report from the Mayo Clinic (Rochester, Minnesota) indicates that by double-blind, placebo-controlled, randomized trial, 4 weeks of treatment with Venlafaxine reduced median hot flash scores (from baseline) by as much as 61%. A daily dose of 75 mg was required to obtain this level of reduction. However, at this dosage, the side effects of dry mouth, decreased appetite, nausea, and constipation were significant. Three randomized studies with related antidepressants are underway. Hopefully, the side effects will decrease, and perhaps the reductions in hot flash scores will increase. However, it would be even more impressive if these studies were of crossover design and longer duration.

William H. Hindle, MD

Moorman PG, Kuwabara H, Millikan RC, et al: Menopausal hormones and breast cancer in a biracial population. *Am J Public Health*: 90:966-971, 2000.

▶ This epidemiolgic study from Yale University used data from the Carolina Breast Cancer Study, which was population-based, case-controlled, and which calculated odds ratios (ORs) by logistic regression. All the women were menopausal (397 cases and 425 controls). The ORs for ever-use hormones was 0.8 (95% CI = 0.5, 1.2) for white women and 0.7 (95% CI = 0.4, 1.2) for black women. Neither longer duration of use nor more recent use increased the risk. Thus, in this study, menopausal hormone use did not increase the breast cancer risk for white or black women although the patterns of use varied considerably. Only carefully designed large, long-term prospective randomized trials, with disease-specific mortality as an end point, will quell the continuous debates about the impact of menopausal hormones on the incidence and outcome of breast cancer.

William H. Hindle, MD

Gao Y-T, Shu X-O, Potter JD, et al: Association of menstrual and reproductive factors with breast cancer risk: Results from the Shanghai breast cancer study. Int J Cancer 87:295-300, 2000.

▶ This population based case-controlled study compared interviews of 1459 women newly diagnosed with breast cancer (ages 25 to 64 years) with 1556 controls. Increased risk of breast cancer was associated with earlier age of menarche, null parity, and later age at first live birth for both pre- and postmenopausal women. Increased risk of breast cancer was associated with never having breast-fed and later age of menopause only for postmenopausal women. A considerable share of breast cancer cases diagnosed in older but not in younger women seemed to relate to older age at first live birth or older age at menopause. The authors suggest that, particularly among young women, these menstrual and reproductive patterns contribute to the increase in breast cancer incidence for Shanghai women.

The statistical power of the Shanghai Breast Cancer Study is impressive. The authors represent 7 medical/epidemiology departments in the US, particularly at the University of South Carolina. Cultural correlations and the impact of changing reproductive behavior in China would be of keen interest.

Using the same Shanghai breast cancer study data base, Mathews et al reported on the lifetime physical activity effect on breast cancer risk in a study group of 1459 newly diagnosed breast cancer cases and 1556 age-matched contols.[1] Exercise only in adolescence reduced the odds ratio (OR) to 0.84 (CI, 95% [0.70-1.0]), whereas exercise only in adulthood had an OR of 0.68 (CI, 95% [0.53-0.88]). Exercise in both adolescence and adulthood produced the greatest risk reduction with an OR of 0.47 (CI, 95% [0.36-0.62]). Graded risk reductions correlated with increasing years of exercise. This adds to other data that physical activity is associated with reduced risk of breast cancer and suggests a potentially beneficial intervention strategy.

Furthermore, can serum steroid hormone assays detect changes, including increased levels, which might correlate with increased cancer risk? Doran et al at the Fox Chase Cancer Center, in Philadelphia, Pennsylvania, reported on results of radio immunoassays of 9 serum steroid hormones collected from 51 healthy postmenopausal women on controlled diets who rotated through 3 8-week consumptions of 15 or 30 g of alcohol per day or placebo beverage.[2] The results showed an increased concentrations of 7.5% estrone sulfate and 5.1% dehydroepiandrosterone (DHEA). The authors speculate that these results (which were not statistically significant) "could suggest a possible mechanism" for an increased risk for breast cancer in women who consume one or two alcoholic drinks a day.

In addition, Lash at the Boston University School of Public Health (Boston, Massachusetts) reported on a case-control study with 334 incident breast cancer cases and found that ". . . any history of drinking alcohol had a risk of breast cancer 1.2-fold greater than women who never drank alcohol (CI, 95% [0.7-1.8])," whereas women with a history of 6 months or more in which they drank "more than average" had an adjusted relative risk of 2.6 (CI, 95% [1.1-5.8]).[3] The multifactorial natural of drinking alcohol and recall bias make epidemiolgic studies of this nature difficult to interpret. However, even with these low levels of relative risk and borderline significance, the authors conclude "Alcohol drinking remains one of the few risk factors for breast cancer amenable to intervention." Prospective randomized trial data documenting the success of such interventions is lacking.

William H. Hindle, MD

References

1. Matthews CE, Shu X-O, Jin F, et al. Lifetime physical activity and breast cancer risk in the Shanghai Breast Cancer Study. *Br J Cancer* 84:994-1001, 2001.
2. Dorgan JF, Baer DJ, Albert PS, et al. Serum hormones and the alcohol-breast cancer association in postmenopausal women. *J Natl Cancer Inst* 93:710-715, 2001.
3. Lash TL, Aschengrau A. Alcohol drinking and risk of breast cancer. *Breast J* 6:396-399, 2000.

Limited Value of Sonohysterography for Endometrial Screening in Asymptomatic, Postmenopausal Patients Treated With Tamoxifen

Bertelli G, Valenzano M, Costantini S, et al (Natl Cancer Inst, Genoa, Italy; Univ of Genoa, Italy)
Gynecol Oncol 78:275-277, 2000

28–2

Background.—Sonohysterography (SHG) appears to be useful for monitoring endometrium in patients receiving tamoxifen therapy. The value of SHG in asymptomatic patients who would have been candidates for biopsy because of abnormal transvaginal US (TVUS) findings was determined.

Methods.—Forty-one postmenopausal patients with breast cancer who had TVUS abnormalities with no symptoms receiving adjuvant tamoxifen were studied. An Aloka SSD 680 (Aloka Tokyo, Japan) system with a 5-MHz vaginal probe was used to perform SHG, with the use of sterile saline solution as a contrast medium.

Findings.—Sonohysterography identified a regular endometrial echo in 21.9% of the patients (Table 1). The 65.8% of patients with a positive SHG underwent histologic assessment, as did the 12.2% in whom SHG was unsuccessful. Benign polyps were found in 36.5%, and endometrial atrophy in 34.1%. In 7.3%, simple hyperplasia was noted.

TABLE 1.—Results of Sonohysterography and Correlation with Pathological Findings in 41 Asymptomatic Patients with Endometrial Thickening (≥ 8 mm) at TVUS During Adjuvant Tamoxifen

| SHG Diagnosis | *n* (%) | Pathology Results (No. of Patients) | | |
		Atrophic	Hyperplastic	Polyp
Polyp	19 (46.3)	5	1	13
Focal thickening	6 (14.6)	4	1	1
Diffuse thickening	2 (4.9)	1	1	0
Failed	5 (12.2)	4	0	1
Normal	9 (21.9)	—	—	—

Note: Endometrial samples were not obtained in 9 patients who had normal SHG results (thin endometrial echo without focal changes.

(Courtesy of Bertelli G, Valenzano M, Costantini S, et al: Limited value of sonohysterography for endometrial screening in asymptomatic, postmenopausal patients treated with tamoxifen *Gynecol Oncol* 78:275-277, 2000.)

Conclusions.—Sonohysterography provides little additional benefit to asymptomatic patients with breast cancer and tamoxifen-associated TVUS abnormalities. More than two thirds of such patients still needed biopsy.

▶ This study from Italy adds to the literature confirming the increased incidence of endometrial abnormalities (polyps and focal thickening) in women on tamoxifen therapy. Abnormal TVUS results were further evaluated by SHG in an effort to decrease the need for endometrial biopsy. However, more than two thirds of these patients still required biopsy. The authors concluded that there is "little additional benefit from SHG."

Clinical questions remain: (1) what is the natural history of these endometrial abnormalities after tamoxifen therapy is completed? (2) Can benign lesions that are premalignant be identified? (3) Can benign lesions that correlate with bleeding be identified?

Generally, the literature supports the 2- to 3-fold increase in endometrial carcinoma occurring in postmenopausal women on tamoxifen therapy, the limited value of any screening procedures in asymptomatic women on tamoxifen, and the occurrence of bleeding as the indication for diagnostic procedures (as it is for postmenopausal women who are not on tamoxifen therapy). The low incidence of endometrial carcinoma (with or without tamoxifen therapy) will require large numbers in clinical trials in order to reach statistical significance.

W. H. Hindle, MD

SUGGESTED READING

Gardner FJE, Konje JC, Abrams KR, et al. Endometrial protection from tamoxifen-stimulated changes by levonorgestrel-releasing intrauterine system: A randomised controlled trial. *The Lancet* 356:1711-1717, 2000.

▶ Multiple published studies on tamoxifen demonstrate dose and duration effects of increasing uterine abnormalities. Some of the endometrial abnormalities can be atypical or malignant. The increased incidence of endometrial cancer associated with tamoxifen therapy is low (two- to threefold) and the baseline incidence of endometrial cancer is small, but the fact that tamoxifen is associated with endometrial cancer creates patient resistance to the therapy and inhibits its use for benign lesions, e.g. mastalgia or myomata uteri. Thus, there has been a search for either another selective estrogen receptor modulator (SERM) without uterine/endometrial stimulation (perhaps raloxifene is such a SERM) or another therapy to counteract the stimulation. The levonorgestrel-releasing intrauterine system in this study from the UK (University of Leicester) was effective in producing a deciduoid endometrium, which was confirmed histologically in 40 of 41 patients. No new polyps formed in the treated group, and the controls had 13% more myomata compared to the treated group. However, vaginal bleeding was a significant adverse side effect, particularly in the first 90 days after insertion of the system. Several women dropped out of the study group due to excess vaginal bleeding. Endometrial surveillance is problematic with the system in place when biopsy and/or hysteroscopy are indicated. Further refinements of the system and long-term follow-up studies are needed.

Bonanni et al at the European Institute of Oncology, Milan, Italy, reviewed the potential benefits and risks of hormone replacement therapy (HRT) combined with tamoxifen therapy and stated ". . . the Italian Tamoxifen Prevention Study showed borderline signficant reductions of breast cancer among women who were on HRT continuously and tamoxifen compared with continuous HRT users who received placebo."[1] The authors note that ". . . in National Surgical Adjuvant Breast Project (NSABP) P-1 trial, women ages 50 or younger had no increased incidence of adverse events." They conclude, "The combination of HRT and tamoxifen at low dose [ed. 10 mg every other day] could thus reduce the risks and side effects while retaining the benefits of either agent."

Mourits et al from the University Hospital Groningen, Groningen, The Netherlands, reviewed 124 references on the effects of tamoxifen, on estrogen receptors, vaginal epithelium, endometrium, endometriosis, mesenchymal tumors of the uterus, ovaries, sexuality, and vasomotor instability.[2] The authors conclude, "The most frequently reported side effect was hot flushes, and the most worrisome gynecologic side effect was a two- to threefold increased risk of endometrial cancer in postmenopausal women." Physicians and other health care providers who care for women on tamoxifen (or those contemplating its use) would do well to carefully read this informative and detailed review.

William H. Hindle, MD

References

1. Bonanni B, Guerrieri-Gonzaga A, Rotmensz N, et al. Hormonal therapy and chemotherapy. *Breast J* 6:317-323, 2000.
2. Mourits MJE, DeVries EGF, Willemse PHB, et al Tamoxifen treatment and gynecologic side effects: a review. *Obstet Gynecol* 97:855-868, 2001.

Benhaim, DI, Lopchinsky, R, Tartter, PI: Lumpectomy with tamoxifen as primary treatment for elderly women with early-stage breast cancer. *Am J Surg* 180:162-166, 2000.

▶ This retrospective analysis from the Mount Sinai Medial Center, New York, NY, included 171 women over 70 years of age with stage I or II invasive breast cancer. The mean follow-up was 58 months (range, 7 to 147 months). Tamoxifen at a dosage of 20 mg daily was given for 5 years after surgery. There were 135 women in the conventional (local treatment with lumpectomy, axillary dissection followed by radiation therapy, or mastectomy) treatment group and 43 in the lumpectomy/tamoxifen group. The demographics varied in that the tamoxifen group was older (mean 80 vs 76 years) and had smaller tumors (mean 1.4 vs 1.8 cm) than the conventional treatment group. The authors report no local recurrence and 1 (2%) distant recurrence in the lumpectomy/tamoxifen group and 4 (3%) local recurrences and 18 (13%) distant recurrences in the conventional treatment group.

Selection bias (patient or physician) may have influenced these results. Furthermore, it would be informative to have separated the mastectomy from the lumpectomy patients in the conventional treatment group. This analysis is interesting and suggestive. What is needed is a long-term randomized clinical trial with adequate numbers.

William H. Hindle, MD

Multicenter Trial of Sentinel Node Biopsy for Breast Cancer Using Both Technetium Sulfur Colloid and Isosulfan Blue Dye

Tafra L, Lannin DR, Swanson MS, et al (Anne Arundel Med Ctr, Annapolis, Md; East Carolina Univ, Greenville, NC; Breast Care Ctr of the Blue Ridge, Roanoke, Va; et al)
Ann Surg 233:51-59, 2001   28–3

Background.—To test the reliability of sentinel node biopsy for detecting breast cancer metastases, a complete lymph node dissection is needed to determine the false-negative rate. This multicenter study investigated the factors associated with such false-negative results in patients with breast cancer undergoing biopsy with a combination technique of isodulfan blue and technetium sulfur colloid (^{99}Tc).

Methods.—Five hundred twenty-nine patients underwent a total of 535 sentinal node biopsy procedures. Isosulfan blue and ^{99}Tc were injected into the peritumoral area.

Findings.—The overall rate of identification of sentinal nodes was 87%. The false-negative rate was 13%. After investigators performed more than 30 procedures, the identification and false-negative rates were 90% and 4.3%, respectively. In a univariate analysis, older patients and inexperienced surgeons had the lowest rates of success. In a multivariate analysis, both patient age and surgeon experience level independently predicted failure. The false-negative rate was consistently higher for older patients, inexperienced surgeons, and patients with 5 or more metastatic axillary nodes.

Conclusion.—Patient age, surgeon experience, and tumor location are important to the success of sentinel node biopsy in patients with breast cancer. Previous surgery, tumor size, and the timing of ^{99}Tc do not appear to be important.

▶ To become standard practice, a new technique must be applicable and proven in multiple diverse settings such as, in the case of this report, at the multiple centers of both private practice and academic surgeons. A series of 529 patients demonstrated an overall identification rate of 87% for sentinel nodes and a false-negative rate of 13%. It is important to note that, according to the authors, "No investigators participated in a learning trial before entering patients," ie, none of the surgeons had begun the learning curve for this procedure prior to beginning this trial. Other reports have indicated that it takes as many as 100 sentinel lymph node biopsy (SLNB) procedures for a surgeon to obtain high efficiency and effectiveness with SLNB. Indeed, in this report, the false-negative rates decreased to 4.3% and the identification rate increased to 90% "after investigators had performed more than 30 cases." This strongly suggests that each surgeon beginning to perform the SLNB procedures should perform surgery on at least 30 patients with direct operating room supervision by an "experienced" (eg, with more than 100 cases) surgeon.

Reintgen et al provided an overview of SLNB and added the H. Lee Moffitt Cancer Center and Research Institute, University of South Florida (Tampa, Florida) SLNB experience.[1] The authors suggest that SLNB (as an outpatient procedure) in association with peripheral blood and bone marrow samples could provide "ultrastaging" for indications of adjuvant chemotherapy through the use of serial sections, immunohistochemical staining, and reverse transcriptase–polymerase chain staining technique ". . . since adjuvant treatments are thought to benefit only 8-12% of the treated population." It is further stated that ". . . the potential annual savings for the American health care system is approximately $695 million . . . "[2]

Tanis et al published a collective review of the biological basis of SLNB with 76 references.[3] Although detailed and often technical, this should be required reading by all SLNB surgeons. Of keen general breast cancer interest are a figure showing the anatomy/lymphatic of the breast and 2 clear and comprehensive tables listing the pertinent literature on SLNB techniques in breast cancer divided into (1) studies using radioactive isotope and (2) studies using radioactive isotope and blue dye.

W. H. Hindle, MD

References

1. Reintgen D, Giuliano R, Cox CE: Sentinel node biopsy in breast cancer, an overview. *Breast J* 6:299-305, 2000.
2. Reintgen D, Joseph E, Lyman GH, et al: The role of selective lymphadenectomy in breast cancer. *Cancer Control J* 4:211-219,1997.
3. Tanis PJ, Nieweg OE, Valdes-Olmos RA, et al: Anatomy and physiology of lymphatic drainage of the breast from the perspective of sentinel node biopsy. *J Am Coll Surg* 192:399-409, 2001.

SUGGESTED READING

Rodier J-F, Routiot T, Mignotte H, et al. Lymphatic mapping and sentinel node biopsy of operable breast cancer. *World J Surg* 24:1220-1226, 2000.

▶ Although this report from Lyon, France, includes only 73 patients, it demonstrates the reliability and reproducibility of sentinel node biopsy in breast cancer cases. Blue dye lymphatic mapping technique was utilized. The node was identified in 82.4% of patients and predicted axillary status (compared to level I and II axillary dissections) in 96.7%. The false-negative rate was 8.0%. Cancer involved the sentinel node in 37.7% of patients and was the only axillary involvement in 30.4% of patients. The calculated sensitivity was 92% (CI, 95% [74%-99%]), and the specificity was 100%.

William H. Hindle, MD

Schrenk P, Rieger R, Shamiyeh A, et al. Morbidity following sentinel lymph node biopsy versus axillary lymph node dissection for patients with breast carcinoma. *Cancer* 88:608-614, 2000.

▶ This objective and qualitative study from the Ludwig Boltzmann Institute for Surgical Laparoscopy (Linz, Austria) compared 35 patients with level I and II axillary lymph node dissections (ALND) with 35 patients with sentinel lymph node biopsy (SLNB) for edema of the arm, effect on arm strength, impairment of arm mobility, numbness, pain, sensory disturbances, shoulder stiffness, subjective lymphadema, and upper arm and forearm circumferences. Postoperative subjective lymphadema was present in 54% of the ALND patients and none of the SLNB patients. The ALND patients had statistically significant morbidity of numbness, pain, decreased arm mobility, subjective lymphadema, and increased upper and forearm circumference compared to the SLNB patients.

These results are not surprising but give promise of the potential elimination of lymphadema as a complication of breast cancer surgery when sentinel node biopsy obviates the standard (routine) axillary lymph node dissection.

William H. Hindle, MD

Olson JA, Fey J, Winawer J, et al. Sentinel lymphadenectomy accurately predicts nodal status in T2 breast cancer. *J Am Coll Surg* 191:593-599, 2000.

▶ This is the Memorial Sloan-Kettering Cancer Center (New York, NY) data covering 1627 sentinel lymph node biopsy (SLNB) patients (1996-1999) of which 223 were T1-T2NO and had lymphatic mapping procedures followed by axillary lymph node dissection (ALND). The SLNB technique has been previously described and utilized both unfiltered technetium 99 sulfur colloid and isosulfan blue dye.[1] With a median tumor size of 2.0 cm (range 0.2 − 4.8 cm) the SLNB was successful in 91%. There were 204 T1 lesions and 59 T2 lesions. The false-negative rates and accuracy were similar for the 2 groups (lesions). Neither SLNB nor intraoperative clinical examination identified 5 (5%) of the 92 pathologically positive axillae. This is consistent with multiple other published studies. The authors state that ". . . patient age, prior surgical biopsy, upper-outer quadrant tumor location, and tumor lymphovascular invasion were not associated with a higher incidence of false-negative SLNB in either T1 or T2 tumors" and recommend that ". . . all patients with T1-2NO breast cancer should be considered candidates for the procedure" (SLNB).

William H. Hindle, MD

Reference

1. Hill AD, Tran KN, Akhurst T, et al. Lessons learned from 500 cases of lymphatic mapping for breast cancer. *Ann Surg* 229:528-535, 1999.

Cohen LF, Breslin TM, Kuerer HM, et al. Identification and evaluation of axillary sentinel lymph nodes in patients with breast carcinoma treated with neoadjuvant chemotherapy. *Am J Surg Path* 24:1266-1272, 2000.

▶ This report from the M. D. Anderson Cancer Center (Houston, Texas) evaluates sentinel lymph node (SLN) biopsy in 38 patients with stage II or III locally advanced breast cancer treated with neoadjuvant chemotherapy comparing SLN with subsequent axillary dissection. Of the 20 patients who with initial hematoxalin and eosin sections were thought to be tumor free, 20% (4 of 20) were found to have occult metastases upon further sectioning. The occult metastases were confirmed by keratin immunohistochemical staining.

The SLN was identified in 82% (31of 38) and accurately predicted the axillary status in 90% (28 of 31) with 3 false negative SLN predictions. These results indicate that SLN technique can be used in patients treated with neoadjuvant chemotherapy and that the serial sections and immunohistochemical staining aids in the identification of occult lymph node metastases.

William H. Hindle, MD

Bass SS, Cox CE, Salud CJ, et al. The effects of postinjection massage on the sensitivity of lymphatic mapping in breast cancer. *J Am Coll Surg* 192:9-16, 2001.

▶ Sentinel lymph node (SLN) biopsy holds the promise of eliminating the scourge of lymphedema after axillary lymph node dissection. This study from the H. Lee Moffitt Cancer Center (Tampa, Florida) covering 594 consecutive patients, evaluated post injection massage on the efficiency of SLN biopsy in the identification of the sentinel lymph node. Compared to controls, the identification increased from 73.0% to 88.3% with blue dye technique and from 81.7% to 91.3% with the radiocolloid technique. The authors state, "The overall rate of SLN identification increased from 93.5% to 97.3%." These are excellent results consistent with other reports from large volume centers. Long-term disease-specific survival results are needed. Now that autologous bone marrow and stem cell replacement survival value are in question, the number of lymph nodes involved with cancer is not as critical as before (except in chemotherapy clinical trials). Future research should be carried out on the survival value of axillary lymph node dissection when the sentinel node is positive for malignancy. However, a graph in this report based on 1147 patients dramatically illustrates what others have also shown: i.e. that a surgeon requires a learning curve of about 100 patients before the identification failure rate is consistently near 5% with SLN biopsy.

William H. Hindle, MD

Results of Conservative Surgery for Limited-Sized Infiltrating Breast Cancer: Analysis of 962 Tested Patients: 24 Years of Experience
Vitucci C, Tirelli C, Graziano F, et al (Regina Elena Cancer Inst, Rome)
J Surg Oncol 74:108-115, 2000   28–4

Background.—Breast-conserving treatment (BCT) for limited-sized infiltrating breast cancer includes partial exeresis of the breast plus axillary lymph node dissection and radiation to the residual mammary gland. The

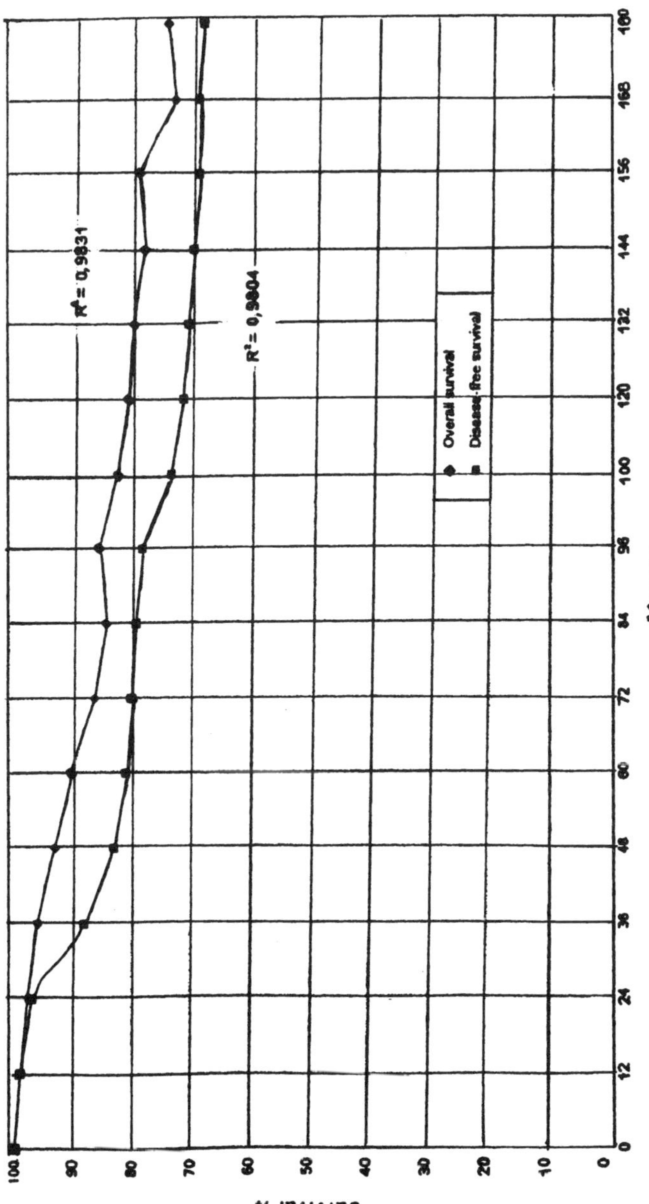

FIGURE 1.—Overall and disease-free survival in conservative surgery for breast cancer. Overall survival was 72% at 15 years (180 months). Disease-free survival was 67% after the same period of follow-up. (Courtesy of Vizucci C, Tirelli C, Graziano F, et al: Results of conservative surgery for limited-sized infiltrating breast cancer: Analysis of 962 tested patients: 24 years of experience. *J Surg Oncol* 74:108-115, 2000. Copyright 2000. Reprinted by permission of Wiley-Liss, Inc., a subsidiary of John Wiley & Sons, Inc.)

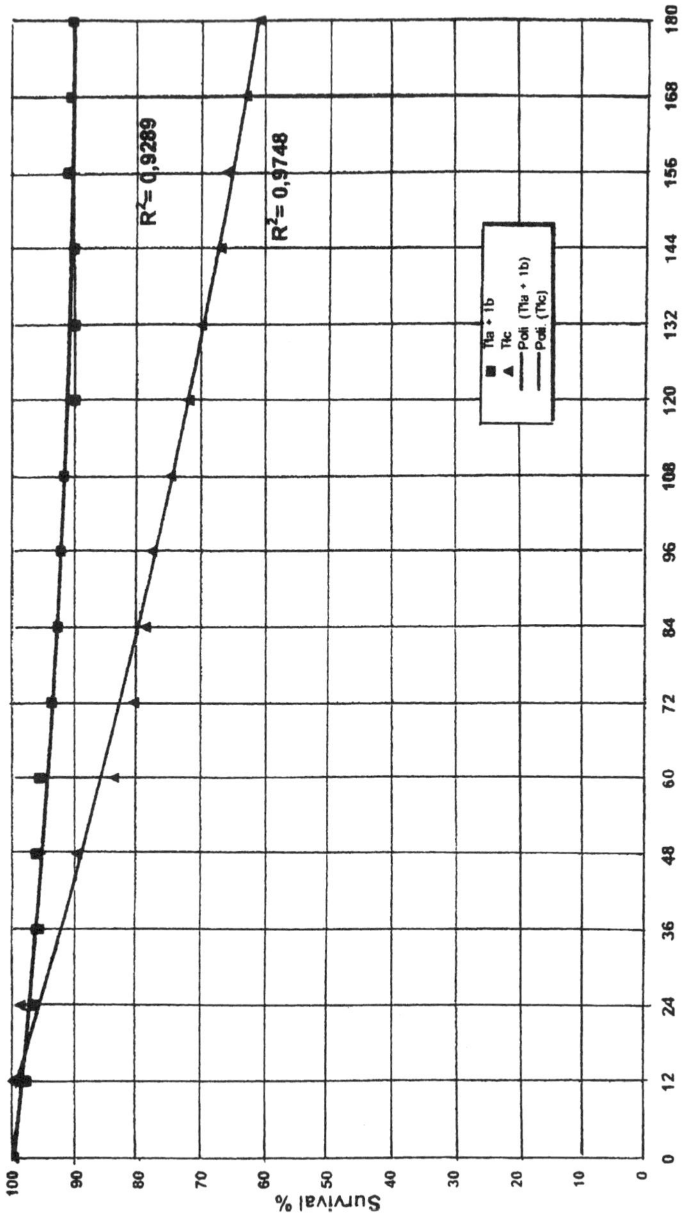

FIGURE 2.—Survival after conservative surgery for breast cancer according to T (1a + 1b vs. 1c). There is a significant difference between group T1a + T1b (90% survival) and group T1c (62% survival) at 15 years. (Courtesy of Vitucci C, Tirelli C, Graziano F, et al: Results of conservative surgery for limited-sized infiltrating breast cancer: Analysis of 962 tested patients: 24 years of experience. *J Surg Oncol* 74:108-115, 2000. Copyright 2000. Reprinted by permission of Wiley-Liss, Inc., a subsidiary of John Wiley & Sons, Inc.)

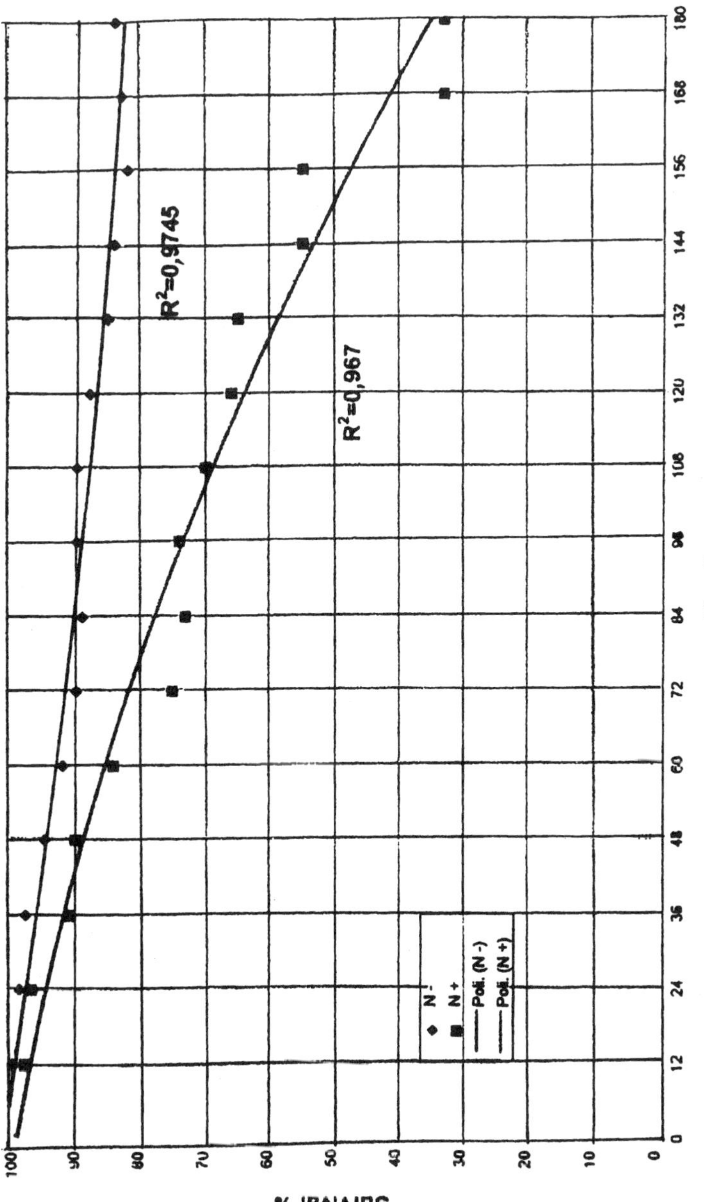

FIGURE 3.—Survival after conservative surgery for breast cancer according to N (negative vs positive). There is a significant difference between group N– (84%) and group N+ (31%) survival at 15 years. (Courtesy of Vitucci C, Tirelli C, Graziano F, et al: Results of conservative surgery for limited-sized infiltrating breast cancer: Analysis of 952 tested patients: 24 years of experience. *J Surg Oncol* 74:108-115, 2000. Copyright 2000. Reprinted by permission of Wiley-Liss, Inc., a subsidiary of John Wiley & Sons, Inc.)

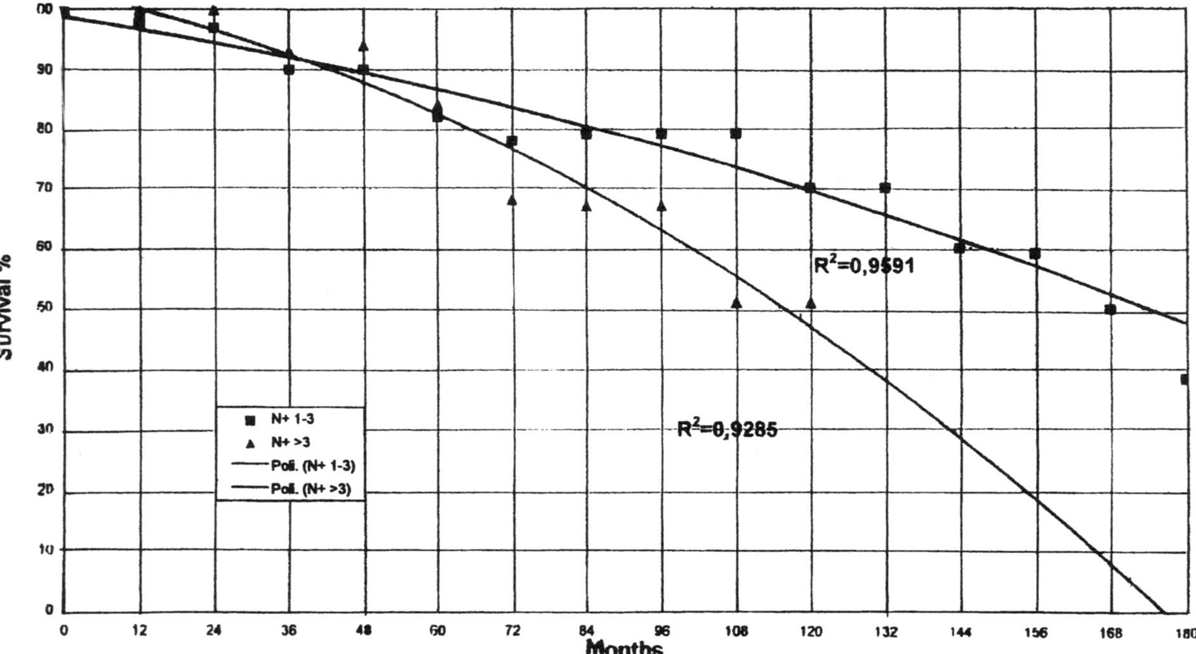

FIGURE 4.—Survival after conservative surgery for breast cancer according to $N+$ with 1 to 3 or with more than 3 involved nodes. There is a significant difference between $N+$ 1 to 3 (39%) and $N+$ more than 3 (0) survival at 15 years. (Courtesy of Vitucci C, Tirelli C, Graziano F, et al: Results of conservative surgery for limited-sized infiltrating breast cancer: Analysis of 962 tested patients: 24 years of experience. *J Surg Oncol* 74:108-115, 2000. Copyright 2000. Reprinted by permission of Wiley-Liss, Inc., a subsidiary of John Wiley & Sons, Inc.)

extent of this procedure varies. A 24-year experience with BCT for limited-sized infiltrating breast cancer was reported.

Methods.—Nine hundred sixty-two patients underwent a total of 980 conservative surgical procedures between 1975 and 1998 at the authors' center. All had T1 to "small" T2, N0-N1, M0 disease. Treatment consisted of a local wide excision, axillary diseection, and 50 Gy of radiation therapy postoperatively to the whole breast. Most of the patients also had an adjuvant systemic treatment, such as chemotherapy and/or hormono-therapy. Twenty-nine percent of the patients were node positive.

Findings.—At 15 years, the overall survival rate was 72%, and the disease-free survival rate was 67% (Fig 1). Survival for those with T1a + T1b and with T1c were 90% and 62%, respectively (Fig 2). Survival was 84% for node-negative patients and only 31% for node-positive patients (Fig 3). In the node-positive group, outcomes were poorest for those with more than 3 involved nodes, none of whom survived to 15 years (Fig 4). Overall, the rate of local relapse was 3.4%. Cosmetic outcomes were judged to be excellent or good in more than 80% of the patients.

Conclusion.—These outcomes confirm the validity of BCT in the treatment of limited-sized infiltrating breast cancer, given appropriate patient selection. T and N status appear to affect survival rates.

▶ This report from the Regina Elena Cancer Institute, Rome, Italy, covers 962 treated patients with breast cancer staged T1-T2 and has 15-year follow-up data. Both the number of patients and length of follow-up are remarkable. Although this is an observational report and selection may bias the results, it does give an overall picture of treated breast cancer. The 15-year overall survival rate was 72%, and the disease-free survival rate was 67%. Breast cancer disease specific mortality would have been of keen interest. The data confirm that tumor size and node involvement are important prognostic factors. Survival for T1a + T1b cancers was 90% compared with 62% for T1c. The survival for node-negative patients was 84% compared with 31% for node-involved patients. No patient with more than 3 nodes involved survived for 15 years. The local relapse rate was an admirably low 3.4% for 980 treated patients. These are excellent long-term (15-year) results for breast conserving therapy.

How extensively is BCT being utilized in the United States? One example is the report of Kelemen JJ et al from the Department of Defense Automated Central Tumor Registry.[1] During the 1986 to 1996 study period, a total of 7815 stage I and II breast cancer cases had complete data for analysis. There was a steady increase from 16% to 47% in use of BCT over the 11 years of the study. In 1996, 54% of women with T1 (less than 2cm) tumors were treated with BCT, according to the authors. There was wide geographic variation of BCT use from 24% in the southwestern United States, to 36% in the northeastern United States and 40% in hospitals outside the conti-nental United States. "Local availability of radiation therapy did not influence choice of treatment," they pointed out. Based on overwhelming evidence and experience, almost all women with stage I and II breast cancer should be offered BCT as the preferred method of treatment.

W. H. Hindle, MD

Reference

1. Keleman JJ III, Poulton T, Swartz MC, et al: Surgical treatment of early-stage breast cancer in the Department of Defense Healthcare System. *J Am Coll Surg* 192:293-297, 2001.

Lumpectomy Margins, Reexcision, and Local Recurrence of Breast Cancer

Tartter PI, Kaplan J, Bleiweiss I, et al (Mount Sinai Med Ctr, New York)
Am J Surg 179:81-85, 2000
28–5

Introduction.—The diagnosis of breast cancer is frequently made by excisional biopsy without margin examination for mammographic findings or palpable masses. Many patients who undergo breast conservation surgery have re-excision performed to ascertain clear margins, even though the association between clear margins and local recurrences remains controversial. The relation between local control and margin status was examined in patients treated with breast conservation.

Methods.—The medical records of consecutive patients with breast cancer who were evaluated between July 1, 1985, and June 30, 1993, were reviewed retrospectively. There were 296 patients who underwent surgery and radiation therapy without mastectomy. All patients were followed up for more than 5 years. Factors associated with obtaining clear histopathologic margins and re-excision were examined to determine clear margins in relation to the risk of local recurrence.

Results.—Clear biopsy margins were correlated with diagnosis by fine-needle aspiration cytology (fine-needle aspiration 42%, spot localization 11%, excisional biopsy 10%; $P < .001$) (Table 1). Attempts to obtain clear surgical margins by re-excision were performed for 35% (109) of the 308 cancers (Table 2). Re-excision was significantly associated with diagnostic method (spot localization 63%, excisional biopsy 36%, fine-needle aspiration 10%; $P < .001$), first margin status (clear 0%, close 11%, positive

---

TABLE 1.—Relationship of First Margin Status to Diagnostic Method

| | First Margin | | |
| | Clear | Not Clear | |
Diagnostic Method	Number (%)	Number (%)	P
Fine-needle cytology	35 (42)	49 (58)	
Spot localization	8 (11)	63 (89)	<0.001
Excisional biopsy	15 (10)	138 (90)	

(Courtesy of Tartter PI, Kaplan J, Bleiweiss I, et al: Lumpectomy margins, reexcision, and local recurrence of breast cancer. *Am J Surg* 179:81-85, 2000, with permission from Excerpta Medica Inc.)

TABLE 2.—First Margin and Final Margin for Patients with and without Reexcision

First Margin	Number of Patients	Reexcised Number of Patients	Final Margin	Number of Patients
Clear	65	0	Clear	65
Close	21	2	Clear	2
			Close	19
Positive	42	20	Clear	12
			Close	2
			Positive	27
			Unknown	1
Unknown	180	87	Clear	77
			Close	5
			Positive	1
			Unknown	97

(Courtesy of Tartter PI, Kaplan J, Bleiweiss I, et al: Lumpectomy margins, reexcision, and local recurrence of breast cancer. *Am J Surg* 179:81-85, 2000, with permission from Excerpta Medica Inc.)

46%, unknown 48%; $P < .001$), patient age (54 years for re-excision, 58 for non–re-excision; $P < .001$), and tumor size (mean 1.4 cm for re-excision and 1.7 cm for non–re-excision; $P = .003$) (Table 3). Patients undergoing re-excision were significantly more apt to be diagnosed by spot localization, have non-negative excisional biopsy margins, be younger, and have smaller tumors compared with patients not undergoing re-excision. Local recurrence was not significantly associated with margin status (8% clear margins, 7% positive margins, 19% close margins, and 11% unknown margins) or re-excision (10% local recurrence rate for patients with negative final margins after re-excision and 12% with positive, close, or unknown first margin without re-excision). Estrogen receptor status was the only variable associated with local recurrence ($P = .009$). Patients who were estrogen receptor negative and had non-negative margins had a

TABLE 3.—Relationship of Reexcision and Diagnostic Method, First Margin, Age, and Tumor Size

	Reexcision		
	Yes (%)	No (%)	P
Diagnostic method			
Excisional biopsy	51 (36)	90 (64)	
Spot localization	51 (63)	30 (37)	<0.001
Fine-needle cytology	9 (10)	81 (90)	
First margin			
Clear	0 (0)	65 (100)	
Positive	20 (46)	22 (54)	<0.001
Close	2 (11)	19 (89)	
Unknown	87 (48)	93 (52)	
Age (years)	54	58	<0.001
Tumor size (cm)	1.4	1.7	0.003

(Courtesy of Tartter PI, Kaplan J, Bleiweiss I, et al: Lumpectomy margins, reexcision, and local recurrence of breast cancer. *Am J Surg* 179:81-85, 2000, with permission from Excerpta Medica Inc.)

20% rate of local recurrence compared with 10% for patients who were estrogen receptor negative with negative margins and 7% for patients who were estrogen receptor positive regardless of margin status ($P = .021$).

Conclusion.—Clear excision margins were significantly more frequently obtained when the diagnosis was made preoperatively by fine-needle aspiration cytology. In patients with non-negative margins, re-excision was more frequently performed in younger women with small tumors diagnosed by spot localization biopsy. Local recurrence was not significantly associated with margins or re-excision. Estrogen-receptor–negative tumors with non-negative margins had significantly higher rates of local recurrence than estrogen-receptor–positive tumors and estrogen-receptor–negative tumors with clear margins and estrogen-receptor–positive tumors regardless of margin status.

▶ These document that with follow-up of more than 5 years (1) clear biopsy margins were associated with diagnosis by fine-needle aspiration cytology and (2) reexcision was significantly related to diagnostic method. Previous studies have shown similar results for preoperative fine-needle aspiration diagnosis as a facilitator for clear surgical margins.[1,2]

It seems logical that clear surgical margins would be beneficial for patients by avoiding re-excision and potentially decreasing incidence of local recurrence and improving survival rate. However, the conundrum is that there is no convincing evidence, in spite of numerous studies, that clear margins yield increased survival rate or decreased local recurrence rates. The cancer biology is confusing and unexplained. Surgical margin status remains an enigma.

As regards preoperative diagnosis by image-guided core needle breast biopsy versus wire-localized excisional breast biopsy, King et al reported on 211 patients treated with breast-conserving therapy demonstrating no significant difference in local recurrence rates between these 2 techniques, with more than 50 months of median follow-up.[3] However, the authors found that all patients' breast-conserving therapy included histologically negative margins.

W. H. Hindle, MD

References

1. Cox CE, Reintgen DS, Nicosia SV, et al: Analysis of residual cancer after diagnostic breast biopsy: An argument for fine-needle aspiration cytology. *Ann Surg Oncol* 2:201-206, 1995.
2. Tartter PL, Bleiweiss IJ, Levchenko S. Factors associated with clear biopsy margins and clear reexcision margins in breast cancer specimens from candidates for breast conservation. *J Am Col Surg* 185:187-220, 1997.
3. King TA, Hayes DH, Cederbom GJ, et al: Biopsy technique has no impact on local recurrence after breast-conserving therapy. *Breast J* 7:19-24, 2001.

SUGGESTED READING

Paskett ED, Stark N. Lymphedema: Knowledge, treatment, and impact among breast cancer survivors. *Breast J* 6:373-378, 2000.

▶ This study from the Wake Forest University School of Medicine (Winston-Salem, North Carolina) documents the frequency and intensity of lymphedema as a physical and psychological complication of axillary dissections. As many as 60% of women treated for breast cancer have lymphedema symptoms.[1] The onset of lymphedema can be delayed and insidious.[2] Treatment can be frustrating, arduous, and prolonged both for the physician and the patient.

Although the numbers of patients and physicians surveyed in this report are small, the findings are important and merit the attention of the clinician. The authors conclude: (1) "Overall, women knew little to nothing about lymphedema before they developed it;" and (2) "Most physicians reported that they did not routinely counsel women or provide written information on lymphedema prevention to their patients . . ." In another study, Woods et al reported that 90% of women with breast cancer lymphedema had not received information about the risk of developing lymphedema.[3] Certainly women deserve full, accurate, and clear disclosure of possible (sometimes "probable") lymphedema complications before treatment begins. All physicians and other health care providers involved in the treatment of breast cancer should provide this pertinent information.

William H. Hindle, MD

References

1. Passik S, Newman M, Brennan M, et al. Psychiatric consultation for women undergoing rehabilitation for upper-extremity lymphadema following breast cancer treatment. *J Pain Symptom Manage* 8:226-233,1993.
2. Knobf MT. Effects of common adult cancers: breast cancer. In: Baird S, et al, eds. Cancer nursing: a comprehensive textbook. Philadelphia, WB Saunders, 425-451, 1991.
3. Woods M. Patient's perceptions of breast cancer-related lymphedema. *Eur J Cancer Care* 2:125-128, 1993.

Variations in Prognostic Factors in Primary Breast Cancer Throughout the Menstrual Cycle

Kroman N, Thorpe SM, Wohlfahrt J, et al (Rigshospitalet, Copenhagen; Statens Serum Institut, Copenhagen)
Eur J Surg Oncol 26:11-16, 2000   28–6

Background.—The impact of the timing of surgery on prognosis in women with primary breast cancer is still unclear. Menstrual cycle–dependent variations in prognostic factors in women with primary breast cancer were studied.

Methods.—Data on 1060 women self-reporting regular menstruation and with a menstrual period within 6 weeks of surgery were analyzed. All underwent a 1-step procedure. None were using exogenous hormones at the time of surgery. Information on the last menstrual period before surgery and follow-up status were analyzed.

Findings.—Endogenous hormone fluctuations did not correlate significantly with estrogen receptor or progesterone receptor status. In addition,

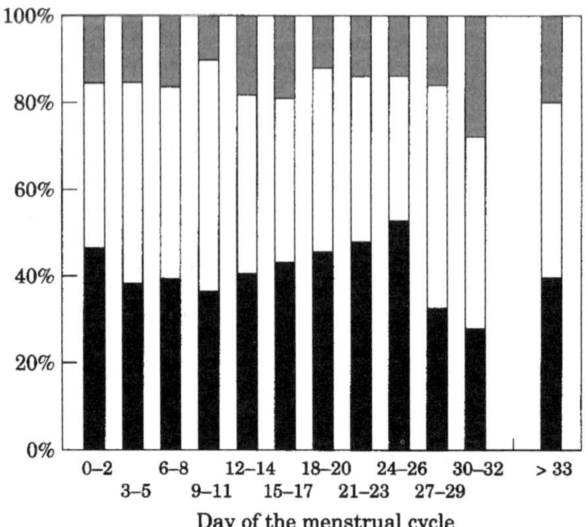

FIGURE 4.—Mitotic scores in relation to day of the menstrual cycle (871 patients). Score 1: less than 5 mitosis per 10 fields of vision. Score 2: 5 to 10 mitosis per 10 fields of vision. Score 3: more than 10 mitosis per 10 fields of vision. *Black bars* indicate score 1; *white bars*, score 2; *shaded bars*, score 3. (Courtesy of Kroman N, Thorpe SM, Wohlfahrt J, et al: Variations in prognostic factors in primary breast cancer throughout the menstrual cycle. *Eur J Surg Oncol* 26:11-16, 2000.)

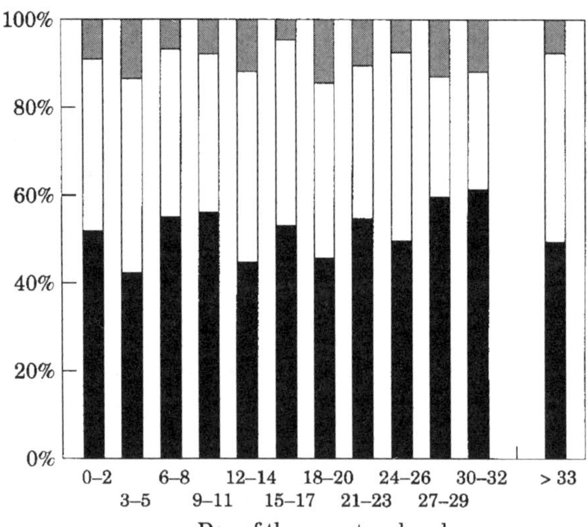

FIGURE 5.—Tumor size in relation to day of the menstrual cycle (909 patients). *Black bars* indicate 0-20 mm; *white bars*, 21-50 mm; *shaded bars*, more than 50 mm. (Courtesy of Kroman N, Thorpe SM, Wohlfahrt J, et al: Variations in prognostic factors in primary breast cancer throughout the menstrual cycle. *Eur J Surg Oncol* 26:11-16, 2000.)

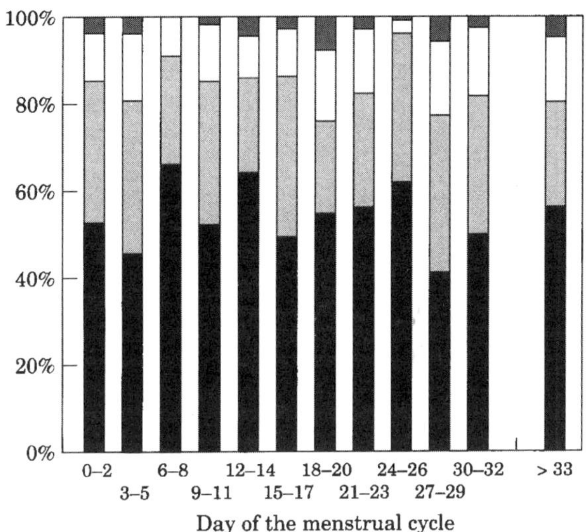

FIGURE 6.—Lymph node status in relation to day of menstrual cycle (1038 patients). *Black bars* indicate negative; *light shaded bars,* 1 to 3 positive nodes; *white bars* 4 to 9 positive nodes; *dark shaded bars,* more than 10 positive nodes. (Courtesy of Kroman N, Thorpe SM, Wohlfahrt J, et al: Variations in prognostic factors in primary breast cancer throughout the menstrual cycle. *Eur J Surg Oncol* 26:11-16, 2000.)

no cycle-dependent variations could be found for mitotic index, lymph node involvement, or tumor size (Figs 4, 5, and 6).

Conclusion.—In this study, prognostic factors did not vary significantly in relation to the timing of surgery relative to the last recorded menstrual cycle. Thus, these data do not support the hypothesis of a cycle-dependent prognostic effect of surgery in women with breast cancer.

▶ These data are reassuring and contrary to some reports indicating adverse effects of breast cancer surgery (and even biopsies, including fine-needle aspirations) performed in the luteal phase of the menstrual cycle. Outcome studies would be invaluable and should settle this debated issue. Hopefully, in the future, this Danish group with large numbers of patients and long-term data will provide a clear-cut answer.

W. H. Hindle, MD

SUGGESTED READING

Margolese RG, Lasry J-C M. Ambulatory surgery for breast cancer patients. *Ann Surg Onc* 7:181-187, 2000.

▶ Anxiety, fear, health assessment, pain, quality of life, and recovery were found to be essentially the same for inpatients and outpatients in this interview analysis from McGill University (Montreal, Canada). Better emotional adjustment and fewer psychological distress symptoms occurred in the ambulatory group. Most of the 90 patients in the study (55 outpatients and 35 inpatients) had level I and II axillary lymph node dissections combined with breast surgery under general anesthesia. It is fascinating that the inpatients took about 10 days longer than the outpatients to return to their usual activities and to feel that they had recovered from the surgery. Inpatients took an average of 27 days to feel recovered. Statistics are quoted that from 1986 to 1995 the incidence of outpatient mastectomies increased from 0% to 11% in the US (and is probably much higher currently). Certainly, comorbidity limits the use of ambulatory mastectomies, but the trend toward outpatient surgery continues. This psychosocial data supports that trend.

William H. Hindle, MD

Ferrante J, Gonzalez E, Pal N, et al. The use and outcome of outpatient mastectomy in Florida. *Am J Surg* 179:253-260, 2000.

▶ Although far removed from a prospective randomized clinical trail, these statistical observations reported by the University of South Florida (Tampa, Florida) give some data about the utilization and readmission rate for outpatient mastectomies. In 1994, in Florida, state discharge abstracts and the state tumor registry revealed 5418 mastectomies, of which 20% were performed on an outpatient basis. The readmission rate was 1.3% compared to 0.6% for the inpatient mastectomies. However, the readmission numbers are small, 14 and 24 respectively. In addition, "mastectomies" includes both simple and modified radical. More would be learned from this data if the subsets had been identified and the reason for the readmission was available for tabulation and analysis. Furthermore, readmission rates do not necessarily correlate with postoperative complications, major or minor, as most complications can be managed on an outpatient basis. More detailed data needs to be collected and published.

William H. Hindle, MD

Factors Influencing the Use of Breast Reconstruction Postmastectomy: A National Cancer Database Study
Morrow M, Scott SK, Menck HR, et al (Northwestern Univ, Chicago)
J Am Coll Surg 192:1-8, 2001   28–7

Objective.—Although a variety of techniques make breast reconstruction an option for women with early-stage breast cancer, little is known about the proportion of mastectomy patients who undergo immediate or early postoperative reconstruction. National patterns of breast reconstruction use, time trends, and factors that predict the use of reconstruction were determined by a large convenience sample from the National Cancer Data Base.

Methods.—A convenience sample of patients listed as undergoing mastectomy between 1985 and 1990 (n = 155,463) and between 1994 and 1995 (n = 68,348) was used. The 2 time periods were compared with respect to patient and tumor factors (Table 1).

Results.—Average patient age in the 2 time periods was 61.2 and 60.8 years. The respective percentage of Caucasian patients was 87.7% and 85%. National Cancer Institute–designated treatment centers accounted for 16.5% and 14.6% of all patients. The respective combined incidences of stage I and in situ carcinoma were 35% and 39.7%. The percentage of patients with unknown tumor grades declined from 57% to 28.5%

TABLE 1.—Patient Population

Variable	1985-1990 n	1985-1990 %	1994-1995 n	1994-1995 %
Age (y)				
0-29	1,095	0.7	450	0.7
30-39	9.945	6.4	4,386	6.4
40-49	25,914	16.2	12,519	18.3
50-59	30,088	19.4	13,867	20.3
60-69	41,555	26.7	15,514	22.7
70-79	33,627	21.6	15,022	22.0
80+	13,959	9.0	6,590	9.6
Geographic region				
Northeast	10,396	6.7	5,809	8.5
Southeast	28,438	18.3	14,570	21.4
Midwest	44,980	28.9	18,487	27.0
South	19,230	12.4	12,129	17.7
Mountain	14,036	9.0	5,151	7.5
Pacific	38,383	24.7	12,202	17.9
Income ($)				
<20,000	14,661	9.4	6,664	9.8
20,000-46,999	115,392	74.2	49,020	71.7
47,000+	17,975	11.6	7,184	10.5
Unknown	7,435	4.8	5,480	8.0
Ethnicity				
Non-Hispanic Caucasian	136,302	87.7	58,127	85.0
Hispanic	3,752	2.4	2,015	3.0
African-American	10,386	6.6	5,878	8.6
Asian	2,259	1.5	951	1.4
Other/unknown	2,764	1.8	1,377	2.0
Type of hospital				
National Cancer Institute-recognized	4,042	2.6	1,640	2.4
Teaching	21,609	13.9	8,338	12.2
Large community	62,807	40.4	24,949	36.5
Government	8,084	5.2	3,622	5.3
Medium/small community	39,954	25.7	14,900	21.8
Profit	6,063	3.9	3,212	4.7
Other/nonapproved	12,904	8.3	11,687	17.1
Pathologic American Joint Committee on Cancer stage				
0	9.773	6.2	5,789	8.5
I	44,775	28.8	21,336	31.2
II	50,960	32.8	25,270	37.0
III	12,123	7.8	6,636	9.7
IV	3,355	2.2	1,401	2.0
Unknown	34,477	22.2	7,916	11.6
Grade				
1	6,848	4.4	6,815	10.0
2	27,431	17.6	20,084	29.4
3	29,600	19.0	20,517	30.0
4	3,065	2.0	1,455	2.1
Unknown	88,519	57.0	19,477	28.5

(Courtesy of Morrow W, Scott SK, Menck HR, et al: Factors influencing the use of breast reconstruction postmastectomy: A National Cancer Database study. *J Am Coll Surg* 192:1-8, 2001. By permission of the Journal of the American College of Surgeons.)

(Table 2). During the 2 periods, 3.4% and 8.3%, respectively, of mastectomy patients had breast reconstruction. Of the variables evaluated for their influence on early reconstruction, 6 factors were identified by multivariate analysis as influencing the use of reconstruction in the second study period (Table 3). Age was the most important determinant of recon-

TABLE 2.—Variables Influencing the Use of Reconstruction

Variables	1985-1990 (n = 155,463)		1994-1995 (n = 63,348)	
	n	%	n	%
Patients reconstructed	5,361	3.4	5,671	8.3
Age (y)				
<50	2,951	8.1	3,106	17.9
50-69	2,154	3.0	2,285	7.8
≥70	256	0.5	280	1.3
Geographic region				
Northeast	146	1.4	451	7.8
Southeast	821	2.9	1,090	7.5
Midwest	1,031	2.2	1,228	6.6
South	586	3.0	773	6.4
Mountain	574	4.1	588	11.4
Pacific	2,203	5.7	1,541	12.6
Income ($)				
<20,000	248	1.7	282	4.2
20,000-46,999	3,932	3.4	3,862	7.9
≥47,000+	1,204	6.7	1,048	14.6
Unknown	242	3.3	479	8.7
Ethnicity				
Non-Hispanic Caucasian	4,849	3.6	5,005	8.6
Hispanic	171	4.6	175	8.7
African-American	184	1.8	341	5.8
Asian	67	3.0	96	7.0
Other/unknown	90	3.3	54	5.7
Hospital type				
National Cancer Institute-recognized	225	5.6	187	11.4
Teaching	756	3.4	851	10.2
Large community	2,033	3.2	2,087	8.5
Government	214	2.6	227	6.3
Medium/small community	1,206	3.0	964	6.5
Profit	321	5.2	306	5.0
Nonapproved	606	4.4	1,026	8.8
Pathologic stage				
0	854	8.7	895	15.5
I	1,535	3.4	1,713	8.0
II	1,561	3.1	1,991	7.9
III	234	1.9	348	5.2
IV	43	1.3	46	3.3
Unknown	1,134	3.3	678	8.6
Histologic grade				
1	283	4.1	473	6.9
2	1,010	3.9	1,469	7.3
3	1,009	3.4	1,565	7.6
4	107	3.5	166	11.4
Unknown	2,952	3.3	1,998	10.3

(Courtesy of Morrow W, Scott SK, Menck HR, et al: Factors influencing the use of breast reconstruction postmastectomy: A National Cancer Database study. *J Am Coll Surg* 192:1-8, 2001. By permission of the Journal of the American College of Surgeons.)

struction, with women aged 50 years and younger 4.3 times more likely to choose reconstruction.

Conclusion.—Immediate breast reconstruction is being chosen infrequently. Factors that influence the decision for early reconstruction include patient age, geographic location, and tumor stage. Patients and physicians need to be educated to take advantage of this breast cancer management option.

TABLE 3.—Multivariate Analysis of Factors Influencing the Use of
Reconstruction 1994-1995 (n = 55, 728)

Variable	Odds Ratio	95% Confidence Interval
Age: ≤ 50 vs > 50 y	4.3	4.2-4.4
PAJCC* stage: 0 vs I-IV	2.1	2.1-2.2
Family income: ≥ $40,000 vs < 40,000	2.0	2.0-2.1
Ethnicity: Non-African-American vs African-American	1.6	1.5-1.7
Hospital type: NCI-recognized vs other	1.4	1.3-1.7
Geographic region: Northeast, Southeast, Mountain, and Pacific vs Midwest and South	1.3	1.2-1.3

*Pathologic American Joint Committee on Cancer.
(Courtesy of Morrow W, Scott SK, Menck HR, et al: Factors influencing the use of breast reconstruction postmastectomy: A National Cancer Database study. *J Am Coll Surg* 192:1-8, 2001. By permission of the Journal of the American College of Surgeons.)

▶ This detailed analysis has impressive numbers and gives a picture of breast surgery practice patterns in the United States. Recent federal legislation mandating insurance coverage for breast reconstruction in cancer treatment should potentially eliminate most patient financial considerations, which previously restricted the use of breast reconstruction. However, overall cost and use of medical resources remain important issues. In this study by univariate analysis, patient age, ethnicity, income, geographic location, type of hospital, and tumor stage influenced breast reconstruction use. Overall, the use of early/immediate reconstruction for mastectomy patients increased from 3.4% (1985-1990) to 8.3% (1994-1995), a modest increase compared with the 35% of those who were offered reconstruction and had the procedure in a single-institution study (1988-1993).[1]

Mastectomy (with the potential of breast reconstruction) will continue to be appropriate treatment for many women with breast cancer because even 10% of women with stage I and 30% of women with stage II breast cancer are not candidates for breast-conserving surgery.[1]

It is of interest in the 1994 to 1995 data of the mastectomy patient population (Table 1), that 25% of the women were less than 50 years of age. Age younger than 50 years was found to be the single best predictor of breast reconstruction use.

The authors conclude that "Many of the factors that influence the use of breast reconstruction, such as age, geographic location, and tumor stage, also predict the use of breast-conserving therapy, and are reflections of physician attitudes that are not supported by available clinical data." Clearly surgeon and patient education is needed.

W. H. Hindle, MD

Reference

1. Morrow M, Bucci C, Rademaker A. Medical contraindications are not a major factor in the underutilization of breast-conserving therapy. *J Am Coll Surg* 186:269-274, 1998.

Reduction Mammaplasty Provides Long-term Improvement in Health Status and Quality of Life

Blomqvist L, Eriksson A, Brandberg Y (Karolinska Hosp, Stockholm)
Plast Reconstr Surg 106:991-997, 2000   28–8

Background.—Women with heavy breasts often experience pain in the upper part of the body, back pain, poor posture, and headache (Table 1). The health status and quality of life in patients with macromastia undergoing reduction mammaplasty were documented.

Methods.—Forty-nine women, aged 20 to 71 years, were treated at 1 center between January and June 1997. The prospective study included a 4-part questionnaire administered preoperatively as well as 6 and 12 months postoperatively.

Findings.—Postoperatively, the women reported significant reduction in pain in all areas assessed: the head, neck, shoulders, back, breast, and bra strap indentation. (Fig 1). The patients also reported improvement in body posture, choice of clothing, sexual relations, and working capacity (Fig 2). No improvements in sleep were reported. Reduction mammaplasty also significantly increased patients' quality of life (Fig 3). At 1 year, health-related quality of life in the patient group was as good as that of an age-matched control group. All improvements were maintained at 12 months.

Conclusions.—Reduction mammaplasty can significantly alleviate pain in women with macromastia. Such treatment improves the quality of life of affected women, who report a below-normal quality of life before reduction mammaplasty.

▶ With the intense emphasis on breast cancer in the United States, there are a limited number of articles on benign breast disease and even fewer on breast symptoms unassociated with histologic pathology. Our Swedish colleagues often lead the way in researching these nonmalignant areas. Clinicians need to be sensitive to and informed about nonmalignant breast problems. Breast concerns are often overshadowed by fear of breast cancer (both on the part of patients and their physicians).

This prospective questionnaire study from Stockholm carefully documents the improvement in symptomatic and quality of life issues for reduction mammaplasty in 49 women. The pertinent literature of similar studies is summarized in Table 1. The data here support the surgical approach to the symptoms associated with macromastia. Clinicians would do well to initiate

TABLE 1.—Review of Improvements of Macromastia Associated Physical and Psychological Problems after Reduction Mammaplasty

Parameter	Atterhem et al., 1998 % Relief 3 Years Postoperative	Boschert et al., 1996 Improvements (p < Values) 6 Months Postoperative	Brühlmann and Tschopp, 1998 % Relief ca 8 Years Postoperative	Gonzalez et al., 1993 % Improved or Relieved 9 Months Postoperative	Kinell et al., 1990 % Improved or Relieved 5 Years Postoperative	Maxwell Davis et al., 1995 % Relief 3 Years Postoperative	Miller et al., 1995 % Improved 1-6 Years Postoperative	Schnur et al., 1997 % Problems Resolved 5.7 Years Postoperative
No. of Patients	214/288	72/200	132/156	33/39	136/161	406/780	163/282	328/363
Breast pain				81	100	86	82-89	73
Neck pain	87	0.0001	.98	100	83	84	95	73
Back pain	95	0.0001	75	97	91	84	92-96	71,73
Shoulder pain	91	0.0001	98	100	85	94	99	83
Bra groove pain	96		99	94	98	85	93	82
Headache	86			94	100	86	86	78
Intertrigo	94			94		97	82	92
Sport	91	0.001	98					89
Running								83
Clothing				86				86
Comfortable with body	88							
Satisfied with body	78				98			81
Posture				81				
Sleeping				61				
Hand numbness					100	91		

(Courtesy of Blomqvist L, Eriksson A, Brandberg Y: Reduction mammoplasty provides long-term improvement in health status and quality of life. *Plast Reconstr Surg* 106:991-997, 2000.)

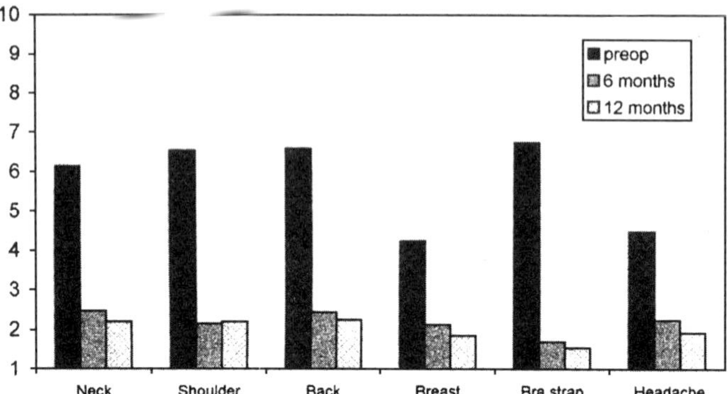

FIGURE 1.—Scored mean pain (1 = no pain, 10 = extreme pain) in 6 locations preoperatively, and 6 and 12 months postoperatively. Values are P less than 0.001 for all locations (paired t test). (Courtesy of Blomqvist L, Eriksson A, Brandberg Y: Reduction mammoplasty provides long-term improvement in health status and quality of life. *Plast Reconstr Surg* 106:991-997, 2000.)

open discussion with their patients about such breast concerns and symptoms.

W. H. Hindle, MD

SUGGESTED READING

Hatcher MB, Fallowfield L, A'Hern R. The psychosocial impact of bilateral prophylactic mastectomy: Prospective study questionnaires and semistructured interviews. *BMJ* 322:76-79, 2001.

▶ Psychosocial/sexual data is difficult to obtain and interpret, and many articles about such data are confusing to clinicians and offer little guidance for practical management. This article from the Royal Free and University College Medical School, London, is an exception that is best summarized by the following direct quotations: (1) "Bilateral prophylactic mastectomy reduces psychological mor-

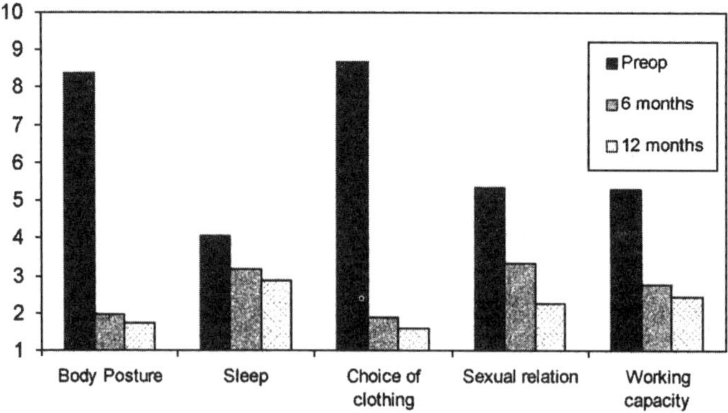

FIGURE 2.—Scored mean of problems (1 = not at all, 10 = very much) related to the size and weight of the breasts preoperatively and 6 and 12 months postoperatively. Values are P less than 0.001 for all items except sleep (paired t test). (Courtesy of Blomqvist L, Eriksson A, Brandberg Y: Reduction mammoplasty provides long-term improvement in health status and quality of life. *Plast Reconstr Surg* 106:991-997, 2000.)

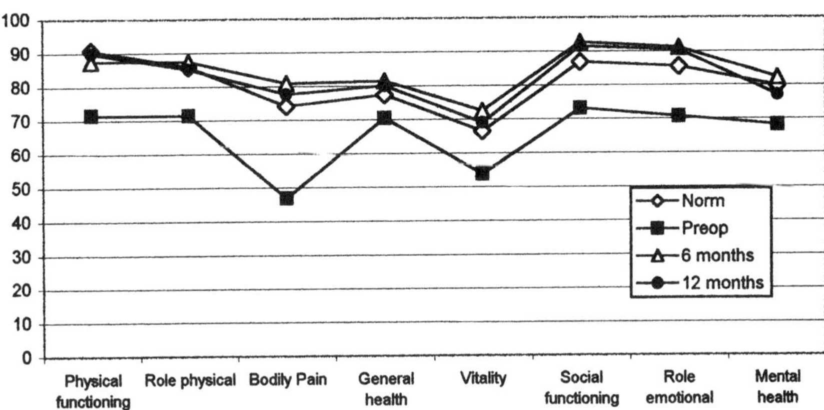

FIGURE 3.—Scored mean of short-form 36 norm data (age group 35 to 44 years) and macromastia patients preoperatively and 6 and 12 months postoperatively. (Courtesy of Blomqvist L, Eriksson A, Brandberg Y: Reduction mammoplasty provides long-term improvement in health status and quality of life. *Plast Reconstr Surg* 106:991-997, 2000.)

bidity and anxiety and does not have a detrimental impact on women's body image or sexual function." (2) "Women who chose such surgery have a higher, often inaccurate, perception of their risk of developing breast cancer." (3) "Genetic counselors need to ensure that women's decisions to have surgery are based on accurate perceptions."

Certainly each case should be evaluated individually, and the decisions not made hastily. In my experience, women considering such surgery benefit from psychological counseling before and after the surgery in order to better handle the emotional aspects of their decision, the surgery itself, and their postoperative adjustment.

William H. Hindle, MD

Favourable and Unfavourable Effects on Long-term Survival of Radiotherapy for Early Breast Cancer: An Overview of the Randomised Trials

Early Breast Cancer Trialists' Collaborative Group (Radcliffe Infirmary, Oxford)
Lancet 355:1757-1770, 2000

28–9

Background.—Many randomized trials have assessed the effects of radiotherapy for early breast cancer on outcomes such as local and distant recurrence, breast cancer mortality, and overall survival. Meta-analyses of these trials suggest that radiotherapy significantly reduces local recurrence risk, but has little impact on overall survival through the first 10 years. The current meta-analysis evaluates the very long-term effects of radiotherapy for early breast cancer.

Methods.—The analysis included 10- and 20-year follow-up data from 40 trials comparing radiotherapy plus surgery and other treatments with the sample treatments without radiotherapy. Data were available on

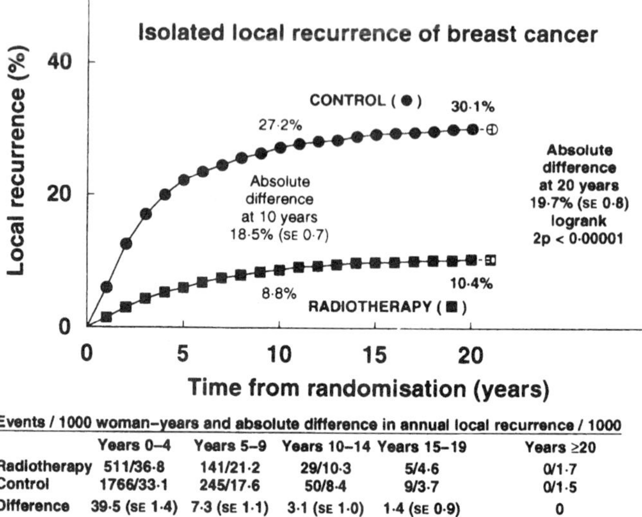

Events / 1000 woman–years and absolute difference in annual local recurrence / 1000				
	Years 0–4	Years 5–9	Years 10–14	Years 15–19	Years ≥20
Radiotherapy	511/36·8	141/21·2	29/10·3	5/4·6	0/1·7
Control	1766/33·1	245/17·6	50/8·4	9/3·7	0/1·5
Difference	39·5 (SE 1·4)	7·3 (SE 1·1)	3·1 (SE 1·0)	1·4 (SE 0·9)	0

FIGURE 3.—Absolute effects of radiotherapy on isolated local recurrence (as first event). *Note*: Format as for Fig 2. Excludes 3 trials without data on site of first recurrence. (Courtesy of Early Breast Cancer Trialists' Collaborative Group: Favourable and unfavourable effects on long-term survival of radiotherapy for early breast cancer: An overview of the randomised trials. *Lancet* 355:1757-1770. Copyright 2000 by The Lancet Ltd.)

19,5782 women over 178,000 woman-years of follow-up, including 2756 local recurrences and 9838 deaths. About half of the patients had "node-positive" disease. The studies tested various radiotherapy approaches, including irradiation of the breast/chest wall irradiation, axilla and fossa, and internal mammary chain.

Results.—The 10-year local recurrence rate was about 9% with radiotherapy versus 27% without (Fig 3). The effect was largely independent of patient characteristics and type of radiotherapy. Radiotherapy was associated with a significant reduction in mortality from breast cancer, but significant increases in mortality from other causes, specifically vascular causes. Thus, by 20 years, the overall survival rate was about 37% with radiotherapy versus 36% without (Fig 2). Early mortality was little affected by radiotherapy. On log-rank analysis, the annual breast cancer mortality rate was about 13% lower with radiotherapy, while the mortality rate from other causes was about 21% higher (Fig 6). Factors significantly affecting the ratio of breast cancer mortality versus other causes included lymph node status, patient age, and decade of follow-up. As a result, these factors also affected the ratio of absolute benefit to absolute hazard associated with radiation.

Conclusions.—This large meta-analysis confirms that radiotherapy for early breast cancer by about two thirds, but increases the overall risk of mortality from other causes. If some radiotherapy regimen could produce a similar reduction in local recurrence without the long-term hazard, it would yield a 2% to 4% improvement in 20-year survival. With current

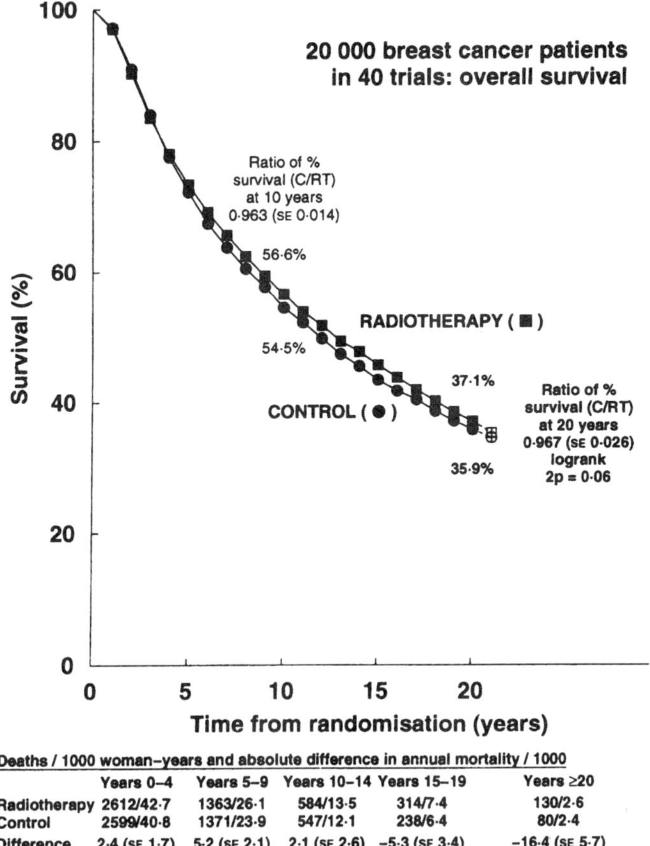

Deaths / 1000 woman–years and absolute difference in annual mortality / 1000

	Years 0–4	Years 5–9	Years 10–14	Years 15–19	Years ≥20
Radiotherapy	2612/42·7	1363/26·1	584/13·5	314/7·4	130/2·6
Control	2599/40·8	1371/23·9	547/12·1	238/6·4	80/2·4
Difference	2·4 (SE 1·7)	5·2 (SE 2·1)	2·1 (SE 2·6)	−5·3 (SE 3·4)	−16·4 (SE 5·7)

FIGURE 2.—Absolute effects of radiotherapy on 20-year survival. *Note*: Proportions surviving at 10 years and 20 years are given, with the ratio (control [C] to radiotherapy [RT]) of the survival probability. Deaths per 1000 woman-years are given for particular periods of follow-up, with the difference in the annual rate per 1000 (control minus radiotherapy). *Open symbols* after year 20 indicate the effects by year 21 of the annual rates in years 20 and later. (Courtesy of Early Breast Cancer Trialists' Collaborative Group: Favourable and unfavourable effects on long-term survival of radiotherapy for early breast cancer: An overview of the randomised trials. *Lancet* 355:1757-1770. Copyright 2000 by The Lancet Ltd.)

regimens, the risk-benefit ratio is likely to be favorable only for younger women at relatively higher risk of local recurrence.

▶ These long-term, disease-specific, survival data collected by meta-analysis of 20,000 women in 40 unconfounded randomized trials clearly demonstrate the effectiveness of radiation therapy in controlling local recurrences of breast cancer. However, the counter-balancing principle applies, with documented increases in risk of death from vascular disease.

This decreased survival resulting from vascular disease has also been demonstrated in trials of postoperative radiotherapy for lung cancer and in 40-year follow-ups of atomic bomb explosion survivors. One hopes that the current sophisticated methodology of breast cancer radiation therapy with

FIGURE 6

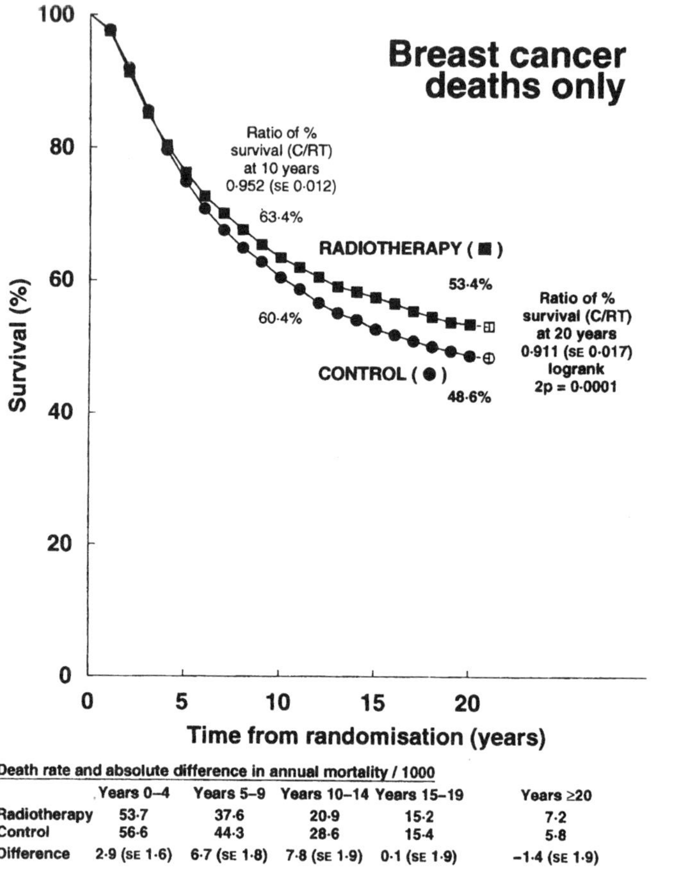

Death rate and absolute difference in annual mortality / 1000

	Years 0–4	Years 5–9	Years 10–14	Years 15–19	Years ≥20
Radiotherapy	53·7	37·6	20·9	15·2	7·2
Control	56·6	44·3	28·6	15·4	5·8
Difference	2·9 (SE 1·6)	6·7 (SE 1·8)	7·8 (SE 1·9)	0·1 (SE 1·9)	−1·4 (SE 1·9)

(Continued)

precise targeting of fields and protection of the heart and major vascular vessels will result in fewer long-term adverse survival effects of irradiation.

W. H. Hindle, MD

SUGGESTED READING

MacKarem G, Roche CA, Hughes KS. The effectiveness of the Gail model in estimating risk for development of breast cancer in women under 40 years of age. *Breast J* 7:34–39, 2001.

▶ This carefully designed (though with small numbers) analysis from the Lahey Hitchcock Medical Center (Burlington, Massachusetts) based on questionnaires, demonstrates lack of correlation with age at menarche, age at first live birth, and the number of first degree relatives with breast cancer. There was correlation between higher numbers of breast biopsies in patients with a benign breast biopsy. "The RR (relative risk) calculated was the RR that existed at the time of the surgical consultation for a suspicious breast lesion." These findings are

FIGURE 6 (cont.)

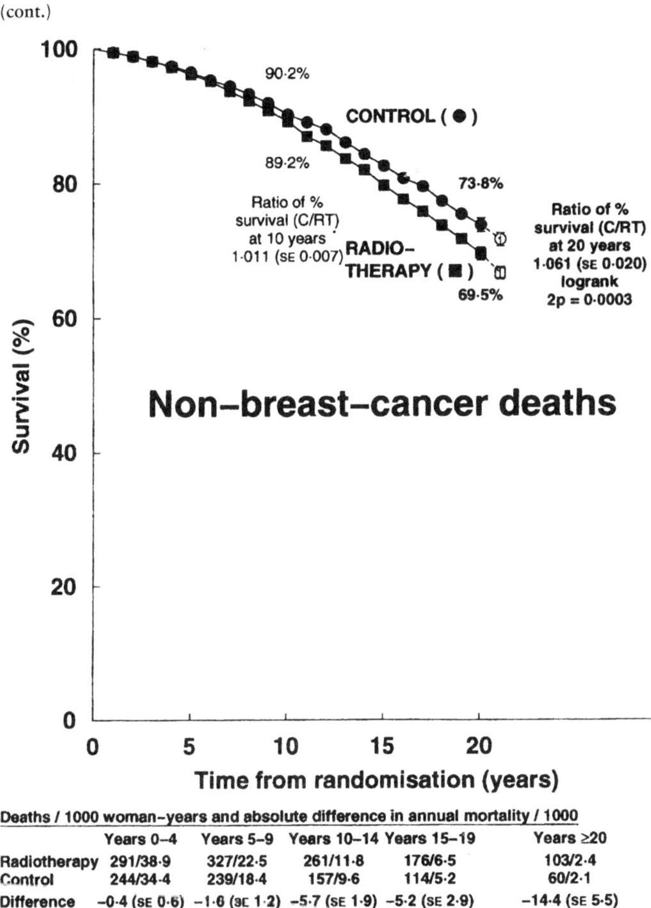

Deaths / 1000 woman-years and absolute difference in annual mortality / 1000				
	Years 0–4	Years 5–9	Years 10–14	Years 15–19	Years ≥20
Radiotherapy	291/38·9	327/22·5	261/11·8	176/6·5	103/2·4
Control	244/34·4	239/18·4	157/9·6	114/5·2	60/2·1
Difference	−0·4 (SE 0·6)	−1·6 (SE 1·2)	−5·7 (SE 1·9)	−5·2 (SE 2·9)	−14·4 (SE 5·5)

FIGURE 6.—Absolute effects of radiotherapy on cause-specific survival. *Note*: Format as for Fig 2. Breast cancer mortality includes all deaths, irrespective of cause, after recurrence. The breast cancer death rate during particular periods of follow-up is calculated by subtraction of non-breast-cancer mortality from the all-cause mortality rate. (Courtesy of Early Breast Cancer Trialists' Collaborative Group: Favourable and unfavourable effects on long-term survival of radiotherapy for early breast cancer: An overview of the randomised trials. *Lancet* 355:1757-1770. Copyright 2000 by The Lancet Ltd.)

contrary to the estimation of RR in the Gail model.[1] The authors conclude, "The Gail model is not useful in identifying immediate risk of breast cancer in women under 40 and should not be used for that purpose." Perhaps the authors could take a similar approach in analysis of the women ages 40 to 49 and ascertain if that age group is accurately predicted by the Gail model.

William H. Hindle, MD

Reference

1. Gail MH, Brinton LA, Byar DP, et al. Projecting individualized probability of developing breast cancer for white females who are being examined annually. *J Natl Cancer Inst* 81:1879-1886, 1989.

One Stop Breast Clinics—Victims of Their Own Success? A Prospective Audit of Referrals to a Specialist Breast Clinic
Patel RS, Smith DC, Reid I (Victoria Infirmary, Glasgow, Scotland)
Eur J Surg Oncol 26:452-454, 2000
28–10

Background.—One-stop breast clinics, initially designed to provide rapid diagnosis for persons with malignant disease, may be receiving unnecessary referrals of the "worried well," who demand access to these clinics and expect the same level of care as persons at high risk of malignancy. The number of unnecessary referrals to specialist breast clinics was investigated.

Methods.—New patient referrals from primary care to specialist breast clinics were audited prospectively. The total number of referrals, proportion of urgent and nonurgent referrals, proportion of unnecessary referrals (as judged by published guidelines), waiting times for outpatient appointments, and patient outcomes were analyzed. Data were obtained on 321 referrals.

Findings.—Thirty-five percent of the referrals were urgent. According to published guidelines, 28% of urgent referrals and 37% of nonurgent referrals were not appropriate (Tables 1, 2, and 3). Ten percent of the patients referred had breast cancer, whereas the remainder had benign or no disease.

Conclusion.—Increasing numbers of patients with minimal or no disease are being referred to specialist breast clinics. One third of the current series had been referred inappropriately. Such referrals inevitably decrease the efficiency of these services for patients with significant symptoms.

TABLE 1.—Principal Symptom According to Referral Letter

Presenting Complaint	Number	%
Breast lump	204	64
Breast pain	55	17
Family history	12	4
Nipple discharge	24	8
Anxiety	3	1
Miscellaneous	23	7

(Courtesy of Patel RS, Smith DC, Reid I: One stop breast clinics—Victims of their own success? A prospective audit of referrals to a specialist breast clinic. *Eur J Surg Oncol* 26:452-454, 2000.)

TABLE 2.—Main Presenting Complaint in Patients With Breast Cancer

Presenting Complaint	Number	%
Breast lump/nodularity	29	91
Nipple change	2	6
Axillary lump	1	3

(Courtesy of Patel RS, Smith DC, Reid I: One stop breast clinics—Victims of their own success? A prospective audit of referrals to a specialist breast clinic. *Eur J Surg Oncol* 26:452-454, 2000.)

▶ Although the medical legal climate, health care compensation, and "organization" of health care services are distinctly different in the United Kingdom and in the United States, the data in this prospective audit study of new patient referrals are of clinical interest. Breast cancer was diagnosed in 10% of the total referrals. Patients with breast cancer did not have pain or nipple discharge as their main presenting complaints. More than 90% presented with breast lump/nodularity. The median age of the cancer patients was 62 years (range 35-91 years). Overall, almost 60% of the patients were discharged from the clinical after 1 appointment.

According to National Health Service referral guidelines,[1] based on both national breast disease management[2] and regional breast cancer[3] guidelines, 28% of the urgent referrals were judged "inappropriate" as were 34% of the nonurgent referrals. Apparently, this study was done before an active program of mammographic breast cancer screening was instituted, as there is no category of mammographic abnormalities or of nonpalpable lesions. Those data are limited to "symptomatic" women. Furthermore, the figures for nipple discharge would be more meaningful if broken down to spontaneous versus elicited nipple discharge and if "nipple change" (both of the 2 cases cited were apparently cancer) were further identified and kept separate from nipple discharge.

W. H. Hindle, MD

References

1. Austoker J, Nansel R, Baum M, et al: Guidelines for referral of patients with breast problems. NHS Breast Screening Programme on behalf of the Department of Health Advisory Committee on Breast Screening. 1995.

TABLE 3.—Main Presenting Complaint in Noncancer Patients

Presenting Complaint	Number	%
Breast lump	175	60
Breast pain	55	19
Nipple discharge/nipple change	22	8
Family history only	12	4
Anxiety only	3	1
Other miscellaneous	22	8

(Courtesy of Patel RS, Smith DC, Reid I: One stop breast clinics—Victims of their own success? A prospective audit of referrals to a specialist breast clinic. *Eur J Surg Oncol* 26:452-454, 2000.)

2. British Association of Surgical Oncology: Guidelines for surgeons in the management of symptomatic breast disease in the United Kingdom. *Eur J Surg Oncol* 21(Suppl A):1-13,1995.
3. Scottish Intercollegiate Guidelines Network: Breast cancer in women—A national clinical guideline. 1998.

Population-Based Study of BRCA1 and BRCA2 Mutations in 1035 Unselected Finnish Breast Cancer Patients

Syrjäkoski K, Vahteristo P, Eerola H, et al (Tampere Univ, Finland; Helsinki Univ; Uppsala Univ, Sweden; et al)
J Natl Cancer Inst 92:1529-1531, 2000

28–11

Background.—Previous research on whole-gene mutation screening demonstrates that 11 mutations account for 84% of all detected BRCA1 and BRCA2 mutations . These 11 mutations offer a rapid method for analyzing the impact of BRCA1 and BRCA2 mutations at the population level without bias toward any individual founder mutation.

Methods and Findings.—This population-based study of BRCA1 and BRCA2 mutations included 1035 unselected Finnish women with breast cancer. The patients were screened for all 11 BRCA1 and 8 BRCA2 mutations detected previously in the Finnish population. In this population, the frequency of BRCA1 and BRCA2 mutations was only 1.8% (Table 1).

Conclusion.—Screening for BRCA1 and BRCA2 mutations in the general breast cancer population is not warranted. Strict criteria for BRCA1 testing in breast cancer are needed.

▶ The crux of this brief communication from the Helsinki University Central Hospital is essentially that, in the words of the authors, "The results illustrate that BRCA1 and BRCA2 mutation screening is not warranted in the general breast cancer population and substantiate the suggested strict criteria for BRCA1 testing in breast cancer." Those criteria are (1) a family history of ovarian cancer, (2) early age at diagnosis of breast cancer, and (3) a family history of 2 or more breast cancers.[1]

For breast cancer patients with BRCA1 or 2, Schrag et al have pointed out that contralateral prophylactic mastectomy may increase life expectancy and they also reviewed other strategies for life expectancy gain.[2] In addition, Shih et al reported that BRCA1 and 2 mutations were twice as common when a second nonovarian cancer was present in the breast cancer patient or her relatives with breast cancer.[3] Furthermore, the Anglian Breast Cancer Study Group reported on a population-based series of 1220 breast cancer cases with identification of BRCA1 in 8 (0.7%) and BRCA2 in 16 (1.3%).[4] Only 17% of the familial breast cancer risk was attributable to BRCA1 and 2.

W. H. Hindle, MD

TABLE 1.—Number of BRCA1 and BRCA2 Mutations in Distinct Groups of Patients With Breast Cancer Characterized by Family History of Breast and/or Ovarian Cancers

Family History (No. of Affected Relatives in Addition to Index Case Subject)	No. of Case Subjects Tested	No. With Mutation					Two-sided *P* Compared With the Group With No Family History
		BRCA1	BRCA2	BRCA1 or BRCA2	%	95% CI	
None	677	1	3	4	0.6	0.2-1.5	
1	256	0	4	4	1.6	0.4-4.0	.23
Breast cancer	236	0	3	3	1.3	0.3-3.7	.38
Ovarian cancer	20	0	1	1	5.0	0.1-24.9	.14
2	78	1	5	6	7.7	2.9-16.0	<.0005
Breast cancer only	67	0	4	4	6.0	1.7-14.6	.003
Breast and ovarian cancers	11	1	1	2	18.2	2.3-51.8	.003
≥3	24	2	3	5	20.8	7.1-42.2	<.0005
Breast cancer only	15	0	0	0	0	0-21.8	1.0
Breast and ovarian cancers	9	2	3	5	55.6	21.2-86.3	<.0005
Total	1035	4	15	19	1.8	1.1-2.9	

(Courtesy of Syrjäkoski K, Vahteristo P, Eerola H, et al: Population-based study of BRCA1 and BRCA2 mutations in 1035 unselected Finnish breast cancer patients. *J Natl Cancer Inst* 92:1529-1531, 2000. By permission of Oxford University Press.)

References

1. Newman B, Mu H, Butler LM, et al: Frequency of breast cancer attributable to BRCA1 in a population-based series of American women. *JAMA* 279:915-921, 1998.
2. Schrag D, Kuntz KM, Garber JE, et al: Life expectancy gains from cancer prevention strategies for women with breast cancer and BRCA1 or BRCA2 mutations. *JAMA* 283:617-624, 2000.
3. Shih HA, Nathanson KL, Seal S, et al: BRCA1 and BRCA2 mutations in breast cancer families with multiple primary cancers. *Clin Cancer Res* 6:4259-4264, 2000.
4. Anglian Breast Cancer Study Group: Prevalence and penetrance of BRCA1 and BRCA2 mutations in a population-based series of breast cancer cases. *Br J Cancer* 83:1301-1308, 2000.

SUGGESTED READING

Papelard H, de Bock GH, van Eijk R, et al. Prevalence of BRCA1 in a hospital-based population of Dutch breast cancer patients. *Br J Cancer* 83:719-724, 2000.
▶ This study covers 642 Dutch unselected breast cancer patients tested for BRCA1 mutations. It is concluded that ". . .the estimated prevalence of breast cancer in the general population in the Netherlands attributable to BRCA1 mutations is 2.1%." However, the figure was 9.5% for age at diagnosis under age 40, and 6.4% for under age 50. In fact, "All mutation carriers were under 50 years-of-age at diagnosis of the first breast cancer and five did not have any relatives with breast cancer." The proportion of bilateral disease in the mutation carriers was the same as found in noncarriers. Slowly the role of BRCA in breast cancer is being elucidated, but the natural history of the origin and progression of breast cancer remains a mystery.

William H. Hindle, MD

Miron A, Schildkraut JM, Rimer BK, et al. Testing for hereditary breast and ovarian cancer in the southeastern United States. *Ann Surg* 231:624-634, 2000.
▶ This genetic study from Duke University Medial Center (Durham, North Carolina) of 213 women tested for hereditary breast/ovarian cancer showed 20.6% to have 29 separate mutations; 11 Jewish women had 3 founder mutations, 13.1% had uncharacterized variants of BRCA1 or BRCA2 of which 9 had not previously been reported. Most of the identified mutants were seen only once. In general the women overestimated their chances of having deleterious gene mutations contrary to statistical estimates of carrier risk.

Preventative surgery questionnaires were given at the beginning of the study and follow-up questionnaires were given after testing results and counseling. The patient's intention to have preventative surgery was reinforced by the positive test results. However, women who had shown little interest in preventive surgery continued to be reluctant after receiving their test results and counseling. It seems that the women had usually made their decision before the study, the testing and the counseling. The clinical conundrum of BRCA1 and BRCA2 testing continues.

William H. Hindle, MD

Breast Carcinoma Presents a Decade Earlier in Mexican Women Than in Women in the United States or European Countries
Rodríguez-Cuevas S, Macías CG, Franceschi D, et al (Hosp de Oncología, México City; Secretary of Health, Mexico, Mexico City; Sylvester Comprehensive Cancer Ctr, Miami, Fla)
Cancer 91:863-868, 2001   28–12

Background.—Breast cancer is the second most common malignancy in Mexico. Mortality from this disease has increased from 3.6 per 100,000 women in 1985 to 6 per 100,000 in 1994. Most breast cancers are not diagnosed until an advanced stage, when cure is unlikely. In this study, patient age at presentation was investigated.

Methods and Findings.—Data were obtained on 29,075 patients registered in the Histopathological Registry of Malignant Neoplasms in Mexico between 1993 and 1996. The overall median age was 51 years. Forty-six percent of all breast carcinomas developed before the age of 50 (Fig 1). The age group most frequently affected was 40- to 49-year-olds, in whom 29.5% of the cancers occurred. The percentage was 14% in women

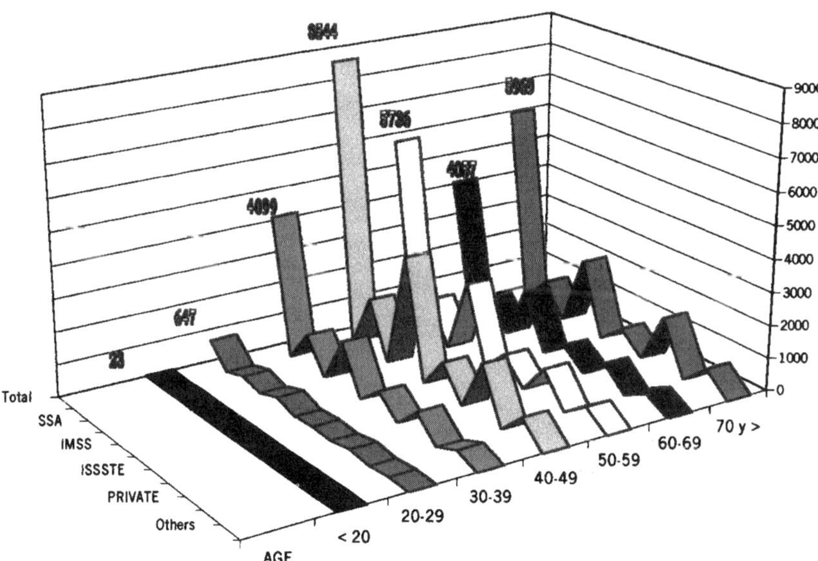

FIGURE 1.—Distribution by age and institution of Mexican patients with breast carcinoma *Abbreviations*: IMSS, Instituto Mexicano del Seguro Social ISSSTE, Instituto de Seguridad Social al Servicio de los Trabajadores del Estado (Courtesy of Rodríguez-Cuevas S, Macías CG, Franceschi D, et al: Breast carcinoma presents a decade earlier in Mexican women than in women in the United States or European countries. CANCER Vol. 91, No. 4, 2001, pp 863-868. Copyright 2001, American Cancer Society. Reprinted by permission of Wiley-Liss, Inc., a subsidiary of John Wiley & Sons, Inc.)

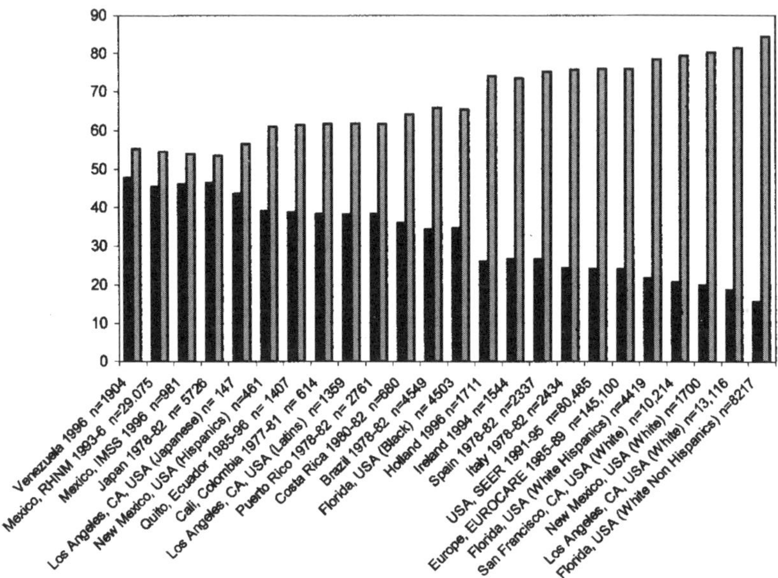

FIGURE 2.—Breast carcinoma in women younger and older than 50 years of age. (Courtesy of Rodríguez-Cuevas S, Macías CG, Franceschi D, et al: Breast carcinoma presents a decade earlier in Mexican women than in women in the United States or European countries. CANCER Vol. 91, No. 4, 2001, pp 863-868. Copyright 2001, American Cancer Society. Reprinted by permission of Wiley-Liss, Inc., a subsidiary of John Wiley & Sons, Inc.)

aged 30 to 39 years as well as in those aged 60 to 69 years (Fig 2 and Table 1).

Conclusion.—Breast carcinoma occurs a decade earlier in Mexican women than in women in the United States or European countries, where

TABLE 1.—Age Distribution by Stage of Women With Breast Carcinoma at the Hospital de Oncología, Mexico City, 1995

Stage	Mean Age (yrs)	Median Age (yrs)	SD (yrs)	Range (yrs)	n
I	50.0	48.0	13.5	19-83	128
II	48.0	50.9	13.0	24-92	748
III	48.6	48.0	10.7	25-80	370
IV	56.3	58.0	9.0	36-69	11
Total	50.1	49.0	12.5	19-95	1257

Abbreviation: SD, Standard deviation.

(Courtesy of Rodríguez-Cuevas S, Macías CG, Franceschi D, et al: Breast carcinoma presents a decade earlier in Mexican women than in women in the United States or European countries. CANCER, Vol. 91, No. 4, 2001, pp 863-868. Copyright 2001, American Cancer Society. Reprinted by permission of Wiley-Liss, Inc., a subsidiary of John Wiley & Sons, Inc.)

the median age at presentation is 63 years and only one fourth of the patients are younger than 50 years. Similar to the situation in Mexico, nearly half the women with breast carcinoma in Venezuela and Japan are younger than 50 years. Breast cancer screening guidelines must be changed in Mexico to improve rates of early diagnosis and survival.

▶ This report from the Hospital de Oncología, Mexico City presents impressive numbers (29,075 cases) and multiple source comparisons (Fig 2) of clinical importance, particularly for the border states of the United States and for other areas wherein the Hispanic population is increasing. Perhaps the American Cancer Society and American College of Radiology breast cancer screening guidelines should be amended based on these remarkable data (when they are verified by other reports). A median age at diagnosis of 51 years, with 29.5% of the cases in the 40- to 49-year of age group and 14% in the 30 to 39 age group, is in striking contrast to incidence/age data for the United States.

The authors reported increased mortality rates of 3.6/100,000 in 1985 to 6/100,000 in 1994 and state, "Most of the tumors are diagnosed in advanced stages with little chance of cure." This is clinically alarming and certainly a call to action by health care authorities in Mexico. Breast cancer screening beginning at an earlier age (perhaps 30 years) than is advised in the United States would seem to be urgently needed.

W. H. Hindle, MD

Suggested Reading

Silverstein MJ, Parker S, Grotting JC, et al. Ductal carcinoma in situ (DCIS) of the breast: Diagnostic and therapeutic controversies. *J Am Coll Surg* 192(2):196-214, 2001.

▶ This state-of-the-art symposium with 62 references covers the following topics: (1) "Minimally invasive biopsy of DCIS: transition from diagnosis to treatment;" (2) "Treatment controversy: do all conservatively treated patients require postexcisional radiation therapy?" (3) "Skin sparing mastectomy and immediate autologous reconstruction for extensive DCIS;" (4) "Axillary micrometastases: fact or artifact?" and (5) "Tamoxifen/hormone replacement therapy after treatment for DCIS: good medicine or malpractice?"

All of these are indeed controversial and complex issues without any current consensus or definite conclusions. This 18-page symposium, by acknowledged authorities in DCIS, should be read and reflected upon by those who are interested and involved in the diagnosis and treatment of DCIS.

William H. Hindle, MD

Jenkinson AD, Al-Mufti RAM, Mohsen Y, et al. Does intraductal breast cancer spread in a segmental distribution? An analysis of residual tumour burden following segmental mastectomy using tumour bed biopsies. *Eur J Surg Onc* 27:21-25, 2001.

▶ Understanding the glandular anatomy of the breast is essential to effective breast surgery. This report from St. Bartholomew Hospital, London, of 101 patients undergoing segmental mastectomy and multiple biopsies of the tumor bed (of which 24 had tumor in the biopsies, i.e. incomplete excision) adds to the data that carcinoma, invasive and in situ, spreads following the branching ductal pattern. Visualization of the separate ductal systems as branches of a tree gives a picture that is helpful, although as with a tree, the major branches spread to intertwine. This is contrary to the historic diagrams of the lobes of the breasts as distinctly separate from the other lobes. In fact, the ducts do branch and intertwine. The classical concept of distinct breast quadrants and freely separated lobes (non-intertwined) is an outdated paradigm unfounded in fact. Certainly surgical excisions should conform to the known segmental pattern of a ductal system. However, the unrestricted extent of a single ductal system and intertwining with other ductal systems currently prevent what would be ideal, i.e. the excision of a single ductal system without trauma to the other ductal systems. Hopefully, new methods of treatment, as yet undiscovered, will come closer to fulfilling this potential therapeutic goal. Of course, there are still those who would argue that mastectomy avoids this branching ductal system problem—at least for the surgeon.

William H. Hindle, MD

Hynynen K, Pomeroy O, Smith DN, et al. MR imaging-guided focused ultrasound surgery of fibroadenomas in the breast: A feasibility study. *Radiology* 219:176-185, 2001.

▶ This is cutting-edge clinical research from the Brigham and Women's Hospital, Boston, Massachusetts. Eight of 11 (73%) of the fibroadenomas showed complete or partial lack of contrast material uptake after the treatment. Focused US surgery has been a known treatment for more than 50 years, but difficulties of controlling focal spot position, precise target definition, and beam dosimetry have limited its use. Currently available MR specially modified for use in the breast is capable of overcoming these difficulties. The problem of patient motion has been addressed but can still be bothersome. Pain during the procedure and 1 case of postoperative pectoralis muscle edema are the reported complications with this technique. Temperature-sensitive phase-difference-based MR was utilized for monitoring the focused US surgery. The authors state, "The ultimate goal of this therapeutic development is to establish the feasibility, safety, and effectiveness of noninvasive therapy for the treatment of malignant breast tumors." Future major hurdles to achieving this goal are: (1) defining the extent of invasion and (2) confirming that all malignant tissue has been destroyed (or "sonicated" as the authors prefer to say). This fascinating research and technology is undergoing continuous improvement. Someday it may have clinical application.

William H. Hindle, MD

Krishnamurthy S, Ashfaq R, Shin HJC, et al. Distinction of phyllodes tumor from fibroadenoma. *Cancer* 90:342-349, 2000.

▶ This careful analysis from the M. D. Anderson Cancer Center, Houston, Texas, of 14 cytologic criteria of fine-needle aspiration samples of 33 fibroadenomas and 12 phyllodes tumors revealed that the presence of more than 30% long spindle nuclei dispersed in the background was only identified in phyllodes tumors. However, this discriminating characteristic occurred in both fibroadenoma and phyllodes tumors at the 10% to 30% level. Thus, an "intermediate" category is proposed for the 10% to 30% lesions. When the long spindle nuclei were less than 10% in the background, all the neoplasm were fibroadenomas. No other discriminating cytologic criteria demonstrated statistical significance between the two neoplasms.

It is of clinical interest that the mean age of the women with fibroadenomas was 34 years, and the average size of the fibroadenomas was 2.0 cm. For phyllodes tumors, the mean age was 44 years and the average size was 4 cm.

Thus, strict cytologic criteria failed to definitively differentiate fibroadenomas from phyllodes tumors. Being graded as histologically benign, borderline, and malignant further complicates the phyllodes tumors. Hopefully, biologic markers will be discovered that differentiate these neoplasms and the subsets of phyllodes tumors.

William H. Hindle, MD

Primary Treatment of Cystosarcoma Phyllodes of the Breast

Chaney AW, Pollack A, Mcneese MD, et al (Univ of Texas, Houston)
Cancer 89:1502-1511, 2000
28–13

Introduction.—Surgery is the primary mode of treatment for cystosarcoma phyllodes of the breast. Uncertainty exists, however, over the need for tumor excision versus mastectomy and the need for radiotherapy or other forms of local therapy. The outcomes of surgery alone for treatment of cystosarcoma phyllodes, including local and distant failure rates and potential prognostic factors, were evaluated.

Methods.—The analysis included 101 patients undergoing primary treatment for cystosarcoma phyllodes at the authors' cancer center from 1944 to 1998. On the basis of accepted histologic criteria, the tumors were classified as benign in 58% of patients, malignant in 30%, and indeterminate in 12%. Twenty-nine percent of tumors were associated with stromal overgrowth. Surgery consisted of mastectomy in 53% of patients and local excision in 47%. Ninety-nine percent of patients had negative surgical margins on microscopic examination. Adjuvant radiotherapy was used in 6% of patients. Outcomes, including the rates of local and distant recurrence, were analyzed at a median follow-up of 47 months.

Results.—The overall survival rate was 88% at 5 years, 79% at 10 years, and 62% at 15 years. For patients in the benign and intermediate histologic categories, the survival rate was 91% at 5 years and 79% at 10 years. For those with malignant tumors, the 5-year survival rate was 82% and the 10-year survival rate was 42%. Analysis-based separate analysis of stromal overgrowth yielded similar results. Four patients had local recurrences, for an actuarial 10-year rate of 8%; distant metastases occurred in 8 patients, for an actuarial 10-year rate of 13%. The only independent predictor of distant failure was stromal overgrowth (Fig 4B,C,D).

Conclusions.—Breast-conserving surgery appears to be appropriate primary therapy for patients with cystosarcoma phyllodes of the breast. With negative surgical margins, the local failure rate is low and adjuvant irradiation appears unnecessary. The risk of distant failure is increased for patients with stromal overgrowth, particularly if tumor size is greater than 5 cm; adjuvant systemic therapy may be considered in this group.

FIGURE 4

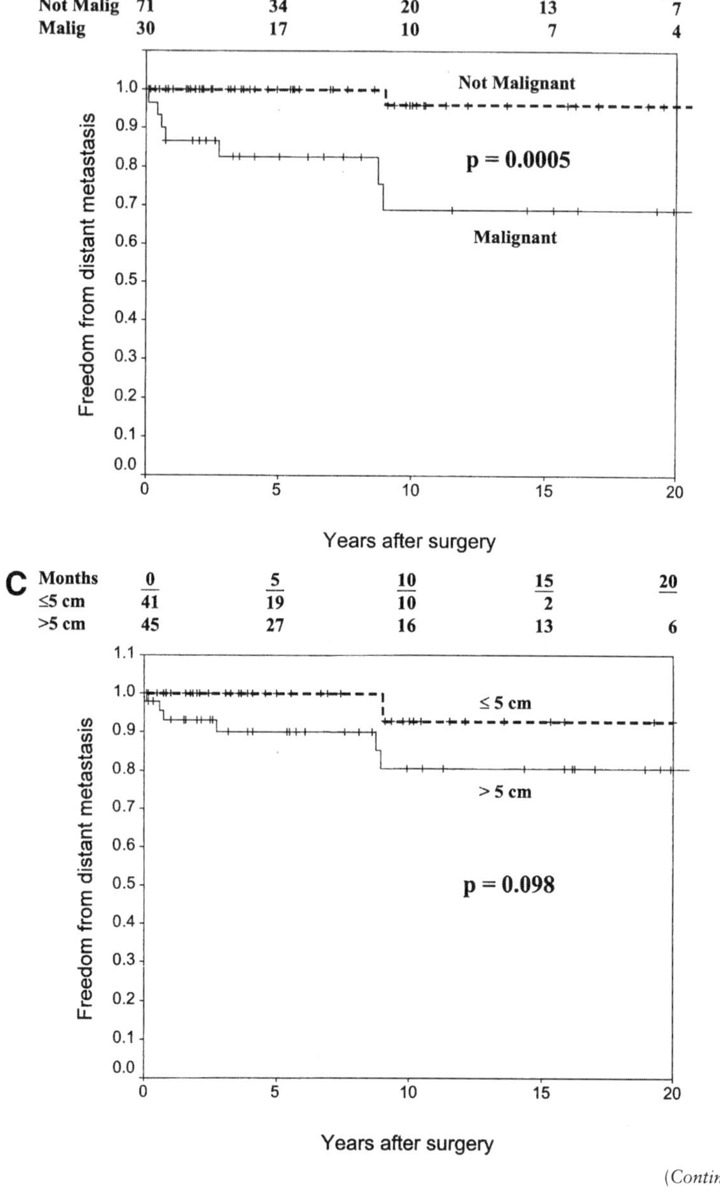

(*Continued*)

FIGURE 4 (cont.)

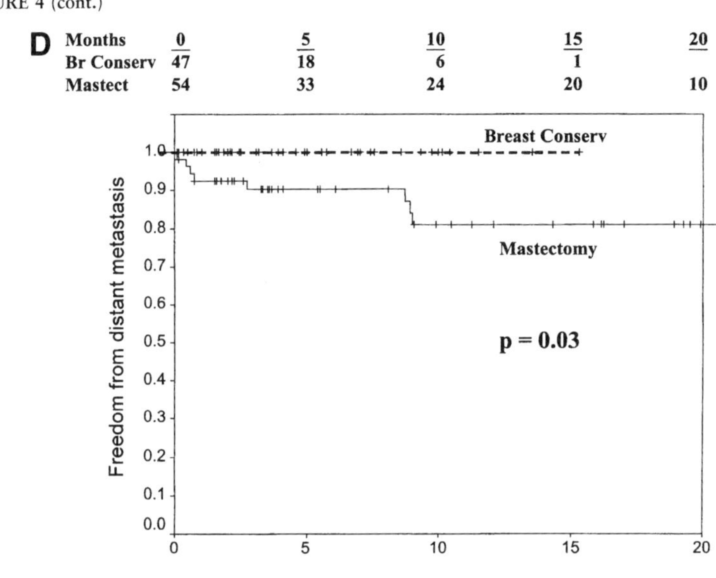

FIGURE 4.—Actuarial freedom from distant metastases subdivided by B, histotype; C, tumor size; and D, surgical procedure. *Abbreviations: Malig,* Malignant; *breast conserv,* breast-conserving surgery. (Courtesy of Chaney AW, Pollack A, Mcneese MD, et al: Primary treatment of cystosarcoma phyllodes of the breast. *Cancer* 89:1502-1511, 2000, American Cancer Society. Reprinted by permission of Wiley-Liss Inc., a subsidiary of John Wiley & Sons, Inc.)

▶ Historically, phyllodes tumors have been an enigma. The occurrence of phyllodes tumors is relatively rare, so no large series have been available for analysis. Subsequently, treatment for these tumors has not been uniform, which makes correlation with the final outcome difficult. The histology is variable and not closely correlated with outcome. Even bilateral phyllodes tumors with malignant histology and contralateral benign histology are reported.[1] Phyllodes tumors were thought to have a high local recurrence rate, which suggested aggressive surgical excision (eg, mastectomy) as treatment. The impact and indications for axillary lymph node dissection, radiation therapy, and chemotherapy were mostly anecdotal and unfounded by evidence-based medicine. Even at the M. D. Anderson Cancer Center (University of Texas, Houston) it took more than 50 years to accumulate the 178 phyllodes tumor patients (including 101 previously untreated) analyzed in this study. The current concept of clear surgical margins and recent criteria for histologic diagnosis has yielded interesting results, which vary from most historical reports. Selection of therapy was based on tumor size and histology. The mean follow-up was 81 months (range 1-442 months), and the median age was 41 years. The authors observe that "No relation between tumor size and histology was observed." Only one local recurrence among the 68 non-malignant histology cases occurred. Local control was obtained by wide local excision with clear surgical margins in 90% of cases. Of the 26 axillary lymph node dissections (performed at the discretion of the operating surgeon), no positive (malignant) nodes were identified. Metastases (mostly to the lung) developed in 23% (7 of 30) of the patients with malignant histology. Stromal overgrowth was the only variable to correlate with outcome on multivariate analysis. Distant metastasis occurred in 1 patient with a histologic benign tumor. On the basis of this analysis of phyllodes tumors, the authors conclude: (1) breast-conserving surgery with appropriate margins is the preferred primary therapy and should be used whenever cosmetically feasible; (2) with clear surgical margins, adjuvant radiation therapy is not indicated; and (3) axillary lymph node dissection is not indicated.

W. H. Hindle, MD

Reference

1. Mrad K, Driss M, Maalej M, et al: Bilateral cystosarcoma phyllodes of the breast: A case report of malignant form with contralateral benign form. *Ann Diagn Pathol* 4:370-372, 2000.

SUGGESTED READING

Chen C-M, Chen C-J, Chang C-L, et al. CD 34, CD 117, and actin expression in phyllodes tumor of the breast. *J Surg Res* 94:84-91, 2000.

▶ Microbiology seems to be the avenue to understand malignancy and the potential to truly differentiate tumors with metastasis potential. Is this study a glimpse of the future? CD117 expression and actin expression did statistically correlate with malignant potential of phyllodes tumors in this report. Actin expression also significantly correlated with frequent mitotic activity. The immunophenotypic markers did not correlate with tumor size. CD34 correlated with benign phyllodes tumors. However, none of the correlations was significant enough to be clinically useful. In addition, with the current methodology, the results of immunohistologic analyses were all mixed to some extent in both benign and malignant phyllodes tumors. Perhaps the methodology of assigning histologic grade to phyllodes tumors adds to these seemingly conflicting results. Hopefully, at some stage in the future, specific microbiology will define cellular biologic behavior.

William H. Hindle, MD

Darling MLR, Smith DN, Rhei E, et al. Lactating adenomas: Sonographic features. *Breast J* 6:252-256, 2000.

▶ This article from the Brigham and Women's Hospital (Boston, Massachusetts), illustrated with black and white photos of typical breast USs, points out that most lactating adenomas have characteristic benign features (circumscribed borders, smooth lobulations, or an echogenic pseudocapsule). Five of the 15 lactating adenoma cases had some features associated with malignancy (irregular, angulated or ill-defined margins, or posterior acoustic shadowing.). However, all 15 lesions had an ovoid shape with the long axis parallel to the chest wall, which is typical of a benign lesion. The pathologic diagnosis was confirmed by surgical excision or US-guided large-core needle biopsy. Since all of these lesions were palpable, fine-needle aspiration (FNA) potentially could have resolved the diagnosis without US or surgery (as in 90% of similar cases). In the Breast Diagnostic Center at Women's and Children's Hospital, Los Angeles

County and University of Southern California Medical Center, our protocol for such lesions would be FNA as the initial procedure of choice. In the rare case when the cytology specimen is inadequate or suggests the possibility of malignancy, US-guided tissue core-needle biopsy would be the next procedure. Except for diagnosed malignancy, surgery (if indicated or requested by the patient—both of which circumstances are rare in our clinical practice) is deferred until after the pregnancy and lactation are completed.

William H. Hindle, MD

Hindle WH, Arias RD, Florentine B, et al. Lack of utility in clinical practice of cytologic examination of nonbloody cyst fluid from palpable breast cysts. *Am J Ostet Gynecol* 182:1300-1305, 2000.

▶ This retrospective study of the medical records (1988-1999) and fluid cytology reports of 689 women who had palpable breast cysts aspirated in the Breast Diagnostic Center (BDC), Women's and Children's Hospital, Los Angeles County and University of Southern California Medical Center (Los Angeles, California) demonstrated the absence of abnormal and malignant cells in the nonbloody cyst fluid and no clinical evidence of associated neoplasm (benign or malignant) in the area of concern upon follow-up examination. However, the follow-up in the BDC clinic setting is imperfect. The initial return appointments are kept by about 60% of patients and an additional 25% subsequently are seen for follow-up at a later date. Thus, no follow-up information is available for 15%.

The protocol of the BDC is: (1) aspirate all palpable breast cysts; (2) palpate the area of the cyst post aspiration to be certain there is no residual mass (cyst or otherwise); (3) repeat the aspiration (with US guidance when necessary) if there is a residual mass; (4) send all bloody cyst fluid to Cytopathology for evaluation, (5) give the patient an appointment to return in 2 months for palpation of the area where the cyst was aspirated to be certain there is no recurrent mass. If the cyst refills, the protocol is repeated. Mammography and US are not routinely performed for palpable cyst. However, mammograms are obtained on all women 30 years of age or older as part of the breast evaluation protocol of the BDC.

William H. Hindle, MD

Hadi MSAA. Sports brassiere: Is it a solution for mastalgia? *Breast J* 6:407-409, 2000.

▶ This study from the King Fahd Hospital of the University, Saudi Arabia, covers 200 women with mastalgia who were alternately treated with danazole or with wearing a sports bra. In the danazole group, 58% had relief of their symptoms but 42% experienced side effects. In the bra group, after some initial discomfort, 85% had relief of their symptoms. For the less than 25% of women who are not satisfactorily managed with reassurance that there is no evidence of malignancy (after complete evaluation, including mammography for women 30 and older in the US), mechanical measures such as described in this study are an underutilized treatment of persistent mastalgia.

William H. Hindle, MD

A Simple Intraductal Aspiration Method for Cytodiagnosis in Nipple Discharge

Hou M-F, Tsai K-B, Lin H-J, et al (Kaohsiung Med Univ, Taiwan, ROC)
Acta Cytol 44:1029-1034, 2000

28–14

Background.—Cytologic evalutaion of nipple discharge has long been considered useful for detecting breast disease, but the diagnostic accuracy of spontaneous discharge is lower than that of aspiration cytology for other breast lesions. The utility of a simple intraductal aspiration technique to increase cytodiagnostic accuracy in women with spontaneous nipple discharge was investigated.

Methods and Findings.—One hundred forty-six women with spontaneous nipple discharge in a single duct without a mass were included in the study. The specimens collected by intraductal aspiration were adequate in 96.6% of the sample, compared with 76% obtained by the conventional squeezing method. With samples obtained by the squeezing method, the cytologic diagnosis was positive in 9 women, suspicious in 10, negative with atypical findings in 59, and negative in 33. With the intraductal aspiration method, the smears were positive in 17 women, suspicious in 14, negative with atypical findings in 78, and negative in 32 (Tables 1 and 2). The sensitivity and specificity of the intraductal aspiration method were 92.3% and 93.9%, respectively, compared with 52.9% and 89.3%, respectively, for the squeezing method (Table 4).

Conclusion.—The intraductal aspiration technique is useful for cytodiagnosis in women with spontaneous pathologic nipple discharge. Compared with the conventional squeezing method, cytologic detection of breast cancer improved from 68.6% to 93.7% and the absolute positive rate from 28.8% to 62.5%.

TABLE 1.—Histologic Findings in Cases of Pathologic Nipple Discharge

Finding	No. of Cases	%
Carcinoma	27	18.5
Infiltrating ductal carcinoma	15	
Intraductal carcinoma	11	
Colloid carcinoma	1	
Ductal hyperplasia	11	7.5
Papillomatosis	21	14.4
Papilloma	60	41.1
Other benign diseases	27	18.5
Fibrocystic diseases	14	
Ductal ectasia	8	
Sclerosing adenosis	3	
Sebaceous cyst fistula	1	
Total	146	100.0

(Courtesy of Hou M-F, Tsai K-B, Lin H-J, et al: A simple intraductal aspiration method for cytodiagnosis in nipple discharge. *Acta Cytol* 44:1029-1034, 2000.)

TABLE 2.—Correlation Between Types of Nipple Discharge
and Histologic Findings

| | Types of Discharge | | | |
Finding	Serous	Bloody	Other	Total No.
Carcinoma	5	22	0	27
Ductal hyperplasia	2	7	2	11
Papillomatosis	8	13	0	21
Papilloma	23	34	3	60
Other benign diseases	7	12	8	27
Total	45	88	13	146

(Courtesy of Hou M-F, Tsai K-B, Lin H-J, et al: A simple intraductal aspiration method for cytodiagnosis in nipple discharge. *Acta Cytol* 44:1029-1034, 2000.)

▶ Preliminary reports of various techniques of nipple canalization and cytologic (even histologic) sampling are beginning to appear. This particular report from Kaohsiung Medical University, Taiwan, compares their intraductal aspiration technique with "the squeezing method." By every measure, the intraductal aspiration produced superior results. Although 100% success in canalizations is reported, the authors also state, ". . .the procedures were performed repeatedly until the specimen was seen in the intra-[ductal] catheter."

Commercial canalization/lavage kits are in the process of approval by the US Food and Drug Administration and may be available in the United States in the near future. In general, other methods of cytodiagnosis of nipple discharge are not clinically useful, and even this "simple intraductal aspiration method" may find limited use, except in specialized breast centers. Furthermore, an experienced dedicated nipple discharge cytopathologist is essential for useful cytology evaluation. Papanicolaou wrote a landmark paper on cytopathology of the breast in 1958.[1]

W. H. Hindle, MD

Reference

1. Papanicolaou GN, Holmquist DG, Bader GM, et al: Exfoliative cytology of the human mammary gland and its value in the diagnosis of cancer and other diseases of the breast. *Cancer* 11:377-409, 1958.

TABLE 4.—Accuracy of Cytodiagnosis for Nipple Discharge With 2
Collection Methods

| | Collection Methods | |
Cytodiagnosis	C	A
Sensitivity (%)	52.9	92.3
Specificity (%)	89.3	93.9
Accuracy (%)	83.7	93.6
Inadequate smears (%)	23.9	3.4

(Courtesy of Hou M-F, Tsai K-B, Lin H-J, et al: A simple intraductal aspiration method for cytodiagnosis in nipple discharge. *Acta Cytol* 44:1029-1034, 2000.)

Galactography and Exfoliative Cytology in Women With Abnormal Nipple Discharge

Dinkel H-P, Gassel AM, Müller T, et al (Univ of Würzburg, Germany; Univ of Giessen, Germany; Univ of Bern, Switzerland)
Obstet Gynecol 97:625-629, 2001

28–15

Purpose.—Abnormal nipple discharge is feared as a sign of breast cancer, however, other causes are more common. An experience with galactography and exfoliative cytology for diagnostic evaluation of abnormal nipple discharge is presented.

Methods.—The 12.5-year experience included 384 women with spontaneous, non-milky nipple discharge who were referred to a university hospital for galactography and smear cytology. Excisional biopsy was performed in patients with clinical or mammographic evidence of tumors. Three hundred fourteen patients underwent galactography, and biopsy was recommended in 189 of these. Biopsy was recommended on the basis of the mammographic or cytologic findings in 11 patients.

Findings.—Among all patients undergoing biopsy, the malignancy rate was 8.8%. The overall tumor rate—including malignancies, papillomas, and papillomatous proliferations—was 59.9% (Table 1). Malignancy was detected at biopsy in 5% of women with nonhemorrhagic nipple discharge versus 13% of those with hemorrhagic discharge (Table 2). Exfoliative discharge had a diagnostic sensitivity of 31% with a specificity of 97%. Among patients with suspicious findings on galactography, the rate of biopsy-detected malignancy was 6%. Galactography was 83% sensitive in the detection of malignancy, with a specificity of 41%. Its sensitivity for detection of any benign or malignant neoplasms was 94%, with a specificity of 55%. Of all cancers detected, one half were found by galactography exclusively.

Conclusions.—In women with abnormal nipple discharge, a positive result on exfoliative cytology provides useful diagnostic information. Galactography is useful in localizing the source of discharge. Biopsy should be performed directly for women who have nipple discharge with clinical or mammographic evidence of tumor. Those with suspicious results on cytologic examination or galactography should also undergo biopsy.

TABLE 1.—Histologic Diagnoses

Biopsy Result	n	%
Normal	2	1.1%
Secretory disease	71	39.0%
Papilloma	70	38.5%
Papillomatous proliferation	23	12.6%
Malignant	16	8.8%
Total	182	100%

(Reprinted with permission from The American College of Obstetricians and Gynecologists courtesy of Dinkel H-P, Gassel AM, Müller T, et al: Galactography and exfoliative cytology in women with abnormal nipple discharge. *Obstet Gynecol* 97:625-629, 2001.)

TABLE 2.—Type of Discharge by Diagnosis

Pathologic Diagnosis	Nonhemorrhagic		Hemorrhagic		
	n	%	n	%	P
Fibrocystic change or normal	22	39%	35	36%	
Papillomas and intraductal proliferations	31	55%	49	51%	
Carcinoma	3	5%	13	13%	.26
All patients with biopsy	56	38%	97	60%	
Patients without biopsy	92	62%	64	40%	<.001

(Reprinted with permission from The American College of Obstetricians and Gynecologists courtesy of Dinkel H-P, Gassel AM, Müller T, et al: Galactography and exfoliative cytology in women with abnormal nipple discharge. *Obstet Gynecol* 97:625-629, 2001.)

▶ This evaluation of 384 women (mean age, 47.5 years, range 15-85 years) with recent-onset, spontaneous non-milky discharge referred for galactography/cytology to 3 radiology departments in Germany over a 12.5 year period revealed malignancy in 3.2% of the entire study group and in 8% of women undergoing biopsy. Carcinoma was diagnosed in 5% of those with non-bloody discharge and in 13% of those with bloody discharge.

The essential clinical questions are: (1) is the discharge pregnancy or lactation related? (2) is the discharge spontaneous or elicited? and (3) is the discharge bloody?

If galactography with an experienced radiologist is available, the procedure offers the advantage of potentially demonstrating the precise location and extent of the intraluminal lesions. Then microdochetomy can be performed through a small circumareolar incision with complete removal of the intraductal lesion and conservation of the surrounding normal tissue. However, with a sensitivity of 83% and specificity of 41% (in this report), galactography alone does not detect all intraductal cancers or reliably rule out malignancy. Histologic verification is necessary to establish a definitive diagnosis, malignant or benign.

In the United States, reliable diagnostic nipple cytology is available in some breast centers but generally is not clinically useful or cost-effective.

The authors wisely conclude: "Biopsy is indicated when palpation, mammography, cytology, or galactography is suspicious."

W. H. Hindle, MD

A Simple Approach to Nipple Discharge

King TA, Carter KM, Bolton JS, et al (Ochsner Clinic and Alton Ochsner Med Found, New Orleans, La)
Am Surg 66:960-965, 2000   28–16

Introduction.—Nipple discharge is a common symptom that is most often related to a benign process. Numerous tests and referral to a breast specialist may be used in an attempt to identify the cause. A more focused approach to the diagnostic evaluation of nipple discharge is described (Fig 1).

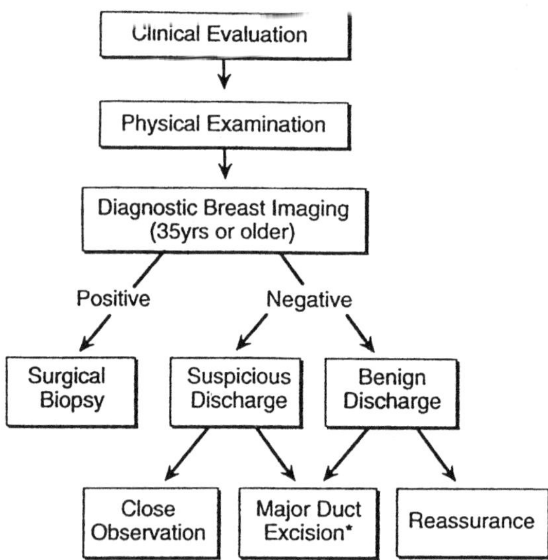

FIGURE 1.—Algorithm for the clinical management of patients with nipple discharge. *Excludes malignancy and stops the discharge. (Courtesy King TA, Carter KM, Bolton JS, et al: A simple approach to nipple discharge. *Am Surg* 66:960-965, 2000.)

Methods.—Over a 2.5-year period, the authors evaluated 104 patients with nipple discharge, average age 49 years. Duct excision was proposed for patients with clinical signs suspicious for malignancy (ie, persistent clear or bloody discharge) or for those who found the discharge bothersome. Patients with a breast abnormality on mammography US underwent biopsy. The treatment plans and outcomes were reviewed for all patients to identify diagnostic tests helpful in distinguishing between benign and malignant disease.

Results.—The mammographic findings led to biopsy in 11 patients, which revealed malignancy in 3, 2 in situ and 1 infiltrating. Duct excision for nipple discharge without mammographic findings was performed in 39 patients, only 1 of whom had malignancy, ductal carcinoma in situ

TABLE 2.—Causes of Nipple Discharge (ND) in Patients Having
Major Duct Incision

Histology	ND Plus Abnormal Mammogram (N = 11)	Suspicious ND (N = 32)	Benign ND (N = 7)	All Patients (N = 50)
Intraductal papilloma	3	17	1	21 (42%)
Duct ectasia or fibrocystic change	5	14	6	25 (50%)
Ductal carcinoma *in situ*	2	1	0	3 (6%)
Infiltrating cancer	1	0	0	1 (2%)

(Courtesy King TA, Carter KM, Bolton JS, et al: A simple approach to nipple discharge. *Am Surg* 66:960-965, 2000.)

TABLE 3.—Diagnostic Tests in Patients with Nipple Discharge (ND)

Test	ND Plus Abnormal Mammogram (N = 11)	Suspicious ND (N = 38)	Benign ND (N = 55)	All Patients (N = 104)
Mammogram	11	37	43	91 (87.5%)
Ultrasound	3	7	5	15 (14.4%)
Ductogram	1	12	4	17 (16.3%)
Fluid cytology	1	4	15	20 (19.2%)
Serum prolactin	1	4	9	14 (13.5%)
Serum TSH	0	1	1	2 (1.9%)
IGCNBB	0	1	3	4 (3.8%)
Nipple biopsy	0	1	0	1 (0.01%)

(Courtesy King TA, Carter KM, Bolton JS, et al: A simple approach to nipple discharge. *Am Surg* 66:960-965, 2000.)

(Table 2). Clinical follow-up showed no cases of breast cancer in any of the 54 nonoperatively managed patients, including 6 with suspicious discharge. A total of 164 tests were performed in the 104 patients—including ductography, cytologic study of the discharge fluid, serum prolactin and thyroid-stimulating hormone levels, and image-guided biopsy (Table 3).

Conclusions.—Among women with nipple discharge and negative results on imaging studies, the rate of malignancy is low. The authors recommend a simplified algorithm for evaluation of nipple discharge. Breast imaging should be performed; if the results are negative, the patient should be offered duct excision. Other tests, such as ductography, cytology, or laboratory studies, are of little help.

▶ This "simple approach" is aggressive surgical management (nonselective complete excision of the central ducts) for nipple discharge unassociated with mammographic or US findings. Patients with imaging findings underwent wire-localized surgical excision, and 3 of the 11 were malignant.

Nipple discharge was classified as suspicious ". . .if it was unilateral; spontaneous; persistent; and described as clear, yellow (serous), pink (serosanguineous), or bloody." Patients with suspicious discharge were offered major duct excision. The surgical technique is described in detail and includes carrying the dissection down "several centimeters beyond any clinical evidence of dilated ducts." Ductal carcinoma in situ was found in one of the 32 suspicious discharges that had central duct excision. The 7 patients with benign discharge showed benign pathology by central duct excision.

The literature supports the judicious limited use of serum prolactin, serum thyroid-stimulating hormone, and cytology for evaluation of nipple discharge. However, ductography is recommended in multiple studies. Even the authors of this report would advise ductography if single-duct excision is contemplated. It would have been of keen interest had the data included the observation of the number of ducts opening on the nipple from which the discharge could be expressed (or noted, if spontaneous).

With such small numbers, it is difficult to draw overall conclusions from this observational retrospective review.

In a similar ductal lavage study on 426 high-risk women,[1] the yield was 15.1% mild atypia/premalignant cells and 5.1% suspicious for malignancy/

unequivocally malignant cells. The ductal lavages were stated to be safe and well tolerated.

W. H. Hindle, MD

Reference

1. Dooley WC et al. Detection of premalignant and malignant breast cells by ductal lavage. *Obstet Gynecol* 97:28, 2001.

SUGGESTED READING

Kim A, Lee J, Choi JS, et al. Fine needle aspiration cytology of the breast: Experience at an outpatient breast clinic. *Acta Cytol* 44:361-367, 2000.

▶ This experience with 246 cases with pathologic confirmation from the Korea University College of Medicine, Seoul, Korea, demonstrates the application of fine-needle aspiration (FNA) for the cytologic diagnosis of breast masses in an outpatient clinic setting. Analysis revealed false negative 4.3%, false positive 0.7%, predictive value for malignancy 98.4%, unsatisfactory sample 9.3%, absolute sensitivity for malignancy 64.5%, complete sensitivity for malignancy 90.3%, and cytologic diagnosis likelihood ratios for malignant 98.71, atypical 5.48, benign 1.09 and unsatisfactory 0.55. Similar results should be possible in any clinic or office setting.

In the Breast Diagnostic Center, Women's and Children's Hospital, Los Angeles County and University of Southern California Medical Center (Los Angeles, California), more than 5,500 FNAs (July 1988-June 2000) have been performed as part of the initial evaluation of palpable dominant breast masses. Resident physicians under faculty supervision have performed most of the FNAs. The final cytology reports have been inadequate for cytologic diagnosis in 14%, but clinically useful information has been obtained in the written description of more than 80% of these "inadequate smears." Only 2.5% of the FNAs were acellular. This initial FNA approach expedites the prompt referral for treatment of women with breast cancer and reassurance of those women with benign cytology.

William H. Hindle, MD

Daltrey IR, Kissin MW. Randomized clinical trial of the effect of needle gauge and local anaesthetic on pain of breast fine-needle aspiration cytology. *Br J Surg* 87:777-779, 2000.

▶ This randomized prospective study of the discomfort experienced during fine-needle aspiration (FNA) evaluated the influence of the gauge of the needle and local anesthetic. Patients used visual analogue scales to score the pain during the FNA. Needles of 21 and 23 gauges with and without local anesthesia were compared. FNA samples (116) were obtained from 98 patients who had been assigned to 1 of the 4 subsets. The results of the 2 surgeons doing the FNA were likewise compared. The mean pain scores (for all groups of patients) were 4.0 and 2.8 for the surgeons with a P value of less than 0.01. The FNA technique with 10 needle passes within the lesion has been described elsewhere.[1] The diagnostic accuracy of FNA is not dependent on the needle size or use of local anesthesia.[1,2] The authors recommend the use of a 23 gauge needle without local anesthesia as the first choice for breast FNA. Somewhat paradoxically, the findings show that the combination of the 23 gauge needle with local anesthesia was more painful than the use of the needle alone without anesthesia.

William H. Hindle, MD

References

1. Daltrey JR, Lewis CE, McKee GT, et al. The effect of needle gauge and local anaesthetic on the diagnostic accuracy of breast fine-needle aspiration cytology. *Eur J Surg Oncol* 25:30-33, 1999.
2. Walker SR. A randomized controlled trial comparing a 21G needle with a 23G needle for fine needle aspiration of breast lumps. *J Res Coll Surg Edinb* 43:122-3, 1998.

Wiberg MK, Bone B, Aspelin P. The potential influence of fine-needle aspiration on MR imaging of the breast. *Acta Radiol* 41:222-226, 2000.

▶ This report from the Karolinska Institute, Huddlinge University Hospital (Huddinge, Sweden) concludes that the diagnostic outcome of MR investigation is not impaired by prior fine-needle aspiration (FNA) biopsy. Seventeen lesions in 15 patients were evaluated with MR pre- and post-FNA. When the paired MR images were compared, there was no statistical difference in the contrast enhancement of the lesions, breast parenchyma, or muscle. This is reassuring for clinicians and supports the "early" use of FNA for evaluation of palpable breast lesions prior to other diagnostic procedures.

Similarly, reassuring data has been published regarding the initial use of FNA for evaluation of palpable breast lesions prior to mammography.

William H. Hindle, MD

Reference

1. Hindle WH, Chen EC. Accuracy of mammographic appearance after breast fine-needle aspiration. *Am J Obstet Gynecol* 176:1286-1292, 1997.

Gobbi H, Tse G, Page DL, et al. Reactive spindle cell nodules of the breast after core biopsy or fine-needle aspiration. *Am J Clin Pathol* 113:288-294, 2000.

▶ This report from Vanderbilt University Medical Center, Nashville, Tennessee, describes 18 cases of reactive spindle cell nodules (1.5 to 9mm) associated with breast core needle biopsy or fine-needle aspiration (FNA), which were mostly (15 of 18) taken from complex sclerosing or papillary lesions. Clinicians who follow patients who have these histologic diagnoses and have had a core biopsy or FNA should be aware of the potential occurrence of these benign nodules. The specific characteristics of the nodules are clearly described and illustrated in this article. The nodules are thought to be of myofibroblastic origin. All the nodules were benign and any premalignant potential is currently unknown. However, the diagnosis is histologic and requires excision of the nodules.

William H. Hindle, MD

Fabian CJ, Kimler BF, Zalles CM, et al. Short-term breast cancer prediction by random periareolar fine-needle aspiration cytology and the Gail risk model. *J Natl Cancer Inst* 92:1217-1227, 2000.

▶ This prospective study, from the University of Kansas Medical Center, analyzed fine-needle aspiration (FNA) cellular samples from 480 women at "high risk" for breast cancer for DNA aneuploidy, expression of epidermal growth factor receptor, estrogen receptor, p53 protein, and HER2/NEU protein by immunocytochemistry. With a median follow-up of 45 months, 20 women have developed breast cancer (13 invasive and 5 in situ). Subsequent cancer was predicted by atypical hyperplasia in the initial FNA and a 10-year Gail projected probability of developing breast cancer. Although expression of epidermal growth factor receptor, estrogen receptor, p53 protein, and HER2/NEU protein were associated (statistically significant) with atypical hyperplasia, they were not predictive of breast cancer (during the time frame of this study). The search for clinically applicable predictors of breast cancer continues.

William H. Hindle, MD

Dennis MA, Parker SH, Klaus AJ, et al. Breast biopsy avoidance: The value of normal mammograms and normal sonograms in the setting of a palpable lump. *Radiology* 219:186-191, 2001.

▶ This retrospective review from the Sally Jobe Breast Centers, Radiology Imaging Associates (Englewood, Colorado) covers 600 palpable breast lumps (in 486 patients) with no mass by focal US and no mammogram findings in the area of clinical concern. How should clinicians manage such patients? If the patient or her physician continues to be concerned about malignancy in the lump, consultation with a breast surgeon (or other breast cancer specialists) is appropriate. However, fine-needle aspiration with an adequate cell sample has a 90% potential of establishing a specific cytologic diagnosis of a dominant palpable breast mass. This could be performed before or after breast imaging. If the cytologic diagnosis is benign, the patient can be followed. With a malignant cytologic diagnosis, the patient should be referred to a breast specialist as soon as possible.

With a mean follow-up of 43 months, no patient in this review developed carcinoma in the area of initial concern and those who had breast biopsies (51 women) all had benign diagnostic results. The authors recommend clinical and imaging follow-up instead of open surgical biopsy for women with breast lumps and "negative" imaging (mammography/US) findings. The authors cite recommendations from surgical practice for biopsy in 42% of women who present with a breast lump/thickening and indicate that as many as 92% of women with breast lumps and normal mammograms do not have cancer by biopsy.

It is of interest in this retrospective review that, of the women with adequate data for analysis, 47% initially reported the breast mass themselves, and that 44% of the patients were referred by gynecologists (the majority were initially self referred).

William H. Hindle, MD

Benign Diagnosis by Image-Guided Core-Needle Breast Biopsy

Duncan JL III, Cederbom GJ, Champaign JL, et al (Ochsner Clinic, New Orleans, La)
Am Surg 66:5-10, 2000   28–17

Purpose.—Patients with abnormal findings on screening mammography commonly undergo image-guided core-needle breast biopsy (IGCNBB). This minimally invasive technique is growing in popularity as a cost-effective, less-deforming alternative to surgical biopsy. However, more information on its accuracy is needed, and particularly on the reliability of a benign result. Two-year surveillance data on women undergoing IGCNBB were analyzed to determine the reliability of a benign result.

Methods.—From a prospective database, the investigators retrieved data on 1110 women undergoing IGCNBB between 1993 and 1996. At least 2 years' follow-up were available for each patient. The women's mean age was 55 years; most of the procedures were done by using stereotactic guidance. The results of IGCNBB were benign in 855 patients. Of these, 728 (85%) underwent recommended mammographic follow-up, starting 6 months postbiopsy (Table 1).

Results.—Through 2 years' surveillance, malignancy developed in just 2 of the 728 patients. A benign result on IGCNBB had a diagnostic sensitivity of 100%, with a specificity of 99%.

Conclusions.—This surveillance study supports the reliability of a benign result on IGCNBB in women with abnormal mammographic findings. This is an accurate diagnosis that identifies a group of patients whose status can be safely followed up by mammography. To ensure appropriate follow-up, the researchers emphasize the importance of following the Breast Imaging Reporting and Data System (BI-RADS) of the American College of Radiology (Table 2).

▶ The superb "false-negative" rate of 0.3% (1:364) in this retrospective review of the Ochsner Clinic (New Orleans, La) experience with benign IGCNBBs is in contrast to reports from other centers whose findings range from 1.2 to 2.5% false negatives. Except for the exclusion of the histologic atypia cases (59 of 855) and the utilization of a weekly multidisciplinary core

TABLE 1.—Results From Core Biopsy and From Follow-up
Surveillance or Biopsy

| | Follow-Up Surveillance or Biopsy | |
Core Biopsy	Benign	Malignant
Benign (n = 728)	726	2
Malignant (n = 196)	0	196

Note: Sensitivity of benign result, 100.0%; specificity of benign result, 98.9%; positive predictive value of benign result, 99.7%; negative predictive value of benign result, 100.0%.
(Courtesy of Duncan JL III, Cederbom GJ, Champaign JL, et al: Benign diagnosis by image-guided core-needle breast biopsy. *Am Surg* 66:5-10, 2000.)

TABLE 2.—Breast Imaging Reporting and Data System (BI-RADS)

Category	Significance	Intervention
0	Incomplete assessment	Additional imaging
1	Negative	Yearly mammogram
2	Benign finding	Yearly mammogram
3	Probably benign	Follow-up mammogram in 3-6 months
4	Suspicious abnormality	Biopsy recommended
5	Highly suspicious for malignancy	Biopsy or excision indicated

(Courtesy of Duncan JL III, Cederbom GJ, Champaign JL, et al: Benign diagnosis by image-guided core-needle breast biopsy. *Am Surg* 66:5-10, 2000.)

biopsy conference, the achievement of this low false-negative rate is unexplained. Perhaps a study comparing the details of the Ochsner approach with that of other centers would reveal the factors that would allow others to achieve a similar low false-negative rate.

Table 2 is critically important for clinicians ordering and following mammograms. In the US, Federal legislation/regulations mandate the use of the BI-RADS categories in mammogram reports. This allows clinicians to know the significance of the imaging evaluation and the appropriate intervention (follow-up). Clinicians should obtain a breast specialist consultation before making an exception to the recommended intervention.

The authors state that their indications for biopsy are limited to BI-RADS Categories 4 and 5. Upon recent review (1998) with this restriction, 27% of their biopsies proved to be carcinoma or atypia. This is a commendable rate of malignant/premalignant pathology. A minimum of 2 years follow-up was a criterion for inclusion in this report. The mean follow-up was 38 months. The 2 cases (2:855) of subsequent invasive carcinoma were both demonstrated in 2-year surveillance mammograms. This raises the question of the necessity of the initial 6-month surveillance mammogram. The authors are evaluating this aspect of their follow-up protocol.

The reliability of patient compliance is a critical issue in this follow-up approach for benign lesions. A commendable 85% of patients followed the surveillance mammography protocol. The authors attribute this increase in compliance from their prior 71% to physician education and a computerized appointment system. The demographics/behavior of the patient population being served (eg, a county hospital with a demonstrated low patient compliance) may make the applications of the Ochsner protocol unsuitable.

Other authors have raised additional issues. Dershaw rightly states, "When benign histologies are not concordant with the imaging pattern, when certain high-risk lesions are found at core biopsy, and when the pathologist is unable to make a definite diagnosis based on the small volume of tissue removed, surgical biopsy is necessary".[1] In addition, all tissue core techniques and devices are Food and Drug Administration approved only for diagnosis and not for therapy. Mendez[2] addresses the difficulties of tissue core biopsy histologic diagnosis of ductal carcinoma in situ and atypical ductal hyperplasia. Open surgical excision biopsy is recommended for definitive histologic diagnosis in these cases.

W. H. Hindle, MD

References

1. Dershaw DD. Imaging guided biopsy: An alternative to surgical biopsy. *Breast J* 5:294-298, 2000.
2. Mendez I, Andreu FJ, Saez E, et al: Ductal carcinoma in situ and atypical ductal hyperplasia of the breast diagnosed at stereotactic core biopsy. *Breast J* 7:14-18, 2001.

Cost-Effectiveness of Stereotactic 11-Gauge Directional Vacuum-Assisted Breast Biopsy

Liberman L, Sama MP (Mem Sloan-Kettering Cancer Ctr, New York)
AJR 175:53-58, 2000   28–18

Background.—Based on cost and accuracy, stereotactic core biopsy is an attractive option to diagnose nonpalpable breast lesions, but it has limitations. The 11-gauge directional vacuum-assisted biopsy probe expands the abilities of stereotactic biopsy but may not be cost effective. This study explored the cost effectiveness of this method.

Methods.—Two hundred consecutive solitary nonpalpable breast lesions were reviewed retrospectively, including mammograms, histologic results, and medical records. Each woman had been evaluated by the stereotactic 11-gauge directional vacuum-assisted breast biopsy. Cost savings were determined by Medicare reimbursements (Table 1), and comparison with needle localization and surgical biopsy costs was made.

Results.—In a total of 151 cases, stereotactic 11-gauge directional vacuum-assisted biopsy obviated the need for a surgical procedure. Calcific lesions (n=154) were identified as well as masses (n=46), with surgery being avoided in 112 calcific lesions and 39 masses. The cost of diagnosis was reduced by $264 per case (20%) with the stereotactic method as opposed to surgical biopsy (Table 3). Use of a 14-gauge automated core biopsy would have been impossible in 106 cases because of the small size of the lesion, its superficial location, or inadequate breast thickness. Surgical biopsy was recommended in 35 lesions after stereotactic biopsy.

Conclusions.—Seventy-six percent of the lesions studied required no surgery, which, compared to surgical biopsy, yielded a 20% decline in the cost of diagnosis (Table 6). Thus, for each case the cost was only $1025 rather than $1289. This makes stereotactic 11-gauge directional vacuum-assisted breast biopsy a valuable tool in the diagnosis of nonpalpable breast lesions.

▶ This retrospective review of 200 consecutive patients demonstrates that further surgical procedures were "obviated" in 76% and that the cost

TABLE 1.—Direct Costs of Stereotactic 11-Gauge Directional Vacuum-Assisted Breast Biopsy

Procedure	CPT Code	Cost ($)*
Stereotactic biopsy, mass		
Stereotactic localization	76095	341
Biopsy of breast, incisional†	19101	220
Histologic analysis	88305	63
Total		624
Stereotactic biopsy, calcifications		
Stereotactic localization	76095	341
Biopsy of breast, incisional†	19101	220
Specimen radiography	76098	24
Histologic analysis	88305	63
Total		648
Stereotactic biopsy, mass with clip		
Stereotactic localization	76095	341
Biopsy of breast, incisional†	19101	220
Histologic analysis	88305	63
Placement of localizing clip‡	19290	64
Total		688
Stereotactic biopsy, calcifications with clip		
Stereotactic localization	76095	341
Biopsy of breast, incisional†	19101	220
Specimen radiography	76098	24
Histologic analysis	88305	63
Placement of localizing clip‡	19290	64
Total		712

Abbreviations: CPT, Current Procedural Terminology.

*National Medicare average allowed charges for selected CPT-coded procedures and modifiers, first 2 quarters of 1999 (Dutton B, Health Care Financing Administration, personal communication).

†CPT codes reflect the recommendations published in the October 1997 *ACR Bulletin* of the American College of Radiology. At that time, the ACR suggested that the use of CPT code 19101 ("biopsy of breast, incisional"; current average allowed charge, $220) for all image-guided biopsy (stereotactic or sonographic) of nonpalpable breast lesions regardless of device (eg, core needle, directional vacuum-assisted needle, or Advanced Breast Biopsy Instrumentation [United Sates Surgical, Norwalk, CT]). They suggested that CPT code 19100 ("biopsy of breast, needle core"; current average allowed charge, $76) continue to be used for non–imaging-guided needle core biopsies of palpable lesions.

‡Published recommendations in the October 1997 *ACR Bulletin.*

(Courtesy of Liberman L, Sarna MP: Cost-effectiveness of stereotactic 11-gauge directional vacuum-assisted breast biopsy. *AJR* 175:53-58, 2000.)

TABLE 3.—Mammographic and Stereotactic Biopsy Findings in 200 Lesions

Stereotactic Biopsy Histology	Mammographic Findings		
	Calcifications ± Mass	Mass	Total (%)
Benign and concordant	99	24	123 (62)
Benign, excision suggested	6	2	8 (4)
Discordant	4	3	7 (4)
Atypical	18	2	20 (10)
Malignant	27	15	42 (21)
Ductal carcinoma in situ	20	2	22 (11)*
Infiltrating carcinoma	7	13	20 (10)
Total	154	46	200 (100)

*Among 21 women who had surgery after stereotactic biopsy diagnosis of ductal carcinoma in situ, surgery revealed infiltrating carcinoma in 4 (19%). All 4 of these women had calcifications on mammography, spanning a median of 0.8 cm (range, 0.5-1.2 cm). In these 4 women, the median number of specimens obtained per lesion was 13 (range, 10-17 specimens) and the median histologic size of infiltrating carcinoma was 0.4 cm (range, 0.1-1.5 cm). All 4 women had axillary surgery at a later date (sentinal lymph node biopsy in 3 and axillary dissection in 1); none had axillary metastases.

(Courtesy of Liberman L, Sarna MP: Cost-effectiveness of stereotactic 11-gauge directional vacuum-assisted breast biopsy. *AJR* 175:53-58, 2000.)

TABLE 6.—Percutaneous Breast Biopsy: Frequency of Obviating Surgery and Cost

Study	Method	Frequency of Obviating Surgery (%)	Cost Savings* (%)
Liberman et al.	Stereotactic 14-gauge automated	140/182 (77)	$893/$1626 (55)
Lee et al.	Stereotactic 14-gauge automated	328/405 (81)	$741/$1278 (58)
Hillner et al.	Stereotactic 14-gauge automated	757/1000 (76)	$804/$2000 (40)
Liberman et al.	Sonographic 14-gauge automated	128/151 (85)	$744/$1332 (56)
Present study	Stereotactic 11-gauge vacuum-assisted	151/200 (76)	$264/$1289 (20)

*Cost savings (in dollars) attributable to percutaneous biopsy divided by cost (in dollars) of diagnostic surgical biopsy.
(Courtesy of Liberman L, Sarna MP: Cost-effectiveness of stereotactic 11-gauge directional vacuum-assisted breast biopsy. *AJR* 175:53-58, 2000.)

savings (measured by reimbursement calculations) was 20% compared with open surgical biopsy. Definitive cost-effective analysis would require the factoring of the cost of equipment, supplies, and overhead.

The authors point out that one third of nonpalpable masses "will not be amenable to 14-gauge automated core biopsy" but can be adequately biopsied by the stereotactic 11-gauge directional vacuum-assisted technique. Furthermore, they state that even Breast Imaging Reporting and Data System category 5 calcifications can be biopsied with "high efficacy" with this technique.

Indeed, the vacuum-assisted technique does seem to be on its way to becoming the standard of care in the United States.

W. H. Hindle, MD

Differences in the Quality of Care for Women With an Abnormal Mammogram or Breast Complaint

Haas JS, Cook EF, Puopolo AL, et al (San Francisco Gen Hosp; Univ of California, San Franicisco; Brigham and Women's Hosp, Boston; et al)
J Gen Intern Med 15:321-328, 2000   28–19

Background.—Because the liability associated with breast problems is increasing, it is important to understand the differences in the quality of care for women with an abnormal mammographic result or breast problem. Factors associated with variations in such care were investigated.

Methods.—Five hundred seventy-nine women seen in 10 general internal medicine practices in Boston were enrolled in the cross-sectional survey study. All had had an abnormal result on mammography or had been referred to mammography for a clinical breast problem. Quality of care was measured by whether the patient received an examination in compliance with a clinical guideline, number of days to appropriate resolution of the problem, and the patient's overall satisfaction with care.

Findings.—Sixty-nine percent of the patients received care consistent with the guidelines. Women more likely to receive recommended care and to have a shorter time to resolution of the breast problem were older than

TABLE 1.—Compliance With Algorithm for Common Breast Problems

Clinical Problem	Appropriate Evaluation
Mammograpic abnormality on screening exam with no history or physical exam findings of a breast lump	
Biopsy recommended	Biopsy (open, core)
Additional imaging	Clinical breast exam within the 12 mo prior to the index mammogram and the additional imaging suggested by the radiologist (e.g., magnification views, ultrasound, follow-up mammogram)
Palpable breast mass or lump with normal or probably benign mammogram result	Ultrasound demonstrating a cyst, or aspiration of fluid, and follow-up breast exam or ultrasound to exclude persistence or recurrence of the finding, (if there is recurrence or persistence of the finding, the patient should be referred to a surgeon), or Follow-up breast exam documenting resolution, or Biopsy (i.e., open, core) of any persistent mass or nodularity
Breast pain persisting for more than 1 mo (without lump)	Clinical breast exam within 12 mo of the index mammogram and a normal or probably benign mammogram result

(From Haas JS, Cook EF, Puopolo AL, et al: Differences in the quality of care for women with an abnormal mammogram or breast complaint. *J Gen Intern Med* 15:321-328, 2000. Reprinted by permission of Blackwell Science, Inc. Courtesy of Smith B: Algorithms for management of common breast complaints. Forum: Harvard Risk Management Foundation. July 1995: 1-5.)

TABLE 4.—Patient-Reported Quality of Breast Care

Characteristic	Women Reporting Excellent Overall Quality of Breast Care	
	Baseline Survey (N = 579)	Follow-up Survey (N = 447)
Eligibility criteria		
Abnormal mammogram	46.6	44.9
Clinical breast complaint	47.2	47.5
Age, y		
<50	44.4	46.6
≥50	49.3	44.9
Race/ethnicity		
White	51.9*	49.8†
African American	35.9	35.6
Hispanic	33.3	25.0
Other	18.5	35.7
Family history of breast cancer		
Yes	47.1	52.0
No	46.3	43.4
Payer		
Managed care	42.9†	42.4
Other payer	52.8	50.7
Degree of worry		
Not al all/a little worried	48.2	46.6
Very/somewhat worried	40.7	42.5
Radiologist's recommendation for further care based on index mammogram		
Biopsy	45.7	49.9
Other‡	47.0	45.3

Note: Some categories include missing data.
*Unadjusted *P* <.05 for comparison within characteristic.
†Unadjusted *P* <.005 for comparison within characteristic.
‡Includes recommendation for additional imaging, follow-up as clinically indicated, and routine follow-up.

(Courtesy of Haas JS, Cook EF, Puopolo AL, et al: Differences in the quality of care for women with an abnormal mammogram or breast complaint. *J Gen Intern Med* 15:321-328, 2000. Reprinted by permission of Blackwell Science, Inc.)

50 years and had abnormal mammogram results rather than a clinical complaint (Table 1). In addition, women with a managed care plan were more likely to receive appropriate care and have a more timely resolution. Satisfaction with care did not differ by age or type of breast problem, but patients with a managed care plan were less likely to rate their care as excellent (Table 4).

Conclusion.—A substantial minority of women in this study did not receive care consistent with a clinical guideline. Younger women with a clinical breast problem and normal or benign-appearing mammogram results were less likely to receive appropriate care and to have the problem resolved in a timely manner.

▶ How effectively are primary health care providers following established guidelines for breast care and how satisfied are the patients in their care? Few data exist to answer these questions, but this survey of 10 internal medicine practices in the greater Boston area covering 579 patients gives insightful information. Although all the physicians had received the guidelines (based on local[1] and national[2] multispecialty recommendations prior to the study, the overall compliance was less than 70%. Patient-reported excellent quality of care was about 46% overall. In general, young women (less than 50 years of age), particularly in managed care settings, were less satisfied with their care. Furthermore, the care was less compliant with the guidelines and took longer for resolution of their problems compared with women more than 50 years of age. Young women with these same characteristics are the most frequently involved in breast care medical legal disputes. Clinicians should pay particular attention to the recommended guidelines and timely resolution of problems in this younger age group.

In this study, the median resolution time was 159 days (range, 0-260 days) for abnormal mammogram results and 28 days (range, 0-289 days) for a clinical breast complaint. The authors state, "There were no associations between patient-reported satisfaction with care and compliance with the guideline. Minority women and those with managed care reported being less satisfied." It is clear that primary care providers need to pay stricter attention to the timely application of established guidelines for breast care, increase patient satisfaction with their care, and document the reason for exceptions and delays in the medical record. Appropriate referral to a breast specialist should be considered when there are (1) guideline exceptions, (2) delays in resolution, (3) patient dissatisfaction, and (4) persistent concern (patient or physician) about malignancy.

W. H. Hindle, MD

References

1. Smith B: Algorithms for management of common breast complaints. *Forum*: Harvard Risk Management Foundation. July 1995: 1-5.
2. Cady B, Steele GD Jr, Morrow M, et al: Evaluation of common breast problems: Guidelines for primary care providers. *CA Cancer J Clin* 48:49-63, 1998.

SUGGESTED READING

Lewin JM, Hendrick RE, D'Orsi CJ, et al. Comparison of full-field digital mammography with screen-film mammography for cancer detection: Results of 4,945 paired examinations. *Radiology* 218:873-880, 2001.

▶ This report from the Universities of Colorado (Denver, Colorado) and Massachusetts (Worcester, Massachusetts), Medical Centers, with impressive numbers, indicates a high level of correlation with no statistically significant difference in cancer detection (diagnosis), between these 2 techniques. Except for the marked differential in cost of the equipment, this should lead to widespread use of digital mammography, which allows electronic transfer, manipulation, and storage of the images. Digital radiology has been in extensive use in other areas of imaging for several years.

Digital mammography had a significantly lower recall rate (11.5% vs 13.%) but a higher biopsy rate (30% vs 19%) compared to screen-film mammography. It is of keen clinical interest that of the 35 breast cancers detected, "four were interval cancers that became palpable within 1 year of screening and were considered false-negative with both modalities." Hopefully, the cancer detection rates for mammography of all types will continue to improve with advances in equipment and techniques.

William H. Hindle, MD

Saarenmaa I, Salminen T, Geiger U, et al. The visibility of cancer on previous mammograms in retrospective review. *Clin Radiol* 56:40-43, 2001.

▶ This study from Finland has strong medical legal implications. In the United States the number of lawsuits filed against radiologists alleging a "missed cancer" on a reported "negative" mammogram has increased dramatically in the past several years. Those involved in the evaluation and adjudication of "failure to diagnose" breast cancer lawsuits should carefully review this article.

Of the 320 initial mammograms of consecutive new breast cancer cases, 45 (14%) were retrospectively visible in earlier mammograms and this increased to 95 (29%) when the pre-operative mammogram was available for comparison. "The most common reasons for non-detection were that the lesion was overlooked (55%), diagnosed as benign (33%) or was visible only in one projection (26%)." The odds ratios were 2.9 for effect of age (over 55 vs under 55) and 1.5 for effect of density (fatty vs others).

The authors conclude, "Tumours are commonly visible in retrospect, but few of them exhibit specific signs of cancer, and are recognized only if they grow or otherwise change. It is not possible to differentiate most of them from normal parenchymal densities."

William H. Hindle, MD

Bobo JK, Lee NC, Thames SF. Findings from 752,081 clinical breast examinations reported to a national screening program from 1995 through 1998. *J Natl Cancer Inst* 92:971-976, 2000.

▶ These extensive data from the National Breast and Cervical Cancer Early Detection Program supply informative facts on the effectiveness of clinical breast examination (CBE) in community-based breast cancer detection. Of all the CBEs, 6.9% were coded abnormal, suspicious for cancer. Five cancers were detected per 1000 examinations. The sensitivity of CBE was 58.8% and the specificity was 93.4%. These results are similar to other reported clinical trials.

Women with normal mammograms and abnormal CBE had a 7.4 per 1000 cancer detection rate. Women with a normal CBE and an abnormal mammogram had a 42.0 per 1000 cancer detection rate. Women with both abnormal CBE and mammogram had a 170.3 per 1000 cancer detection rate.

These impressive numbers support the combined use of CBE and mammography for effective breast cancer screening. However, if the available resources limit the screening to only 1 method of detection, it is clear that mammography is the prime choice. Furthermore, other screening studies have repeatedly demonstrated that only mammography is effective in detecting ductal carcinoma in situ.

William H. Hindle, MD

Subject Index

W

Weight
  birth
    blood pressure and, 24-hour
      ambulatory, in nonproteinuric
      hypertensive pregnancy, 256
    decreased, after antenatal
      dexamethasone, 77
    effects of altitude *vs.* economic status
      on, 8
    increasing, as risk factor for third
      degree perineal ruptures during
      delivery, 203
  birth, low, extremely
    adverse effects of early
      dexamethasone treatment in infants
      of, 233
    neurologic and developmental
      disability after, 239

perinatal death and tocolytic
  magnesium sulfate and, 90
body, short-term effects of
  progestational contraceptive drug
  on, in young women, 387
neonatal, hormonal regulation of, 5
Withdrawal
  syndrome, neonatal, after in utero
    exposure to selective serotonin
    reuptake inhibitors, 263

Z

Zidovudine
  regimens, shortened, to prevent
    mother-to-child transmission of
    HIV, 123

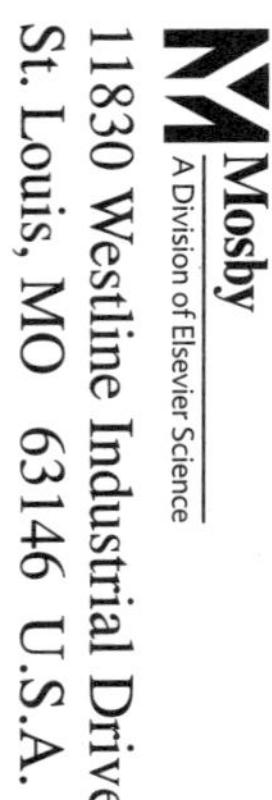

VISIT OUR HOME PAGE!
www.mosby.com/periodicals